ATLAS OF SURGICAL TECHNIQUES

NOTICE

Medicine is an ever-changing science. As new research and clinical experience broaden our knowledge, changes in treatment and drug therapy are required. The author and the publisher of this work have checked with sources believed to be reliable in their efforts to provide information that is complete and generally in accord with the standards accepted at the time of publication. However, in view of the possibility of human error or changes in medical sciences, neither the author nor the publisher nor any other party who has been involved in the preparation or publication of this work warrants that the information contained herein is in every respect accurate or complete. Readers are encouraged to confirm the information contained herein with other sources. For example and in particular, readers are advised to check the product information sheet included in the package of each drug they plan to administer to be certain that the information contained in this book is accurate and that changes have not been made in the recommended dose or in the contraindications for administration. This recommendation is of particular importance in connection with new or infrequently used drugs.

ATLAS OF
SURGICAL
TECHNIQUES

Marvin L. Gliedman, M.D.

PROFESSOR AND CHAIRMAN, DEPARTMENT OF SURGERY
ALBERT EINSTEIN COLLEGE OF MEDICINE
SURGEON-IN-CHIEF, DEPARTMENTS OF SURGERY
MONTEFIORE MEDICAL CENTER/ALBERT EINSTEIN
COLLEGE OF MEDICINE, BRONX, NEW YORK

Illustrations by Charles M. Stern and Lauren Keswick, M.S.

McGRAW-HILL INFORMATION SERVICES COMPANY
Health Professions Division

NEW YORK   ST. LOUIS   SAN FRANCISCO   COLORADO SPRINGS   OKLAHOMA CITY   AUCKLAND
BOGOTÁ   GUATEMALA   HAMBURG   LISBON   LONDON   MADRID   MEXICO   MONTREAL
NEW DELHI   PARIS   SAN JUAN   SÃO PAULO   SINGAPORE   SYDNEY   TOKYO   TORONTO

1234567890   HALKGP   8943209

ISBN 0-07-023491-4

This book was set in Palatino by Compset, Inc.;
camera and film preparation was done by Jay's Publishers Services, Inc.
The editors were Sally J. Barhydt and Peter McCurdy;
the production supervisor was Robert Laffler;
the cover and text design was done by José R. Fonfrias;
the index was prepared by Irving C. Tullar.
Arcata Graphics/Halliday was printer, and Arcata Graphics/Kingsport-Sherwood was the binder.

Library of Congress Cataloging-in-Publication Data

Gliedman, Marvin L., date
  Atlas of surgical techniques / Marvin L. Gliedman.
    p.   cm.
  ISBN 0-07-023491-4
  1. Surgery, Operative—Atlases.   I. Title.
  [DNLM: 1. Surgery, Operative—atlases.   WD 517 G559a]
RD32.G45   1990
617'.91—dc20
DNLM/DLC
for Library of Congress   89-12981
                                                              CIP

Table of Contents

Section Contributors

Scott J. Boley, M.D.

PROFESSOR OF SURGERY, ALBERT EINSTEIN COLLEGE OF MEDICINE
CHIEF OF THE DIVISION OF PEDIATRIC SURGERY, MONTEFIORE MEDICAL CENTER/
ALBERT EINSTEIN COLLEGE OF MEDICINE
BRONX, NEW YORK

Carl E. Silver, M.D.

PROFESSOR OF SURGERY, ALBERT EINSTEIN COLLEGE OF MEDICINE
CHIEF OF THE DIVISION OF HEAD AND NECK SURGERY
MONTEFIORE MEDICAL CENTER/
ALBERT EINSTEIN COLLEGE OF MEDICINE
BRONX, NEW YORK

Frank J. Veith, M.D.

PROFESSOR OF SURGERY, ALBERT EINSTEIN COLLEGE OF MEDICINE
CHIEF OF THE DIVISION OF VASCULAR SURGERY, MONTEFIORE MEDICAL CENTER/
ALBERT EINSTEIN COLLEGE OF MEDICINE
BRONX, NEW YORK

Preface

A surgeon's operating techniques are a continually changing distillation of what he or she has seen, read, and experienced from his or her residency to the present; we add useful nuances and surgical "tricks" and delete those which we find cumbersome. New procedures are added based on descriptions in the literature and on the availability of new instruments that modify steps in a complex operation. This Atlas presents a series of operative procedures which have been found to be appropriate to a particular task. We do not claim priority or newness in these approaches but only that this is the way we do them. What we have observed to be good, useful and workable, for us, has been kept or added to our technique while what is less good or laborious, to us, has been discarded.

Atlases of surgery are available in a spectrum of formats. At one extreme a particular surgeon will describe but one operation in a compendium volume of surgical procedures. At the other extreme one surgeon will describe his experience with every operation. Hopefully, this volume is an appropriate compromise based upon the techniques employed on our surgical service and in the training of our residents. We have relied heavily on a visual presentation—series of detailed drawings. The sections on head and neck surgery, pediatric surgery, and vascular surgery contain procedures described by the Chiefs of those divisions. A few of the procedures in general surgery, namely, gastric bypass for morbid obesity, hemorrhoidectomy, the drainage of perirectal abscesses and the treatment of anal fistula are described by Dr. Peter Wilk who was in the department and shared his expertise with us. We have limited the contributors to the members of our surgical faculty, and have had a single surgeon describe the techniques in a particular area. This allows a continuity of approach and also permits the authors to show alternatives in surgical technique in their area of expertise.

Certainly, every Atlas is incomplete; more procedures and variations could be added—almost endlessly. We have chosen to stop with this representative core.

During the years this volume was in preparation, residents have had the opportunity to review the drawings for a particular procedure prior to carrying out the operation. They have found them instructive and useful. Our hope is that other surgeons, at every stage in their surgical career, similarly will find this Atlas of value.

ACKNOWLEDGMENTS

My sincere appreciation and admiration to Lauren Keswick and Charles Stern who labored long and hard to convert my operative steps and pencil scratchings into sketches and finally finished drawings. Their success was always a source of wonderment to me. My gratitude to the contributors of Sections: Scott J. Boley, M.D., Carl Silver, M.D., and Frank J. Veith, M.D., my colleagues and friends for more than two decades, who have added their expertise to this volume. My sincere thanks to Dr. Ronald Kaleya who reviewed the text and added numerous valuable corrections.

To the Surgical Residents of the Department of
Surgery of Montefiore Medical Center
and the Albert Einstein College of Medicine.
How much the teacher learns from the pupil!

Hemithyroidectomy

1   A nodule in the left lobe of the thyroid gland is depicted. The lesion is well defined, and apparently well encapsulated. The transverse skin incision, placed within a natural skin crease if possible, is made at the level of the thyroid isthmus, approximately a finger-breadth inferior to the palpable cricoid cartilage.

2   After elevation of skin flaps in the subplatysmal plane, a vertical incision is made in the midline, between the sternohyoid muscles, from the level of the hyoid bone to the sternal notch.

3   To expose the left lobe, the left sternohyoid muscle is dissected from the surface of the thyroid gland and, farther laterally, from the sternothyroid muscle. Lateral retraction of the sternothyroid muscle will provide adequate exposure for resection of small or moderate-sized lesions. If additional exposure is required, the muscle may be transversely divided.

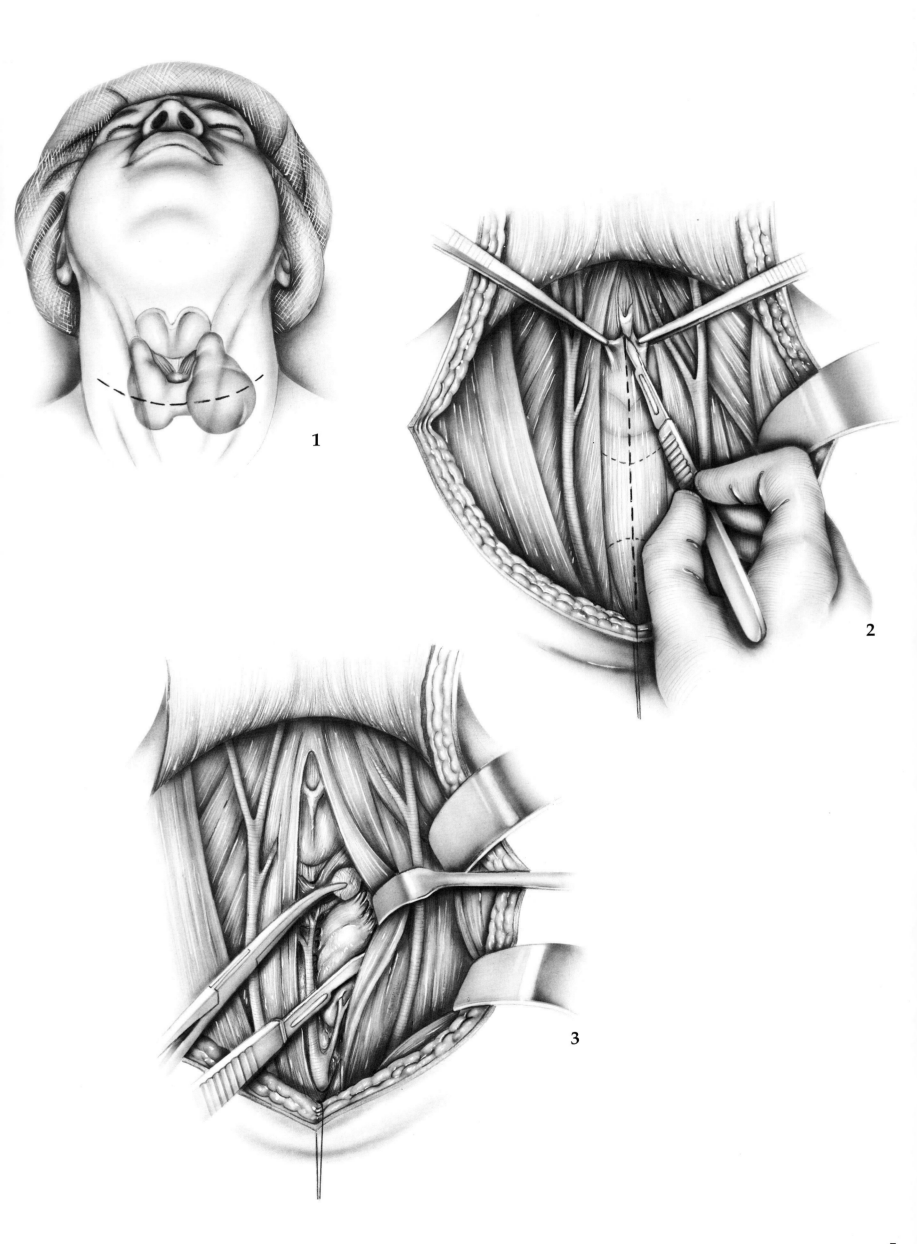

Hemithyroidectomy (*cont.*)

4 With the sternohyoid retracted laterally, the sternothyroid muscle is exposed, covering the left thyroid lobe and nodule. If the muscle is not invaded by tumor, it is separated from the surface of the lobe and either transected, as shown, or retracted laterally.

5 The thyroid lobe is exposed, and retracted medially. One or more middle thyroid veins are divided to permit retraction of the lobe and exposure of the deep paratracheal structures in the space between the thyroid and the carotid vessels. The recurrent laryngeal nerve is seen ascending, and crossing—in this case superficially—the inferior thyroid artery. The veins at the inferior pole are divided.

6 The inferior thyroid artery is divided medial to the recurrent laryngeal nerve. The superior pole is triply clamped, divided, ligated, and transfixed.

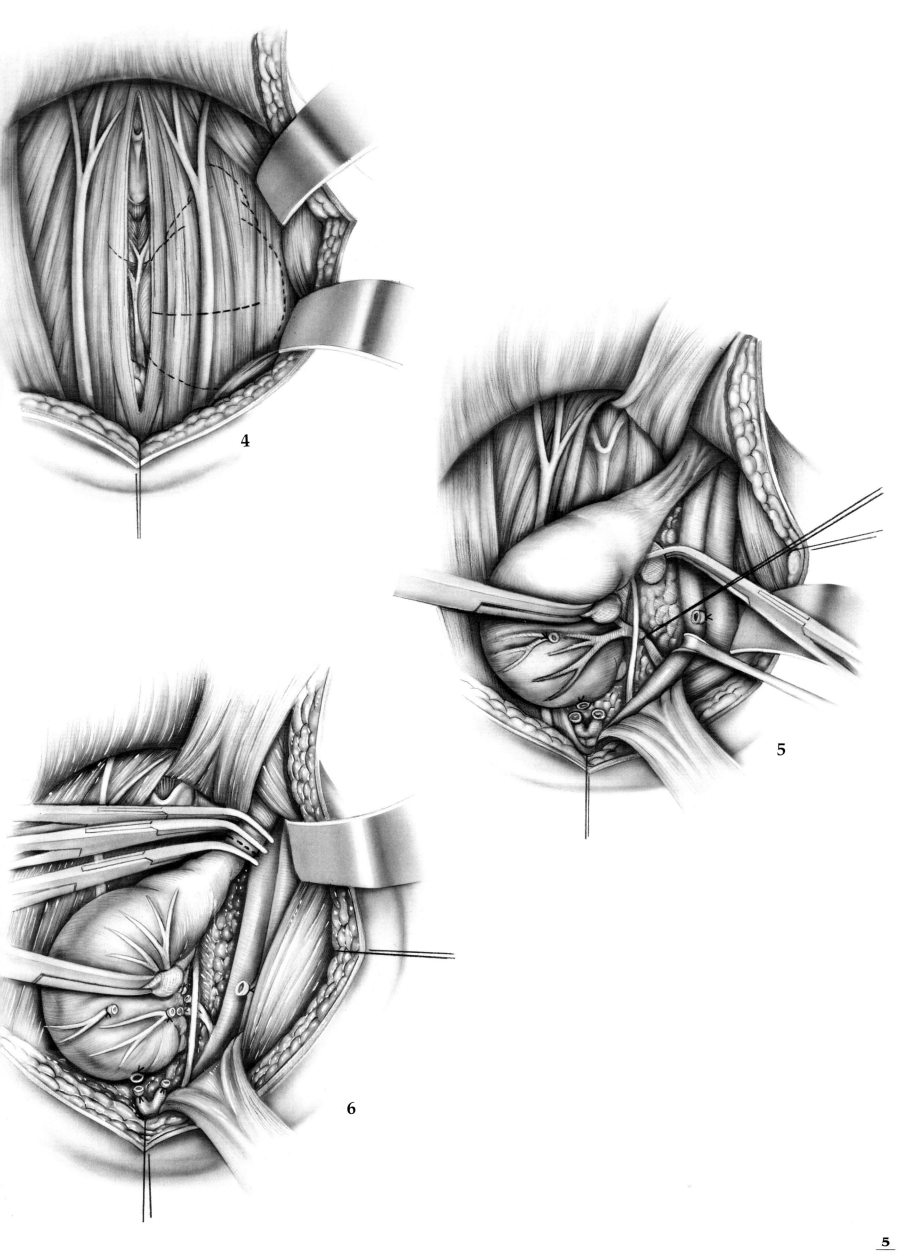

4

5

6

Hemithyroidectomy (*cont.*)

7 With the superior and inferior blood supplies divided, the lateral suspensory (Berry's) ligament, a broad fibrous attachment of thyroid to trachea, is palpated medial to the superior portion of the recurrent laryngeal nerve. After transection of this structure (broken line) the thyroid lobe remains only loosely attached to the trachea. The superior parathyroid gland, situated lateral to the recurrent laryngeal nerve, and the inferior parathyroid gland, situated medial to the nerve, are separated from the thyroid lobe and left *in situ*.

8 The remaining loose attachments of the thyroid lobe to the trachea are sharply divided, reflecting the lobe medially as far as the thyroid isthmus. The isthmus is divided between serially placed clamps, and the surgical specimen, consisting of left lobe and isthmus, is removed.

9 After resection, the junction of the right lobe and the isthmus is transfixed. The recurrent laryngeal nerve, parathyroid glands, reflected sternothyroid muscle, and retracted sternohyoid muscle are demonstrated. It is not necessary to reapproximate the sternothyroid muscle, but the sternohyoid muscle should be resutured if it has been transected. The midline is reconstructed by suturing of the muscles, and the skin flaps are approximated over closed wound suction catheters (not shown).

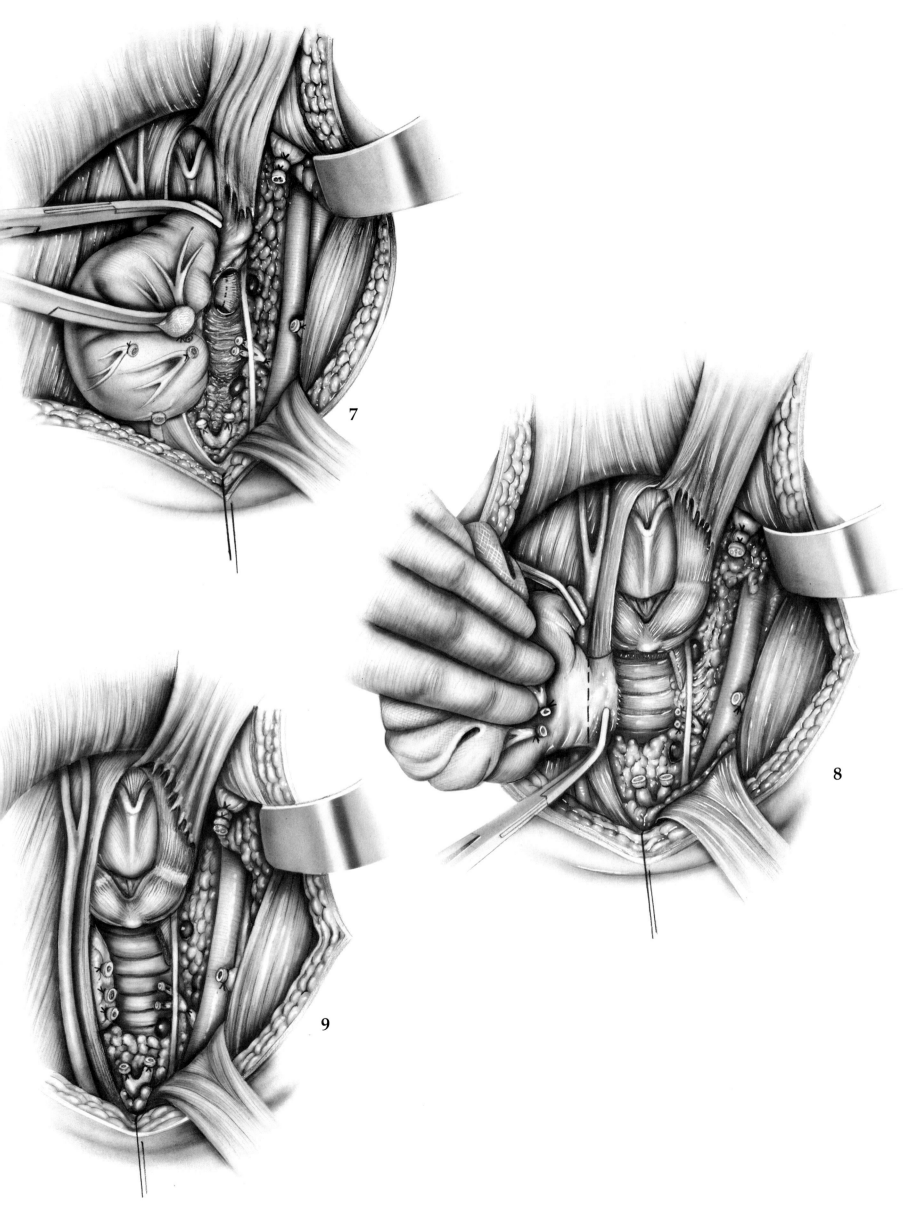

7

8

9

Total Thyroidectomy for Invasive Thyroid Cancer

1 An invasive malignant tumor of the left thyroid lobe is demonstrated in relation to the planned skin incision, which is placed approximately one fingerbreadth inferior to the cricoid cartilage—in a natural skin crease, if possible.

2 A transverse section demonstrates the invasive nature of the tumor, which infiltrates the sternothyroid muscle as well as the thyroid gland.

3 One or both layers of pretracheal muscles are resected in continuity with the thyroid tumor, as indicated by the dotted lines. This portion of muscle will be left attached to the resected specimen.

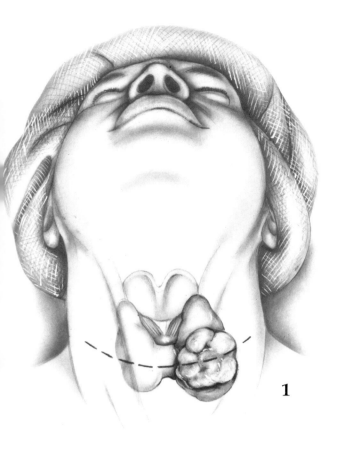

1

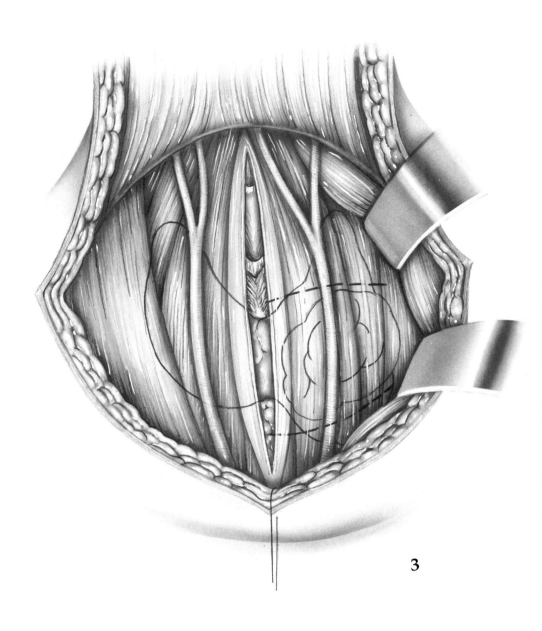

3

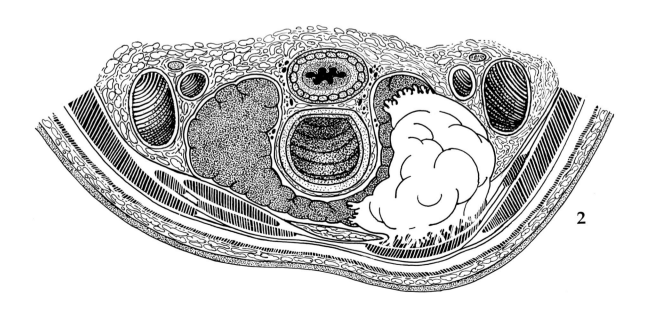

2

Total Thyroidectomy for Invasive Thyroid Cancer (*cont.*)

4 The lateral attachments of the thyroid lobe and the tumor are separated from adjacent structures, particularly carotid vessels. The inferior thyroid artery, passing deep to the carotid artery and the recurrent laryngeal nerve, is ligated in continuity, lateral to the nerve.

5 If the recurrent laryngeal nerve is invaded by tumor, the nerve must be sacrificed (broken lines) and the invaded portion of the nerve resected with the thyroid lobe.

6 The superior pole is triply clamped and divided.

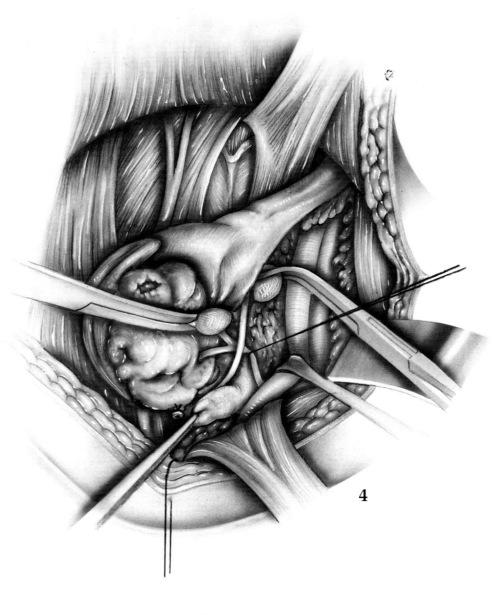

4

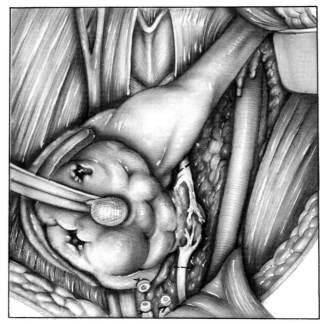

5

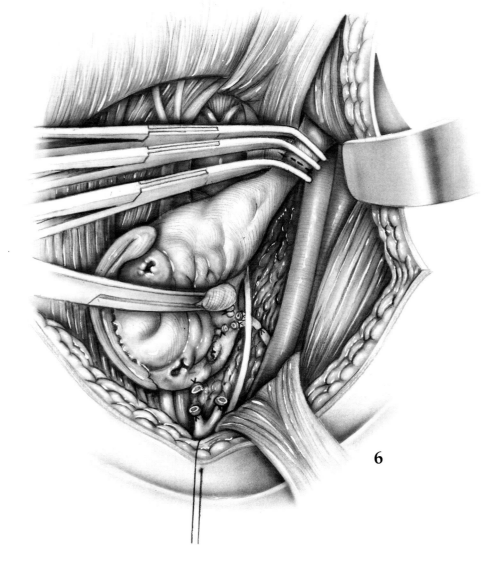

6

Total Thyroidectomy for Invasive Thyroid Cancer (*cont.*)

7 The lateral suspensory (Berry's) ligament is transected, liberating the lobe from the trachea. The superior parathyroid gland (lateral to recurrent nerve) has been preserved, but the inferior gland lies on the surface of the tumor and is included in the resection.

8 The completely mobilized lobe, with attached overlying muscle, is demonstrated. The lobe may be removed, if necessary, to confirm malignancy by frozen section.

9 If total thyroidectomy is considered necessary, the contralateral lobe is mobilized and resected, with care to preserve the parathyroid glands and their blood supply. The branches of the inferior thyroid artery are ligated close to the thyroid lobe. A posterior portion of the lobe may be left *in situ* in order to preserve parathyroid tissue ("near-total lobectomy").

10 At the conclusion of the procedure, the left lobe with overlying muscles has been totally resected. A posterior remnant of thyroid tissue remains on the right side.

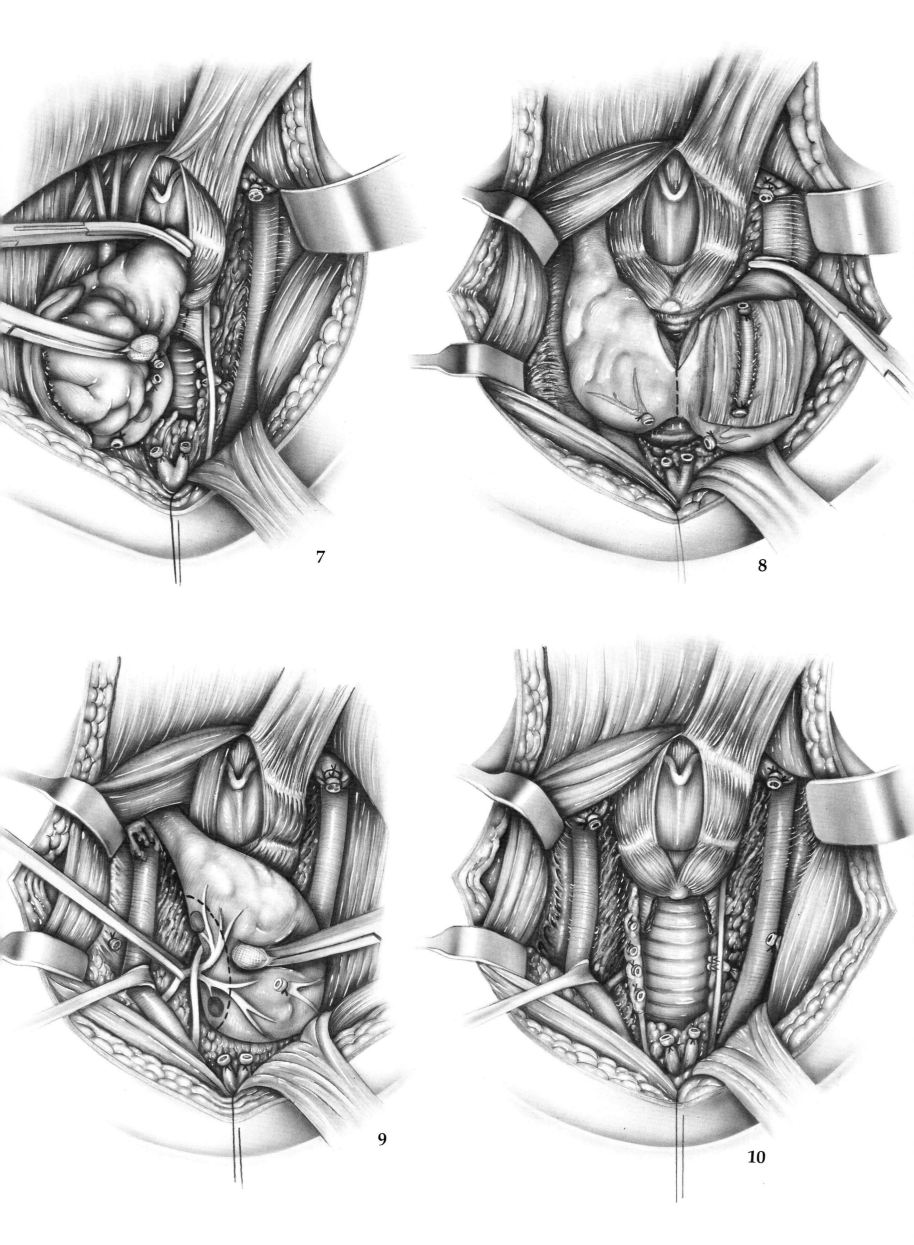

7

8

9

10

Parathyroid Exploration

1 The incision and approach for cervical parathyroid exploration are similar to those for thyroidectomy. A transverse incision one fingerbreadth inferior to the palpable cricoid cartilage provides good exposure of the thyroid and the parathyroid region. The normal locations of the four parathyroid glands are shown. The right superior gland is enlarged, and represents the source of excessive parathyroid hormone production. Skin flaps are elevated in the subplatysmal plane, and each thyroid lobe exposed as shown in **Plate 1, Figs. 2–3,** and **Plate 2, Fig. 4.**

2 The right lobe is exposed (**Plate 2, Fig. 5**). A tape is passed around the inferior thyroid artery. The recurrent laryngeal nerve is seen ascending superficial to the artery. The parathyroid glands are shown in relation to the nerve and artery; the superior gland is lateral to the nerve and superior to the artery, while the inferior gland is medial and inferior. The normal inferior gland is approximately 5 mm in length and weighs between 50 and 75 mg. The enlarged superior gland shown in this example is about 2.5 cm in diameter and weighs approximately 600 mg. Glands that weigh 100 mg or more are enlarged, and invariably demonstrate histologic aberrations. The enlarged gland is excised.

3 The operative field after excision of the parathyroid lesion is shown. Frozen-section confirmation of the excised parathyroid tissue is essential. The "normal" inferior gland is biopsied by resection of a few cubic millimeters of tissue from its free border and corroborated by frozen section. The contralateral side is explored, and the parathyroid glands identified and also histologically verified. Bilateral exploration and biopsy of all parathyroid tissue identified is necessary for adequate surgical examination of the patient.

4 The parathyroid glands often migrate from the "normal" locations indicated in this figure. The inferior glands descend embryologically with the thymus gland, and are often situated within the thymic capsule. In some cases the intrathymic parathyroid glands may descend deep within the anterior mediastinum, requiring manubriotomy or sternotomy for exposure. This situation, if suspected, should be documented by appropriate localization studies before operation (usually after failure of an initial exploration). The superior parathyroid glands tend to descend in a prevertebral, paraesophageal location. Even when quite large they are usually accessible through the cervical incision.

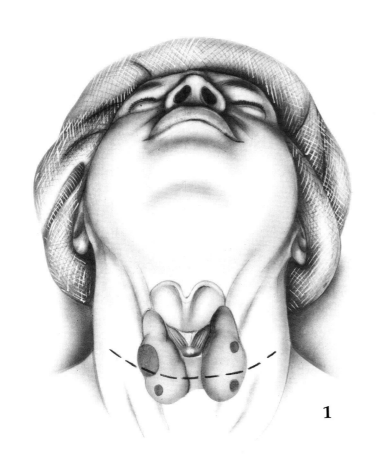

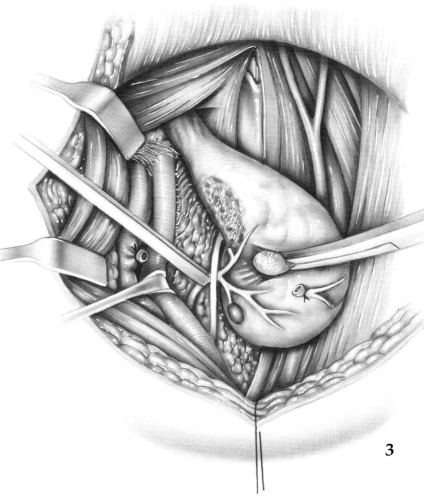

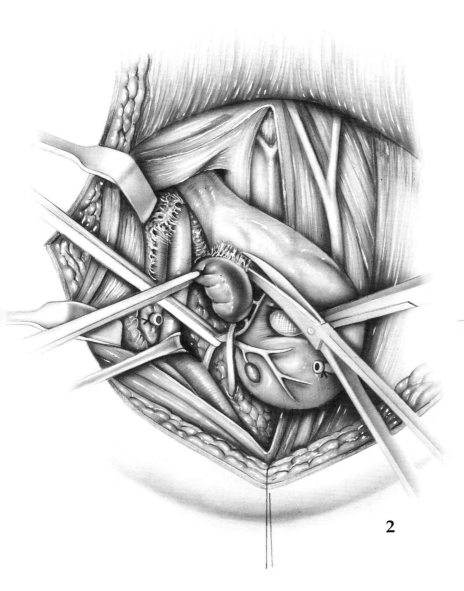

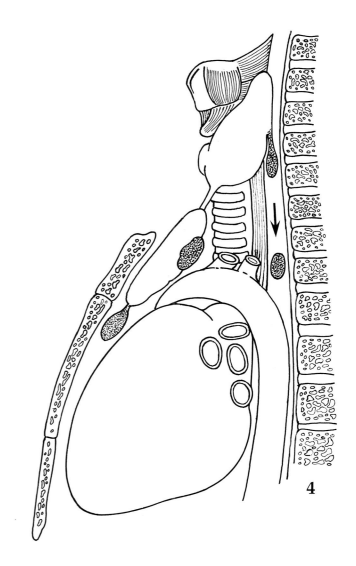

Lateral Parotid Lobectomy

1 The relations of the parotid gland, facial nerve, and skull base are shown. The main nerve trunk emerges from the stylomastoid foramen and is situated a few millimeters inferior to the groove between the mastoid process and the bony ear canal (tympanomastoid groove). The nerve crosses superficial to the styloid process and ramifies within the parotid gland, dividing it into lateral (superficial) and medial (deep) lobes. The main trunk divides into superior (temporofacial) and inferior (cervicofacial) branches, which divide into temporal, zygomatic, buccinator (superior and inferior), submandibular, and cervical branches. The lateral lobe comprises from 70 to 80 percent of the parotid tissue; consequently, most parotid tumors are situated in this portion of of the parotid gland.

2 A sickle-shaped incision placed anterior to the tragus, extending inferiorly to the mastoid tip and then beneath the angle of the mandible, provides adequate exposure for parotid resection and will result in an inconspicuous scar. The incision may be extended superiorly as necessary for resection of large or superiorly situated tumors; or inferiorly to permit cervical lymphadenectomy.

3 Skin flaps are elevated, exposing the parotid tissue, the cartilage of the external ear canal, the sternomastoid muscle, the posterior facial vein, and the greater auricular nerve. The vein and nerve are divided and the posterior inferior (tail) portion of the parotid is separated from the sternomastoid muscle. The parotid tissue is separated from the cartilaginous ear canal until the junction with the bony canal is reached.

4 The posterior belly of the digastric muscle is exposed deep and anterior to the sternomastoid muscle, and the remaining attachments of the parotid to the sternomastoid are divided. The main trunk of the facial nerve is identified at the superior portion of the digastric muscle, just inferior to the tympanomastoid groove, crossing the styloid process, which can be identified by palpation. The nerve is situated deep within the parotid tissue, which must be carefully dissected and retracted until the nerve is clearly exposed.

5 The lateral lobe is liberated from its deep attachments in the plane of the facial nerve, tracing and preserving the individual branches until the lobe containing the tumor has been liberated completely. There is no fascial plane between the lateral and deep lobes; parotid tissue must be transected in order to accomplish the resection. The tumor is removed with as much normal parotid tissue attached as is consistent with facial nerve preservation.

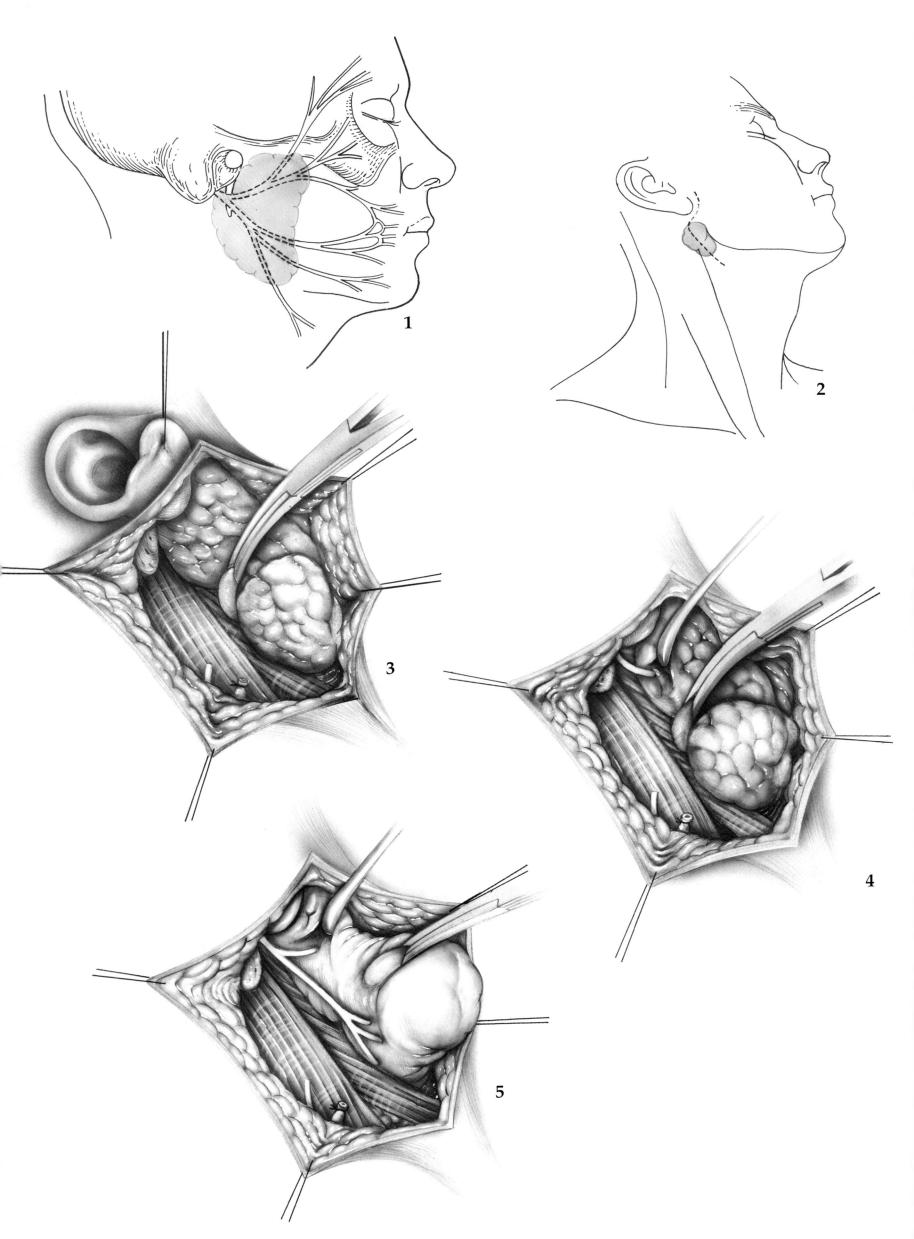

Lateral Parotid Lobectomy (*cont.*)—
Deep Lobe Parotidectomy

6 In this case, with the tumor confined to the inferior parotid, the inferior lateral lobe has been resected, dissecting the branches of the inferior division of the facial nerve as far as necessary. The superior division has been dissected sufficiently to provide an adequate resection margin.

7 The wound edges are approximated with fine suture material, and small closed wound suction catheters are placed subcutaneously, avoiding contact with the facial nerve.

DEEP LOBE PAROTIDECTOMY

8 In order to resect a deep lobe tumor, it is necessary to dissect the facial nerve sufficiently to separate and retract the nerve from the underlying tumor. This usually requires resection of much of the lateral lobe in order to expose and liberate the nerve. With the nerve retracted, the deep lobe tumor is dissected free and removed.

9 If necessary, a buccinator branch may be divided to afford access to the deep lobe tumor. Division of a single buccinator branch will produce no functional deficit.

10 To liberate a tumor situated in the retrostyloid portion of the deep lobe, the stylomandibular ligament is divided and the mandible dislocated anteriorly.

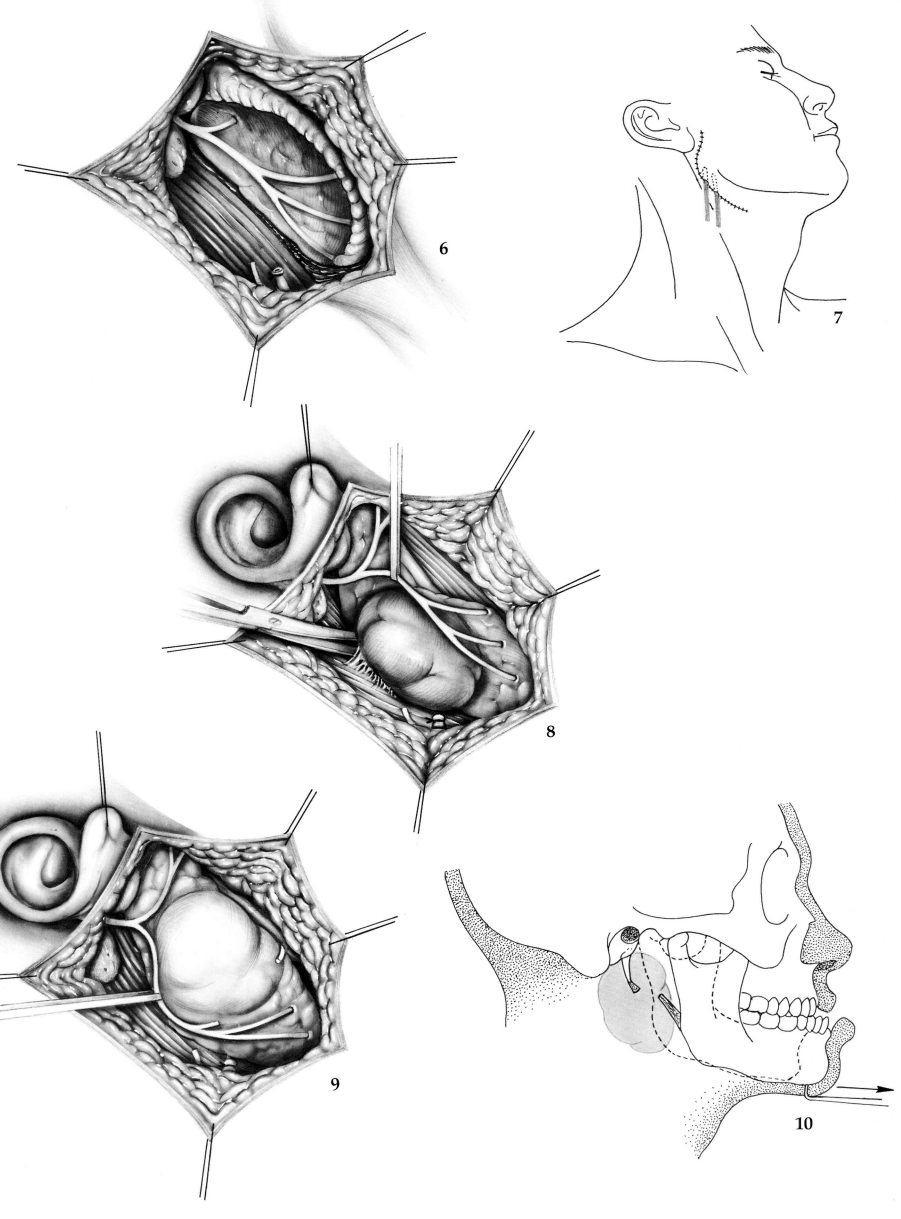

Resection of Facial Nerve with Graft

1 A malignant tumor is demonstrated, invading the bifurcation of the facial nerve. In this case there is sufficient length of uninvolved main trunk of the facial nerve to permit surgical rehabilitation by grafting.

2 After removal of the specimen, the stump of the main trunk of the facial nerve, as well as the various peripheral branches, remain. The greater auricular nerve, situated superficial to the sternomastoid muscle, may be dissected posteriorly toward the spine, where it is joined by one or two branches that emerge from the cervical plexus root. This readily available and naturally bifurcated sensory nerve may be used for grafting relatively short segmental defects. The sural nerve may be used to replace longer defects, or in cases where the greater auricular nerve is not available.

3 The graft is sutured to the nerve ends by microsurgical technique using $10\times$ to $40\times$ magnification. Monofilament nylon sutures of 15- to 30-μm diameter (9-0 to 11-0) are placed in the perineurium of individual fasicles without tension. It is not possible to anastomose all individual branches, but the mandibular and zygomatic branches should be reinnervated whenever feasible.

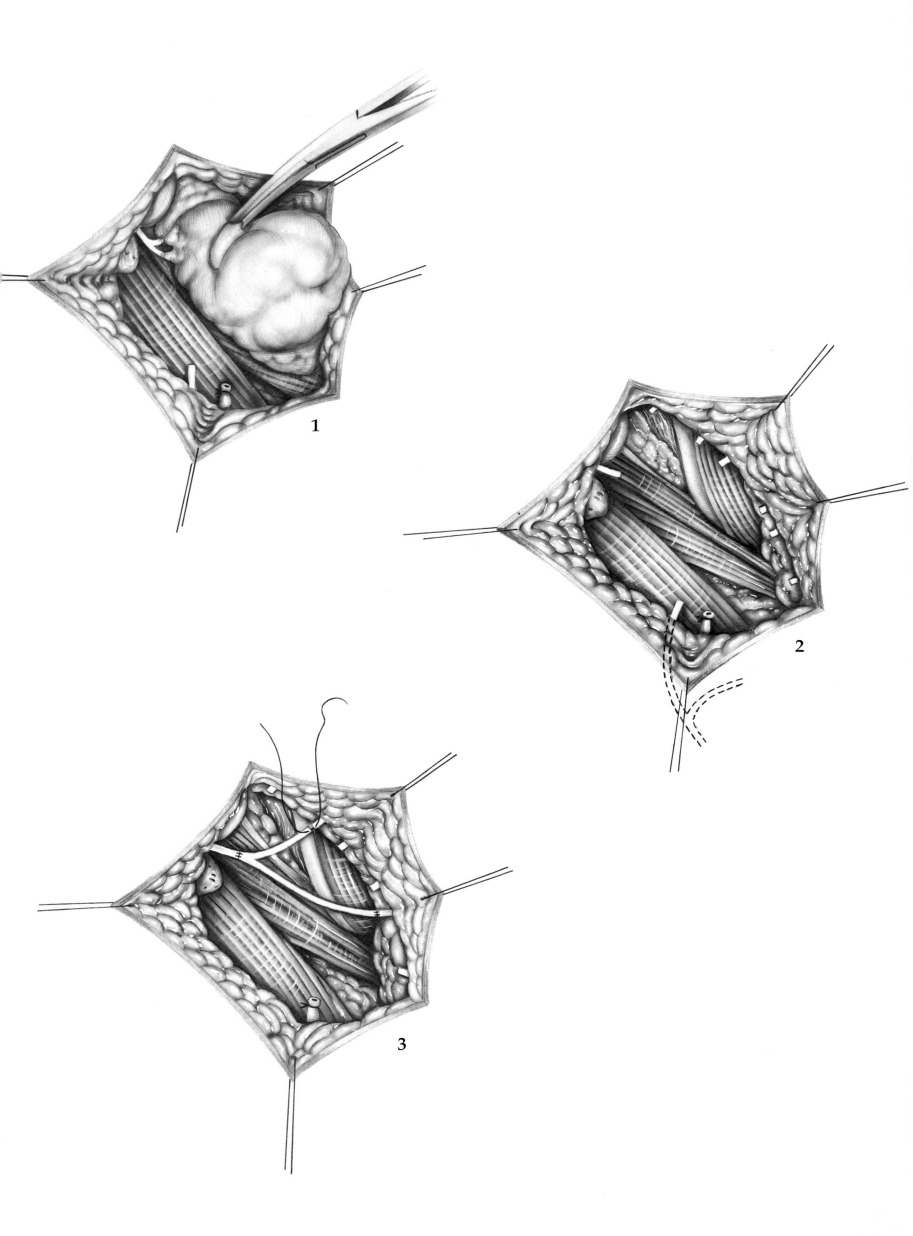

1

2

3

Excision of Thyroglossal Cyst

1 A sagittal section demonstrates the anatomic relationships of the cyst, the hyoid bone, and the potential tract leading to the foramen cecum. Although thyroglossal cysts may descend farther inferiorly than shown, or may be situated in a suprahyoid location, this example depicts the most common situation. The cyst is situated inferior and adjacent to the body of the hyoid bone, deep to the infrahyoid musculature.

2 An incision is made directly over the mass, in a natural skin crease if possible. The incision is slightly longer than the diameter of the cyst.

3 Skin flaps are developed in the subplatysmal plane to expose the entire cyst as well as the superior border of the hyoid bone. The infrahyoid muscles are separated from the cyst, dividing the attachments of the muscle to the body of the hyoid bone. The deep aspect of the cyst is separated from the laryngeal prominence and thyrohyoid membrane.

4 After complete liberation of the cyst from its soft-tissue attachments, the insertions of the suprahyoid muscles are severed from the body of the hyoid bone.

5 The complex of cyst and hyoid bone is retracted sufficiently to expose and sever the synarthrosis between the body and the greater cornu on one side. This process is repeated on the opposite side.

6 After release of the hyoid body, dissection may reveal a tract extending into the musculature of the tongue base. The potential tract follows the path of embryologic descent of the thyroid anlage, illustrated in **Fig. 1.** A portion of this tract, deep to the hyoid bone, may persist and should be excised. Persistence of the entire tract, as far as the foramen cecum, is rare. In many cases, no deep tract may exist. Nevertheless it is important to be certain that an epithelial lined structure is not left *in situ* after resection, as this may result in recurrence of a cyst or a persistent draining sinus.

7 After removal of the cyst-hyoid-tract complex, the defect is repaired by suturing of the infrahyoid to the suprahyoid muscle. Skin flaps are reapproximated and the subcutaneous space drained with a Penrose drain or by closed wound suction catheters.

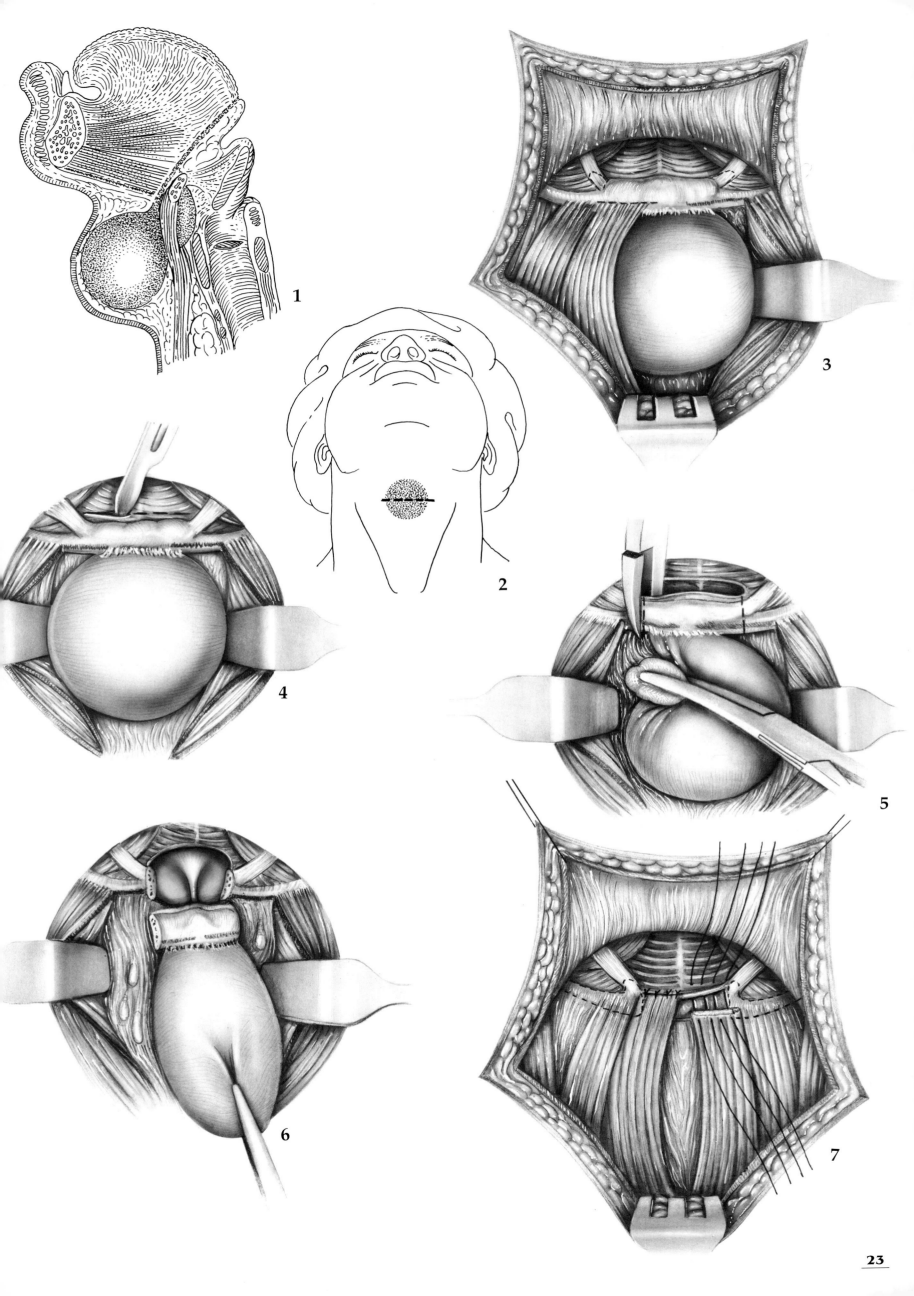

Excision of Pharyngoesophageal Diverticulum (Zenker's Diverticulum)

1 A pulsion diverticulum of the pharyngoesophageal mucosa protrudes through a defect between the oblique fibers of the inferior constrictor muscle and the transverse fibers of the cricopharyngeus muscle. The underlying cause is thought to be dysfunction of the cricopharyngeus. Small diverticula may be treated by cricopharyngeal myotomy alone (**Fig. 5**), but a moderate-to-large diverticulum, as demonstrated, must be resected, or sutured in a permanently inverted position (diverticulopexy). Many surgeons employ an oblique incision along the anterior border of the sternomastoid muscle (*A–A'*). Skin flaps need not be created with this approach. A transverse incision (*B–B'*) at the level of the cricoid cartilage, with elevation of skin flaps in the subplatysmal plane, will provide adequate exposure and a superior cosmetic result. The diverticulum is usually approached from the left side.

2 The sternomastoid muscle is retracted laterally and the carotid sheath vessels are dissected free and separated from the midline structures. The omohyoid muscle and inferior thyroid artery are divided in order to expose the esophagus and diverticulum.

3 The thyroid lobe is retracted anteriorly, permitting exposure of the esophagus and diverticular sac in the prevertebral region. Division of the infrahyoid muscles will facilitate rotation and exposure of the neck of the sac and esophagus. Identification of the recurrent laryngeal nerve (not shown), at the lateral border of the trachea, inferior to the thyroid lobe, is advisable in order to avoid trauma to this structure by retraction or other manipulation. The sac is dissected free from adherent structures and delivered until attached only to the esophagus at its neck. The fibers of the inferior oblique and cricopharyngeus muscles are freed from the sac mucosa.

4 The junction of sac and esophagus is often poorly defined and quite broad. Passage of a mercury-filled rubber bougie, transorally, into the distal esophagus will prevent encroachment on the esophageal lumen when the sac is resected and the esophagus repaired. A stapling device may be employed if the sac's neck is well defined and sufficiently small to fit properly into the jaws of the stapler. A safe method of resecting a broad-based sac, by progressive incision and suture of the mucosa, is demonstrated. No attempt is made to invert the mucosa. Nonabsorbable suture material is preferred.

5 Cricopharyngeal myotomy, to prevent recurrence, is performed by dissecting the mucosa from the overlying muscularis and vertically incising the transverse muscle fibers.

6 In order to reinforce the mucosal closure, the vertically incised inferior pharyngoesophageal muscle is sutured transversely to the inferior constrictor. A nasogastric feeding tube is passed prior to closure of the muscle.

7 The completed closure of the muscularis is shown. Although disruption of the esophagotomy closure rarely occurs, drains should be placed in the region.

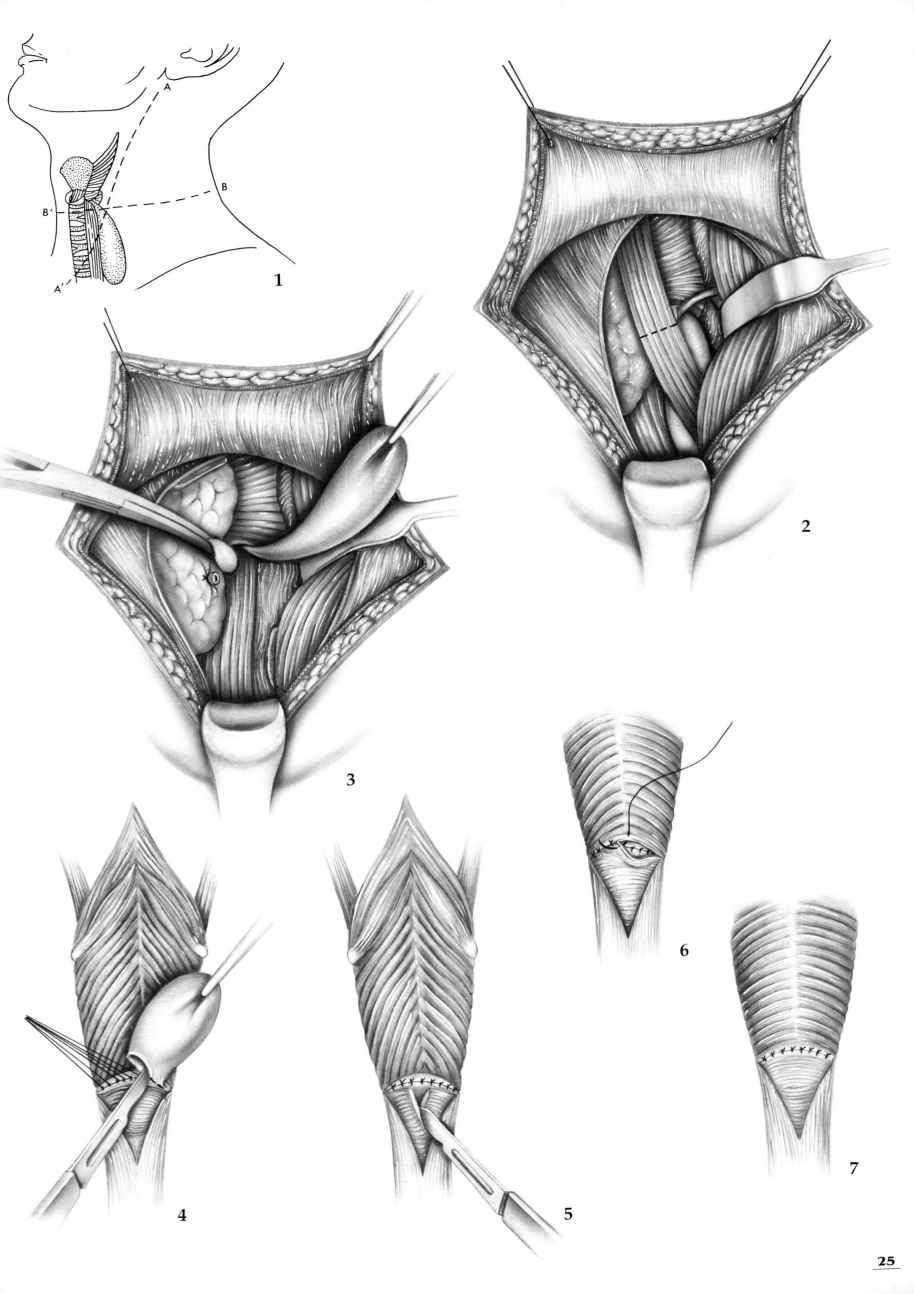

Modified Radical Mastectomy

1 The patient is placed supine on the operating table with the arm extended on an armboard or extension table. The arm is prepped and draped into the operative field, allowing manipulation during surgery. At closure, the ability to adduct the arm may aid the approximation of the skin edges. The tumor is sampled by core-needle or excisional biopsy, or by incisional biopsy if the tumor mass is large. Upon confirmation of malignant histology, a transverse elliptical incision is made because it affords cosmetic advantages and is preferred in the case of subsequent breast reconstruction. The skin incision is made 5 cm above and below the tumor's edges. The nipple and areola are excised.

2 The skin incision is made just deep enough to allow the breast tissue to pout through the wound. Adair clamps are placed on the superior skin edge; the assistant provides steady traction with these clamps while the surgeon applies counterpressure on the breast tissue. Using sharp and blunt dissection techniques, the superior flap is developed from the sternal border medially, to the anterior axillary line laterally, and to the clavicle superiorly. When the dissection is carried out in the appropriate plane, the breast tissue separates easily and relatively bloodlessly from the skin and subcutaneous tissue. No attempt is made to create thin skin flaps. Similarly, the Adair clamps are placed on the inferior skin edge and the lower flap is developed beyond the inferior mammary fold until the rectus and oblique muscles are visible.

3 The superficial pectoral fascia is the deep margin of resection. The pectoralis fascia is incised parallel to the sternum. It is grasped with small clamps and sharply dissected from the pectoralis major muscle underlying it. The perforating branches of the internal mammary artery are ligated carefully, because they tend to retract into the substance of the pectoralis muscle. As the dissection proceeds laterally, the fascia is incised parallel to the clavicle and at the inferior margin of the pectoralis major muscle.

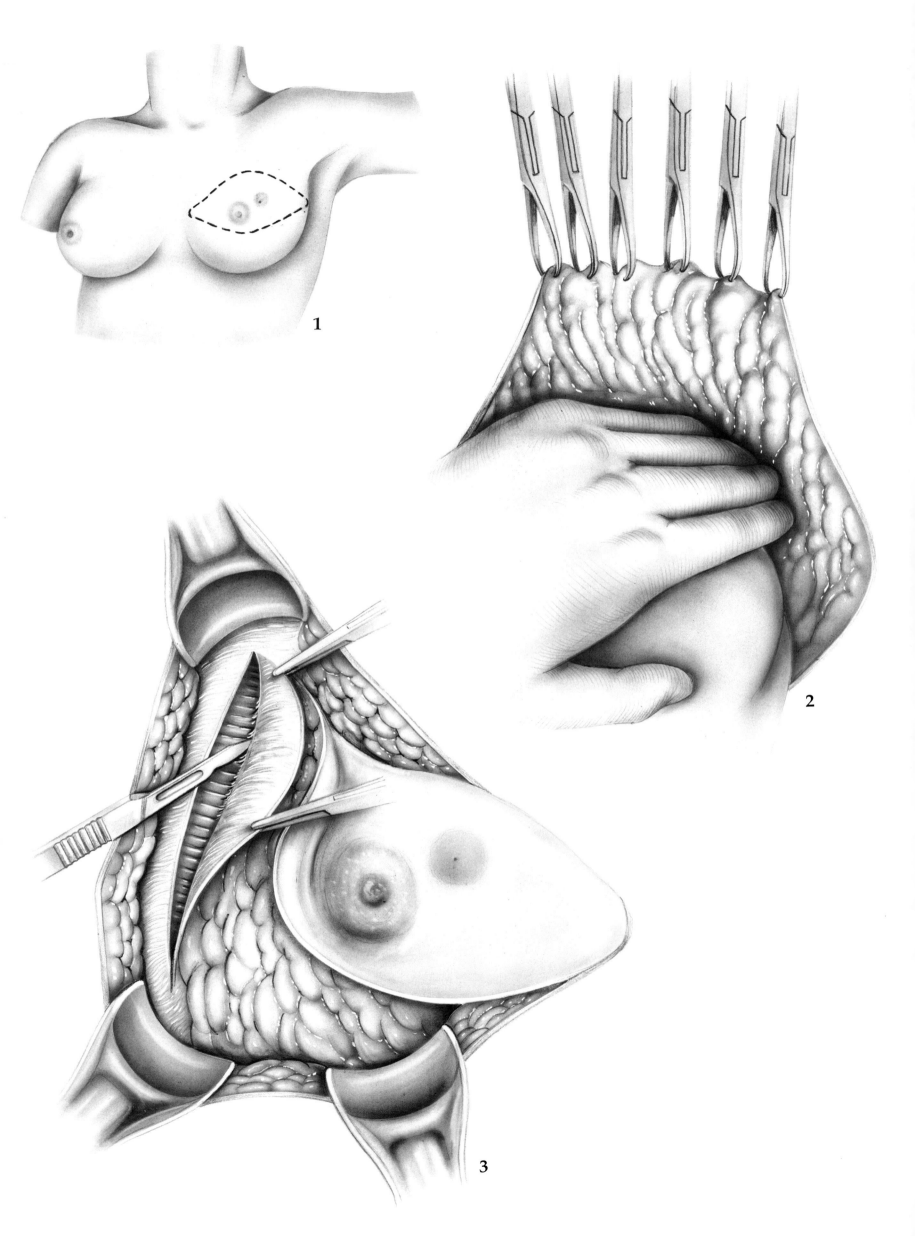

1

2

3

Modified Radical Mastectomy (*cont.*)

4 The pectoral fascia is incised along the lateral border of the pectoralis major, allowing cephalad retraction of this muscle, which exposes the pectoralis minor muscle. The fat between the pectoralis major and minor muscles is dissected bluntly, carrying the specimen laterally toward the remainder of the axillary contents. The nerve innervating the lateral portion of the pectoralis major muscle is present in this plane; an attempt should be made to preserve it.

5 The axillary fascia is then incised at the lateral border of the pectoralis minor muscle. Retraction of this muscle medially exposes the remainder of the axillary contents. The most medial few centimeters of the axillary contents, where the axillary vein enters the chest wall (Level III nodes), cannot easily be cleared without the division of the pectoralis minor muscle. However, our past commitment to the complete exenteration of the axilla has not been shown to be as important as the removal of a significant sample of the Level I and II nodes. Therefore, in recent years, we have not divided the insertion of the pectoralis minor muscle.

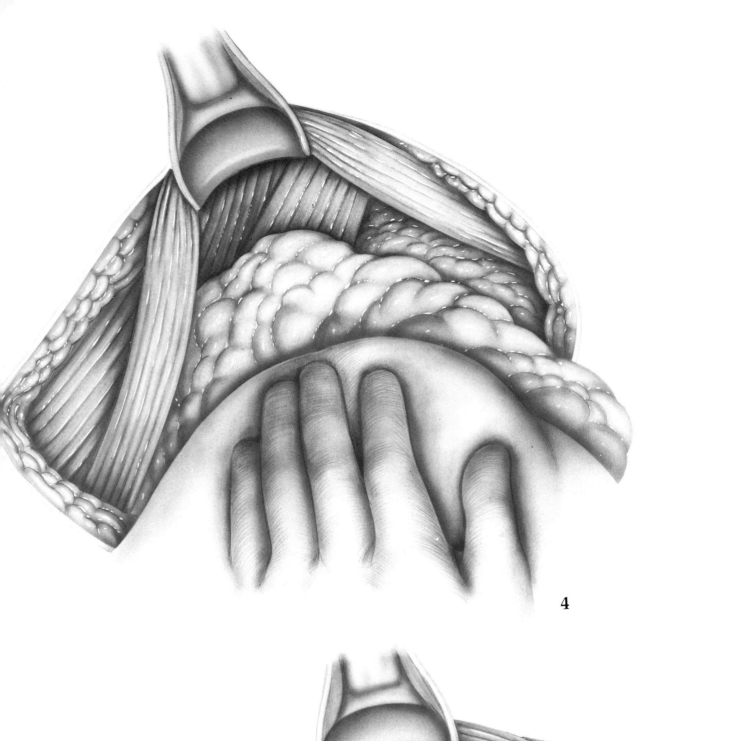

4

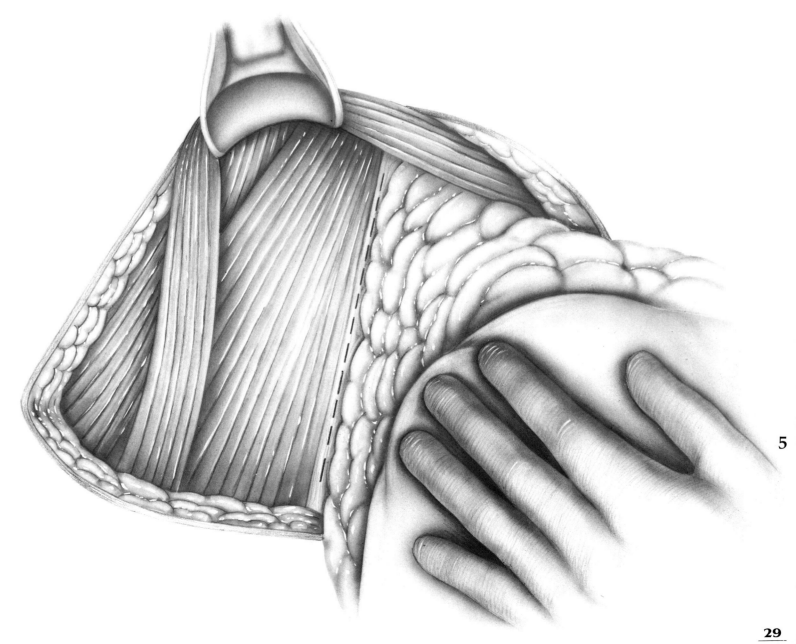

5

Modified Radical Mastectomy (*cont.*)

6 The fascia investing the axillary vein is incised. Lymph node bearing tissue along the inferior margin of the axillary vein is dissected inferiorly. Medially, the long thoracic (Bell's) nerve is identified and preserved. The lymph node bearing tissue surrounding it is dissected and included in the specimen. Because of the risk of brachial plexus injury and subsequent lymphedema of the arm, the dissection should not be carried above the axillary vein.

7 While we used to take all of the venous branches and nerves entering the axilla beneath the axillary vein, preserving only the long thoracic and thoracodorsal nerves, we no longer consider this skeletization an important feature of the axillary dissection. The lateral margin of the dissection is the anteromedial border of the latissimus dorsi muscle.

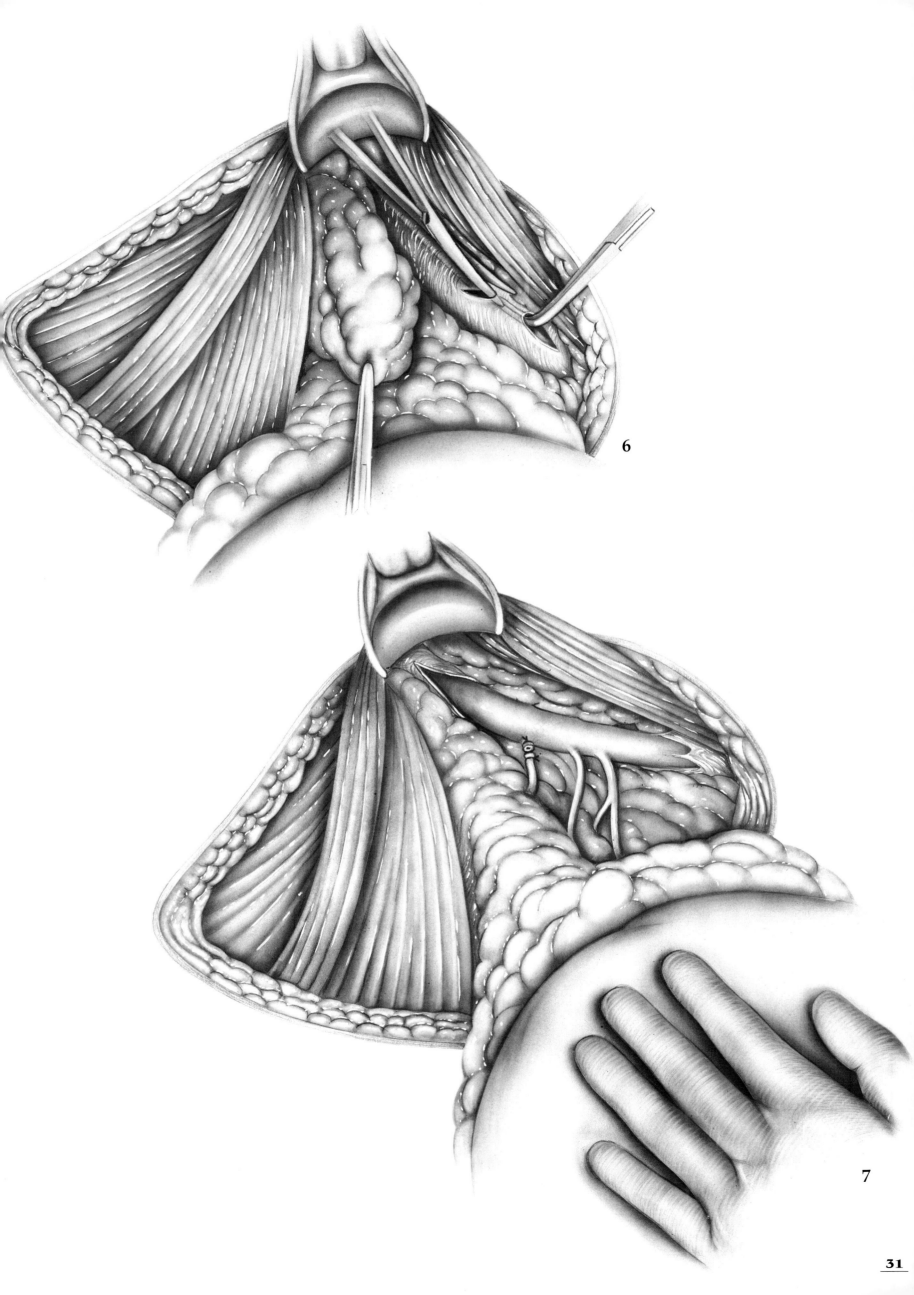

6

7

Modified Radical Mastectomy (*cont.*)

8 The cleared axilla shows the axillary vein superiorly, the pectoral, intercostal, and serratus muscles against the chest wall, and the latissimus dorsi muscle deep and laterally.

9 Meticulous hemostasis is achieved. Two closed suction catheter drains, one under the flaps and one in the axilla, are placed through separate incisions. These drains evacuate any residual blood and lymph from the wound. The wound is closed with interrupted absorbable sutures in the subcutaneous tissues and interrupted #0000 nylon sutures in the skin. The wound must be closed without tension. Should tension be present, the flaps may be further mobilized by freeing the superior flap above the clavicle and dissecting the inferior flap onto the anterior abdominal wall. Once the wound is closed, a pressure bandage is applied to the chest wall.

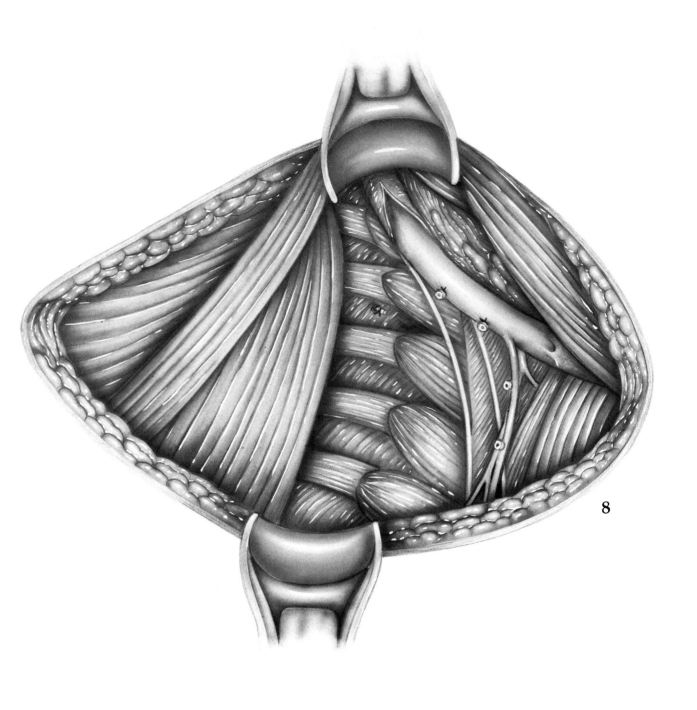

8

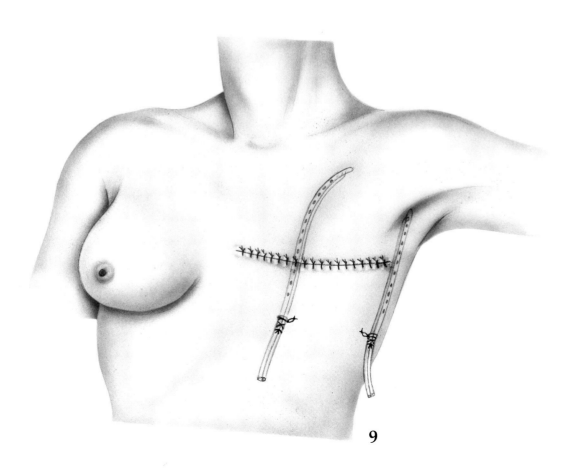

9

Nissen Fundoplication

1 After the induction of general anesthesia, a #34 French Ewald orogastric tube is placed. The abdomen is explored through an upper midline or extended left subcostal incision. The falciform ligament is divided and the left lobe of the liver is retracted toward the patient's right. Beginning above the left gastric artery, the gastrohepatic omentum is incised along the proximal stomach and distal esophagus. The peritoneum overlying the anterior esophagus is cut, allowing complete encirclement of the esophagus above the gastro-esophageal junction. The vagi are identified and preserved. Very rarely several of the short gastric vessels need to be divided to free an adequate portion of the fundus for the subsequent "wrap."

2 Occasionally the lateral segment of the left lobe of the liver will need to be freed from its diaphragmatic attachments, allowing it to be retracted from its position overlying the gastroesophageal junction. The left triangular ligament is carefully divided by either electrocautery or sharp dissection with scissors. The crura are approximated with interrupted nonabsorbable sutures to tailor the size of the esophageal hiatus.

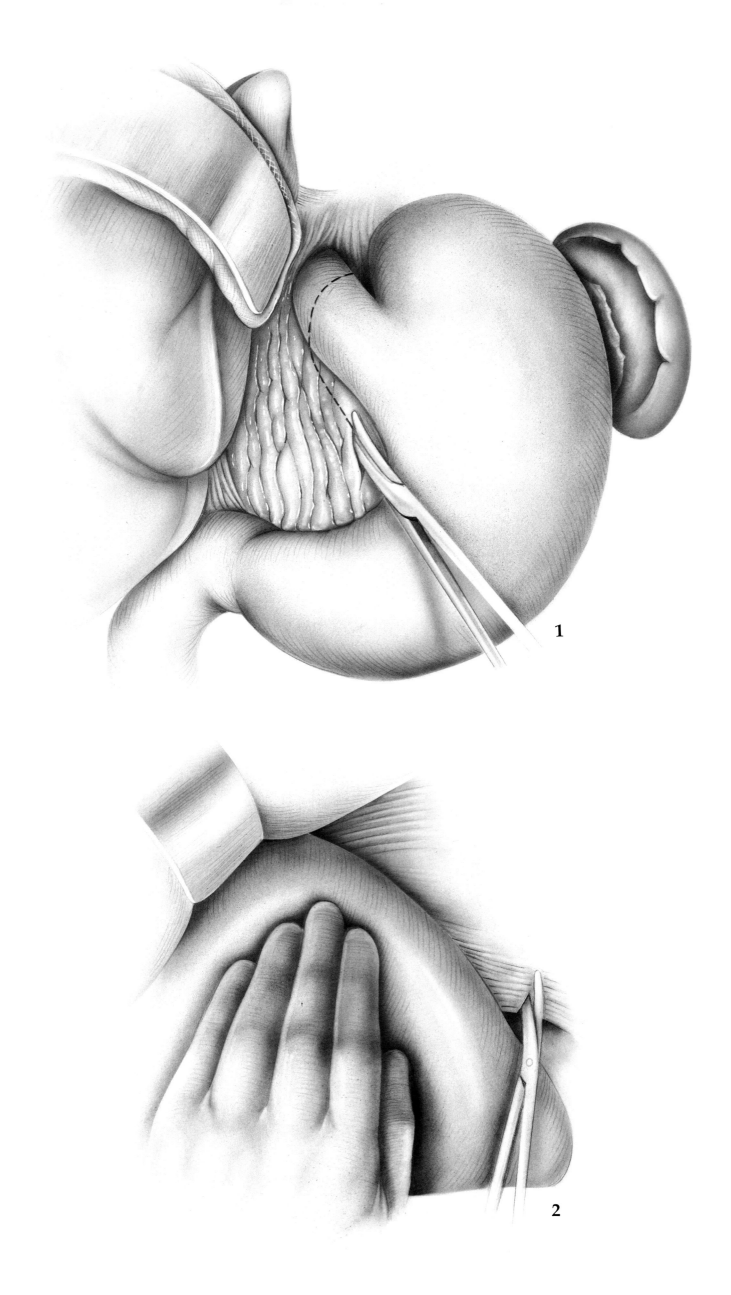

Nissen Fundoplication (*cont.*)

3 The surgeon pushes the fundus posteriorly around the lower esophagus and the most proximal stomach. An Allis clamp placed on either side of the wrapped fundal pouch stabilizes the fundal "horseshoe."

4 A #34 French straight catheter is placed alongside the esophagus within the fundal pouch and three #00 silk sutures are placed through the fundus, the esophagus, and, again, the fundus of the stomach, enclosing the catheter. The use of this catheter, which can be manipulated at surgery, ensures a sufficiently wide fundal collar that the patient will retain ease of eructation and will have no dysphagia postoperatively.

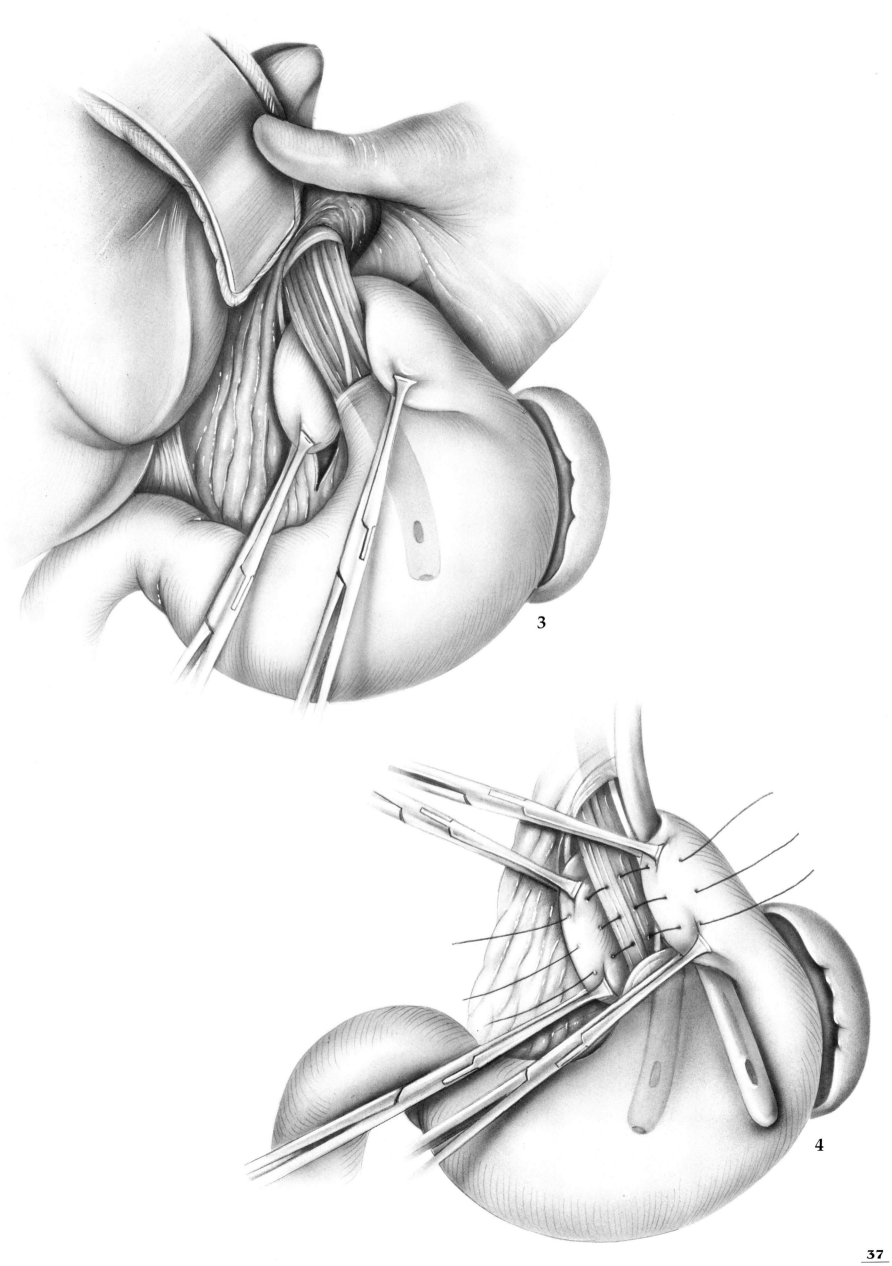

3

4

Nissen Fundoplication (*cont.*)

5 The completed gastric collar overlaps the distal esophagus and the most proximal stomach.

6 Both the straight catheter and the Ewald tube are removed and a sump nasogastric tube is inserted. The anesthesiologist inflates the stomach with saline and air as the surgeon presses on the stomach to test the competence of the plication.

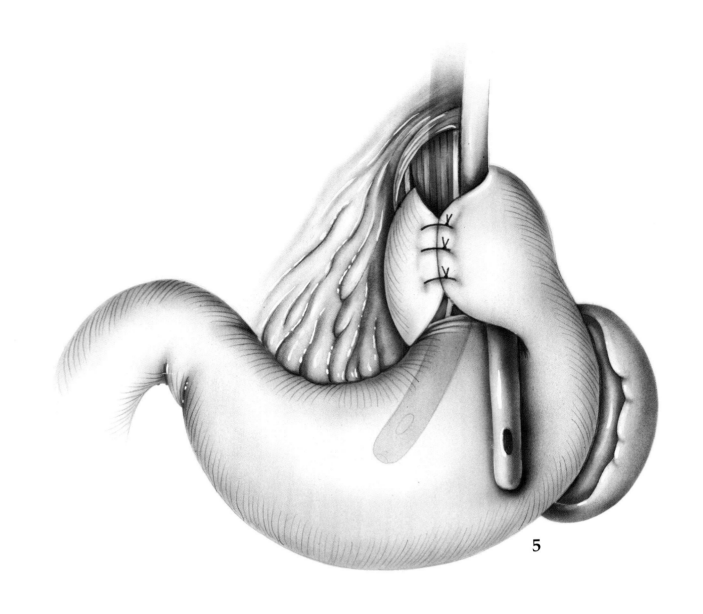

5

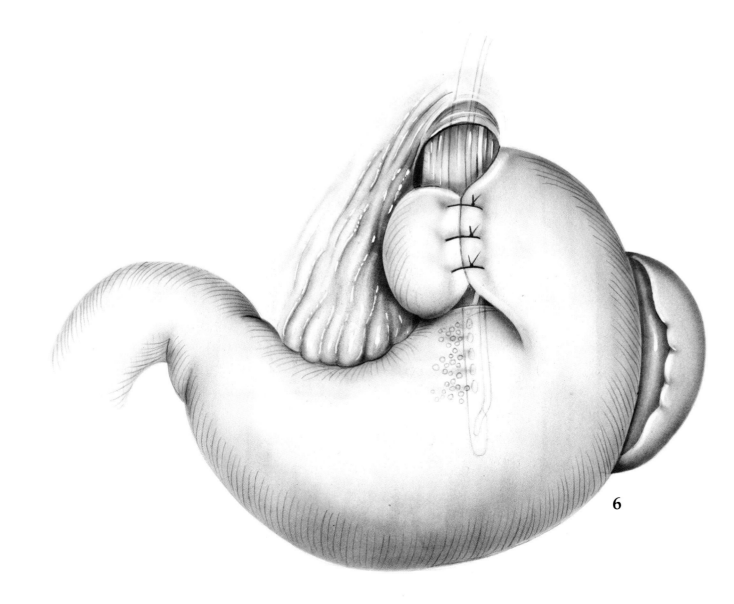

6

Gastroenterostomy (Continuous Suture Technique)

1 The abdomen is explored through an upper midline or left subcostal incision.

2 The transverse mesocolon is elevated into the wound and an incision is made in the bare area of the mesocolon posterior to the vascular arcades.

3 Two Babcock clamps are used to deliver a portion of the stomach, through the defect in the transverse mesocolon, to an infracolic position.

4 The greater omentum is dissected from the stomach at the site of the proposed gastroenterostomy on the greater curvature or posterior gastric wall. A loop of jejunum is approximated to the stomach with two #00 silk stay sutures. The stay sutures (henceforth, *A* and *A'*) are placed approximately 6 to 7 cm apart; the anastomosis is constructed within them.

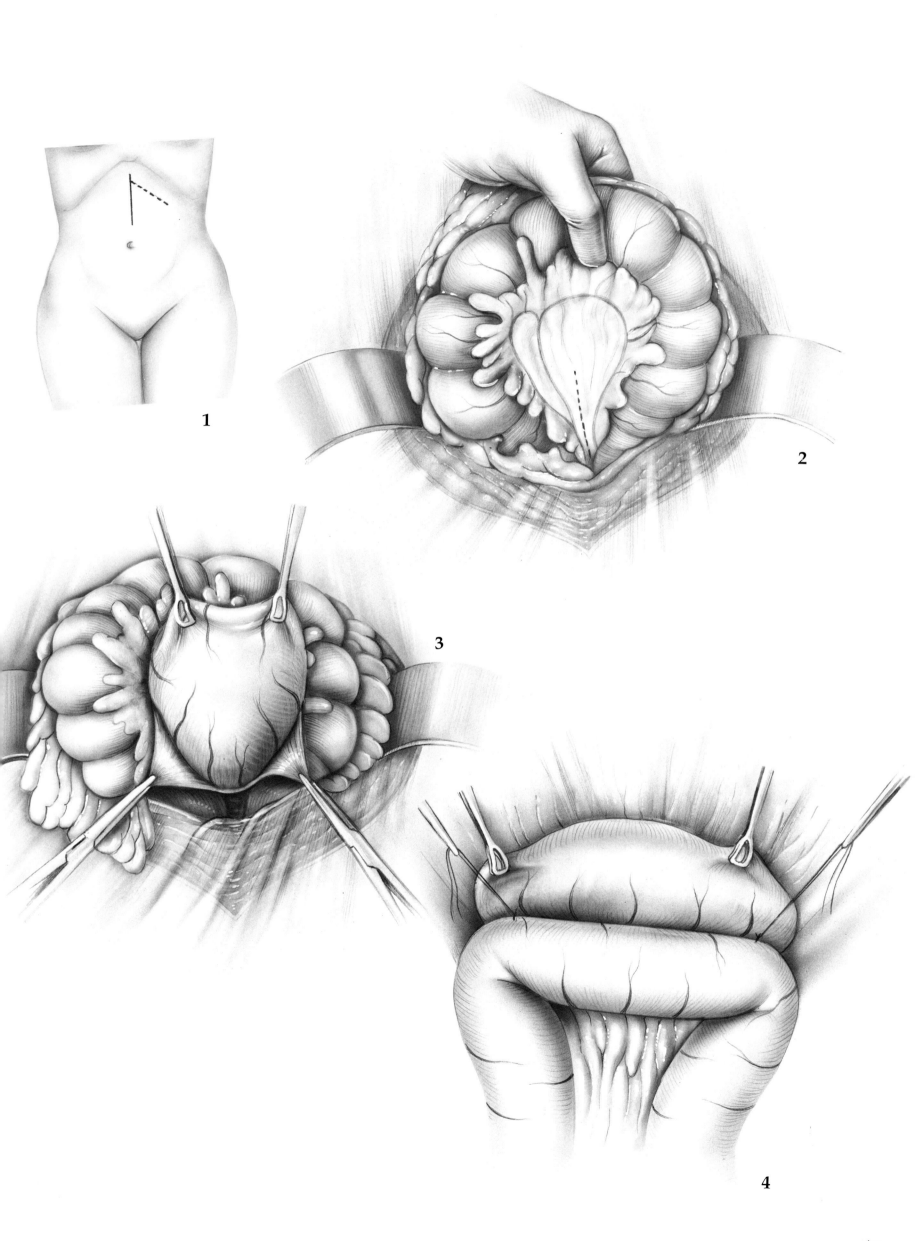

1

2

3

4

Gastroenterostomy (Continuous Suture Technique) (*cont.*)

5 The posterior outer layer of the anastomosis is begun at point *B*. The stomach and jejunum are sewn together in a continuous, seromuscular fashion with a #00 polyglycolic acid suture. When the posterior suture line is completed at point *B′*, this suture is set aside so that it may be used for the anterior outer layer after the completion of the inner layer. Parallel enterotomies are created in the stomach and jejunum with the electrocautery, as indicated by the broken lines (**Fig. 6**).

6–8 The posterior, full-thickness, inner suture line is fashioned with a #00 polyglycolic acid suture run opposite to the direction of the posterior outer suture line. Varying the starting points of the inner and outer suture lines avoids a common defect in the anastomosis at its completion.

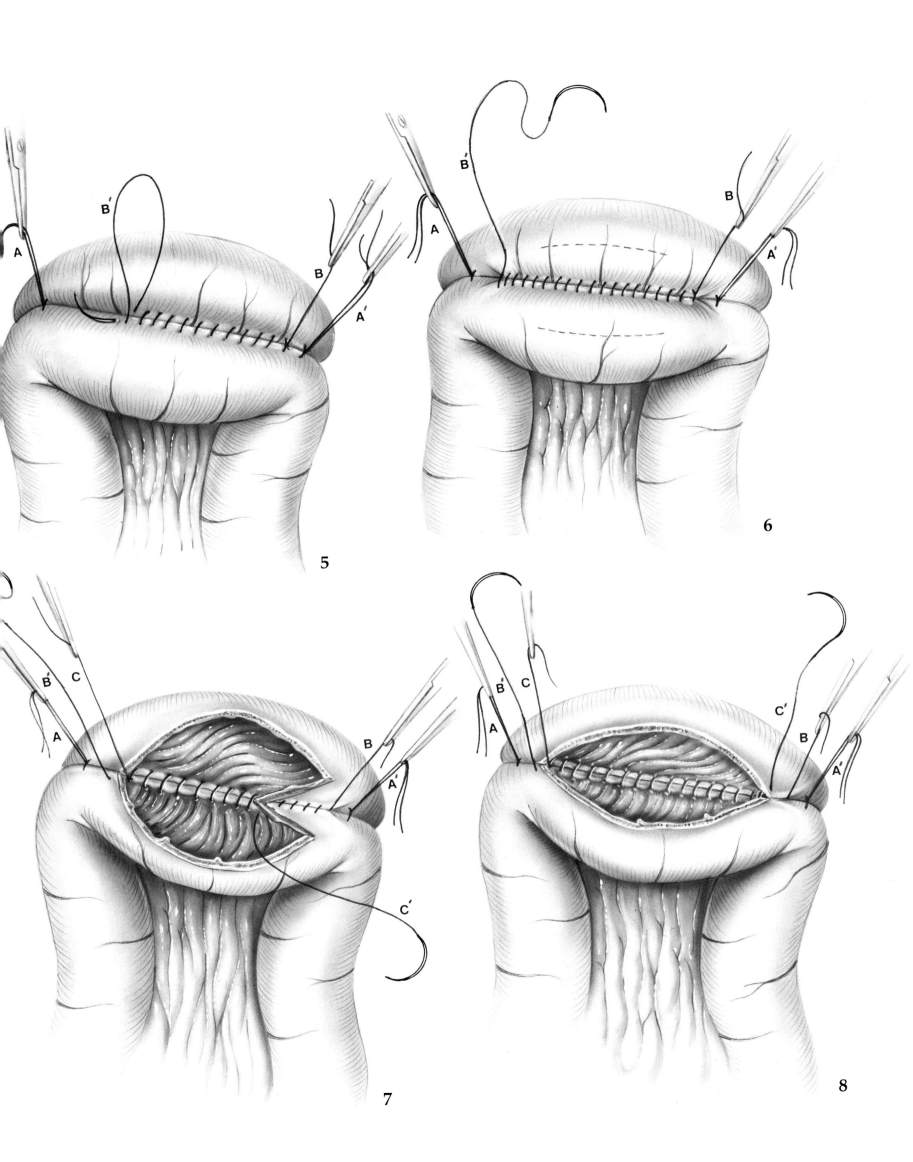

5

6

7

8

Gastroenterostomy (Continuous Suture Technique) (*cont.*)

9 The inner layer is continued anteriorly and tied at its point of origin (C).

10 The original suture is used again to complete the anterior, seromuscular outer layer of the anastomosis. It, too, is tied at its point of origin.

11 The stay sutures are cut and the stomach is allowed to retract into the supracolic position.

12 The mesocolon is fixed to the anastomosis with a series of interrupted #000 silk sutures so that the stomach remains above the mesocolon and the jejunum remains below. This maneuver may be helpful if subsequent surgery is required.

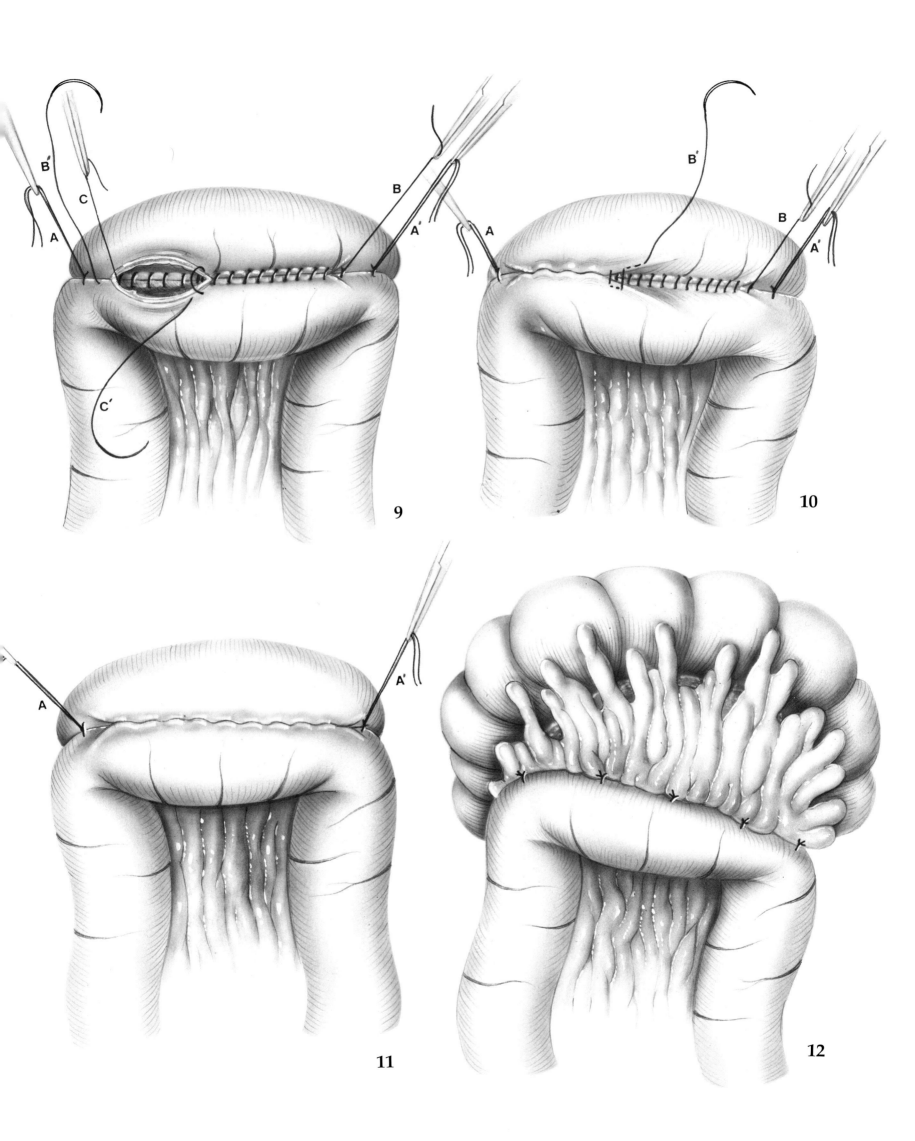

9

10

11

12

Hemigastrectomy (Billroth I Type) and Vagotomy

1 The patient is placed on the operating table in the supine position. A midline incision is made from the xiphoid extending below the umbilicus. Upon entry into the abdomen, the falciform ligament is divided between clamps and ligated.

2 The gastrocolic ligament of the greater omentum is divided outside the gastroepiploic arcade, either between clamps or with the aid of a ligating/dividing stapling instrument. The gastrohepatic ligament is then opened, allowing division of the right gastric artery as well as the branches of the left gastric artery. The left gastroepiploic artery is divided and ligated below its second branch and the greater curvature is cleared of residual omentum at this site. A Payr clamp is placed transversely across the stomach from this level on the greater curvature to a point 4 cm below the gastroesophageal junction on the lesser curvature. A Dennis intestinal anastomosis clamp is placed parallel and proximal to the Payr clamp for a distance of 4 cm. Using electrocautery, the portion of the stomach between these clamps is divided.

3 When the division of the stomach almost reaches the tip of the first Dennis clamp, a second Dennis clamp is placed with its tip at a point 2 cm below the gastroesophageal junction on the lesser curvature.

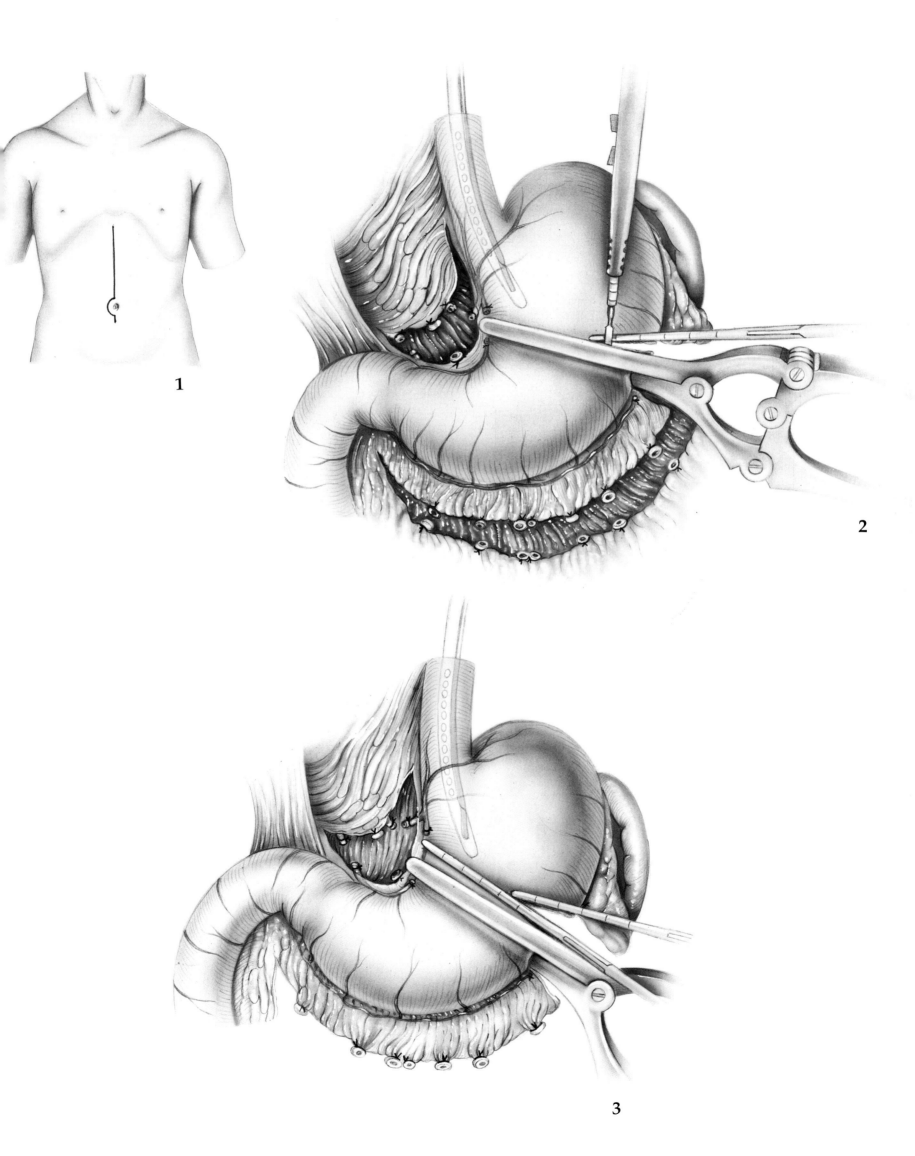

1

2

3

Hemigastrectomy (Billroth I Type) and Vagotomy (*cont.*)

4–5 The remainder of the stomach is divided between the Payr clamp and the second Dennis clamp with electrocautery. Because the anastomosis will be constructed with a single layer of interrupted seromuscular sutures without incorporation of the gastric mucosa, hemostasis is obtained by thoroughly cauterizing the gastric mucosa that extends beyond the anastomosis clamps until a distinct char becomes apparent.

6–9 Using the two Dennis clamps as a handle to draw down on the proximal gastric pouch, the posterior vagus can be identified in its position posterior and medial to the esophagus and can be brought into view with a crooked finger (**Fig. 7**). Drawing a long nerve hook (Smithwick) proximally and distally along the axis of the vagus will clear a 2-cm segment of the right vagus from its overlying areolar tissue (**Fig. 8**). A clamp is placed on the nerve in its midportion (**Fig. 9**).

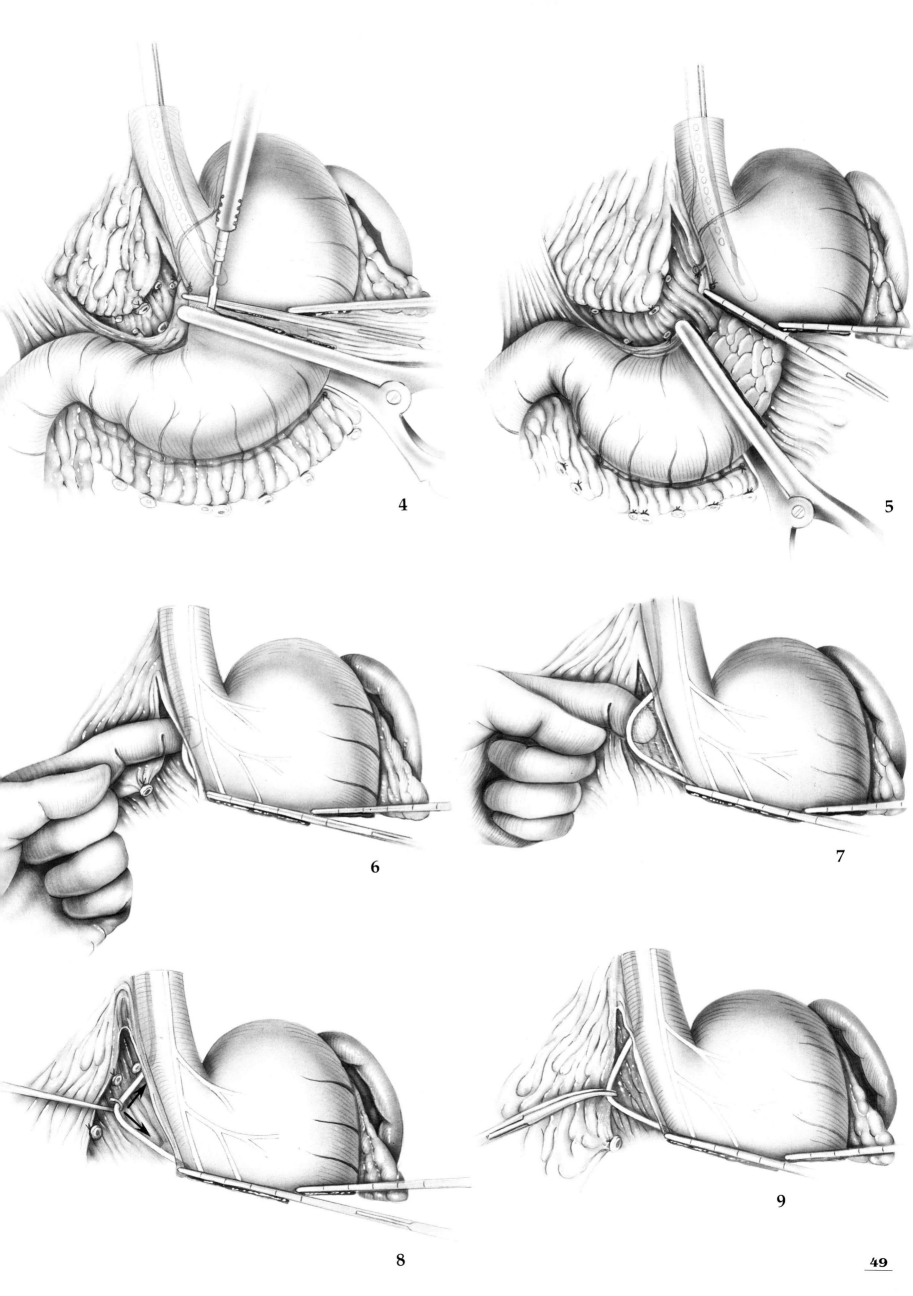

4

5

6

7

8

9

Hemigastrectomy (Billroth I Type) and Vagotomy (*cont.*)

10–12 Hemoclips are applied proximally and distally (**Figs. 10–11**), and a segment of the nerve is excised (**Fig. 12**).

13–16 The surgeon's finger is then interposed between the esophagus and its overlying peritoneum. Tenting the peritoneum anteriorly permits the anterior vagus to be palpated as a taut string against the finger (**Fig. 13**). The nerve hook is again used to clear a segment of the vagus (**Fig. 14**) which is subsequently clipped above and below (**Fig. 15**) and resected (**Fig. 16**). The remainder of the peritoneum overlying the esophagus is divided and the esophagus is inspected for additional vagal fibers.

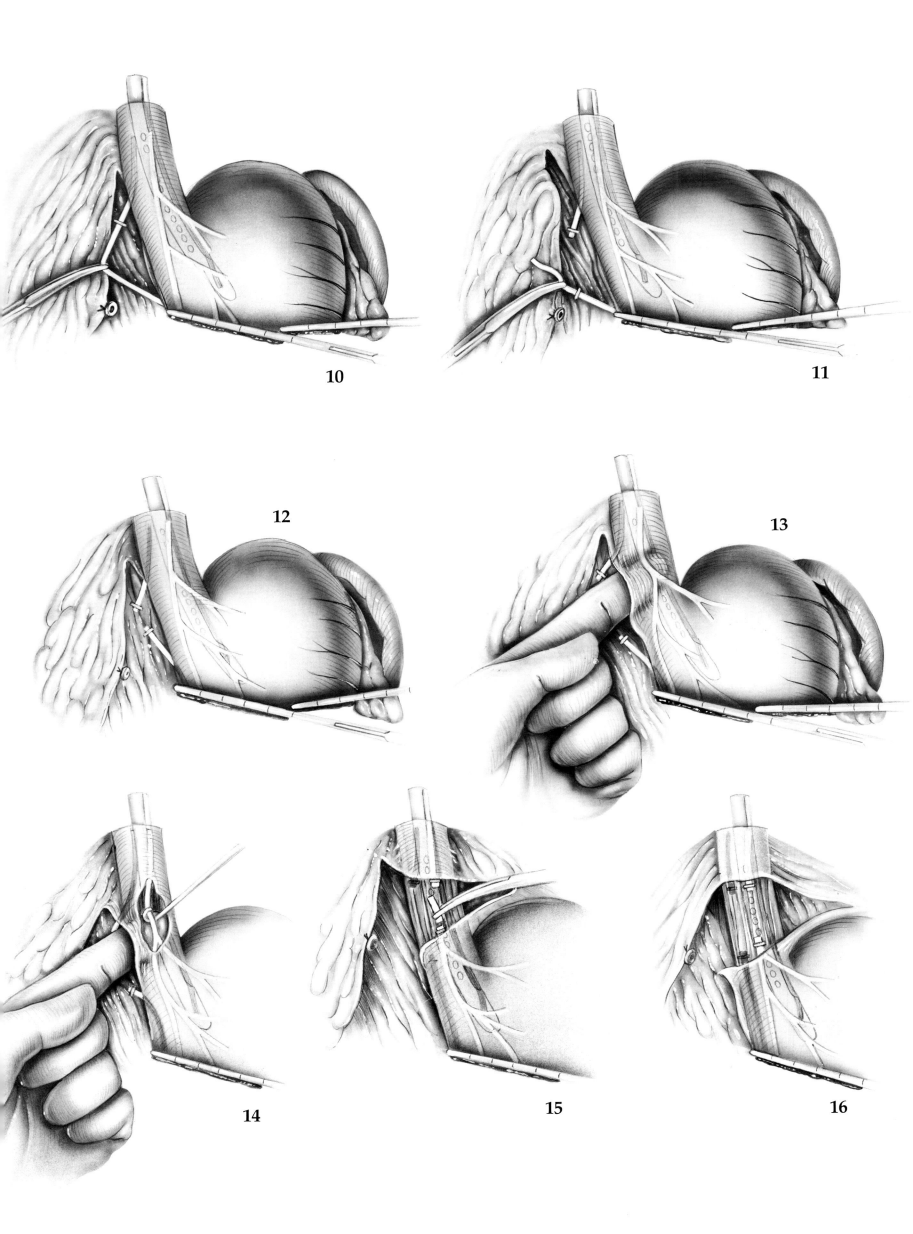

10

11

12

13

14

15

16

Hemigastrectomy (Billroth I Type) and Vagotomy (*cont.*)

17–20 The proximal pouch is tailored by closing the portion of the stomach contained in the second anastomosis clamp. Interrupted seromuscular #000 silk Lembert stitches are placed through the anterior and posterior gastric wall as indicated by the hatched lines (**Fig. 17**). This is facilitated by rotating the Dennis clamp to expose the posterior gastric wall. When a series of these stitches have been placed (**Fig. 18**), traction on them allows the removal of the Dennis clamp and the inversion of the closed, charred gastric stump (**Fig. 19**). The remaining Dennis clamp will be used for the subsequent gastroduodenal anastomosis (**Fig. 20**).

21 The Payr clamp on the distal portion of the stomach is elevated and the gastric remnant is divided between anastomosis clamps placed on the duodenum just distal to the pylorus.

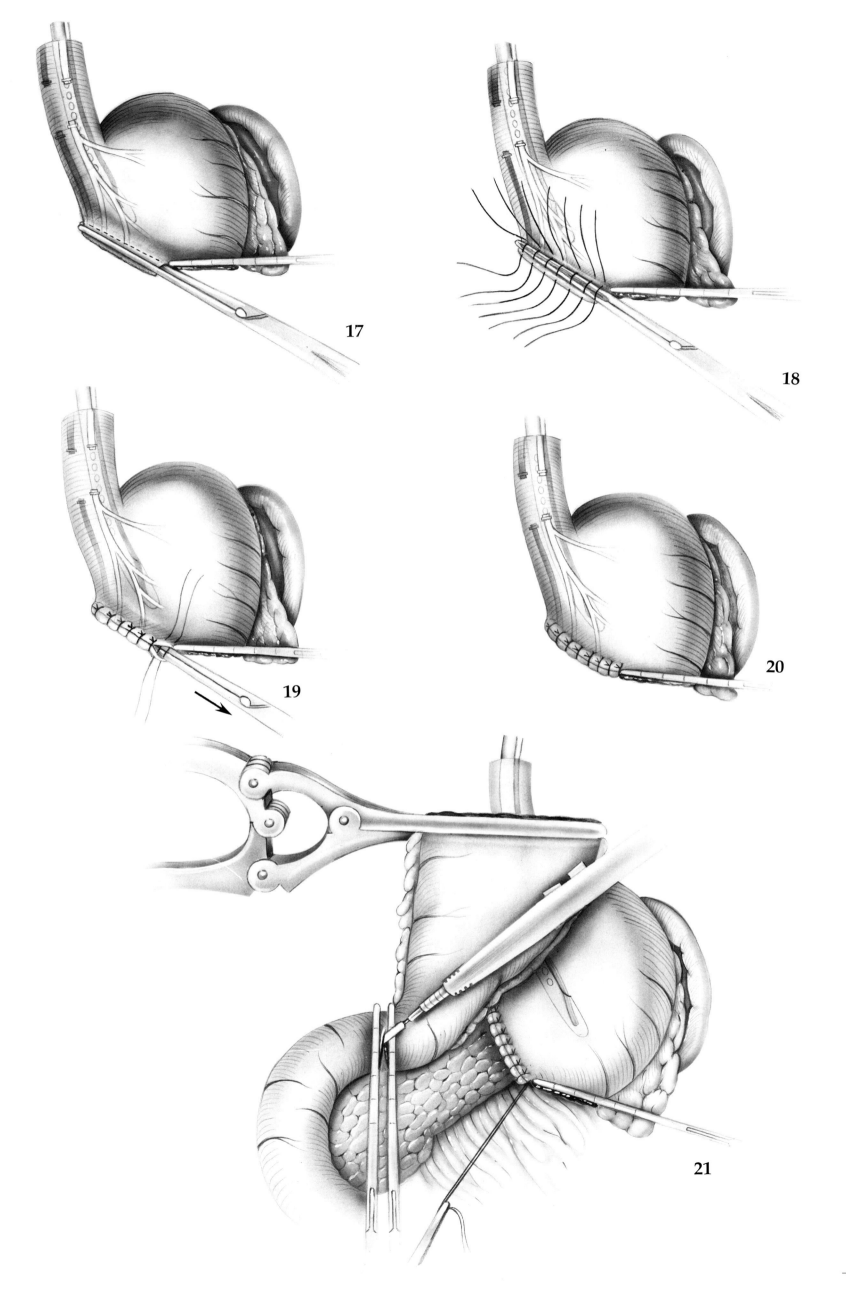

17

18

19

20

21

Hemigastrectomy (Billroth I Type) and Vagotomy (cont.)

22–24 #000 silk corner stitches are placed. The lesser-curvature corner stitch crosses the previously closed lesser-curvature suture line transversely (**Fig. 22**) and then into the duodenal wall along its long axis. The greater-curvature corner stitch is placed through the long axis of both the stomach and the duodenum (**Fig. 22**). A Kocher incision is made lateral to the duodenum to relieve tension on the anastomosis. A "closed" gastroduodenostomy is fashioned by placing interrupted #000 silk seromuscular sutures in the posterior gastric and duodenal walls. The assistant rotates the anastomosis clamps while the surgeon places these sutures (**Fig. 23**). The clamps are held close to one another while the surgeon ties the posterior suture line. The corner sutures are not tied at this time (**Fig. 24**).

25 The anastomosis clamps are rotated so that a similar row of interrupted sutures may be placed in the anterior gastric and duodenal walls. Once positioned, these sutures are elevated and the anastomosis clamps are withdrawn, permitting the anastomosis to invert. The anterior sutures are tied along with the corner sutures.

26 At the point where the lesser-curvature (Hofmeister) suture line meets the gastroduodenostomy suture line, another stitch is placed transversely across the lesser-curvature suture line and through the duodenum distal to the gastroduodenostomy suture line. This maneuver further invaginates the junction between the two suture lines and reduces the risk of leakage from this point.

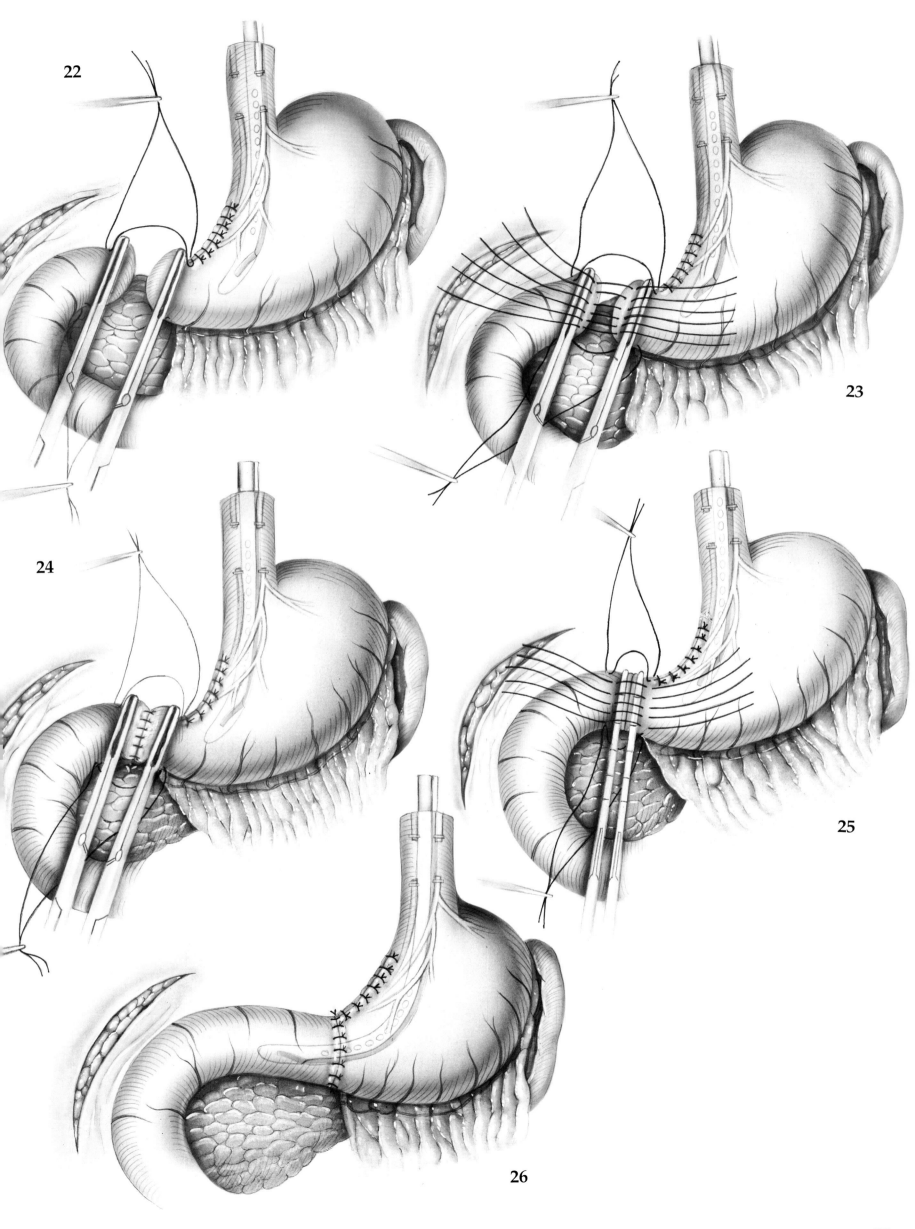

Gastrectomy (Billroth II Type)

1–3 As a variation of the technique described for the Billroth I reconstruction, the Hofmeister closure may be accomplished by using an automatic stapling device to close the lesser-curvature portion of the gastric pouch. The initial operative steps are the same as for the Billroth I (see **Plate 23, Figs. 1–2**). The stapling device is used instead of the second anastomosis clamp. Once it is fired, it is left in place until the stomach is divided between it and the Payr clamp (**Fig. 2**). Again, the protruding mucosa is cauterized liberally to prevent subsequent bleeding (**Fig. 3**).

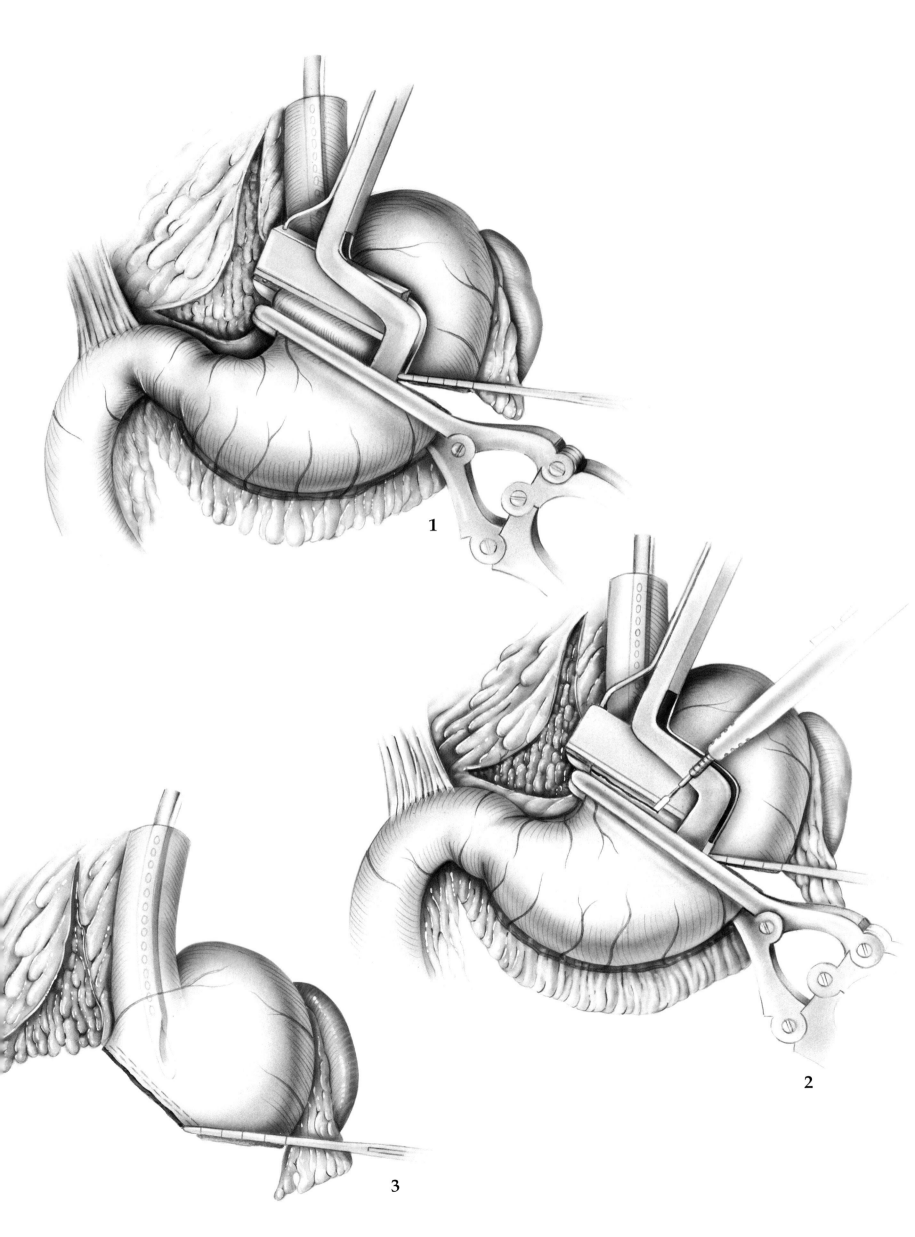

1

2

3

Gastrectomy (Billroth II Type) (*cont.*)

The duodenal closure may be performed either with a single layer of seromuscular sutures (**Figs. 4–7**) or with an automatic stapling device (**Figs. 8–10**).

Sewn Duodenal Closure

4–7 As in the previous procedure, the distal stomach is divided between anastomosis clamps just beyond the pylorus (**Fig. 4**). The duodenal stump is closed with a row of interrupted, seromuscular, #000 silk sutures placed first in the posterior and then in the anterior duodenal walls (**Fig. 5**). The sutures are tied sequentially as the anastomosis clamp is withdrawn (**Fig. 6**). The duodenal stump is inspected to ensure a secure closure (**Fig. 7**).

Stapled Duodenal Closure

8–10 The stapling device may be used to close the duodenum so long as there is no substantial edema or rigidity of the proximal duodenum. (Otherwise there is the risk that the rigid and unyielding staples will cut through the duodenal wall.) The closure is accomplished by dividing the duodenum with electrocautery between the stapling device placed distally and an anastomosis clamp placed proximally.

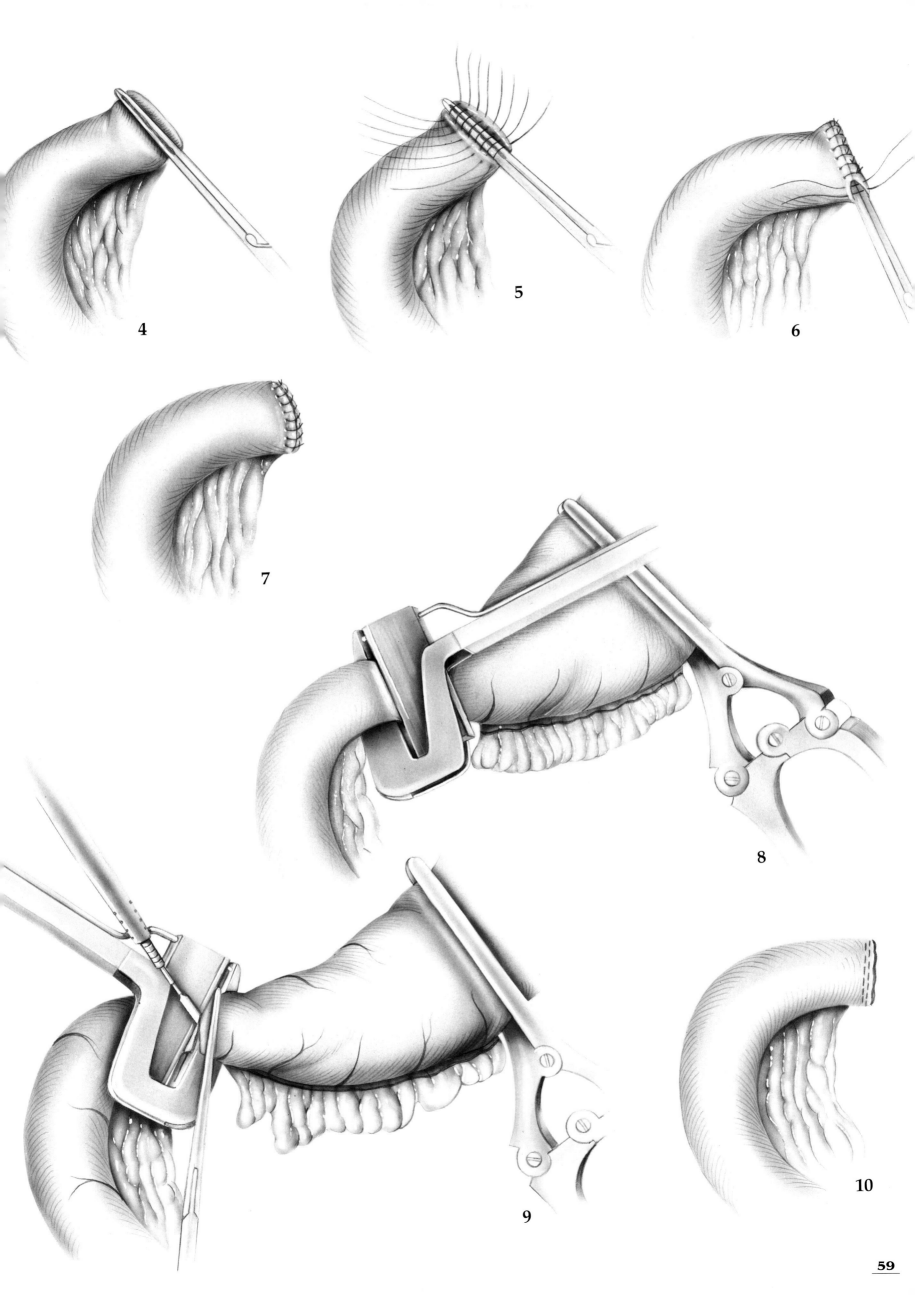

4

5

6

7

8

9

10

Gastrectomy (Billroth II Type) (*cont.*)

11 The Billroth II reconstruction is performed in a retrocolic fashion with a very short loop of proximal jejunum or distal duodenum after mobilizing the ligament of Treitz (as shown by the broken line in **Fig. 11**). The transverse mesocolon is opened immediately adjacent to the mobilized jejunum, avoiding injury to the vascular arcades in the mesocolon.

12 The jejunum is brought through the mesocolon using two Allis clamps placed on the anti-mesenteric border of the intestine.

13–15 The two Allis clamps are held up in the air by the assistant as the surgeon places an anastomosis clamp across the antimesenteric border of the jejunum. The small excluded segment of jejunum is resected sharply (**Fig. 14**). Careful inspection for mucosa in the resected jejunum obviates the risk that the anastomosis clamp has not reached across the lumen of the jejunum. The edge of the jejunum is cauterized to provide a seal and hemostasis (**Fig. 15**).

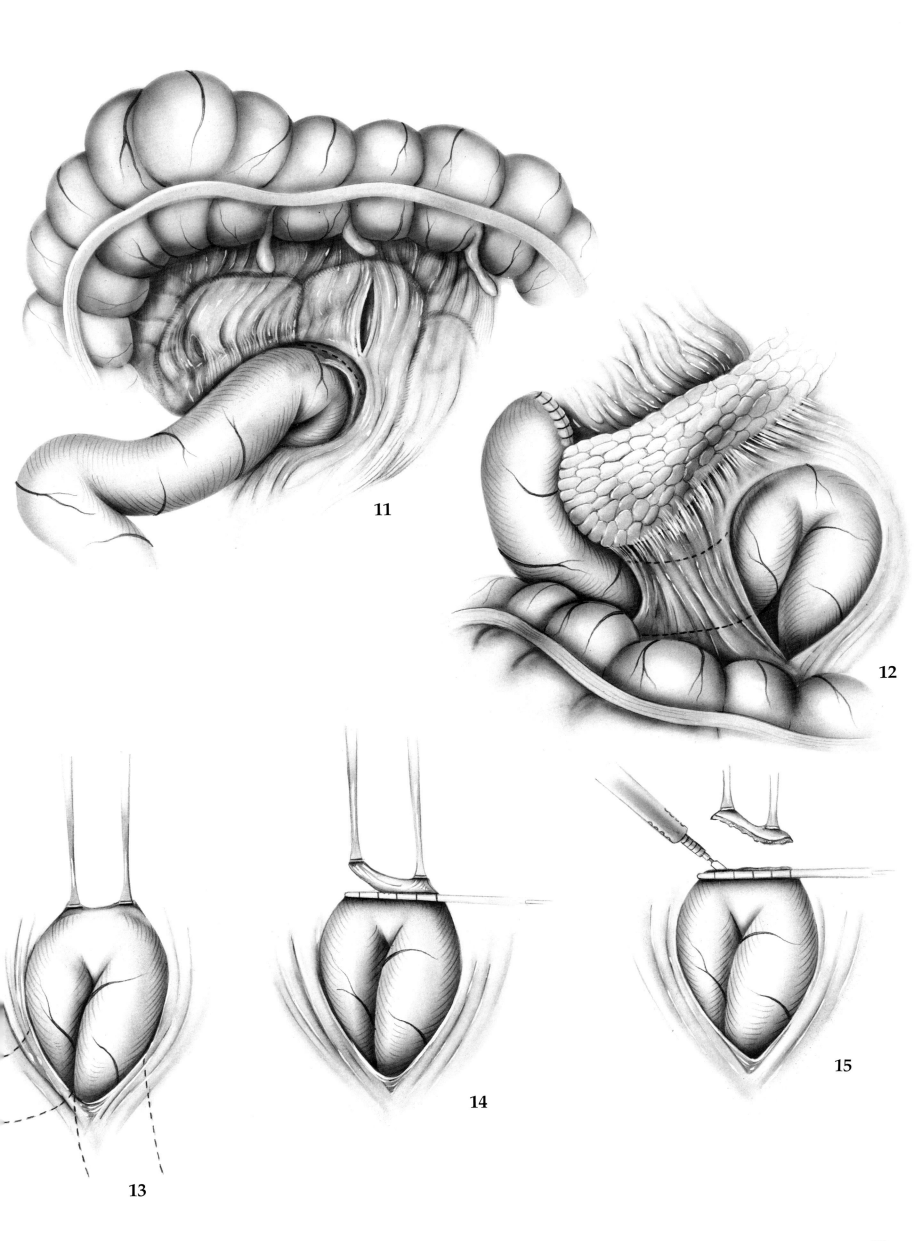

11

12

13

14

15

Gastrectomy (Billroth II Type) (*cont.*)

16 A "closed" gastrojejunostomy is begun by placing a corner suture transversely through the Hofmeister closure of the stomach, just beyond the tip of the anastomosis clamp, and then through the jejunum. The second corner suture is placed on the greater-curvature side of the gastric remnant, proximal to the heel of the anastomosis clamp, and then through the jejunum.

17 The posterior row is accomplished as in the Billroth I, with a series of interrupted seromuscular #000 silk sutures placed in the posterior gastric and jejunal walls.

18 The anastomosis clamps are approximated and the sutures are tied. The corner sutures are not tied at this time.

19 The anastomosis clamps are rotated toward one another to expose the anterior walls of the stomach and the jejunum, and a row of interrupted seromuscular #000 silk sutures is placed. The ends of the sutures are elevated and the sutures are tied as the anastomosis clamps are slowly withdrawn. The anastomosis is palpated to break the seal created by the previous cauterization of the gastric and jejunal walls.

20 An additional transverse suture is placed across the Hofmeister closure and the jejunum on the lesser-curvature side of the gastrojejunostomy, further inverting this junction so as to protect against a leak.

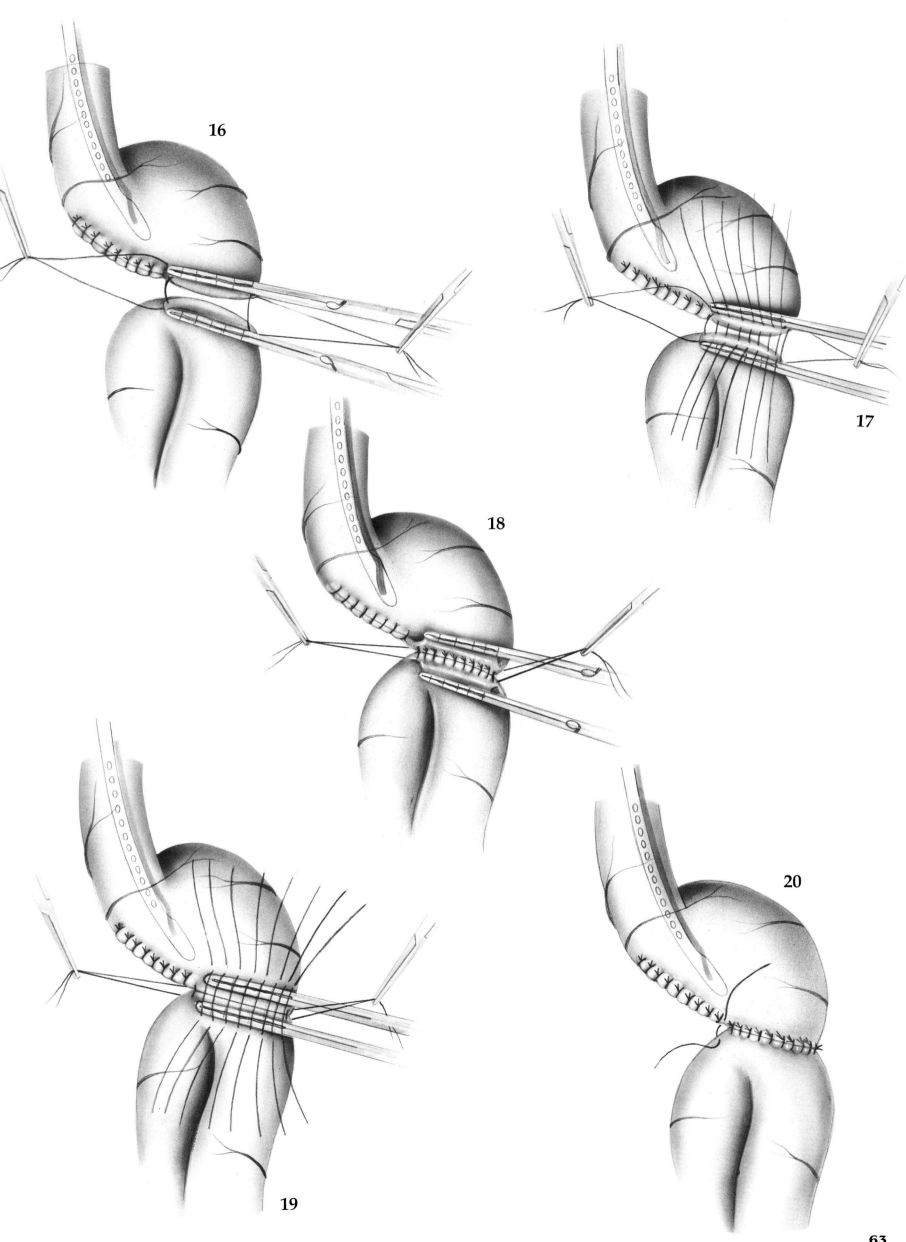

16

17

18

19

20

Gastrectomy (Billroth II Type) (*cont.*)

21–22 The jejunum is brought below the transverse mesocolon and the nasogastric tube is advanced into the afferent limb for postoperative decompression. Sutures are placed to fix the gastrojejunostomy at the level of the mesocolon, thus closing the defect in the mesocolon and securing the stomach above, and the jejunum below, the mesocolon.

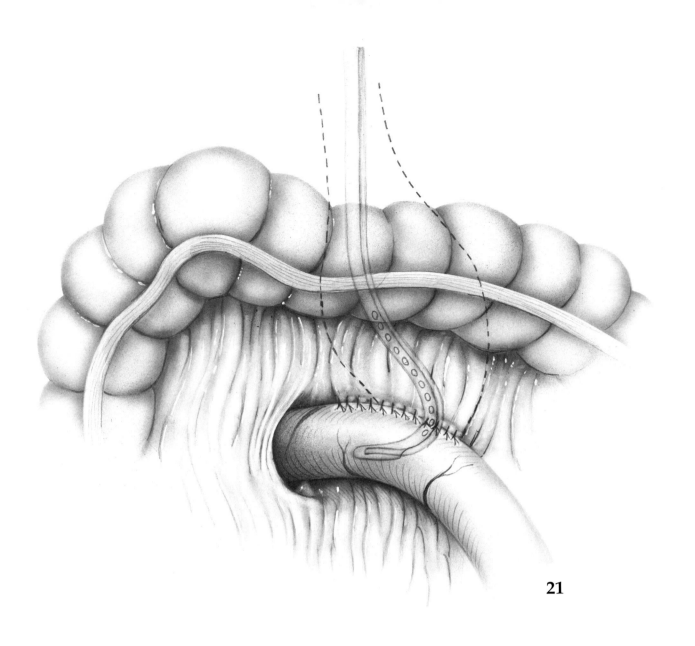

21

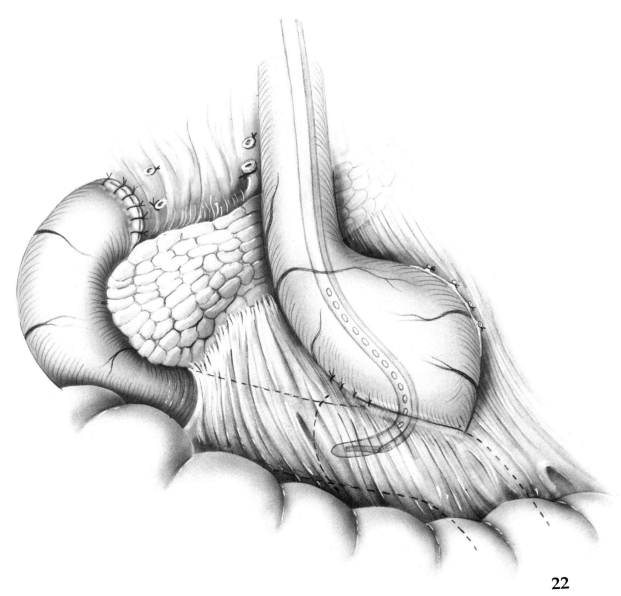

22

PLATE
3 3

Duodenal Stump Closure and T-Tube Duodenostomy

1 The rigid and scarred duodenum with an ulcer in its posterior wall is shown. A Kocher incision is made lateral to the duodenum, mobilizing it and thus lessening the tension on its anterior wall.

2 The closure is accomplished with a row of #00 or #000 silk sutures placed through the capsule of the pancreas, the remnant of the posterior wall or the edge of the ulcer, and then the anterior wall of the duodenum.

3 These sutures are tied, approximating the anterior and posterior walls of the duodenum with the mucosa everted at the cut end. No attempt is made to invert the closure.

4 A #10 French T-tube is tailored with its short arms 2 cm long and a portion removed opposite the long arm.

5 A fine tonsil clamp is applied to a short arm of the T-tube.

6 The T-tube is stretched along the axis of the tonsil clamp.

7 The T-tube is inserted into the duodenal lumen through a spot on the lateral duodenal wall that has been touched with the electrocautery.

8 Several fine silk seromuscular sutures are used to close the duodenal wall around the long limb of the T-tube, establishing a watertight seal between the T-tube and the duodenal lumen. The long arm of the T-tube is tunneled extraperitoneally as far as possible, and then brought out through the abdominal wall. The tube is secured to the skin with a heavy silk suture.

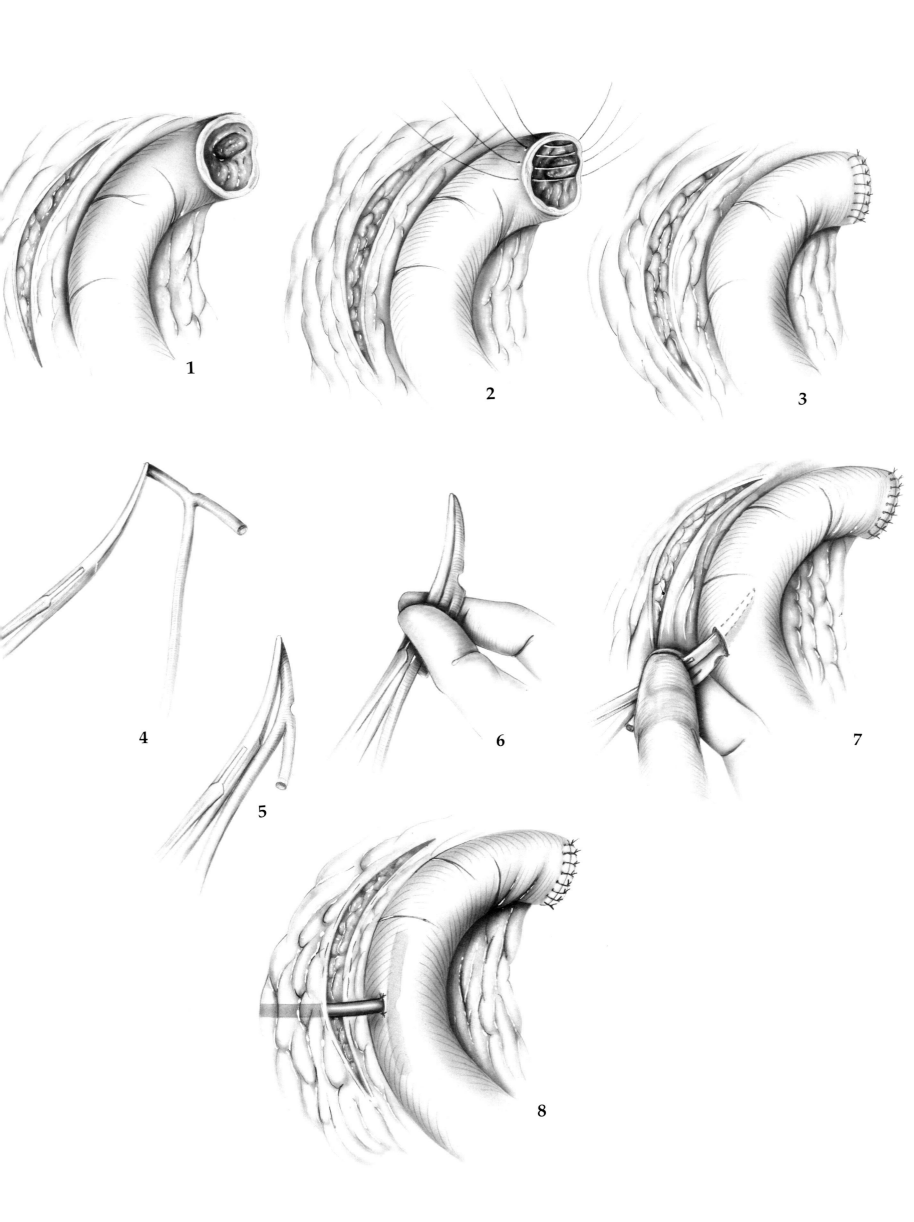

Closure of a Perforated Duodenal Ulcer

1 The abdomen is opened through a midline incision which allows inspection of the upper abdomen and the identification of the perforation in the first portion of the duodenum. Two #000 silk seromuscular Lembert stitches are placed above and below the perforation.

2 A tongue of intact omentum is brought through the two previously placed silk sutures, which are tied over it, without tension, sealing the perforation. A very sizable duodenal perforation may be closed in this fashion, using a broader tongue of omentum.

3 After the placement of the omental patch over the perforation, a third silk suture is placed into the proximal duodenal wall and passed through the omental tongue and, subsequently, the duodenal wall, once again distal to the omentum and perforation.

4 This suture secures the omental patch over the perforation. The abdomen is lavaged, and a decision reached regarding further therapy for the patient's ulcer diathesis.

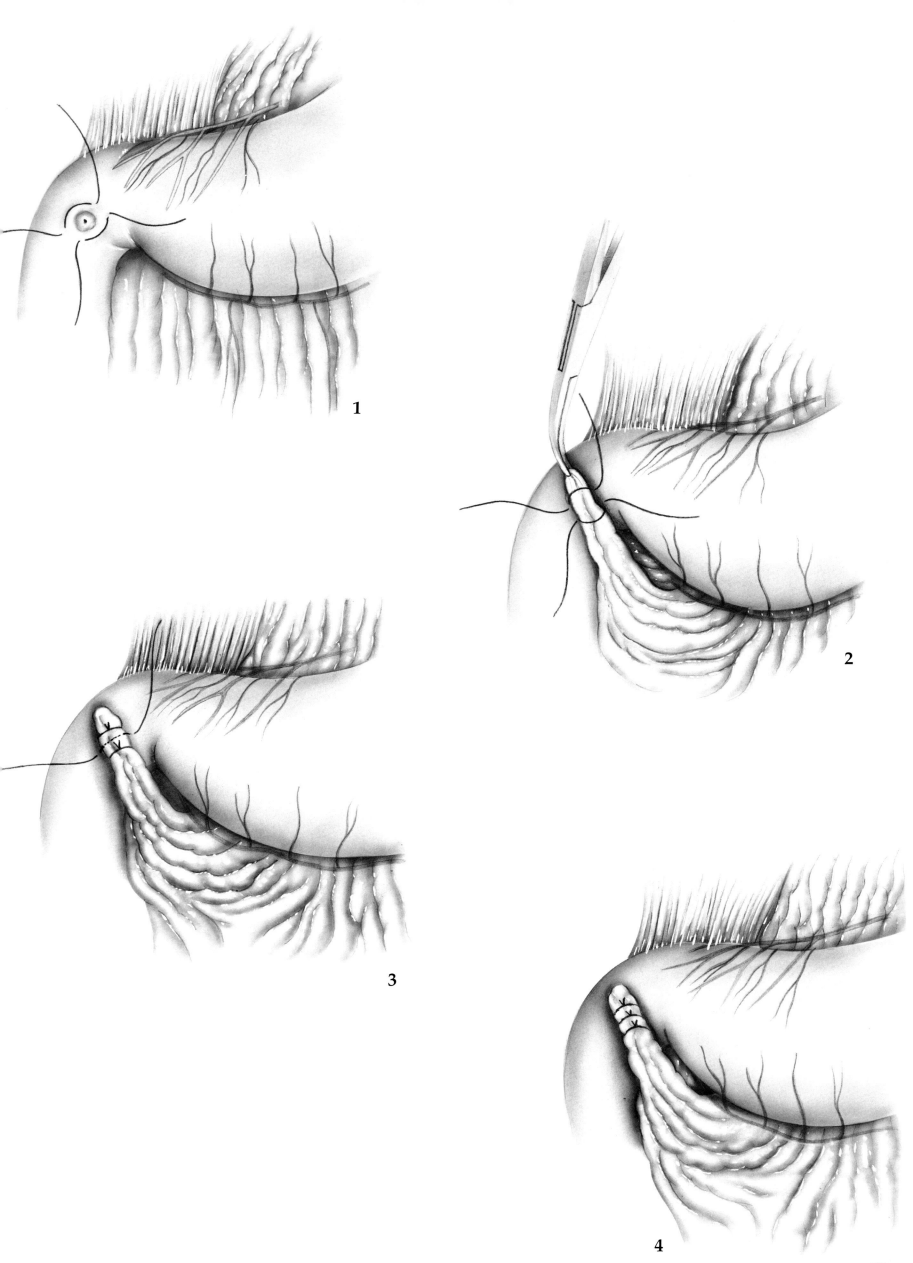

Superselective Vagotomy Following Closure of a Perforated Duodenal Ulcer

1–2 The anterior and posterior vagal trunks are isolated at the esophagus (see **Plate 24, Figs. 6, 7 and Plate 25, Figs. 13, 14**). The trunks are encircled with vessel loops.

3 The gastrohepatic omentum is incised along the broken line, allowing the surgeon's fingers to enter the lesser sac.

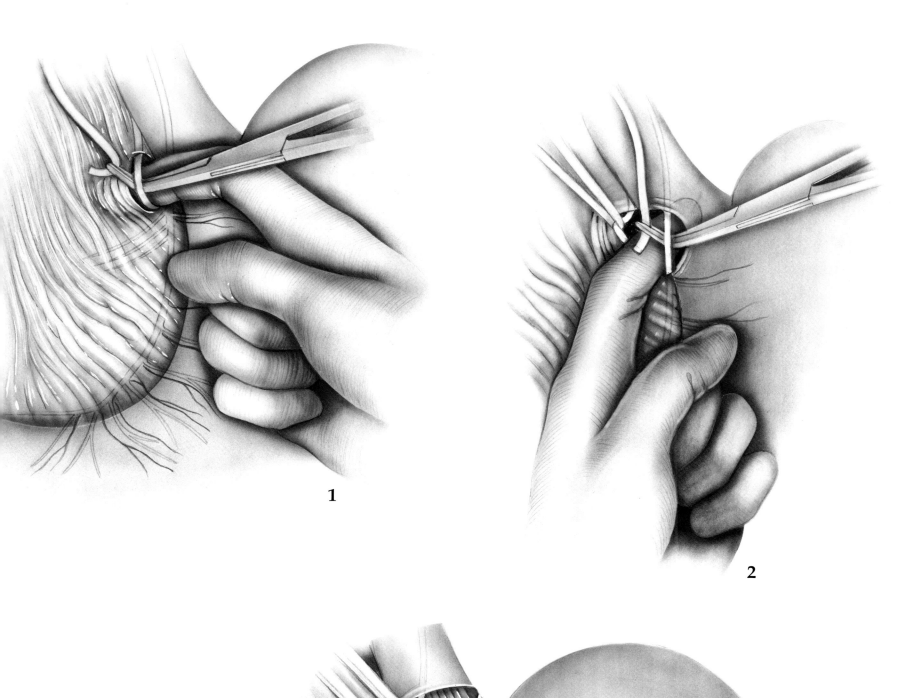

1

2

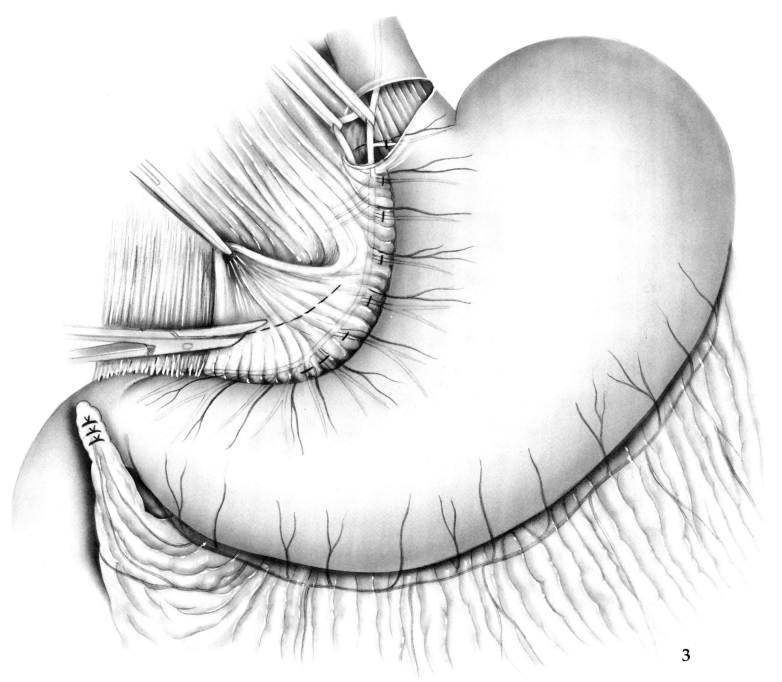

3

Superselective Vagotomy Following Closure of a Perforated Duodenal Ulcer (*cont.*)

4 Starting at the "crow's foot" and proceeding to the gastroesophageal junction, the vessels and accompanying nerve fibers located in the anterior leaflet of the lesser omentum are divided between clamps and tied with #000 silk.

5 Once the anterior leaflet of the lesser omentum has been opened to the gastroesophageal junction, a Penrose drain is placed about the esophagus to provide gentle lateral traction, exposing the posterior leaflet of the lesser omentum. Similarly, the vessels and nerves to the stomach in the posterior leaflet are divided and tied.

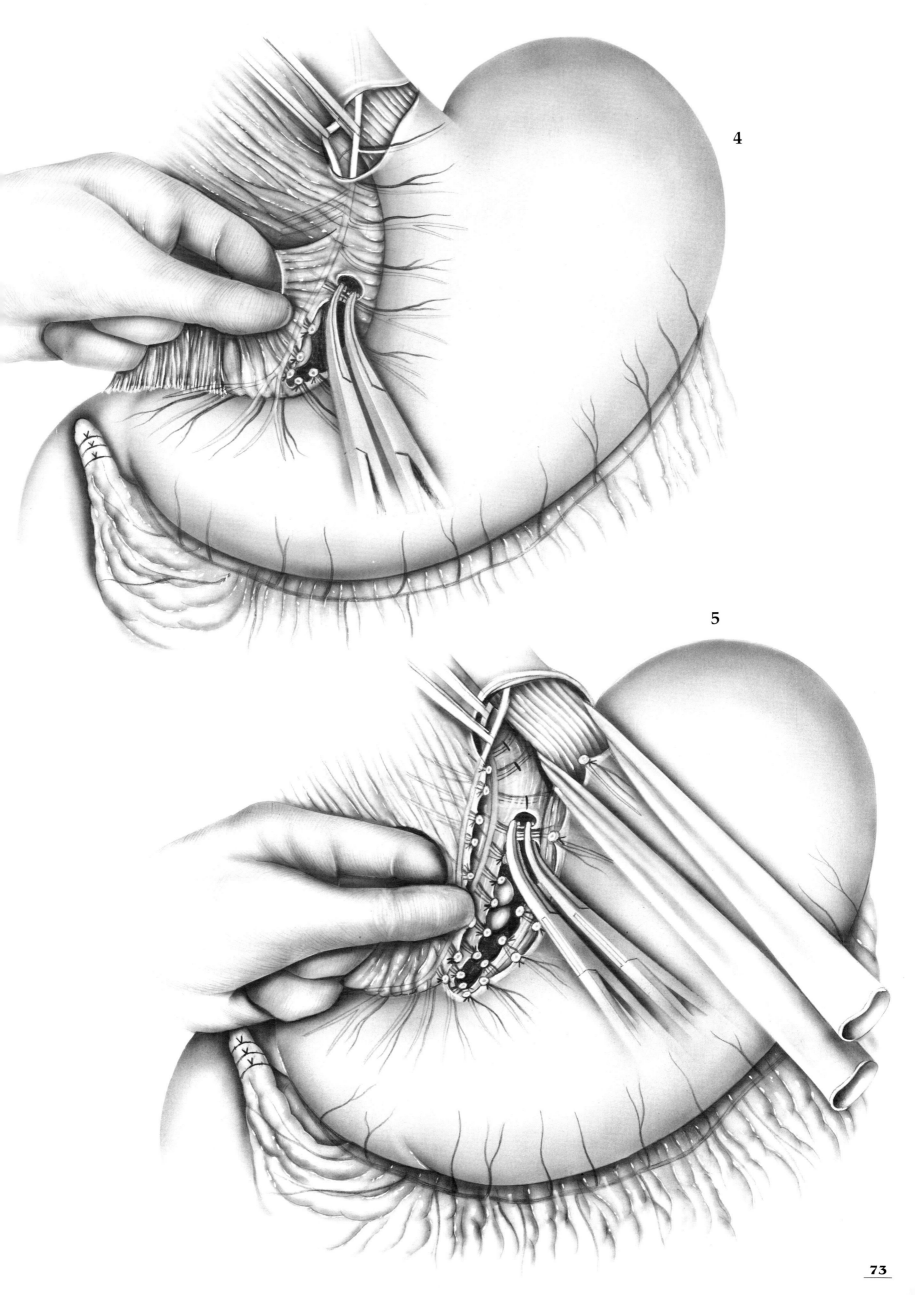

4

5

Superselective Vagotomy Following Closure of a Perforated Duodenal Ulcer (*cont.*)

6 Upon completion of the division of the posterior leaflet, a bare area exists along the lesser curvature from the gastroesophageal junction to the "crow's foot." This is closed with interrupted #000 silk sutures by approximating the gastric sides of the divided anterior and posterior leaflets of the lesser omentum, effectively reperitonealizing this portion of the stomach.

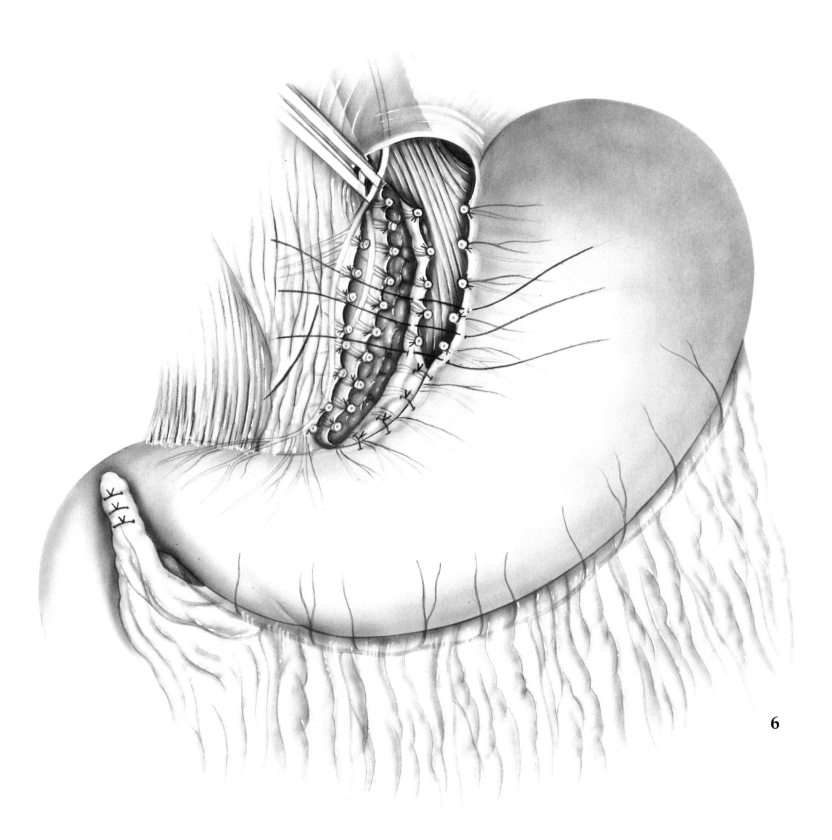

6

Gastric Bypass for Morbid Obesity

1 The abdomen is explored through a midline incision extending approximately 25 cm below the xiphoid. Exposure is achieved with a blade of the Upper Hand retractor placed on each costal margin. If a cholecystectomy is planned, this is done prior to the gastric bypass procedure. Cholecystectomy is performed if stones are present—not for prophylaxis.

2 The left lateral segment of the liver is mobilized by incising the triangular ligaments and is retracted medially. The operation is particularly difficult if the liver is fatty and cannot be retracted easily. The peritoneum overlying the intraabdominal portion of the esophagus is incised transversely (broken line).

3 The esophagus is identified and dissected circumferentially.

4 A wide Penrose drain is passed around the esophagus for retraction.

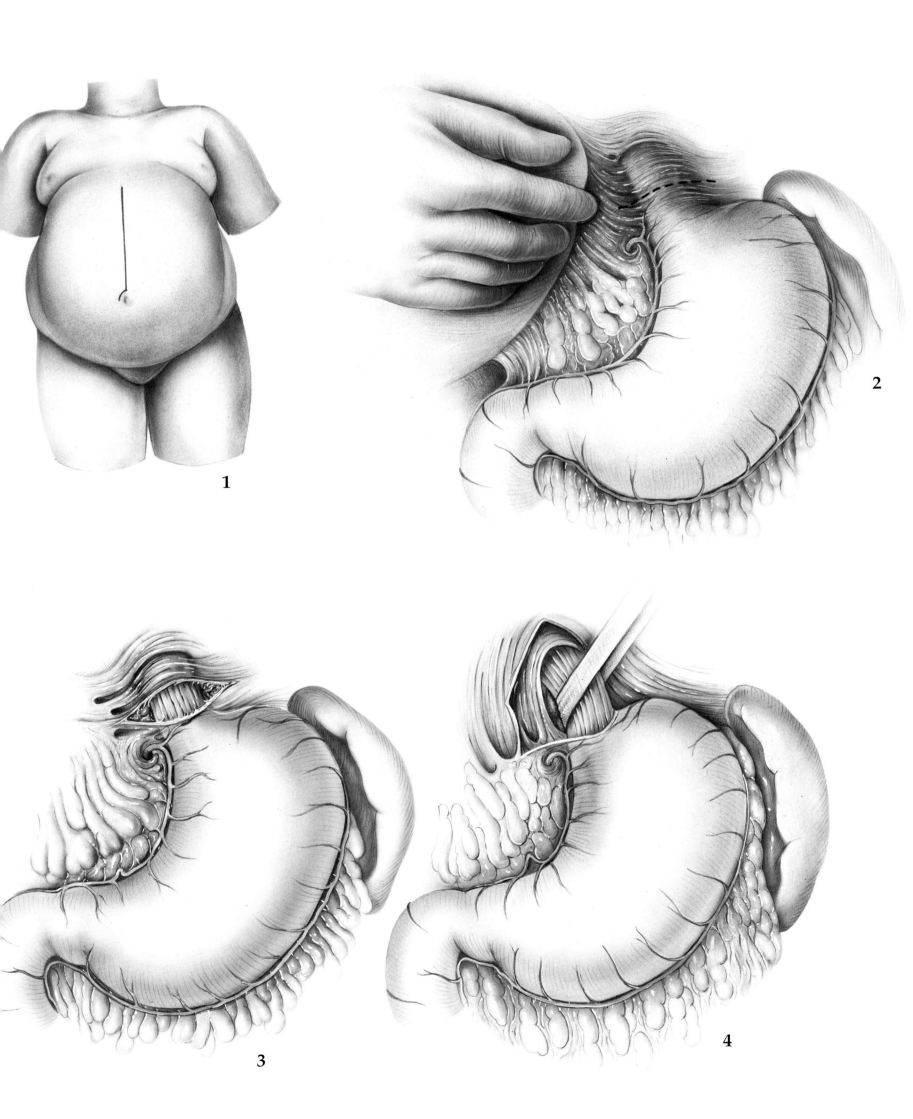

Gastric Bypass for Morbid Obesity (*cont.*)

5 The gastric fundus is mobilized by division and ligation of the vessels of the proximal greater curvature, the short gastric vessels, and the vessels in the gastrohepatic ligament. At least one branch of the left gastric artery is preserved at the cardia to provide blood supply to the proximal gastric pouch. The spleen will fall away from the stomach after the short gastric vessels are divided. The index finger is passed behind the stomach, creating a path through the lesser sac for the placement of the stapling devices.

6 The nasogastric tube is withdrawn into the esophagus. Two linear stapling devices are placed across the stomach. The estimated capacity of the proximal pouch should be 50 mL, or about the size of an egg. The staplers are placed accordingly.

7 The staplers are fired, and the stomach is divided with electrocautery between the two staplers.

8 The proximal gastric pouch, shown here, has a capacity of approximately 50 mL.

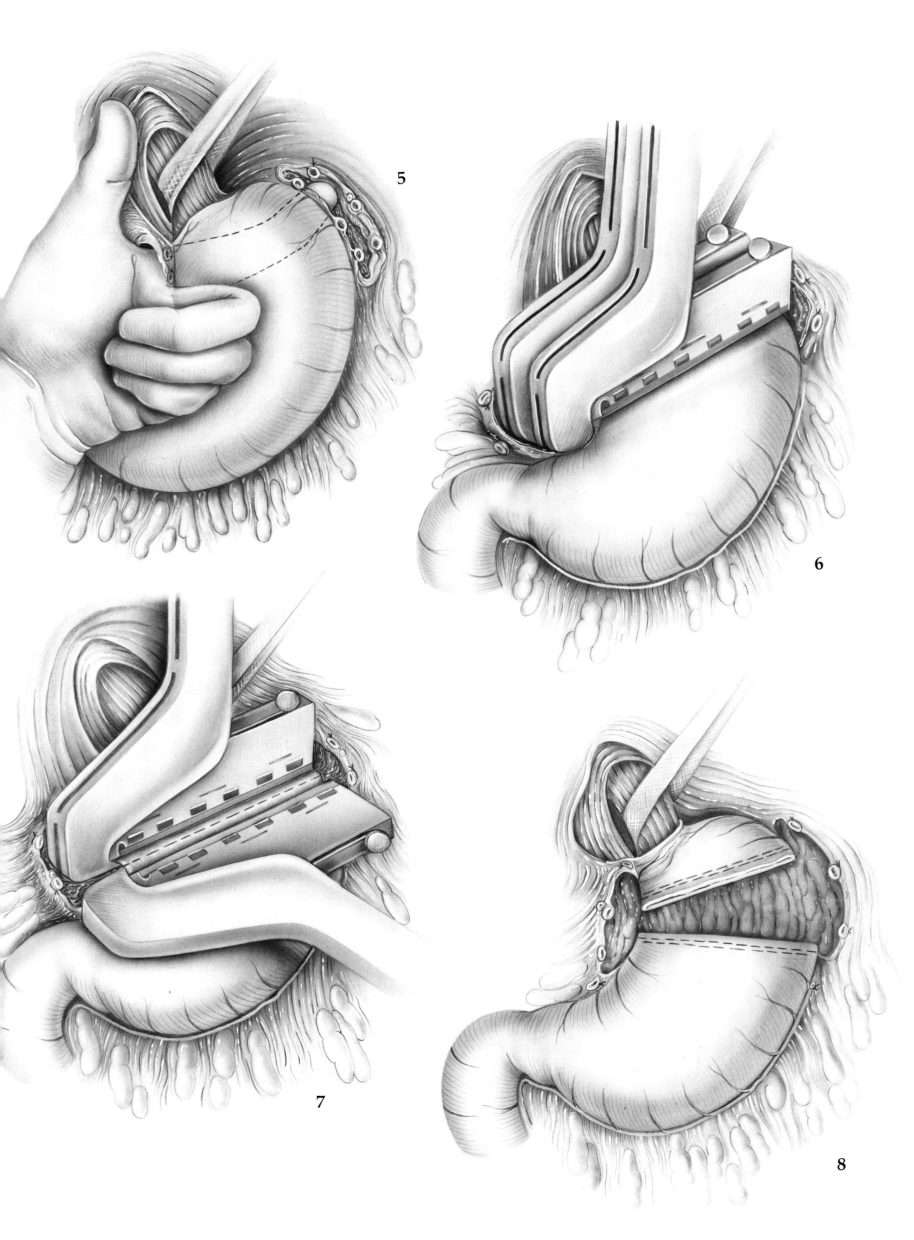

5

6

7

8

Gastric Bypass for Morbid Obesity (*cont.*)

9 A Roux-en-Y loop is constructed with the proximal jejunum, beginning approximately 15 cm from the ligament of Treitz. The mesentery of the jejunum is divided between clamps, retaining an adequate blood supply to the Roux limb.

10 The jejunum is divided between an intestinal anastomosis clamp distally and a linear stapling device proximally.

11 The distal limb of the Roux-en-Y is brought into the supracolic compartment through the bare area of the transverse mesocolon.

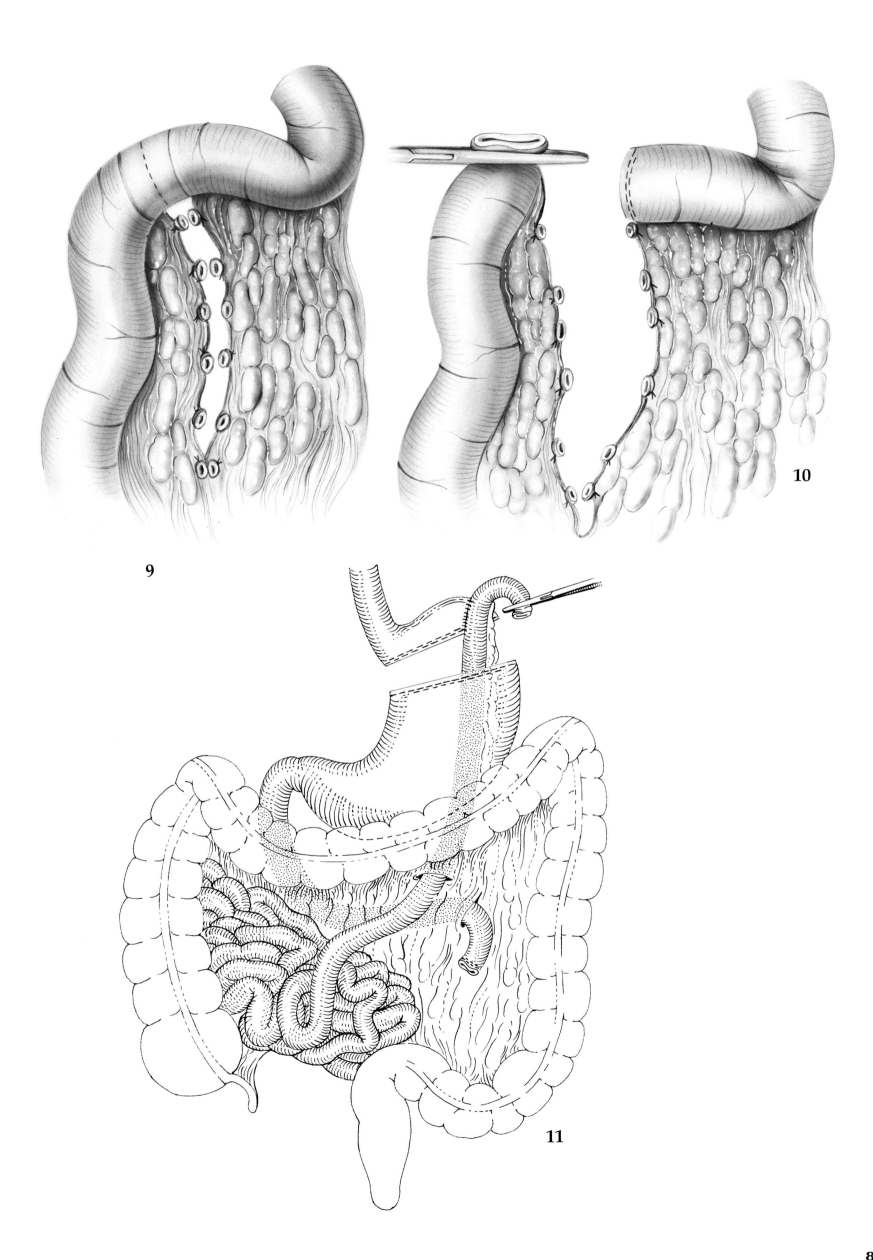

9

10

11

Gastric Bypass for Morbid Obesity (*cont.*)

12 The gastrojejunostomy is accomplished in two layers on the anterior gastric wall. Using interrupted seromuscular #000 silk sutures, the posterior outer layer is fashioned.

13 One-cm enterotomies are created on the anterior gastric wall and the antimesenteric side of the jejunum, as indicated. In order to make these enterotomies measure precisely 1 cm, the serosa of the jejunum and the gastric wall are scored with the electrocautery and a 1-cm uterine sound is bluntly pushed through the remaining mucosa.

14 The posterior inner layer is accomplished with interrupted full-thickness #000 polyglycolic acid sutures placed through the jejunal and gastric walls and tied so that the knots are within the lumen of the anastomosis.

15 A 1-cm uterine sound is placed into the cut end of the jejunum and then through the anastomosis, to prevent inadvertent approximation of the anterior and posterior margins of the anastomosis as the anterior inner layer is sewn.

16 The anterior inner layer of the anastomosis is completed using interrupted full-thickness #000 polyglycolic acid sutures. The knots are tied on the outside of the anastomosis.

17 A row of interrupted seromuscular #000 silk stitches is placed, completing the anastomosis. The uterine sound is removed and the anastomosis can be inspected through the cut end of the jejunum. The anastomosis may also be performed by sewing the cut end of the jejunum to the gastrotomy. In this case, the sound is passed through an enterotomy which is closed following the completion of the anastomosis.

18 A linear stapling device is used to close the stump of the jejunum.

19 The completed gastrojejunostomy lies on the anterior gastric wall.

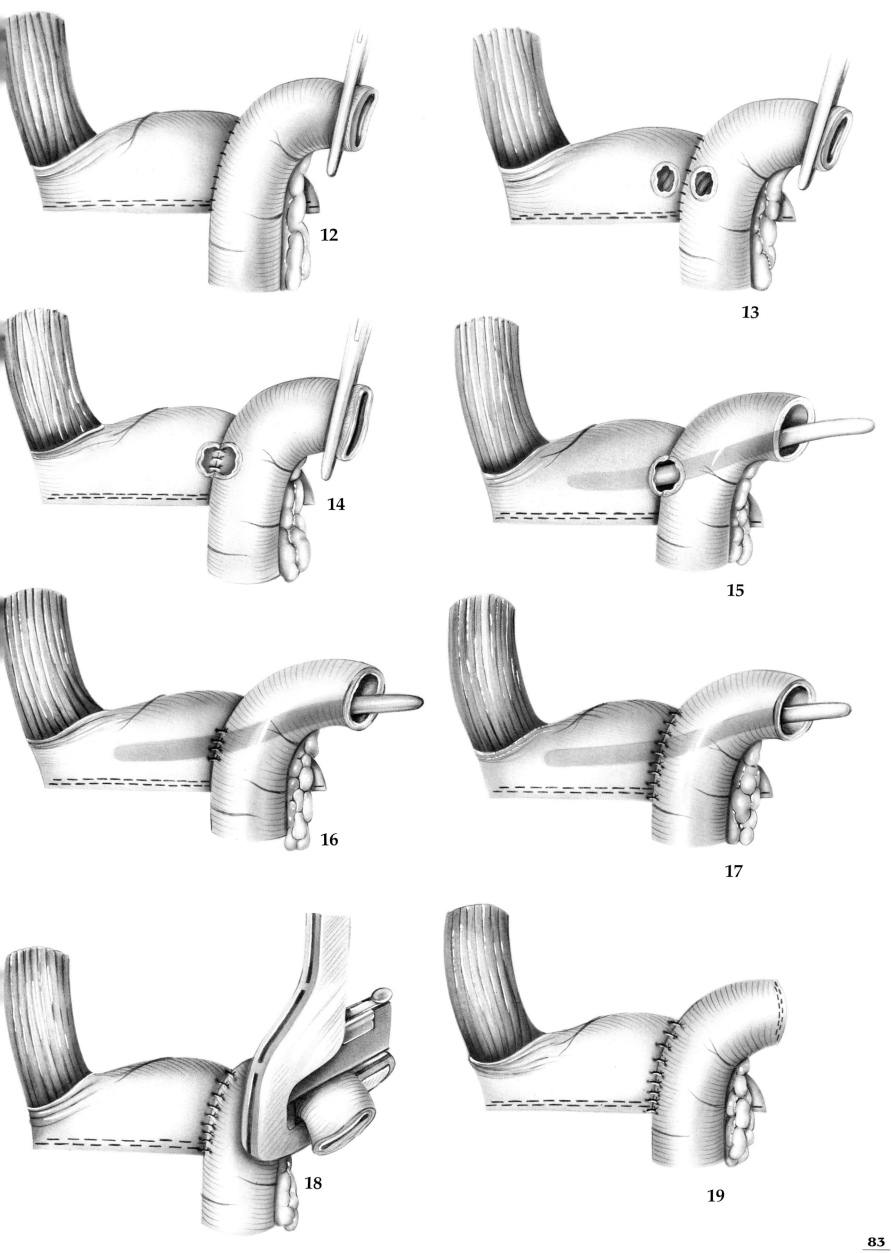

Gastric Bypass for Morbid Obesity (*cont.*)

20 Continuity of the jejunum is reestablished by approximation of the proximal stapled jejunum to a segment 45 cm distal to the gastrojejunostomy with two #000 silk stay sutures. Enterotomies are created on the antimesenteric sides of both loops of jejunum.

21–22 A gastrointestinal anastomosis stapling instrument is introduced into the two limbs of the jejunum through the enterotomies. Once the stapler is fired, a 5-cm jejunojejunostomy is created.

23 The remaining defect in the bowel wall is closed with interrupted #000 silk sutures or a linear stapling instrument.

24 The defect in the transverse mesocolon is closed by approximating its margins to the jejunal wall with interrupted #000 silk sutures. The completed gastric bypass consists of a 50-mL gastric pouch anastomosed to a Roux-en-Y loop of jejunum. The nasogastric tube is placed in the gastric remnant and secured to the patient's nose. A closed suction drain is placed in the left subdiaphragmatic space and brought out to the skin through a separate incision. The wound is closed with #1 polyglycolic acid interrupted and buried retention sutures. A closed suction drain is placed in the subcutaneous tissues and brought out to the skin through another separate incision. The subcutaneous tissues are then closed with #000 plain sutures. The skin is closed with skin staples.

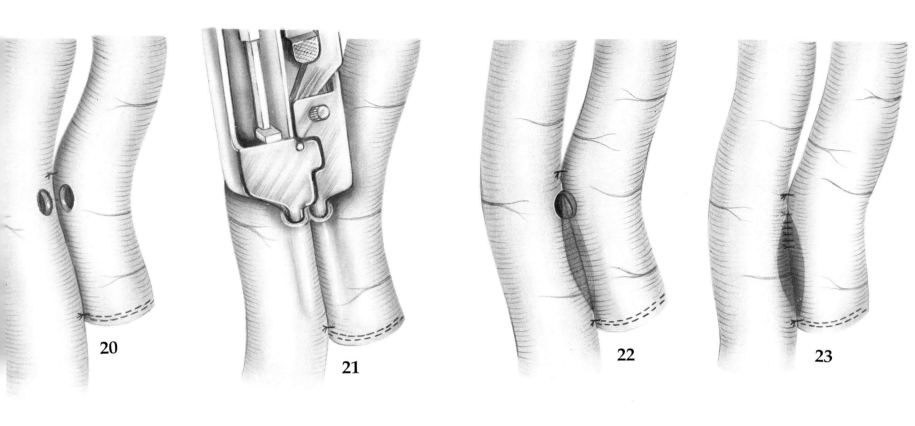

20

21

22

23

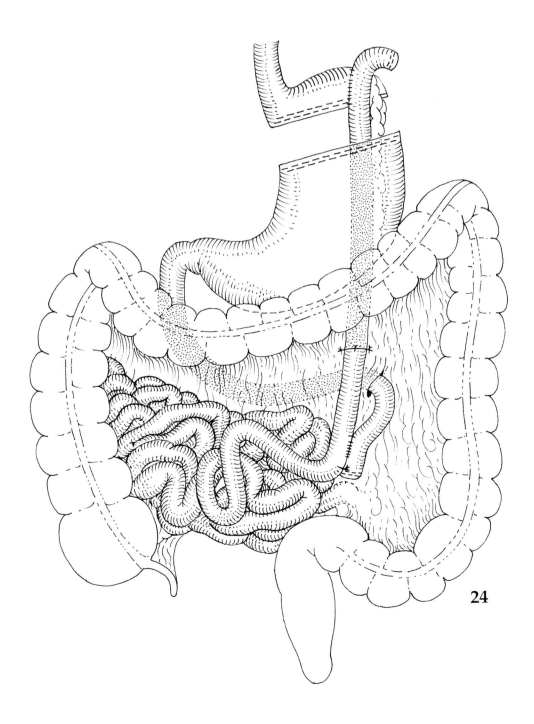

24

Total Gastrectomy for Gastric Cancer

1 The patient is positioned supine on the operating table. A midline incision extending from the xiphoid to below the umbilicus is made. The abdominal contents are inspected to determine whether a radical total gastrectomy will remove all grossly visible tumor.

2 The greater omentum is sharply divided from the entire length of the transverse mesocolon.

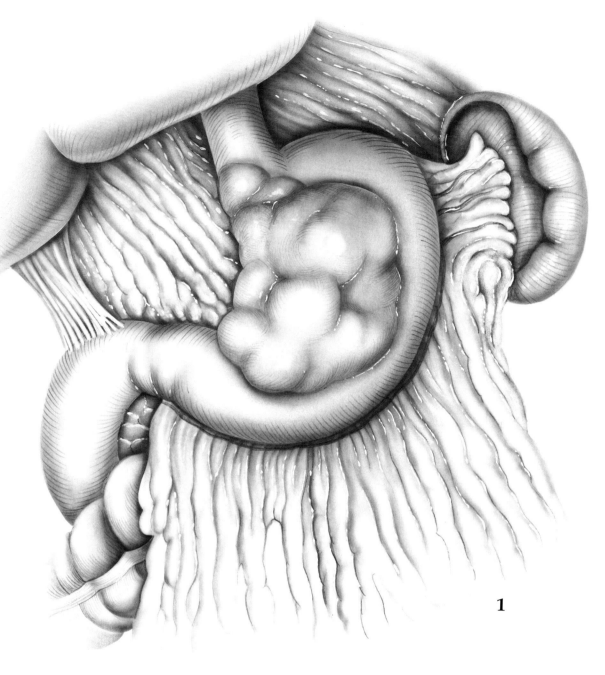

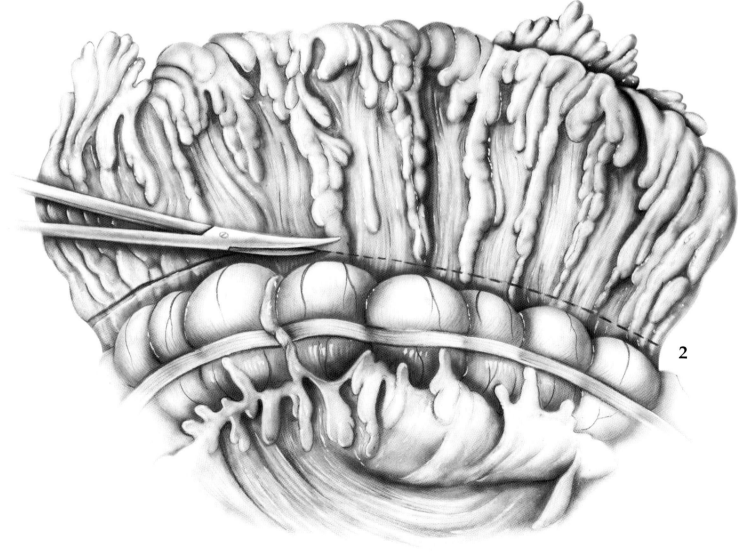

Total Gastrectomy for Gastric Cancer (*cont.*)

3–6 The lesser sac is entered by retracting the stomach and attached omentum cephalad. The left gastric artery is identified at the celiac axis (**Fig. 3**). The overlying lymphatic tissue is dissected toward the specimen, thus exposing the left gastric artery. The left gastric artery is then ligated in continuity with a #0 silk tie immediately above the origin of the common hepatic artery, which can be palpated coursing toward the liver (**Fig. 4**). Two tonsil clamps are placed on the artery (**Fig. 5**), which is divided and tied with #00 silk (**Fig. 6**).

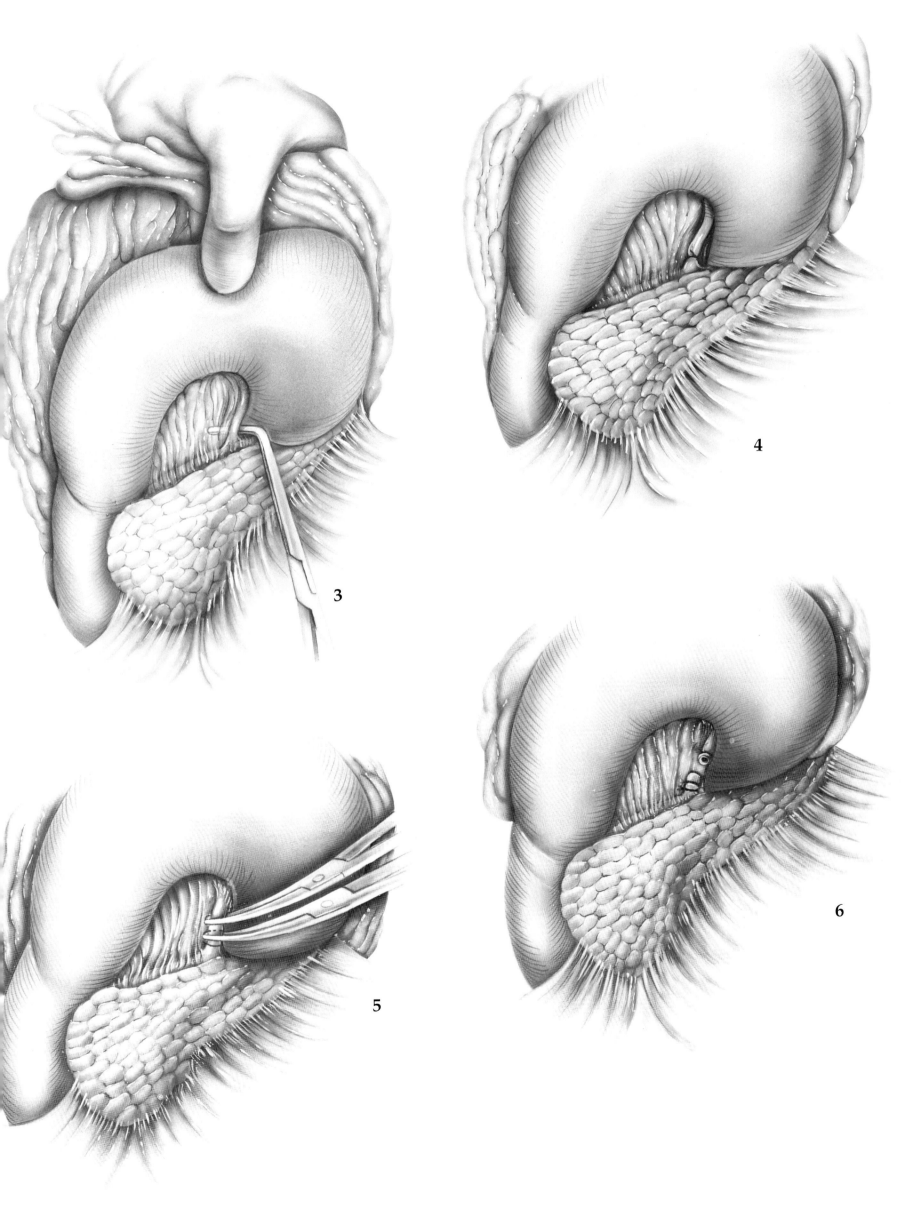

Total Gastrectomy for Gastric Cancer (*cont.*)

7 The short gastric and left gastroepiploic arteries are identified, divided between clamps, and tied with #00 silk, thus preserving the spleen while separating it from the stomach. The dissection is carried above the fundus along the posterior aspect of the diaphragm and around to the esophagus, as indicated by the broken line.

8 The right gastric artery can be easily palpated coursing along the lesser curvature immediately above the pylorus. The right gastroepiploic vessels are identified as they emerge below the pylorus and enter the gastrocolic ligament. These vessels are clamped, divided, and ligated with #000 silk.

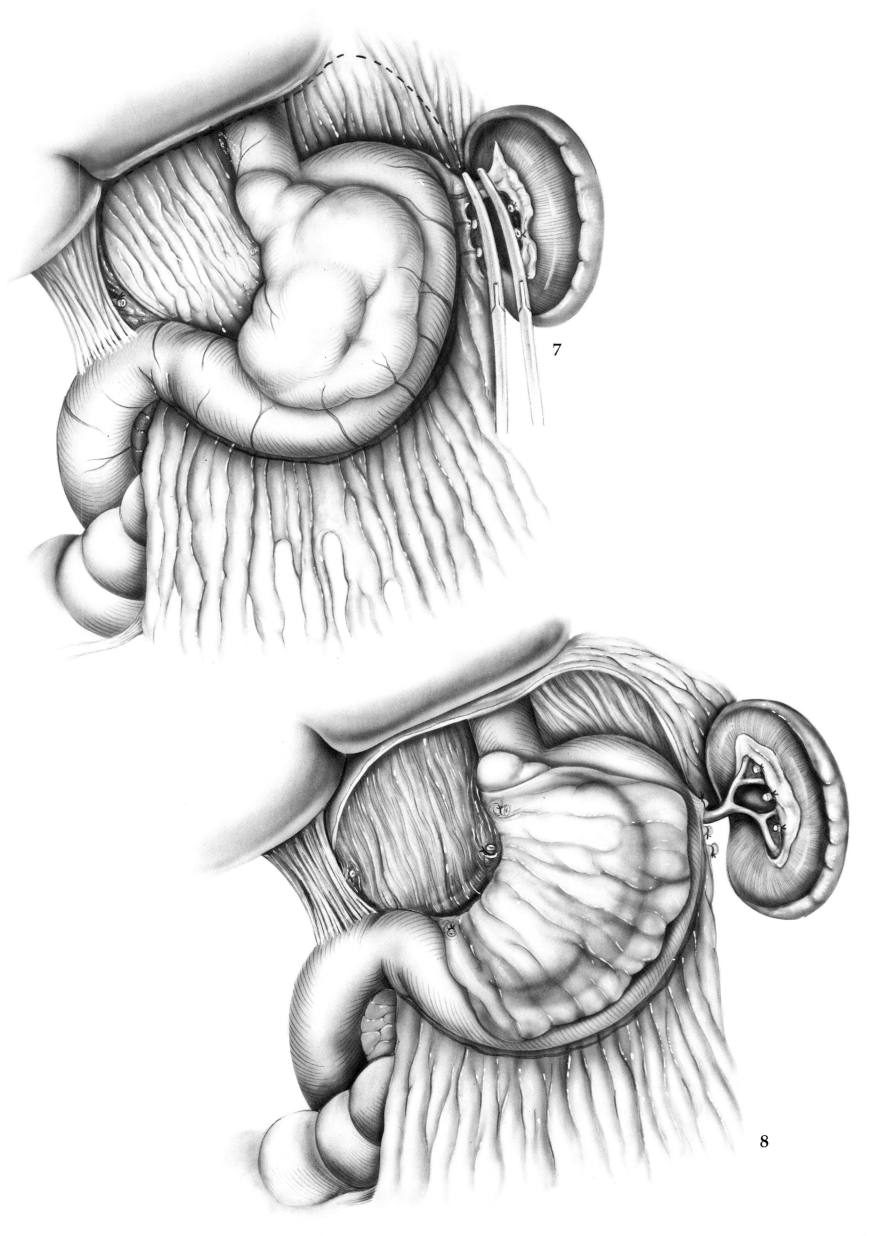

7

8

Total Gastrectomy for Gastric Cancer (*cont.*)

9 The gastrohepatic omentum is freed from the undersurface of the liver and folded anteriorly over the gastric wall. The duodenum is mobilized proximally and closed with a stapling device approximately 2 to 3 cm beyond the pylorus. A Kocher clamp is placed
proximal to the stapling instrument, and the duodenum is divided with electrocautery.
The stomach has been completely freed, except for its attachment to the esophagus.

10 The vagi are divided, providing additional length to the intraabdominal portion of the
esophagus. The esophagus is divided between two Satinsky vascular clamps placed just
below the esophageal hiatus.

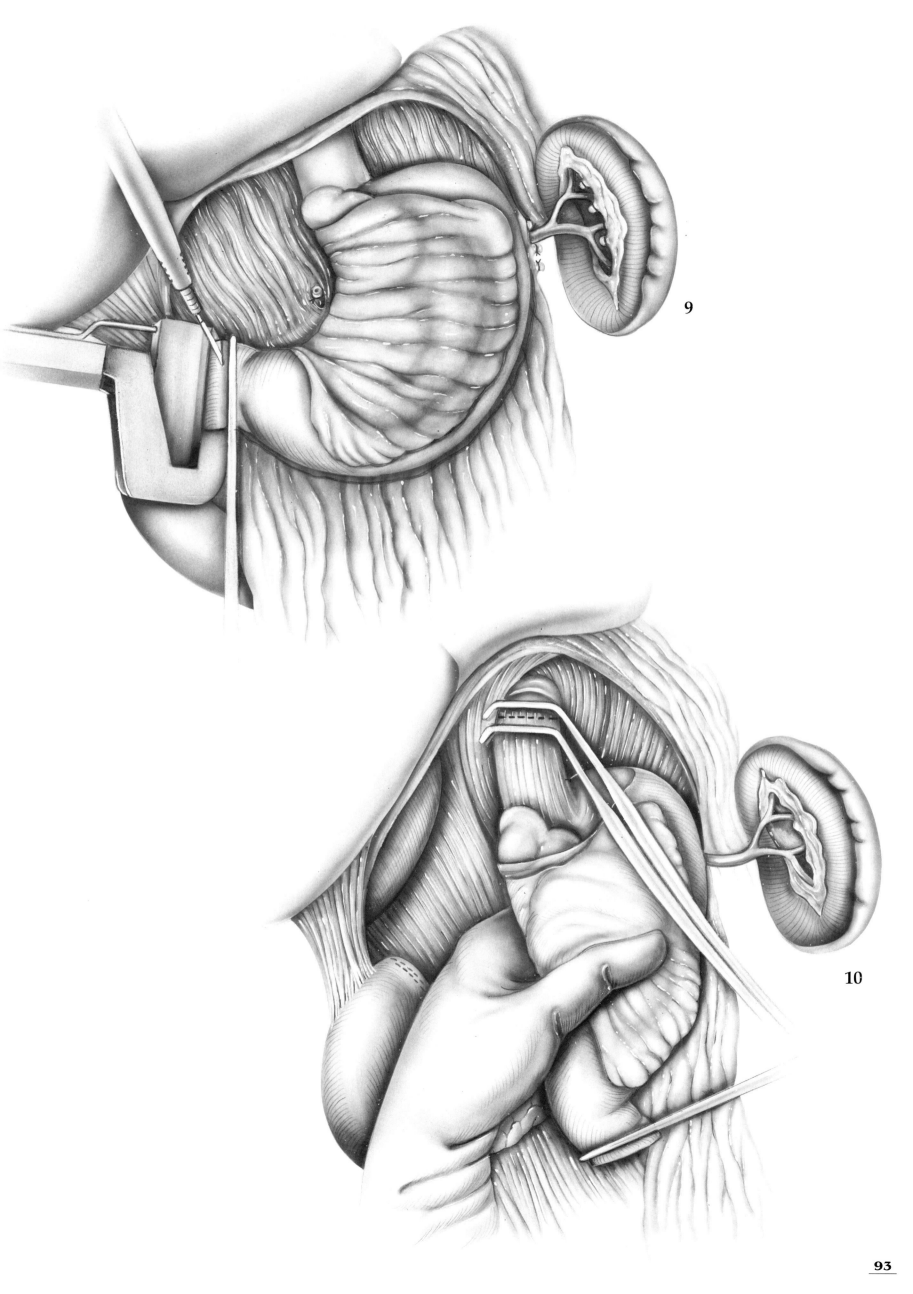

9

10

Total Gastrectomy for Gastric Cancer (*cont.*)

11 Following the removal of the stomach from the operative field (it will be sent to the pathologist for evaluation of the margins of resection), all vestiges of residual celiac or peripancreatic lymphatic tissue or remaining omentum in the retrogastric space are removed.

12 Approximately 25 cm beyond the ligament of Treitz the jejunum is divided between a transecting stapling device and a Kocher clamp, by electrocautery.

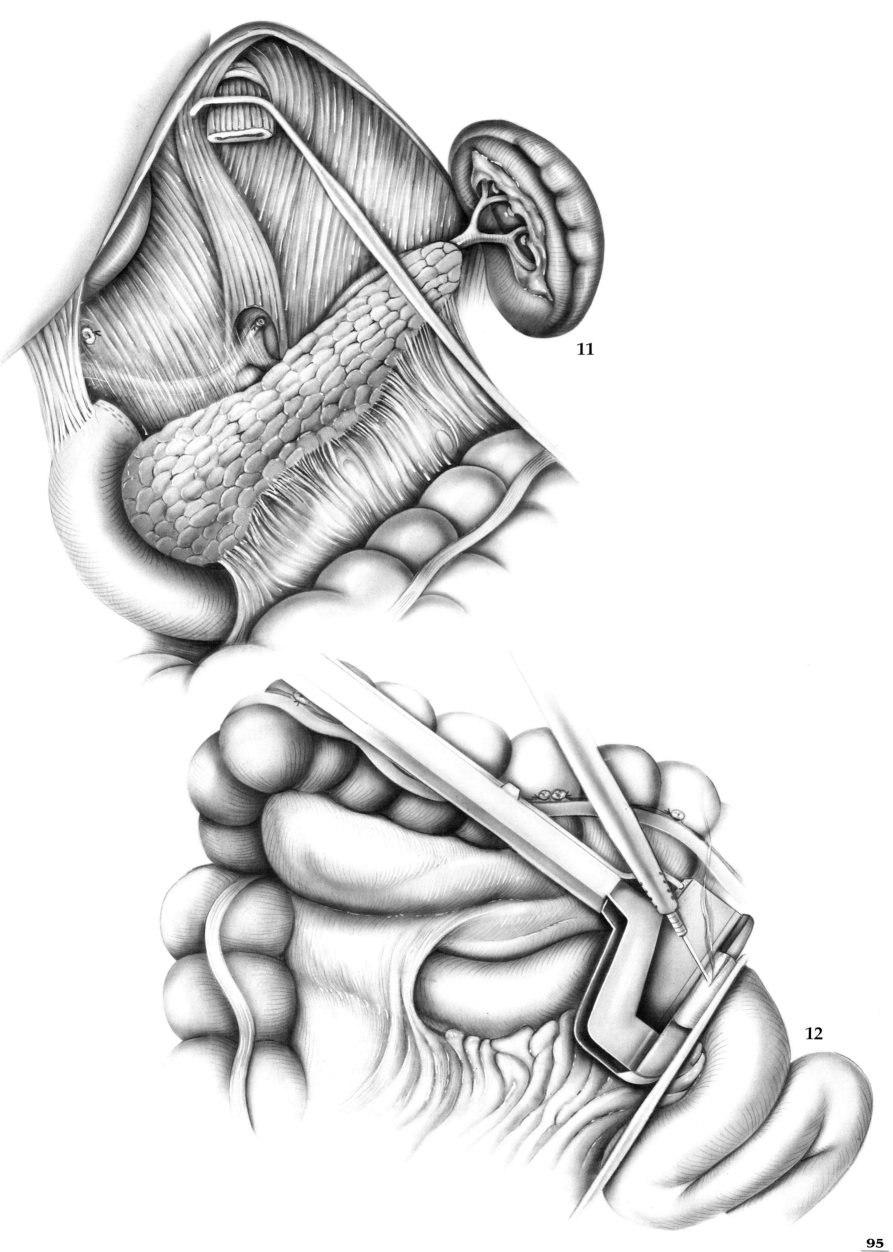

11

12

Total Gastrectomy for Gastric Cancer (*cont.*)

13 The mesentery of the jejunum is divided, mobilizing the distal segment for construction of the Roux-en-Y limb to be used for the esophagojejunal anastomosis.

14–15 The stapled proximal jejunum is approximated to the jejunum 45 cm beyond the level of transection with proximal and distal #000 silk stay sutures. These sutures should be spaced 8 to 10 cm apart. An enterotomy is created with electrocautery on the antimesenteric side of both loops of jejunum (**Fig. 14**), allowing the placement of a gastrointestinal anastomosis stapling device. After the stapler is discharged (**Fig. 15**), the suture lines are inspected for bleeding. If bleeding is present, it is controlled either with electrocautery or with small interrupted silk sutures.

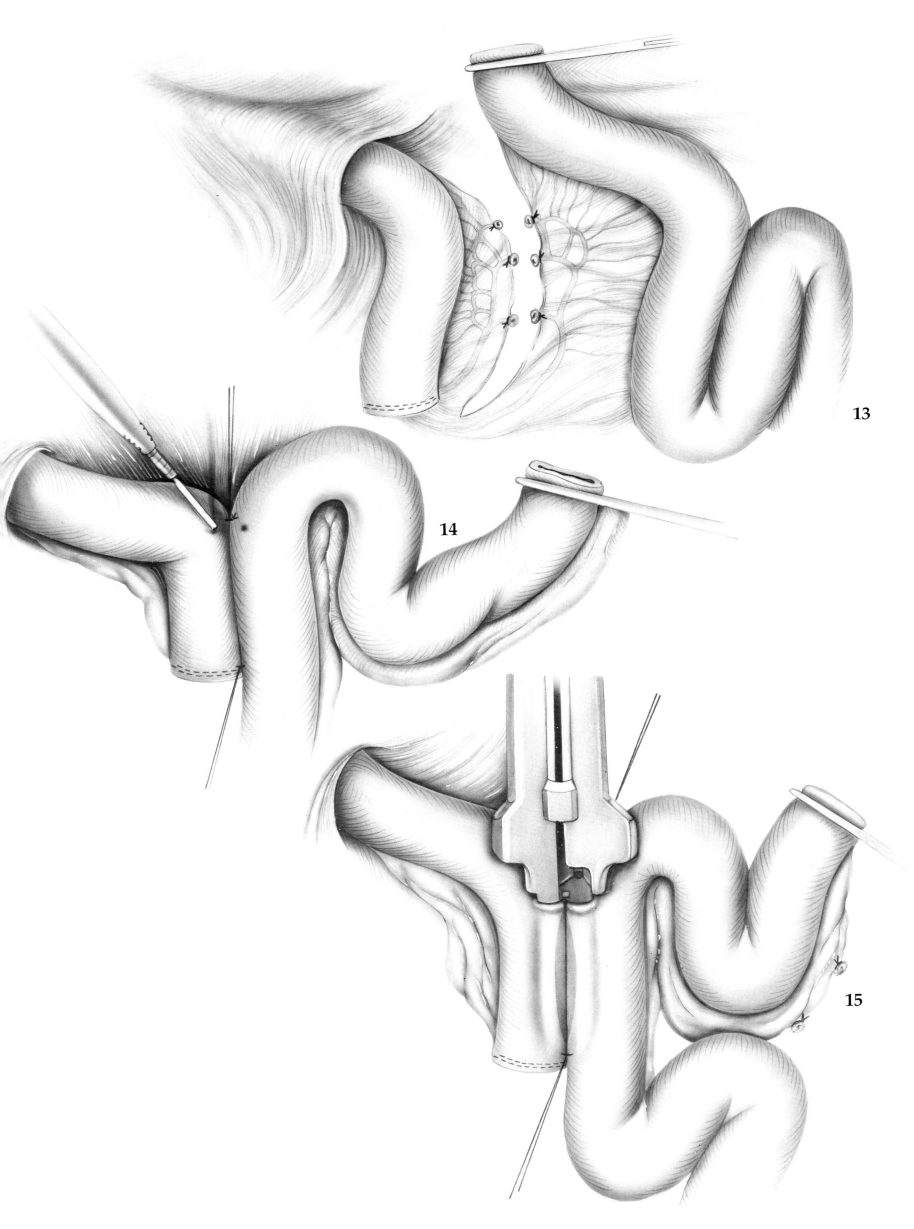

13

14

15

Total Gastrectomy for Gastric Cancer (*cont.*)

16–17 The enterotomy remaining after removal of the stapler is closed with simple, full-thickness, interrupted #000 silk sutures. There is no need to invert this closure.

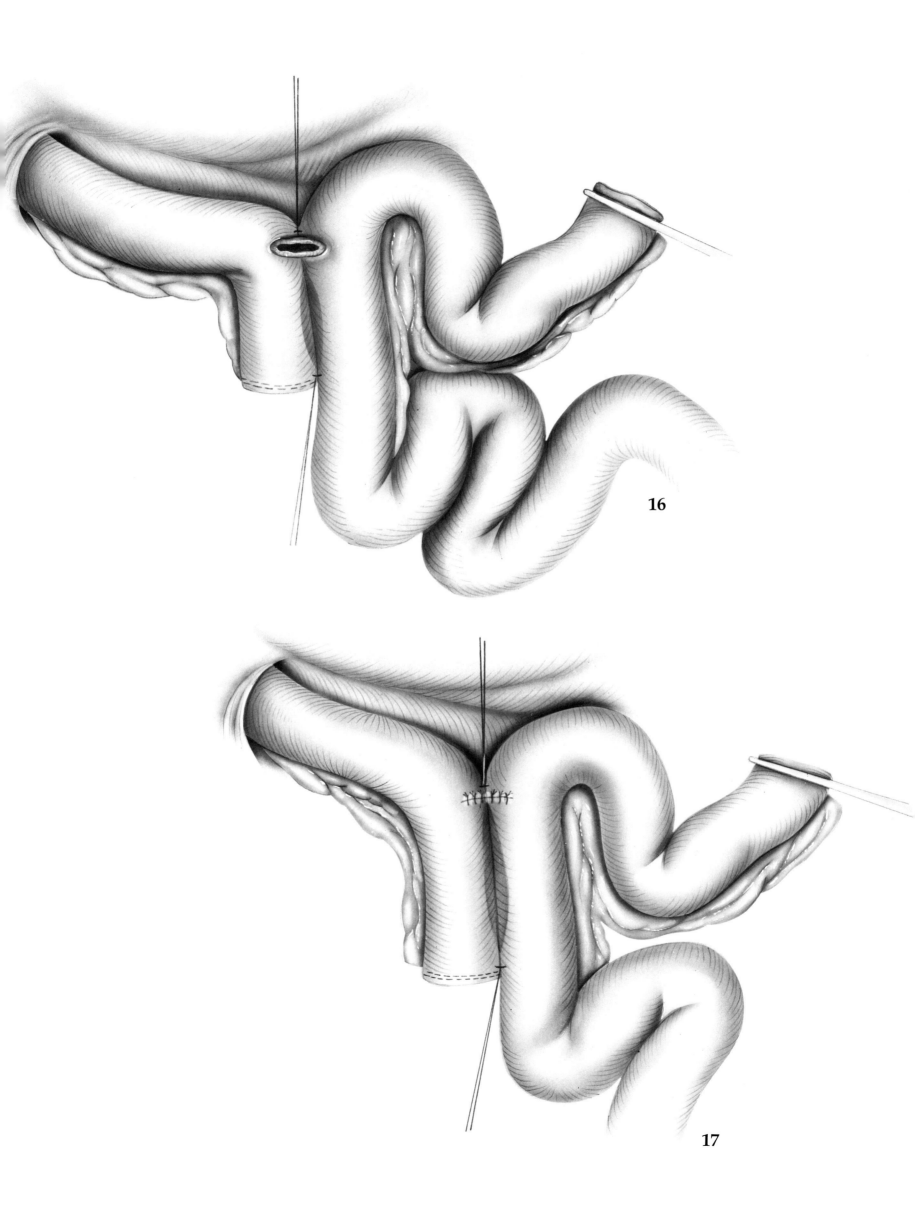

16

17

Total Gastrectomy for Gastric Cancer (*cont.*)

18 The Roux-en-Y limb is brought through a defect created in the bare area of the transverse mesocolon. The end of the jejunum is closed with #000 silk in an inverting, interrupted single-layer fashion, or stapled closed.

Sutured Esophagojejunostomy

19 The posterior esophagus is sutured to the jejunum with interrupted #000 silk sutures, incorporating the submucosa of the esophagus into each stitch. The jejunum is opened along its axis below the posterior outer row.

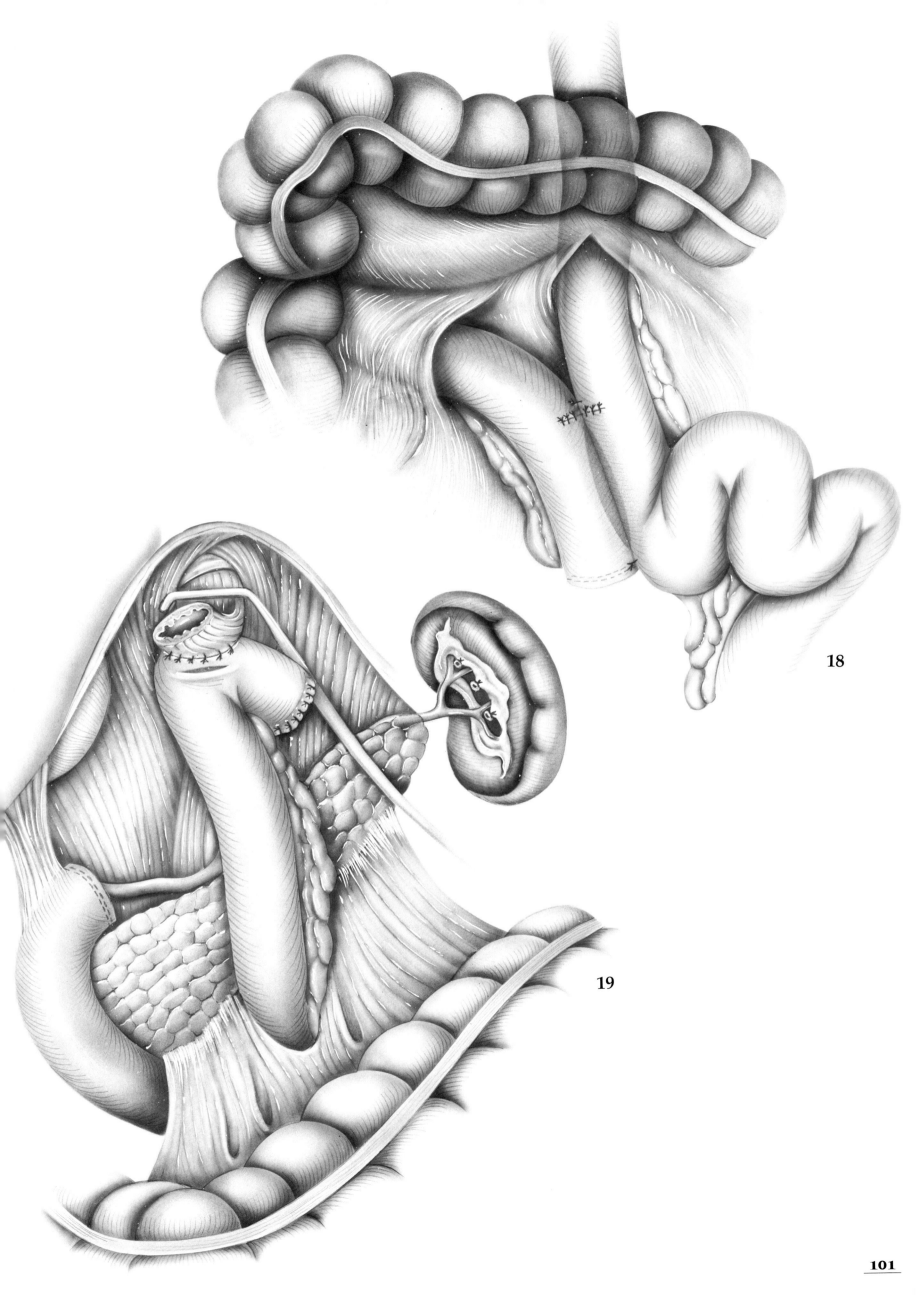

18

19

Total Gastrectomy for Gastric Cancer (*cont.*)

Sutured Esophagojejunostomy (*cont.*)

20–22 The full-thickness inner layer is accomplished, circumferentially, with interrupted #000 silk sutures.

23 An outer row of partial-thickness interrupted #000 silk sutures is placed to invert the anterior portion of the inner layer with the jejunum. On both sides of the anastomosis, the jejunum is sutured to the crura of the diaphragm, reducing tension on the anastomosis. A sump nasogastric tube is advanced through the anastomosis and into the jejunum. The anesthesiologist fixes the tube to the patient's nose and marks the level on the tube itself. The defect in the mesocolon is closed by approximating the margins of the defect to the jejunal wall with interrupted fine silk sutures.

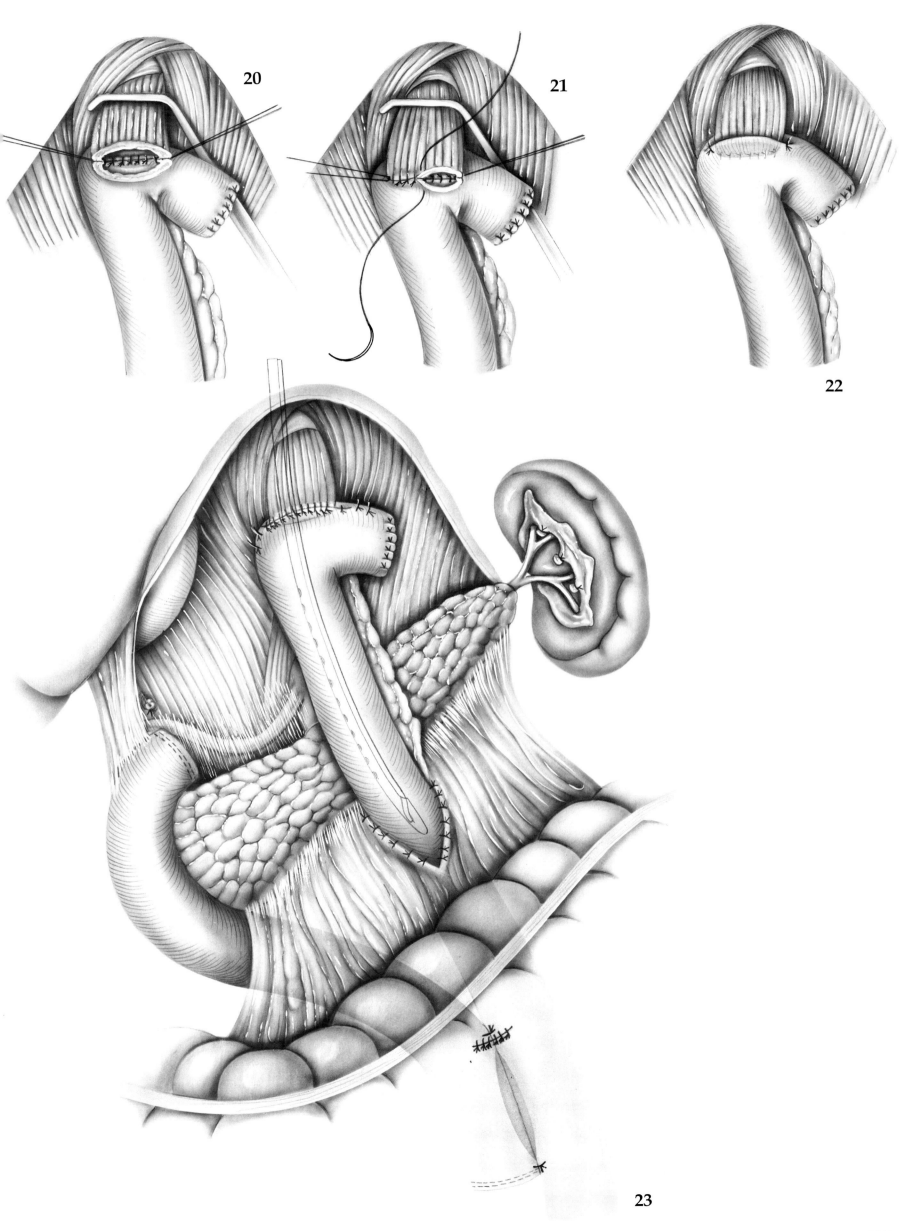

20

21

22

23

Total Gastrectomy for Gastric Cancer (*cont.*)

Stapled Esophagojejunostomy

As the common alternative technique, a circular stapling device may be used to fashion the esophagojejunostomy.

24 A full-thickness, running #0 polyglycolic acid suture is run around the distal esophageal stump, beginning and ending anteriorly. This suture is not tied. Four #00 silk stay sutures are then placed, at 2, 5, 7, and 10 o'clock, through the stump of the esophagus. The circular stapling device, with the anvil removed, is inserted through the open end of the jejunum and then through an enterotomy created on the antimesenteric side of the Roux-en-Y loop, approximately 4 cm from the cut end.

25 The anvil is replaced on the stalk of the stapler. Traction on the stay sutures at the 5 and 7 o'clock positions allows partial introduction of the anvil into the esophagus. Subsequent traction on the sutures at 2 and 10 o'clock will pull the anterior wall of the esophagus over the anvil.

26 The polyglycolic acid purse-string suture is tied, snugging the esophageal stump over the stalk of the stapler. The stay sutures are cut.

27 The stapler is closed and discharged.

28 A suture is placed through the esophagus and jejunum at the anastomosis. The anvil is then extended from the stapler and the stapler is removed from the end of the jejunum. The anvil is removed from the stapler, allowing inspection of the rings of bowel cut during the firing of the stapler. Two complete rings are essential. The proximal ring may be sent to the pathology lab as the most proximal level of resection. The anastomosis is inspected through the open end of the jejunum.

29 The stump of the jejunum is closed with a linear stapling device, and the jejunum is sutured to the crura of the diaphragm to relieve tension on the staple line.

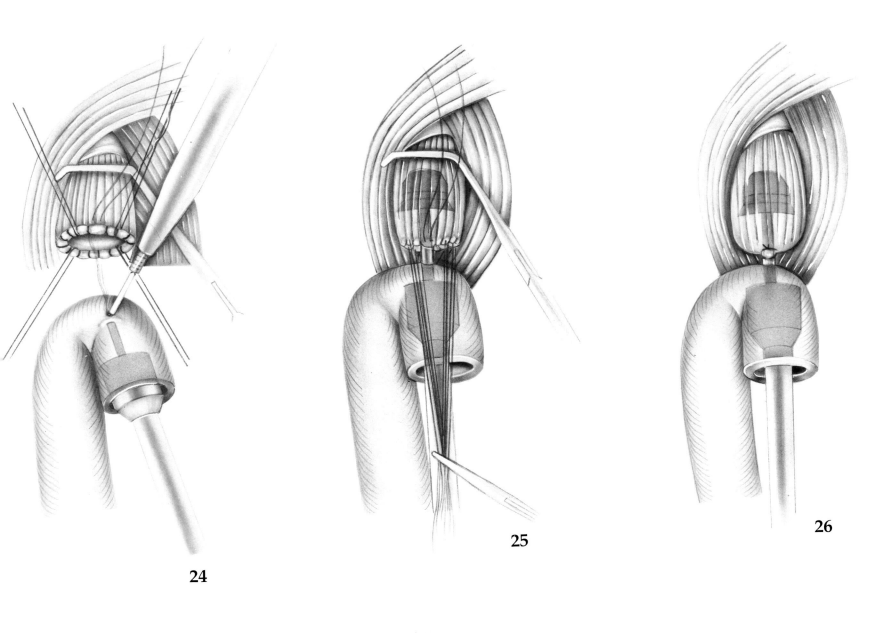

24

25

26

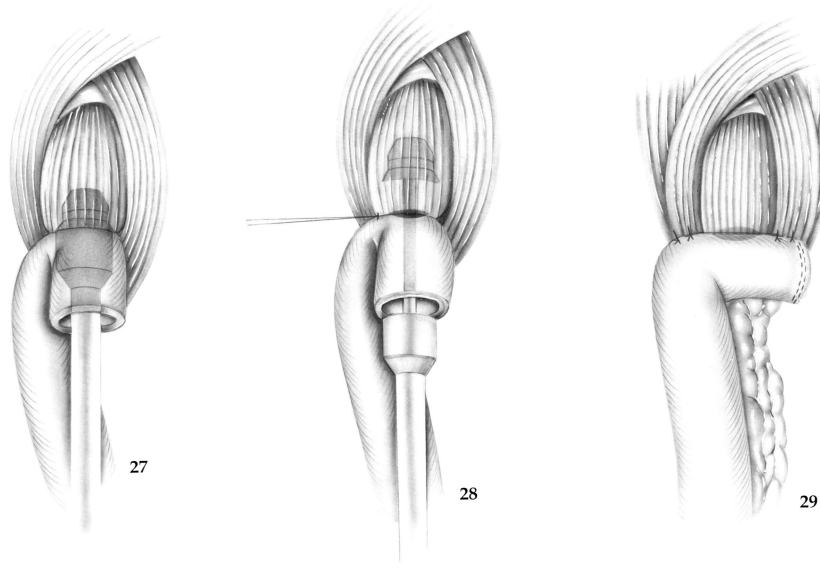

27

28

29

Proximal Gastrectomy for Cancer

1 The abdomen is explored through a midline incision extending from the xiphoid to below the umbilicus. The lesion and viscera are examined to evaluate the local extent of disease and to look for possible distant metastases, as well as to determine whether the proposed radical proximal gastrectomy will be sufficient to clear all local disease with adequate margins.

2 The greater omentum is sharply divided from the entire length of the transverse mesocolon.

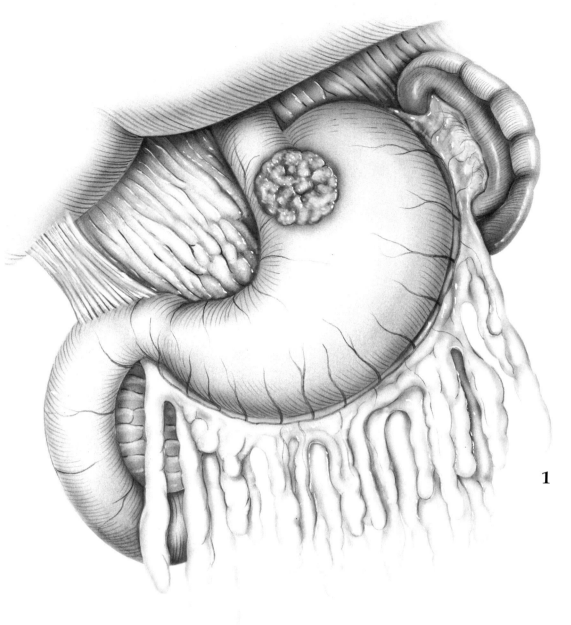

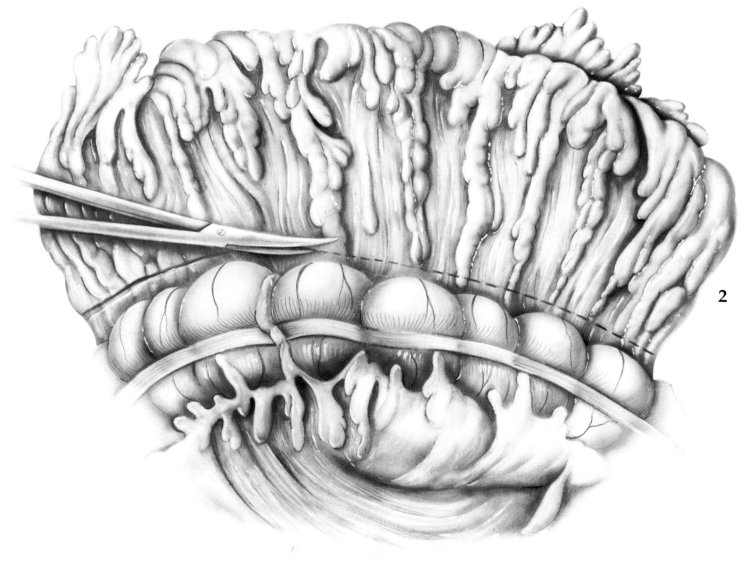

Proximal Gastrectomy for Cancer (*cont.*)

3 The stomach with the attached omentum is elevated cephalad, thus entering the lesser sac. The left gastric artery is identified as it emerges from the celiac trunk just beyond the common hepatic artery, which can be palpated coursing toward the liver. Using a right-angle clamp, the left gastric artery is dissected from its enveloping areolar tissue.

4 The left gastric artery is ligated with a #0 silk tie passed around the artery.

5–6 The left gastric artery is clamped distally and proximally with tonsil clamps, divided, and tied with #00 silk ties.

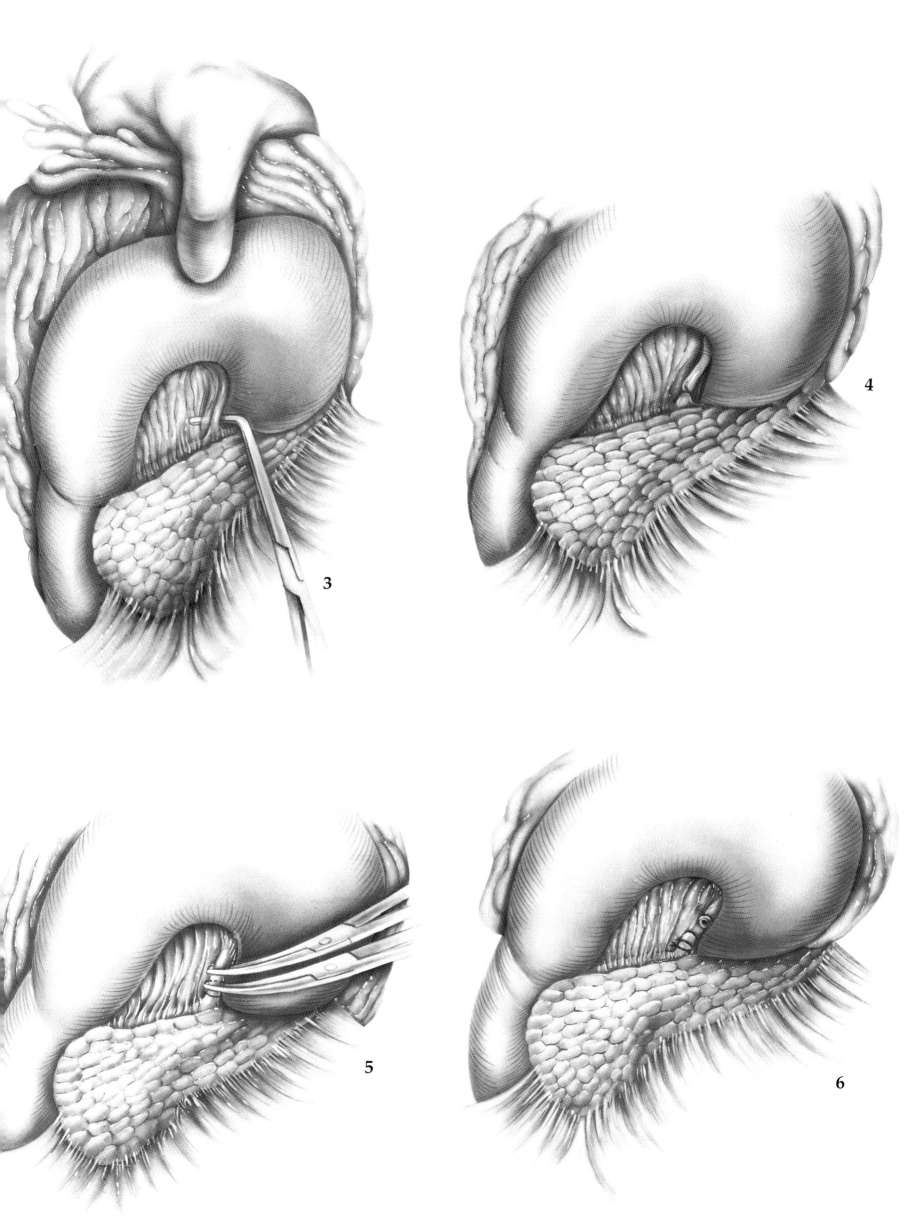

Proximal Gastrectomy for Cancer (*cont.*)

7–8 Beginning at the pylorus, the greater omentum is separated from the greater curvature of the stomach. The right gastroepiploic and right gastric vessels, which are preserved, will provide blood supply to the stomach after the resection of the body and fundus of the stomach.

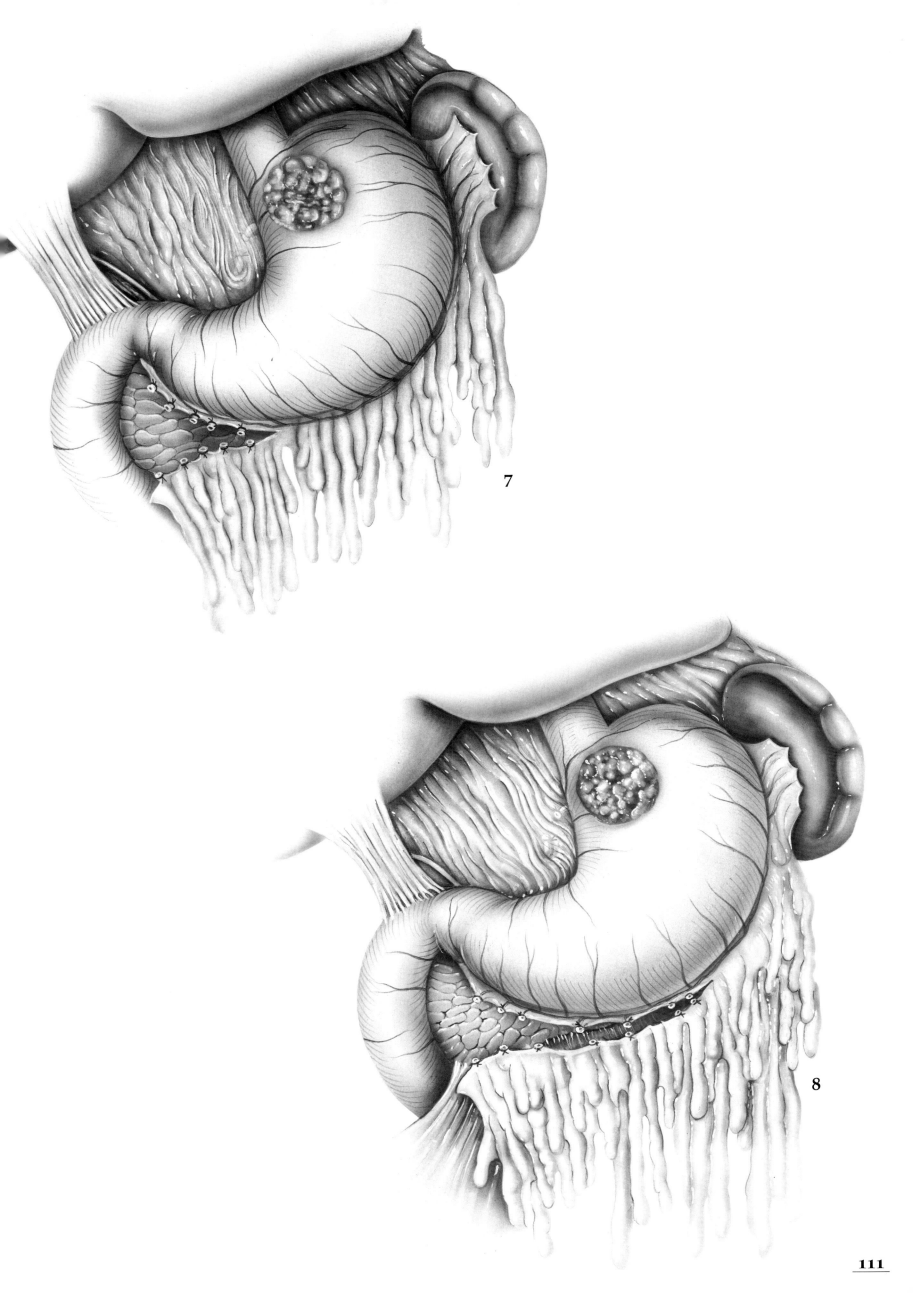

7

8

Proximal Gastrectomy for Cancer (*cont.*)

9 The lesser omentum is divided from the hepatoduodenal ligament on the right, and from the liver superiorly. The dissection is carried to the left, clearing the peritoneum overlying the esophagus and that superior to the fundus of the stomach, as indicated by the broken line.

10 The lesser omentum is folded over the anterior wall of the stomach at the conclusion of this dissection. The posterior vagus is identified along the posteromedial aspect of the esophagus and the anterior vagus is found in the areolar tissue on the anterior esophageal wall.

11–12 Hemoclips are placed on the vagi, proximally and distally, and a segment of each vagus nerve is resected. The division of the vagi will provide additional length to the intraabdominal portion of the esophagus.

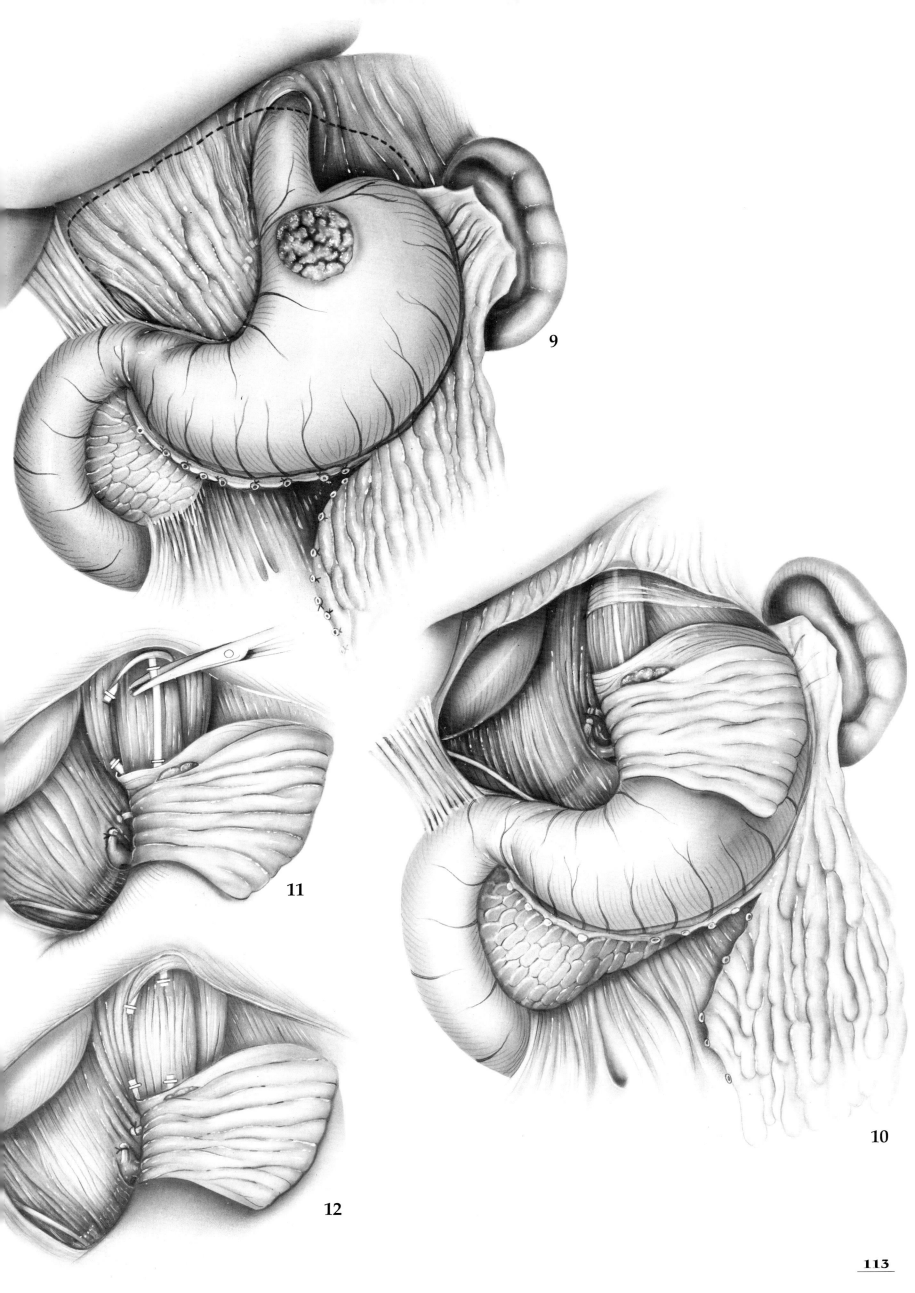

9

11

12

10

Proximal Gastrectomy for Cancer (*cont.*)

13 The short gastric vessels are divided between clamps and tied with #000 silk.

14 The gastroepiploic arcade is divided and tied proximally on the greater-curvature side of the antrum, as are branches of the right gastric artery on the lesser curvature. Residual omentum and fat are cleared at these sites. A Payr clamp is applied at the level of the proposed gastric transection.

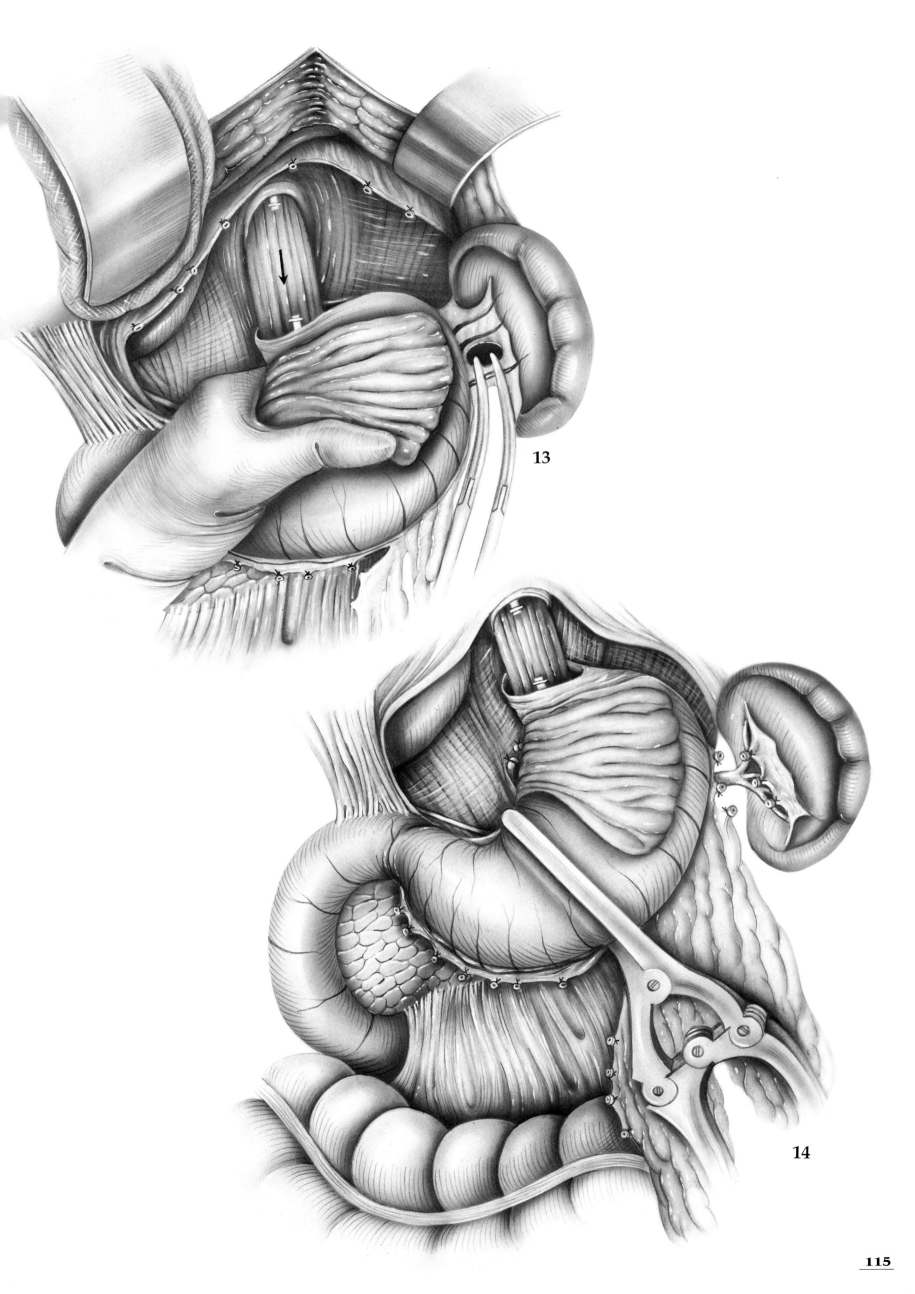

13

14

PLATE
5 8

Proximal Gastrectomy for Cancer (*cont.*)

15–16 A linear stapling device is placed distal to the Payr clamp and discharged. The stomach is transected with electrocautery. The mucosa protruding from the stapler is cauterized to provide hemostasis.

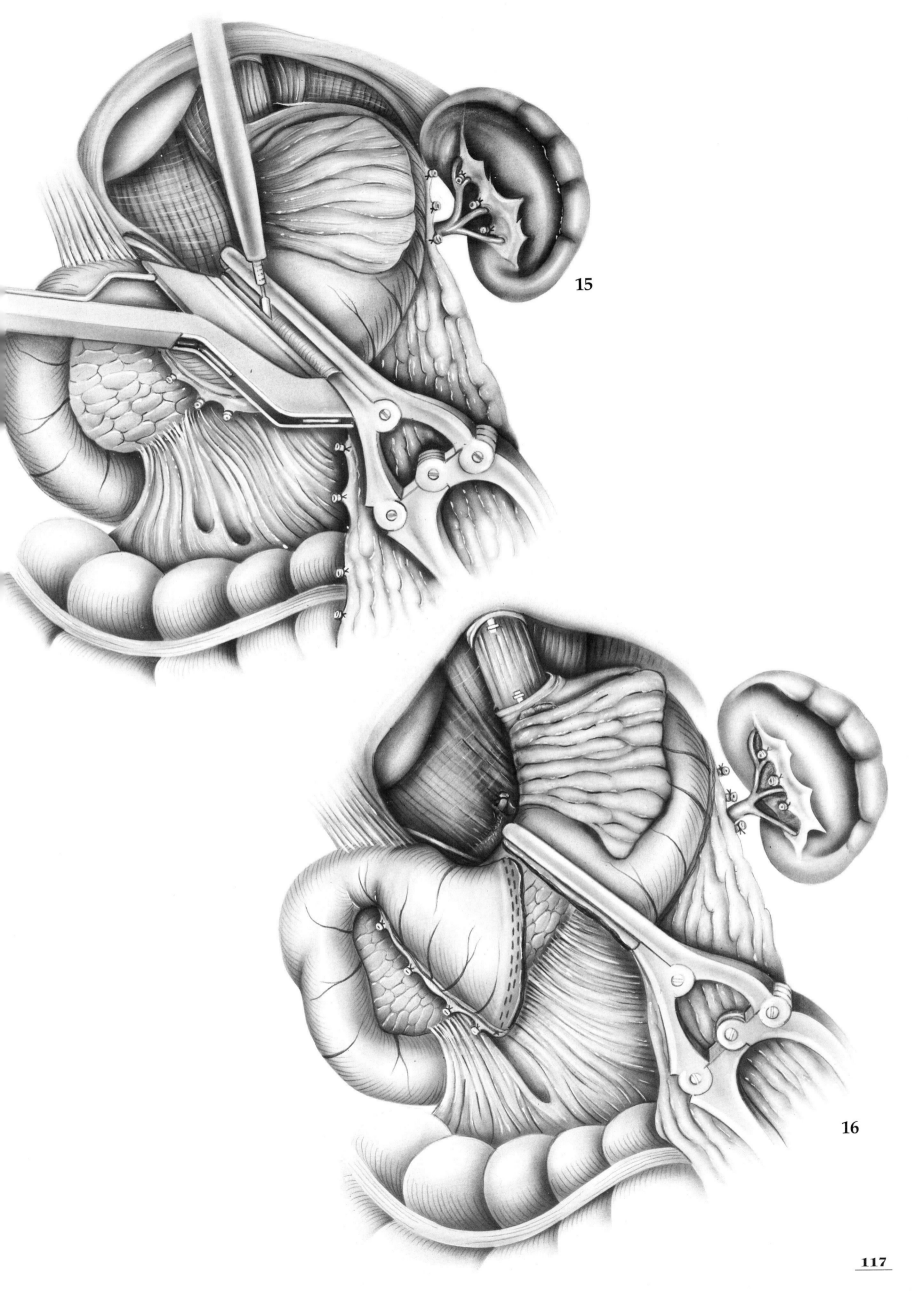

15

16

Proximal Gastrectomy for Cancer (*cont.*)

17–18 After the stapler is opened and removed, the staple line is oversewn with a running #00 polyglycolic acid suture to reinforce the closure.

19 The nasogastric tube is withdrawn into the esophagus and two Satinsky vascular clamps, separated by 10 to 15 mm, are placed across the esophagus. The esophagus is divided between these clamps, leaving a long esophageal stump extending below the upper Satinsky clamp. The specimen is removed from the operative field and sent for pathological examination of the resection margins.

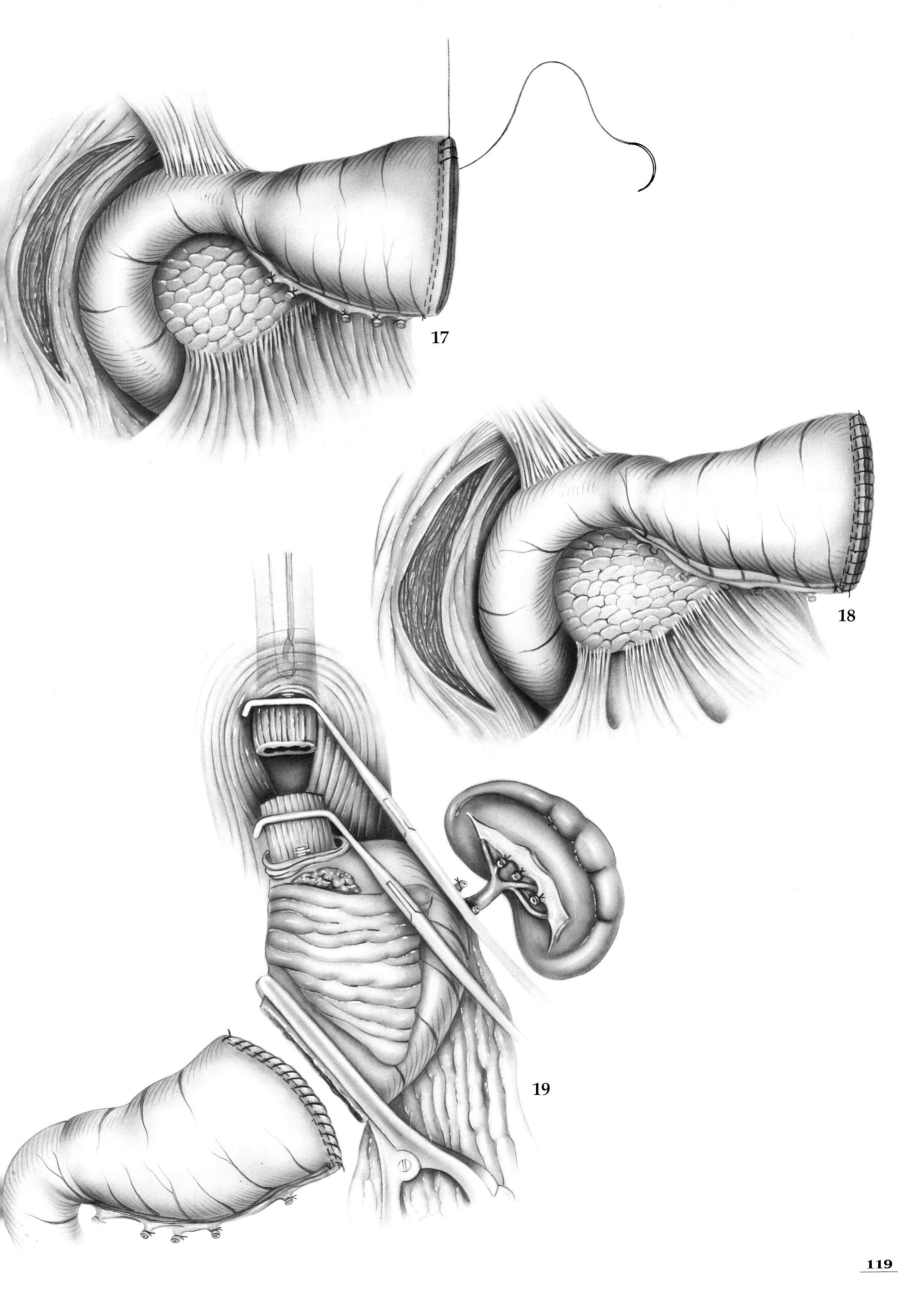

17

18

19

Proximal Gastrectomy for Cancer (*cont.*)

Pyloroplasty

20 A pyloroplasty is created, extending from the anterior wall of the distal antrum to the proximal duodenum.

21–23 Two #00 silk stay sutures are placed superior and inferior to the midportion of the pyloromyotomy. These sutures are distracted and the longitudinal pyloromyotomy is closed transversely with an interrupted layer of full-thickness #000 silk sutures.

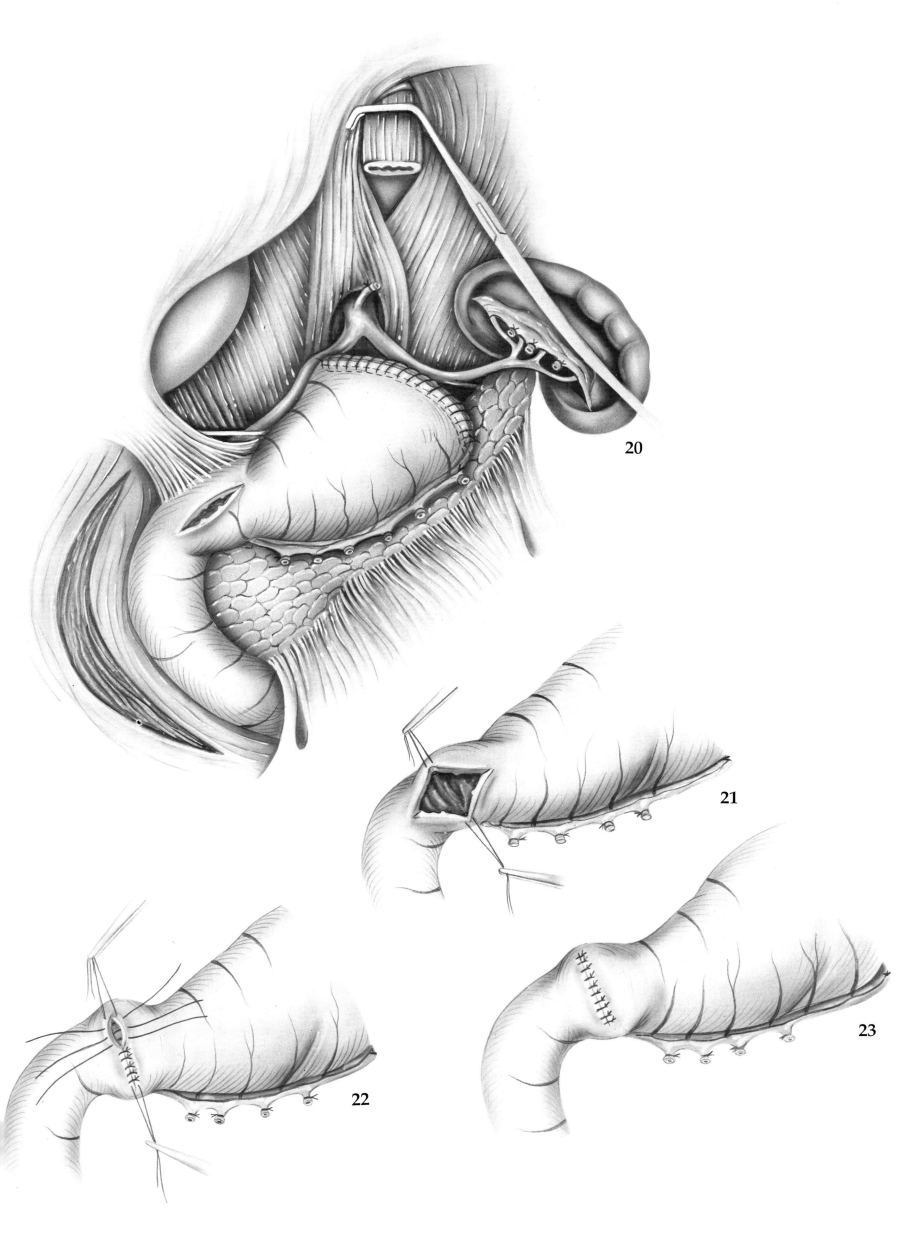

20

21

22

23

Proximal Gastrectomy for Cancer (*cont.*)

Sutured Esophagogastrostomy

24 The residual stomach is placed posterior to the stump of the esophagus. Using interrupted #000 silk sutures, the stomach is suspended posteriorly from the crura surrounding the esophageal hiatus.

25 The posterior outer row of the esophagogastrostomy is accomplished using interrupted #000 silk sutures. The esophageal stitches must reach through the submucosa, so as to include tissue of adequate strength to hold the esophagus to the stomach.

26 An anterior gastrotomy is created with electrocautery, 3 cm below the transected stomach.

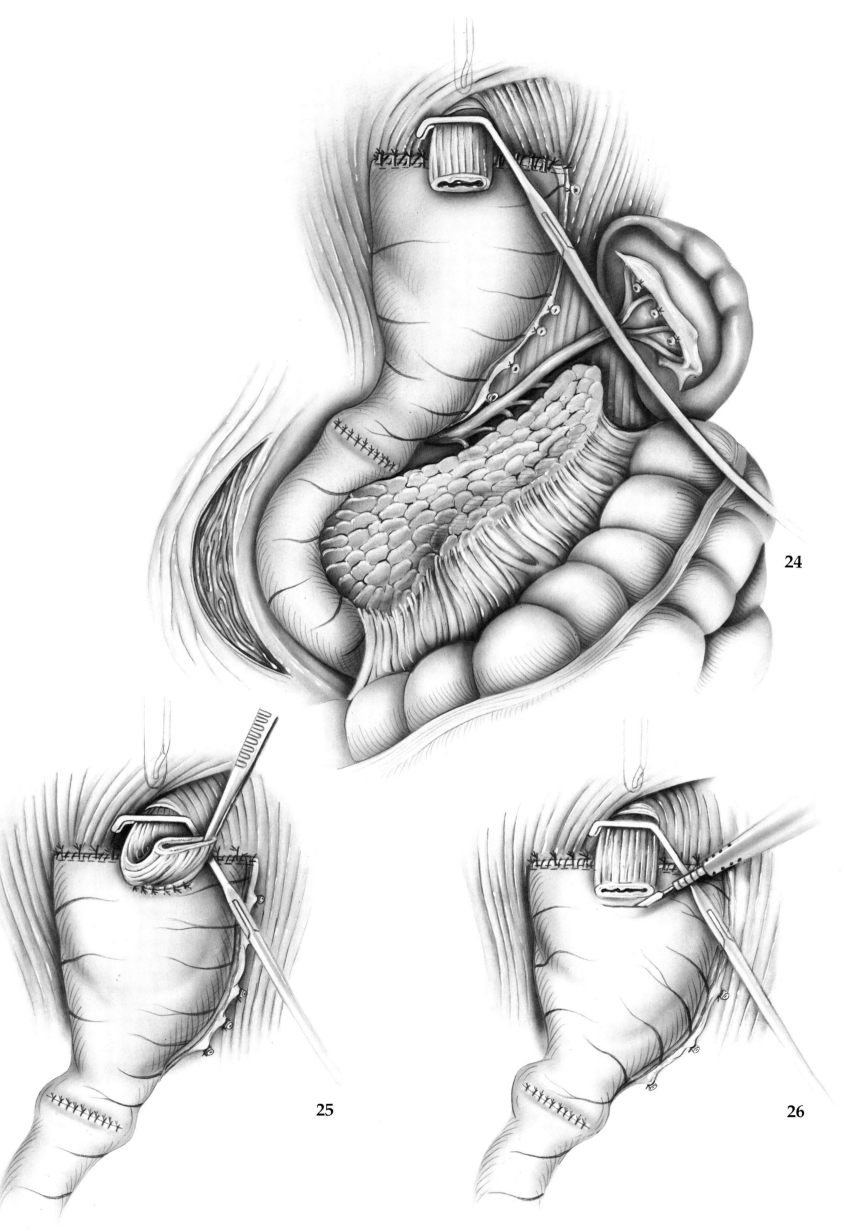

24

25

26

Proximal Gastrectomy for Cancer (*cont.*)

Sutured Esophagogastrostomy (*cont.*)

27–30 The inner layer of the anastomosis is performed with interrupted, full-thickness, #000 poly-glycolic acid sutures. Corner sutures are placed so that the knots are tied on the outside (**Fig. 27**). The posterior row is placed with the knots tied on the inside of the anastomosis (**Fig. 28**). The anterior row is completed with the knots tied on the outside (**Fig. 29**). The Satinsky clamp is removed at the completion of the inner layer (**Fig. 30**).

31–32 A wide Lembert suture is placed on the gastric wall, medial and lateral to the anastomosis. This suture, when tied, will fold the anterior stomach over both itself and the inner layer of the esophagogastrostomy (**Fig. 31**). The anterior layer of interrupted #000 silk sutures is placed, completing the anastomosis. The nasogastric tube is advance by the anesthesiologist, with the guidance of the surgeon's hand, through both the esophagogastrostomy and the pyloroplasty.

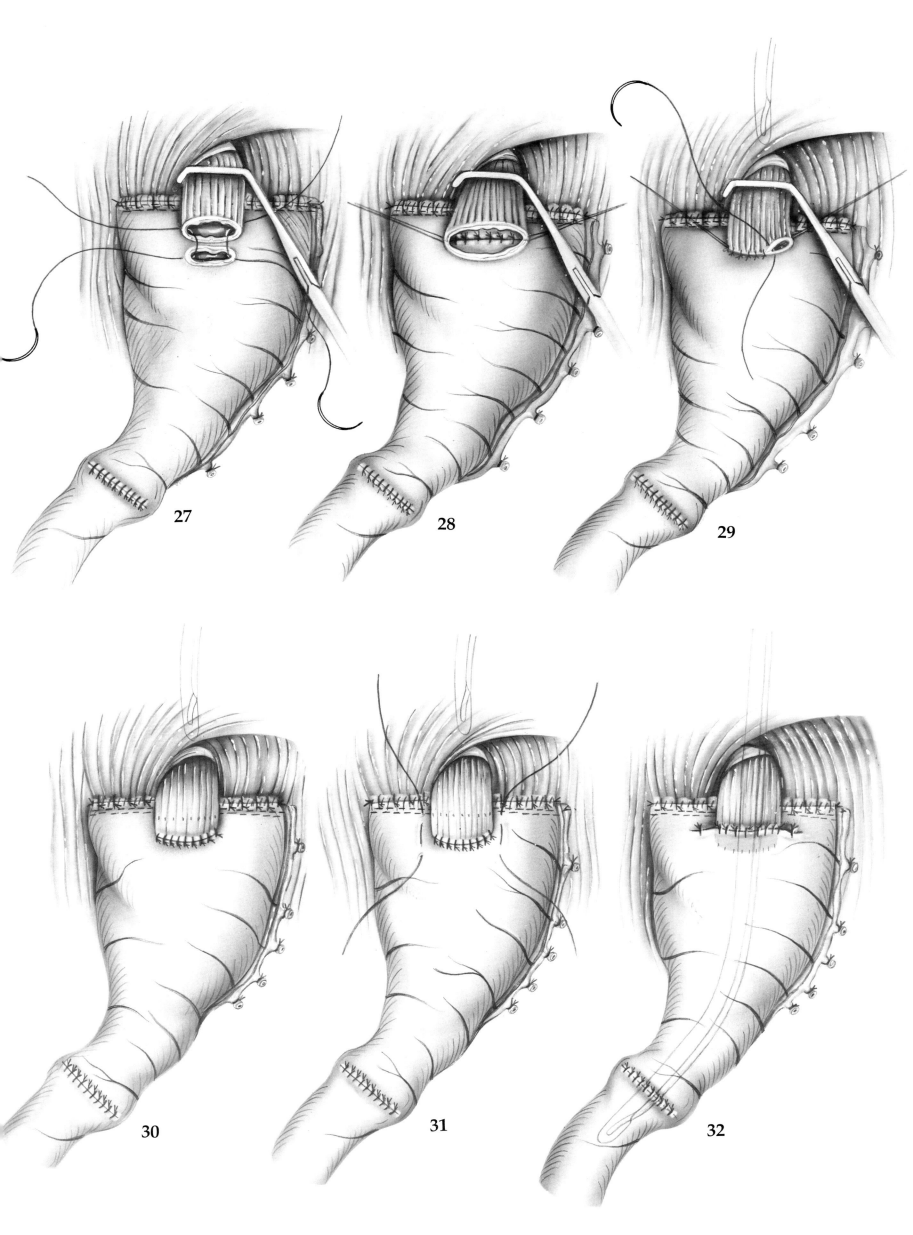

27

28

29

30

31

32

Proximal Gastrectomy for Cancer (*cont.*)

Stapled Esophagogastrostomy

As the common alternative to the hand-sewn anastomosis, a circular stapling device may be used to fashion the esophagogastrostomy.

33–35 The stapler, with the anvil removed, may be inserted through the pyloroplasty (**Fig. 33**) or through a separate gastrotomy (**Fig. 34**). The fully extended stalk of the stapler is used to tent the anterior stomach wall at least 3 cm below the closure of the gastric pouch so that the blood supply to the segment of stomach between the esophagogastrostomy and the proximal stomach is not compromised. A small gastrotomy is made with the electrocautery and the stalk is passed through the stomach wall. The anvil is replaced, firmly and squarely, upon the stalk of the stapler (**Fig. 35**).

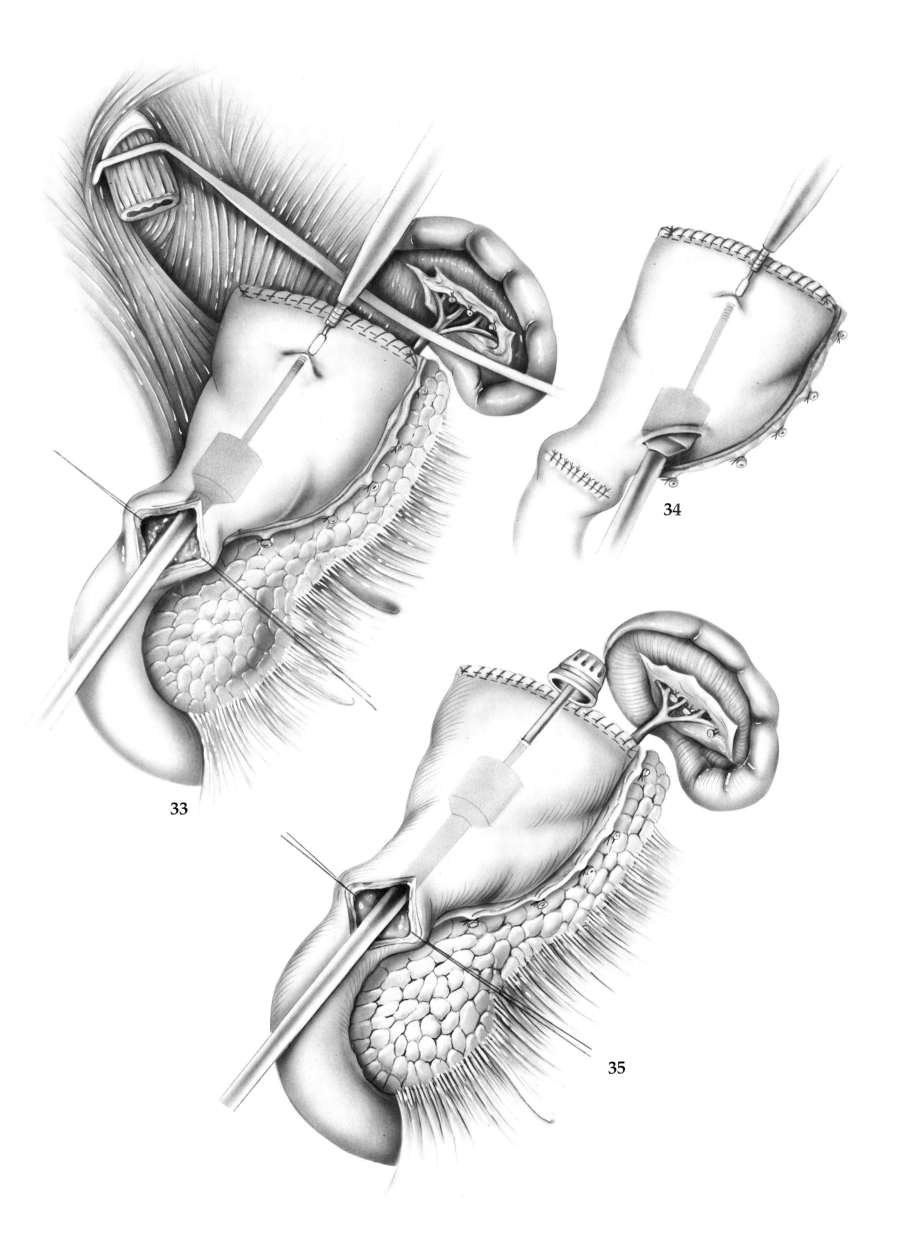

33

34

35

Proximal Gastrectomy for Cancer (*cont.*)

36 The antrum and stapler are set aside, and a full-thickness #0 polypropylene "whip" stitch is run around the esophageal stump. This suture must start and end on the anterior esophagus.

37–38 Four #00 silk stay sutures are placed at 2, 5, 7, and 10 o'clock on the esophageal stump; they include the previously placed polypropylene "whip" stitch.

39–41 The stay sutures at 5 and 7 o'clock are pulled taut, opening the posterior aspect of the esophageal lumen. The assistant gently advances the anvil into the esophagus (**Fig. 39**). The anterior esophageal wall is then pulled over the anvil with the stay sutures placed at 2 and 10 o'clock. All four stay sutures are pulled caudad as the stapler is advanced against the Satinsky clamp (**Fig. 40**). The Satinsky clamp is then removed (**Fig. 41**).

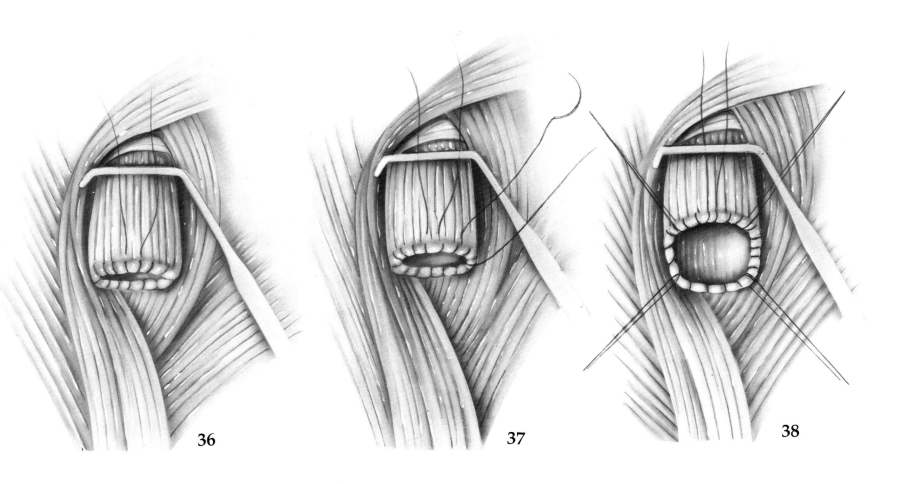

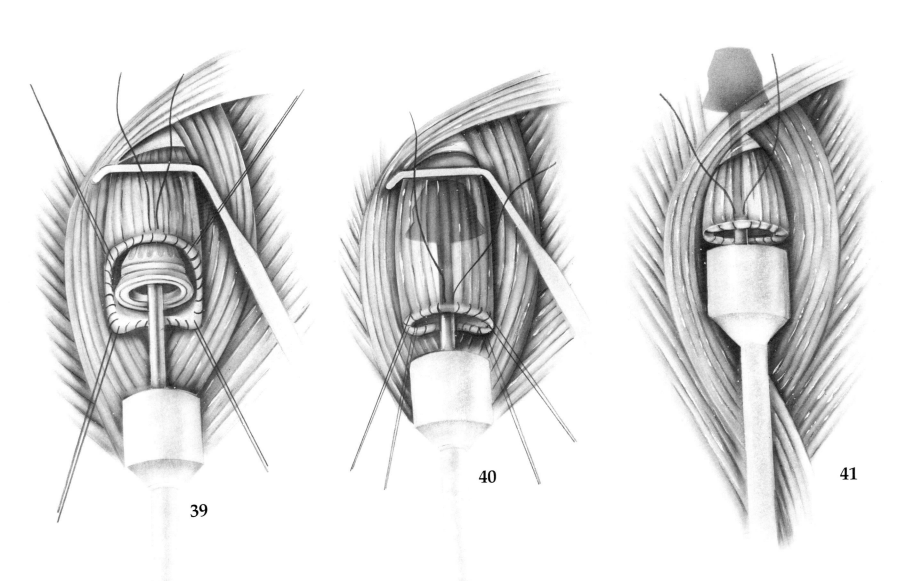

Proximal Gastrectomy for Cancer (*cont.*)

42 The polypropylene "whip" stitch is tied securely around the stapler's stalk. The silk stay sutures are cut and withdrawn.

43 The anvil and body of the stapler are approximated, and the stapler is fired.

44 The stalk is again extended, separating the anvil from the body of the stapler and releasing the esophagogastrostomy.

45 A #00 silk suture is placed across the anastomosis, assisting in the removal of the anvil from the esophageal lumen. The stapler is removed from the stomach and the gastrotomy or pyloroplasty is closed as previously described (**Plate 60, Figs. 20–23**).

46 The nasogastric tube, guided by the surgeon's hand, is passed through the anastomosis and beyond the pyloroplasty. The anterior stomach wall is suspended from the crura of the diaphragm, reducing tension on the anastomosis.

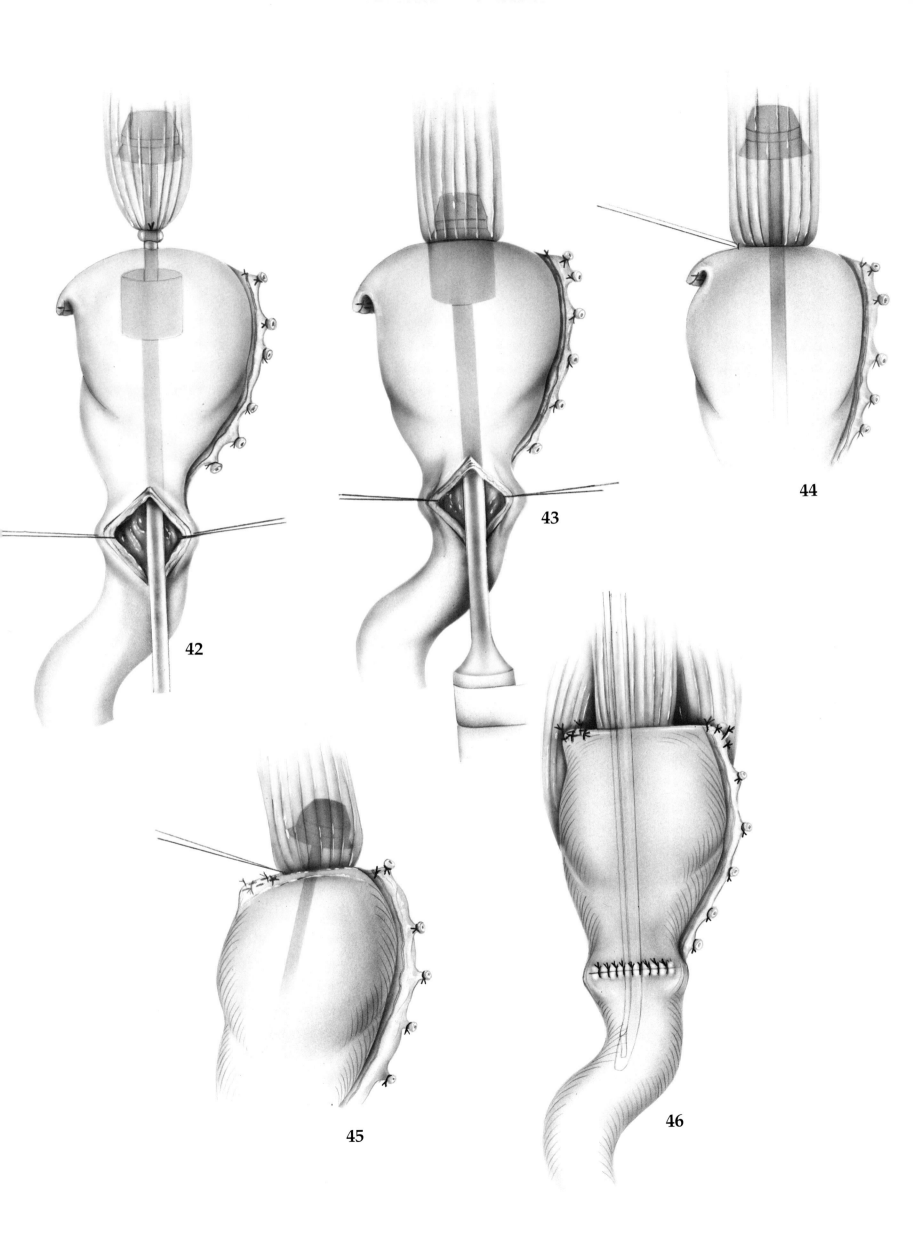

42

43

44

45

46

Esophagogastrointestinal Reconstruction in the Left Chest Following Gastric Resection

Occasionally the esophagogastric or esophagojejunal anastomosis cannot be accomplished in the abdomen because of proximal extension of the tumor along the esophagus requiring resection of the entire intraabdominal portion of the esophagus. In these instances, a limited left anterior thoracotomy may be used to provide the additional length of esophagus required for the anastomosis.

1 After the abdomen is closed, the patient's left arm is abducted and an incision is made in the inframammary fold extending from the sternum to the anterior axillary line. The 6th or 7th intercostal space is opened by the division of the intercostal muscles using the electrocautery, carefully protecting the underlying lung.

2 A Finichietto-Burford retractor, without blades, is used to distract the ribs. The retractor is tied to the upper and lower ribs with two umbilical tapes passed around each rib. This technique provides maximum exposure through this limited incision. The lung is freed inferiorly and retracted medially. The parietal pleura overlying the esophagus is opened, exposing the esophagus.

3 The esophagus is bluntly dissected free with the surgeon's finger.

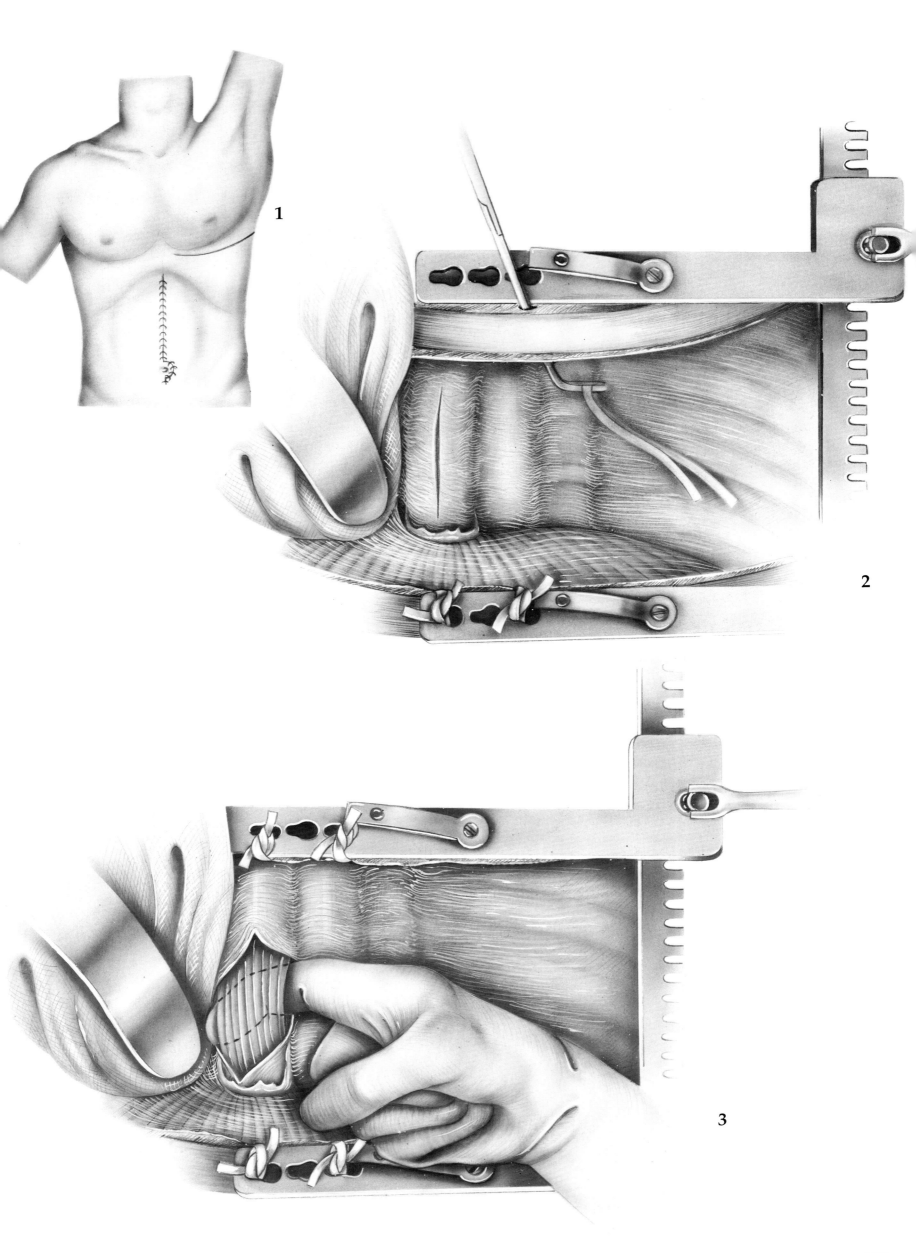

Esophagogastrointestinal Reconstruction in the Left Chest Following Gastric Resection (cont.)

4–5 The surgeon retracts the thoracic esophagus anteriorly and caudally. Two Satinsky vascular clamps are placed across the esophagus. The esophagus is divided safely above the most proximal extent of the tumor.

6 If the specimen was not removed during the intraabdominal portion of the operation, the distal divided specimen tied to the proximal Roux-en-Y limb of jejunum is brought up through the esophageal hiatus, which was widened during the abdominal dissection.

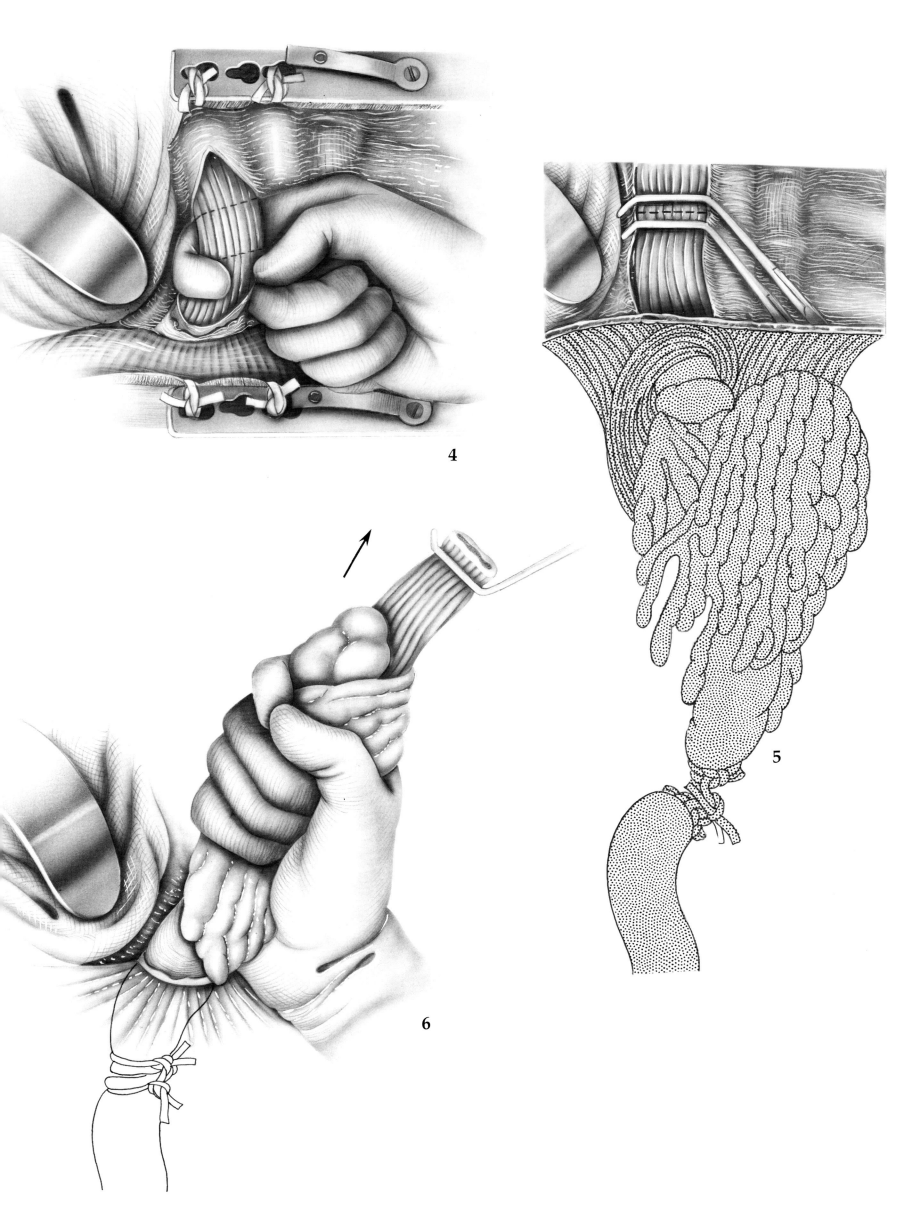

4

5

6

Esophagogastrointestinal Reconstruction in the Left Chest Following Gastric Resection (*cont.*)

7 The posterior esophagus is sutured to the jejunum with interrupted #000 silk sutures, incorporating the submucosa at least 2.5 cm distal to the stapled closure of the jejunal limb. The jejunum is opened along its axis just below the outer posterior row of sutures.

8–9 The full-thickness inner layer is accomplished, circumferentially, with interrupted #000 polyglycolic acid sutures. A #000 silk Lembert suture is placed on either side of the anastomosis, causing the jejunum to fold anteriorly over the anterior inner layer.

10 The interrupted partial-thickness #000 silk outer layer is completed. The jejunum is sutured to the preaortic fascia and parietal pleura to reduce tension on the anastomosis. A posterior chest tube is placed. The rib retractor is removed and the ribs are approximated with two heavy, absorbable pericostal stitches. The muscles are then closed in layers with absorbable sutures.

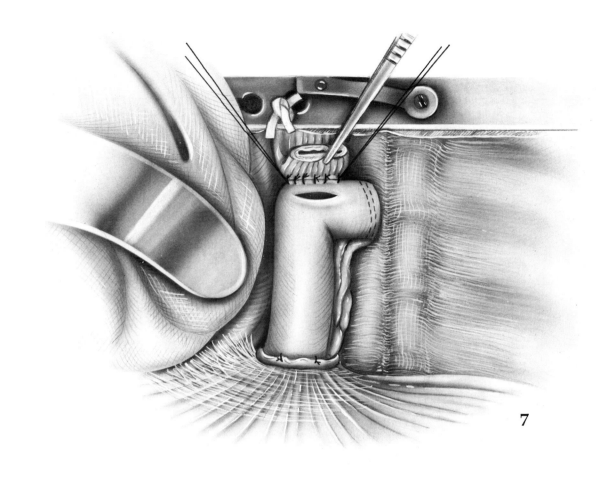

7

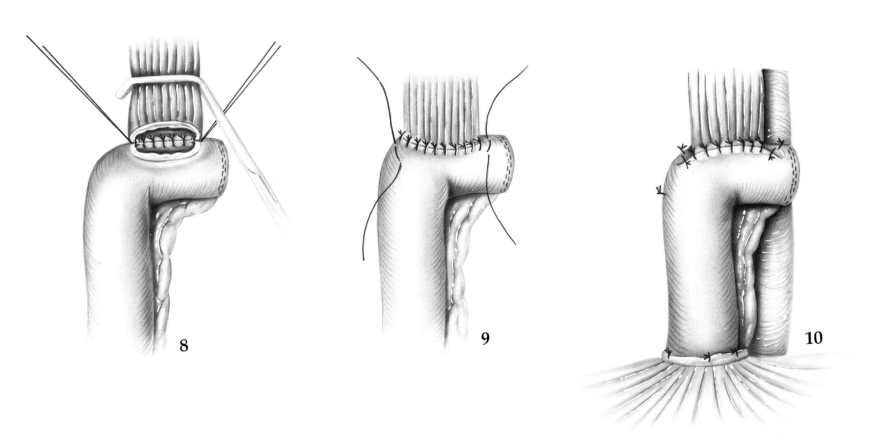

8

9

10

Distal Gastrectomy for Cancer

1 The abdomen is explored through a midline incision extending from the xiphoid to below the umbilicus. The abdominal contents are examined to determine extent of disease and whether a radical distal subtotal gastrectomy will remove all grossly visible tumor. As previously described, the greater omentum is freed from the entire length of the transverse colon (**Plate 53, Fig. 2**). The stomach and the attached omentum are elevated; the left gastric artery is freed, tied with #0 silk, divided between clamps, and tied again (**Plate 54, Figs. 3–6**).

2 The greater omentum is divided from the proximal greater curvature by doubly ligating and dividing the gastroepiploic vessels on the gastric side of the gastroepiploic arch. Because only 25 percent of the stomach will be retained, this dissection is not carried distal to the body of the stomach.

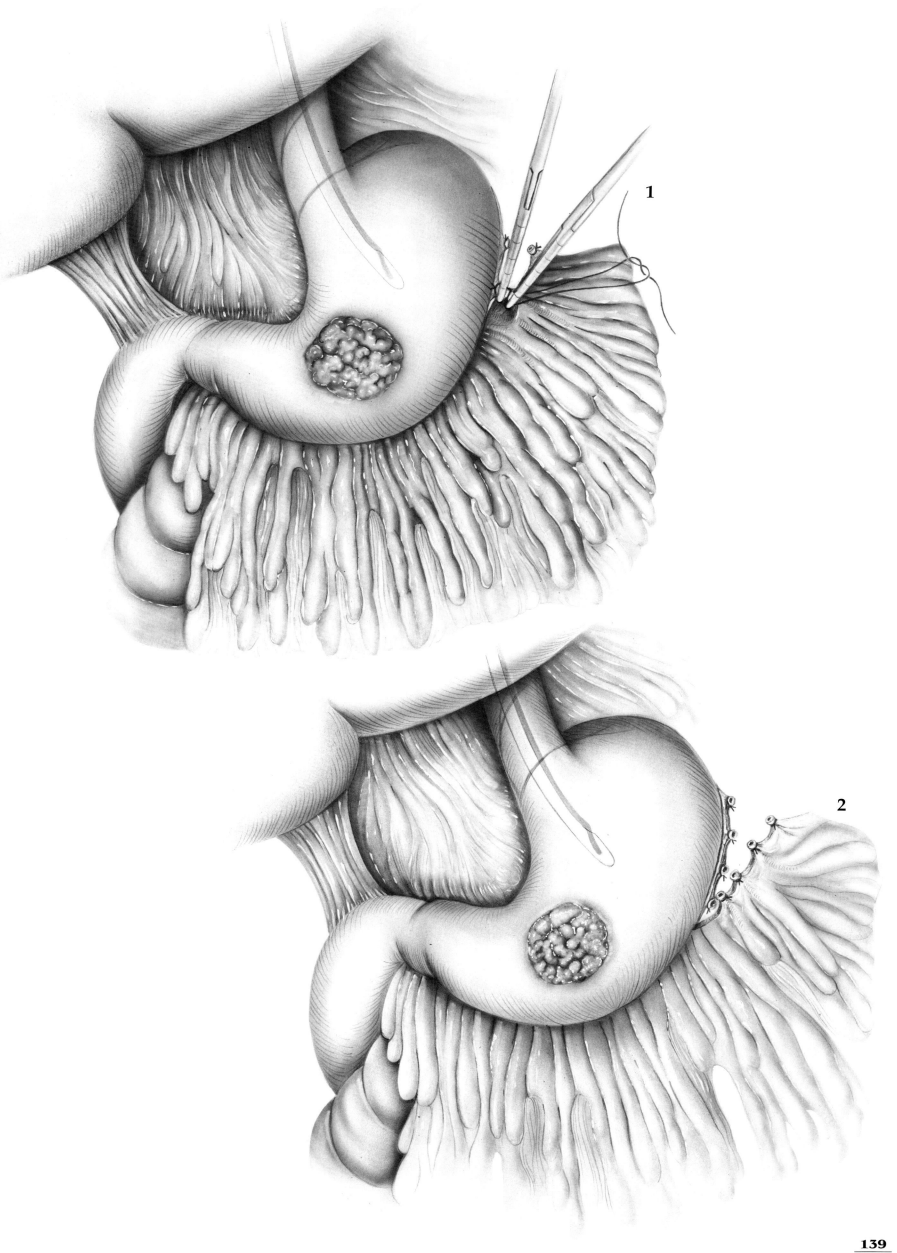

1

2

Distal Gastrectomy for Cancer (*cont.*)

3 The right gastric artery is identified near its origin from the common hepatic artery, divided between clamps, and ligated.

4 The gastrohepatic ligament is freed along the proximal lesser curvature of the stomach. This dissection is carried cephalad along the esophagus 2 cm proximal to the gastroesophageal junction. The lesser omentum, with its accompanying lymph nodes, is dissected from the undersurface of the liver and then caudad along the hepatoduodenal ligament.

5 Once the gastrohepatic ligament is freed, the level of transection is determined as indicated by the broken line.

6 A Payr clamp is placed transversely across the stomach to a point 4 cm below the gastroesophageal junction on the lesser curvature. A Dennis intestinal anastomosis clamp is placed parallel and proximal to the Payr clamp for a distance of 4 cm. Using electrocautery, the portion of the stomach between these clamps is divided (see **Plate 23, Fig. 2**).

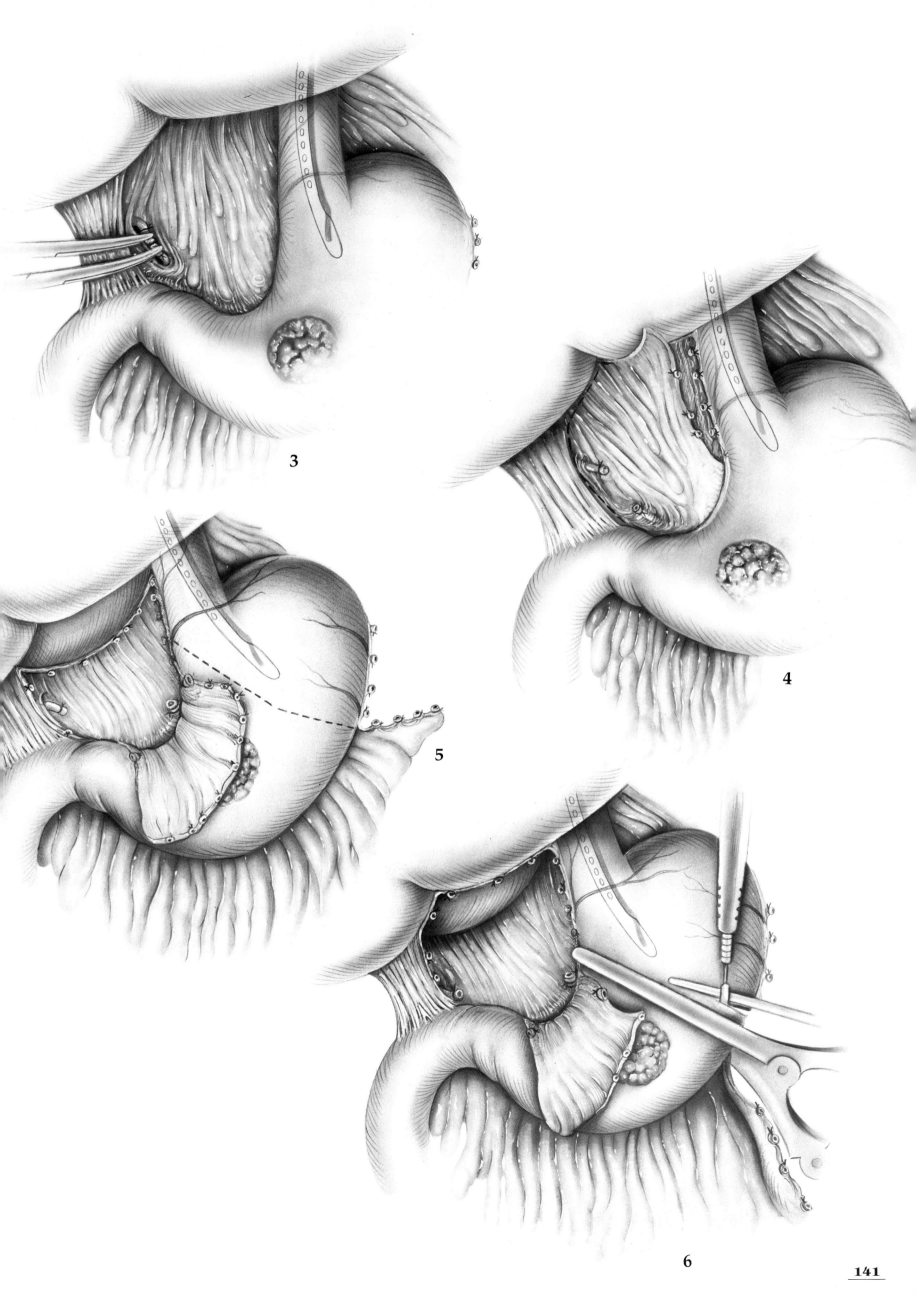

3

4

5

6

Distal Gastrectomy for Cancer (*cont.*)

7 When the division of the stomach almost reaches the tip of the first Dennis clamp, a second Dennis clamp is placed with its tip at a point 2 cm below the gastroesophageal junction. The stomach is divided between the Payr and Dennis clamps with electrocautery (see **Plate 23, Fig. 3**).

8 Because the anastomosis will be constructed with an interrupted single-layer seromuscular suture line, hemostasis is achieved by thoroughly cauterizing the gastric mucosa that extends beyond the anastomosis clamp until a distinct char becomes apparent.

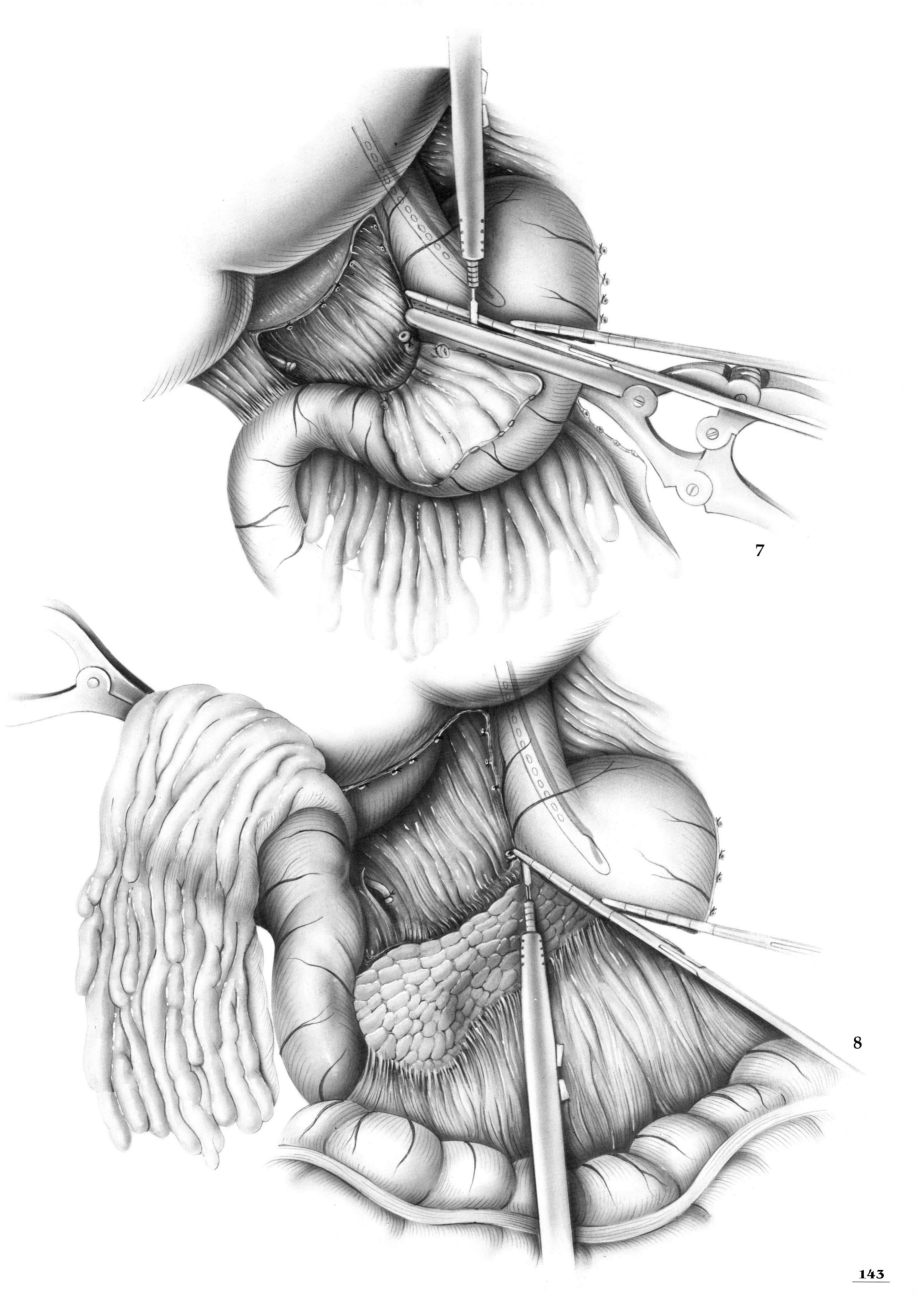

7

8

Distal Gastrectomy for Cancer (*cont.*)

9 The Payr clamp is retracted cephalad with the attached stomach and omentum, exposing the proximal duodenum. Intestinal anastomosis clamps are applied to the duodenum just distal to the pylorus. The duodenum is divided between these two clamps with electrocautery. The specimen is removed from the operative field and sent for pathological examination of the margins of resection.

10 The duodenum is closed with a row of interrupted seromuscular #000 silk sutures placed first in the posterior and then in the anterior duodenal wall. The sutures are tied sequentially as the anastomosis clamp is withdrawn.

11–13 The gastric pouch is tailored with a row of interrupted seromuscular Lembert #000 silk sutures placed over the anastomosis clamp that reaches the lesser curvature. Tying these sutures as the anastomosis clamp is withdrawn inverts the closure. The gastrojejunostomy is constructed in a retrocolic fashion as described previously (see **Plates 23** and **28–32**).

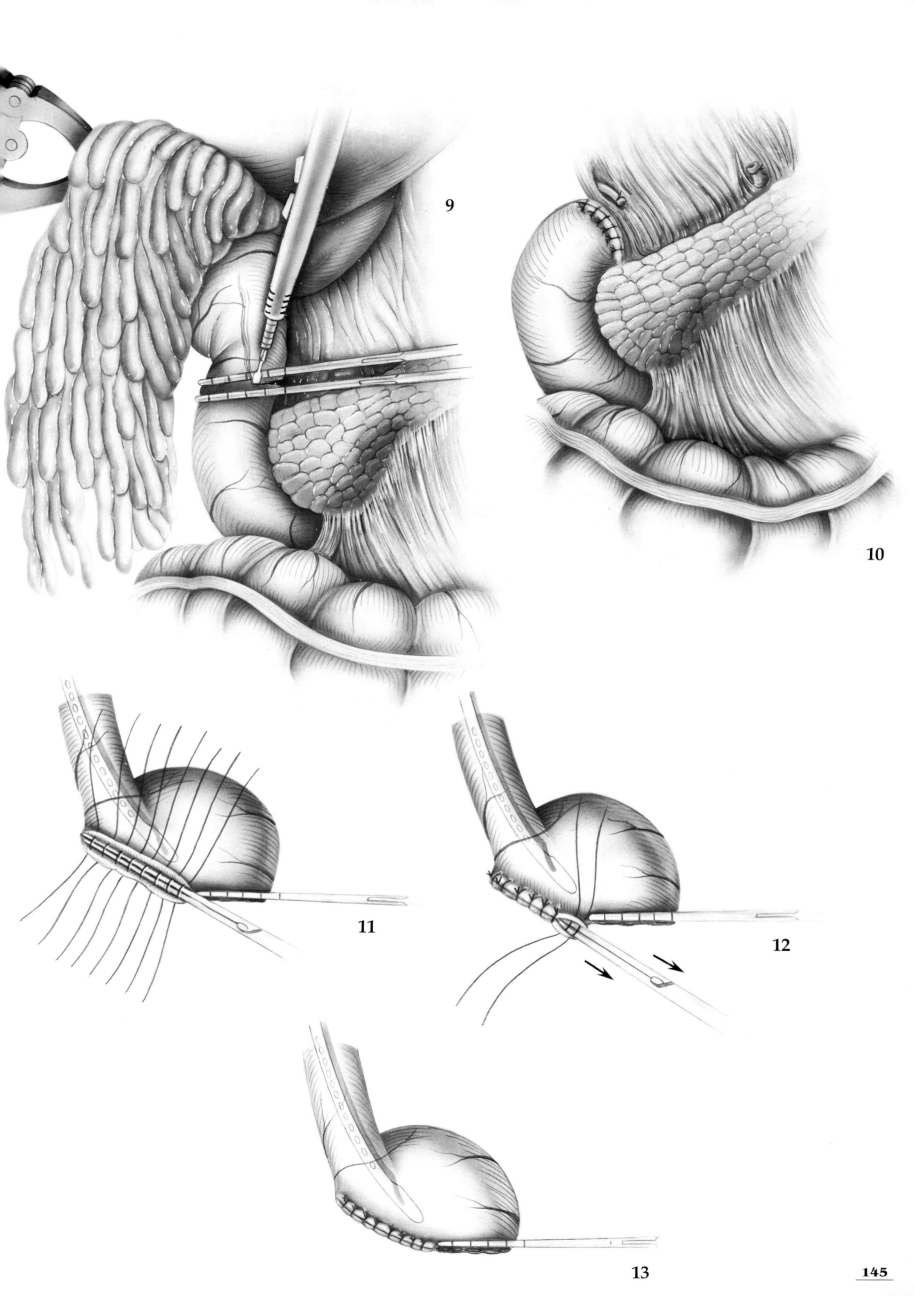

9

10

11

12

13

Cholecystectomy (From Fundus Downward)

1 The patient is placed supine on the operating table. The abdomen is explored through a right subcostal incision. The falciform ligament is divided between Kelly clamps and tied.

2 Exposure is achieved using three laparotomy pads folded into thirds and placed above the hepatic flexure, on the transverse colon and duodenum, and medially where the stomach intrudes into the wound. An open laparotomy pad is placed down to the posterior perito- neum, covering the three previously placed pads.

3 Two Deaver retractors provide downward traction on these laparotomy pads, thus expos- ing the undersurface of the liver, the gallbladder, and the hepatoduodenal ligament. The seal between the liver and the diaphragm is broken by sweeping the hand over the liver's surface. A Kelly clamp is placed on the fundus of the gallbladder and retracted caudally. The peritoneum overlying the gallbladder, approximately 1 cm from the liver, is incised with a scalpel as indicated by the broken line.

4 A plane between the gallbladder and the liver bed in the gallbladder fossa is developed bluntly. Small blood vessels are controlled with small surgical clips or with electrocautery. At the lower end of the dissection, attention is directed toward the junction of the cystic and common bile ducts. The peritoneum overlying the lateral portion of the hepatoduo- denal ligament is incised as indicated by the broken line. The cystic duct and artery are dissected bluntly. Once the cystic duct is identified, a clamp is placed on the ampulla of the gallbladder. Retraction on this clamp exposes the remaining peritoneal investments of the gallbladder, which are divided.

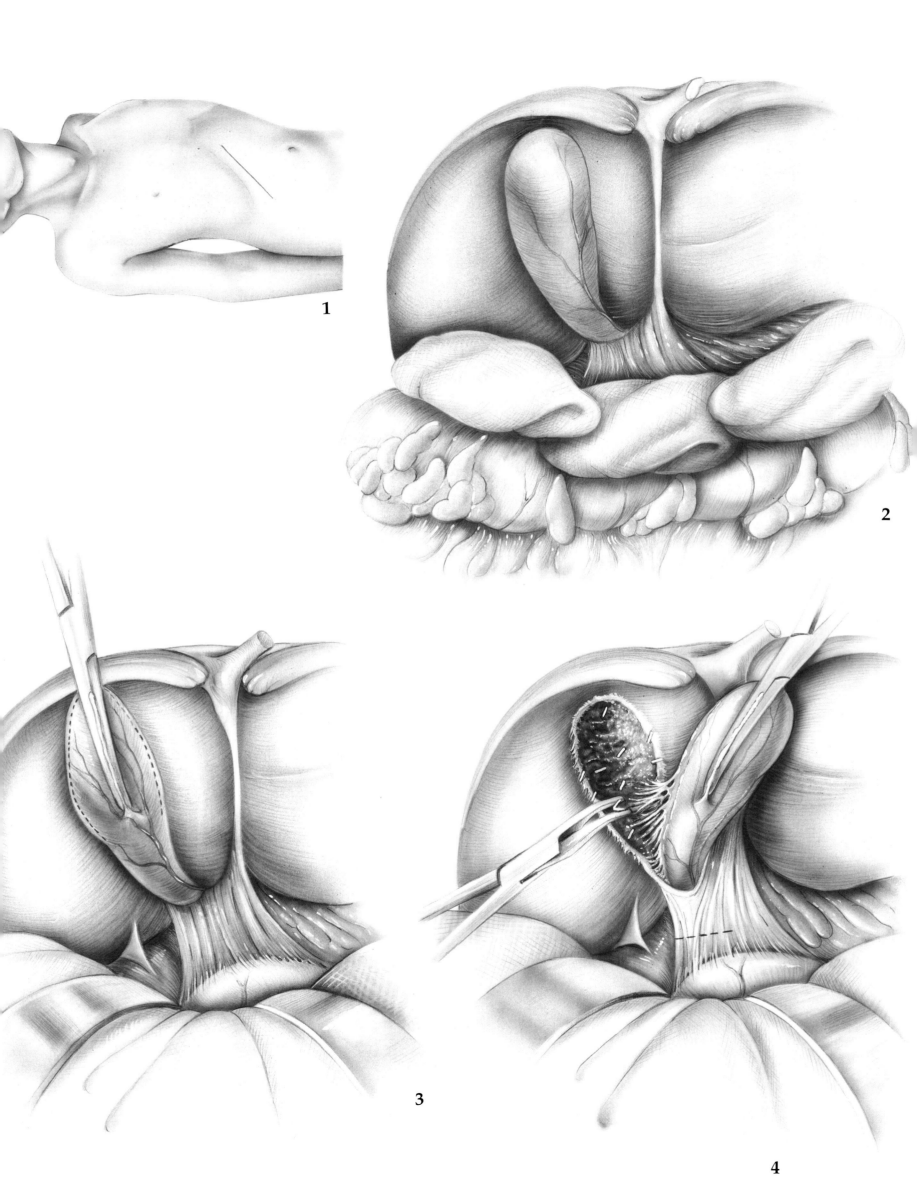

Cholecystectomy (From Fundus Downward) (*cont.*)

5–6 The cystic artery is shorter than, and does not have the elasticity of, the cystic duct. The cystic artery is always divided and ligated prior to the division of the cystic duct. Should the duct be divided before the artery, the greater mobility of the gallbladder increases the risk of avulsion of the cystic artery at its origin from the hepatic artery. The cystic artery is identified coursing onto the gallbladder. A #000 silk tie in a right-angle clamp is passed around the freed artery.

7–9 The cystic artery is tied in continuity prior to division (**Fig. 7**). A tonsil clamp is applied to the distal artery. The artery is divided with a scalpel against the clamp (**Fig. 8**). Once the artery is divided, traction on the gallbladder causes the cystic duct to extend, exposing more clearly the cystic duct–common hepatic–common bile duct junction (**Fig. 9**).

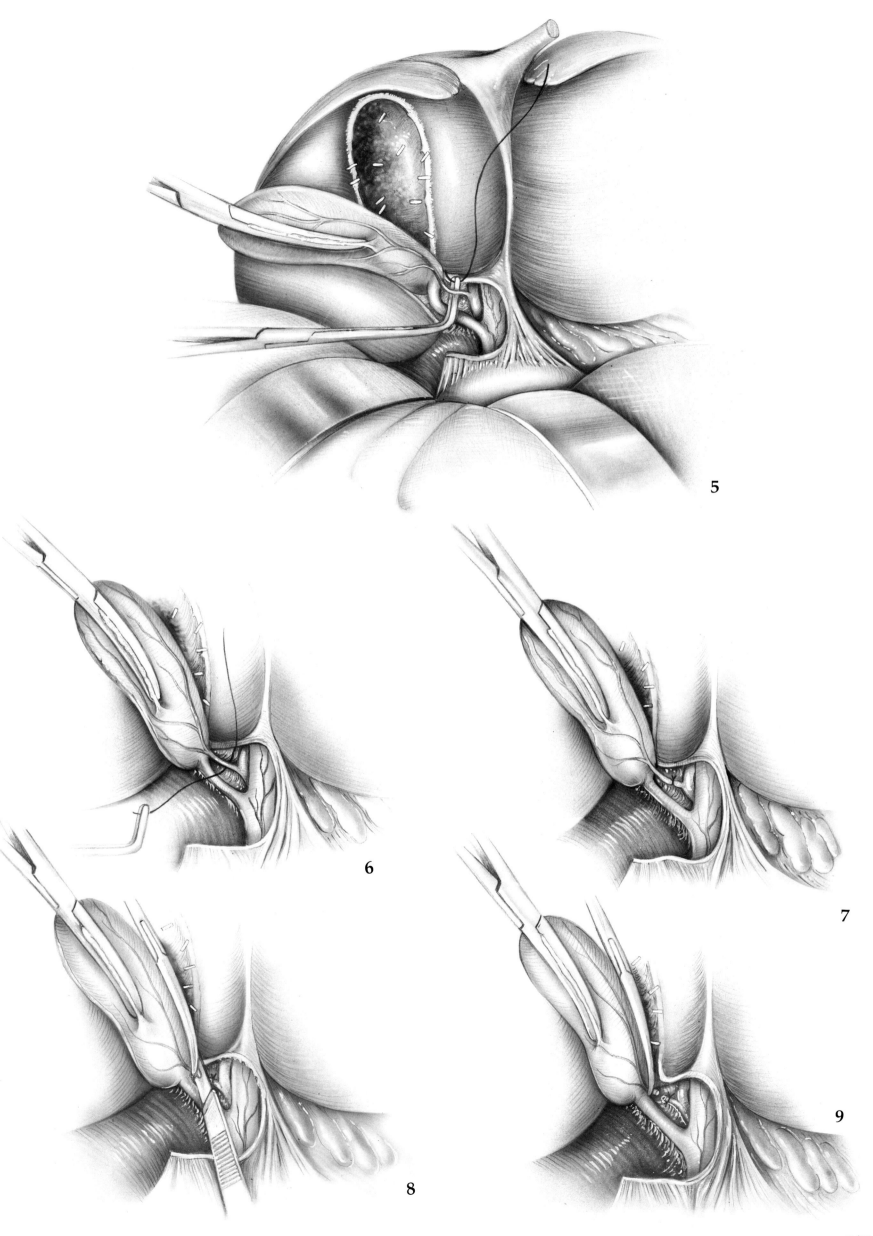

5

6

7

8

9

Cholecystectomy (From Fundus Downward) (*cont.*)

10 The cystic duct is clamped only after the junction of the cystic and common ducts is clearly visualized. This requires clearing of the common hepatic duct as well as the common bile duct distally. The duct is tied in continuity, approximately 1 cm from its junction with the common bile duct, with a #00 silk ligature. A tonsil or Mixter clamp is applied to the duct on the gallbladder side of the tie. The cystic duct is divided as indicated by the broken line.

11 The specimen is removed. The gallbladder fossa is inspected for bleeding, which is controlled with surgical clips or electrocautery. The common duct is palpated between the thumb anteriorly and the forefinger inserted in the foramen of Winslow posterior to the duct. The gallbladder fossa is left open.

12 A drain is not used routinely. If, however, the dissection was difficult and significant moistness in the gallbladder bed persists, a closed suction drain is placed in the gallbladder fossa and brought out through a separate incision in the abdominal wall. The drain is secured to the skin with a heavy silk stitch.

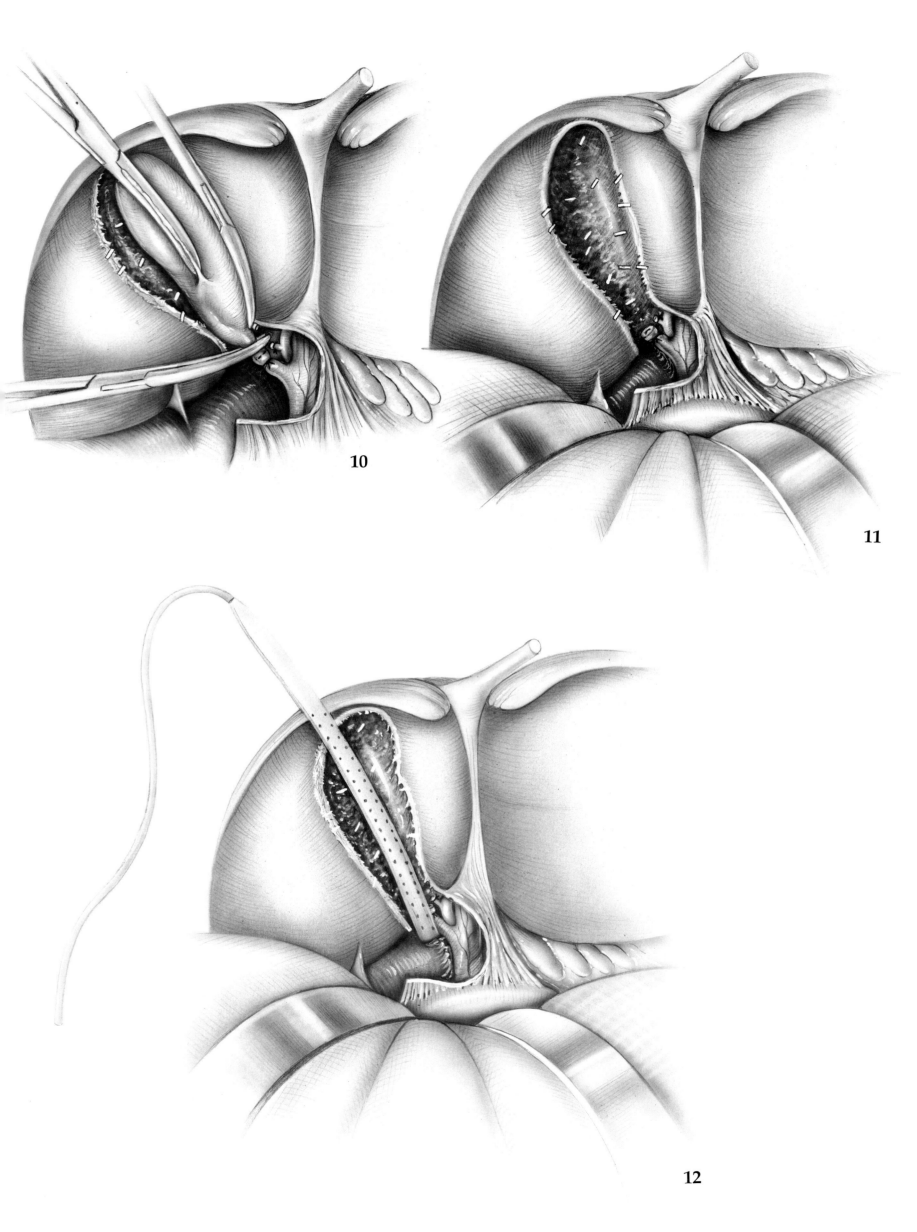

10

11

12

Cholecystectomy (From Below to Fundus)

Some surgeons prefer to dissect the cystic artery and duct prior to removing the gallbladder. The admonition to clearly visualize the junction of the common hepatic, common bile, and cystic ducts, as well as the cystic artery extending onto the gallbladder, applies all the more when this technique is used.

1 The positioning and exposure of the operative field is the same as that described in **Plate 73, Figs. 1–3.** A Kelly clamp is placed on the gallbladder, which is retracted caudally. The peritoneum investing the lateral border of the hepatoduodenal ligament is incised first (see **Plate 73, Fig. 4**). The cystic duct and artery are bluntly dissected well onto the gallbladder. A #000 silk ligature is passed around the cystic artery.

2 The cystic artery is ligated proximally. A tonsil clamp is placed on the cystic artery distally; then the artery is divided sharply between the tie and the clamp. The cystic duct is dissected to its junction with the common hepatic and common bile ducts. The cystic duct is then tied in continuity, approximately 1 cm from this junction, with an absorbable ligature. A tonsil or Mixter clamp is placed on the cystic duct close to the gallbladder, and the duct is divided adjacent to the clamp as indicated by the broken line.

3 The clamp on the fundus is retracted inferiorly, and the peritoneum overlying the gallbladder fundus is incised approximately 1 cm away from the hepatic bed. The gallbladder can be removed as previously described (**Plate 73, Figs. 2–4**) from above downward or, as depicted here, from below upward. Small vessels in the gallbladder bed are divided between surgical clips or with electrocautery to achieve hemostasis.

4 Postoperative drainage is rarely necessary. However, if required, a closed suction drain can be used as previously described (**Plate 75, Fig. 12**).

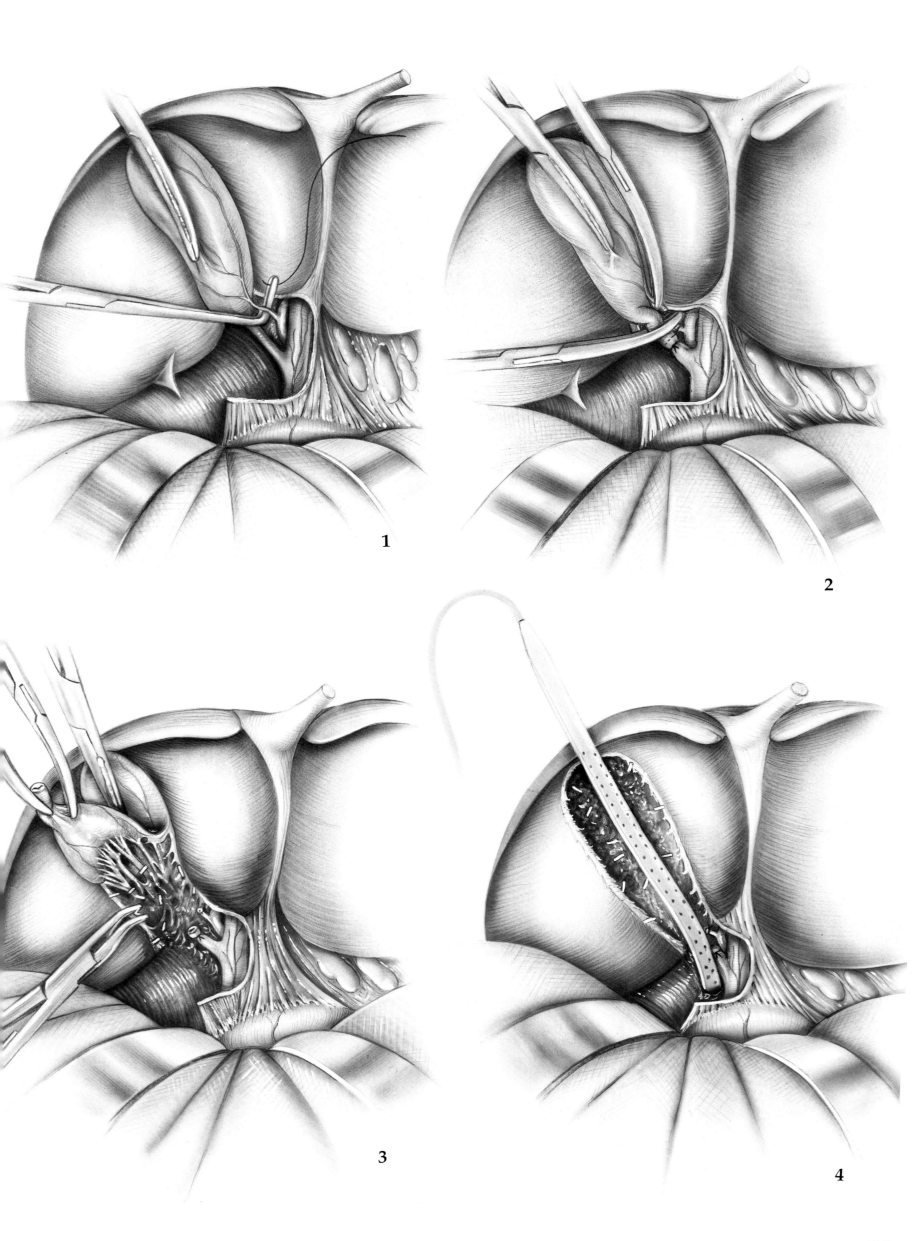

Common Bile Duct Exploration

The common bile duct is explored following cholecystectomy if stones are palpated within the duct or if the cystic duct cholangiogram or preoperative endoscopic retrograde cholangiogram demonstrates stones.

1 The duodenum is mobilized by incising the peritoneum along its lateral border (Kocher maneuver). The surgeon bluntly opens the plane between the duodenum and the retroperitoneal structures. The common bile duct is palpated along its length as it courses behind the first portion of the duodenum and into the pancreas. This maneuver allows manipulation of the duct during the exploration. Two #000 silk sutures are placed, along the axis of the duct, through the anteromedial and anterolateral walls near the junction of the common bile and common hepatic ducts. These sutures are distracted and a choledochotomy is created on the anterior surface of the duct with a #15 scalpel.

2 The choledochotomy is enlarged proximally and distally, using an angled Pott's scissors, as indicated by the broken line.

3 An attempt is made to push the stone manually up the duct to the choledochotomy.

4 The stone forceps is most useful for removal of stones close to the choledochotomy. It is introduced into the duct through the choledochotomy.

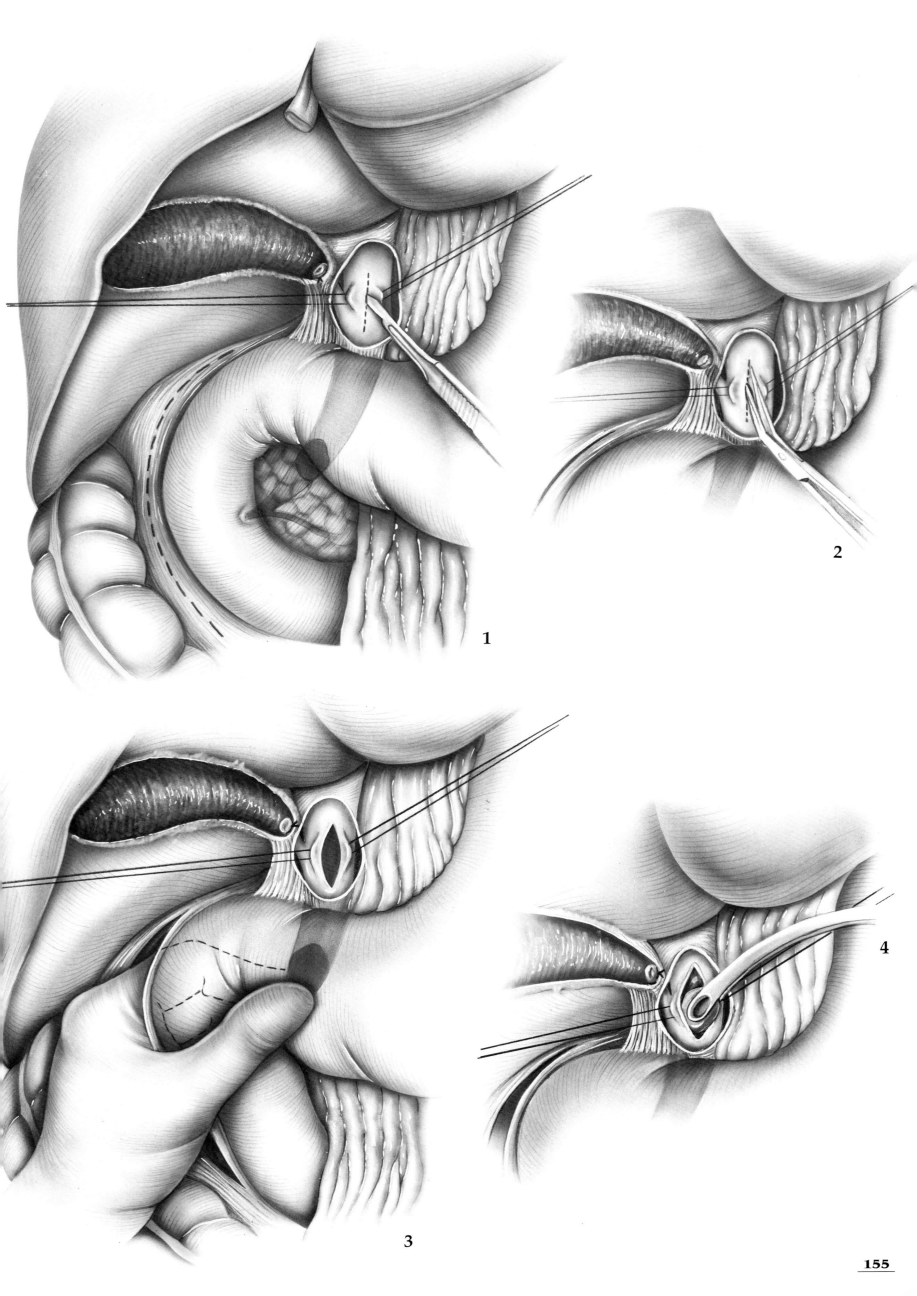

Common Bile Duct Exploration (*cont.*)

5 A #12 or #14 French soft, red, Robinson whistle-tip catheter is introduced into the common bile duct with a right-angle clamp. Saline solution is injected through the catheter under pressure as it is withdrawn. This maneuver is repeated in the distal right and left hepatic ducts, irrigating out smaller stones, stone fragments, and other debris.

6 A 3-mm Bakes dilator is passed distally into the duodenum, ensuring patency of the ampulla of Vater. At no time should a larger Bakes dilator be used for this procedure.

7 A T-tube is tailored by cutting the short arms to 2-cm lengths. The intersection of the "T" is removed, as shown, by applying traction at this point with a clamp and cutting off the tented-up portion. In cases where the duct is small, half or less of the back wall of the "T" may be removed. If postoperative instrumentation of the duct through the T-tube tract is contemplated at the time of surgery, the catheter must be at least #16 French in caliber.

8–9 A short arm of the T-tube is introduced into the common hepatic duct with a right-angle clamp and is held in place while the other short arm is inserted into the common bile duct with a forceps. The forceps is used to hold the tube steady as the right-angle clamp is removed.

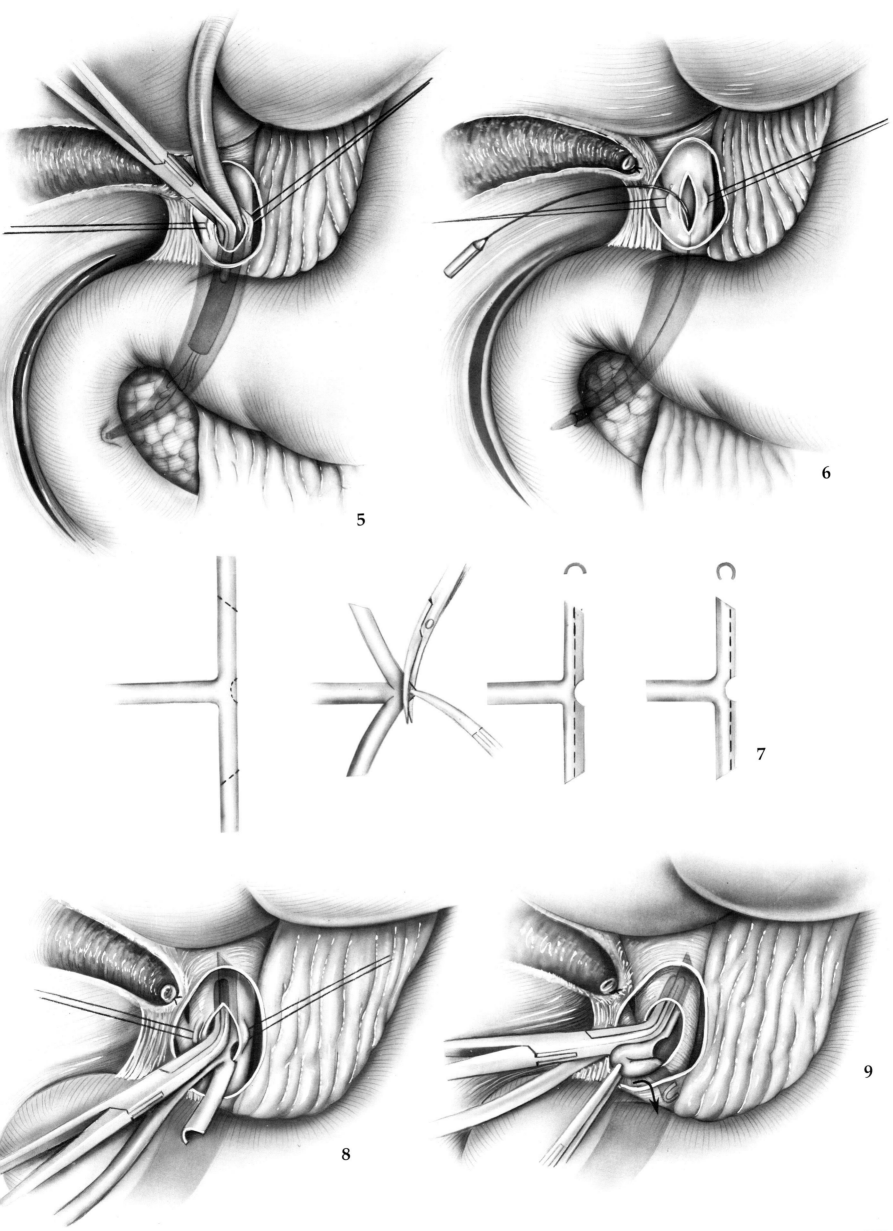

5

6

7

8

9

Common Bile Duct Exploration (*cont.*)

10–11 The lateral and medial traction sutures are removed, and a bile-tight closure of the duct is accomplished with a continuous #000 polyglycolic acid suture begun at the inferior corner of the choledochotomy. The suture is tied to itself at the completion of the distal suture line.

12 Despite a snug closure from below, the long arm is pushed inferiorly and another simple #000 polyglycolic suture is placed proximal to the tube, forming a collar around the tube as it emerges from the choledochotomy. A completion cholangiogram is performed to exclude residual stones.

13 A closed suction drain is placed behind the common bile duct through the gallbladder bed. This catheter is brought out to the skin through a separate incision. The drain is secured to the skin with a heavy silk stitch.

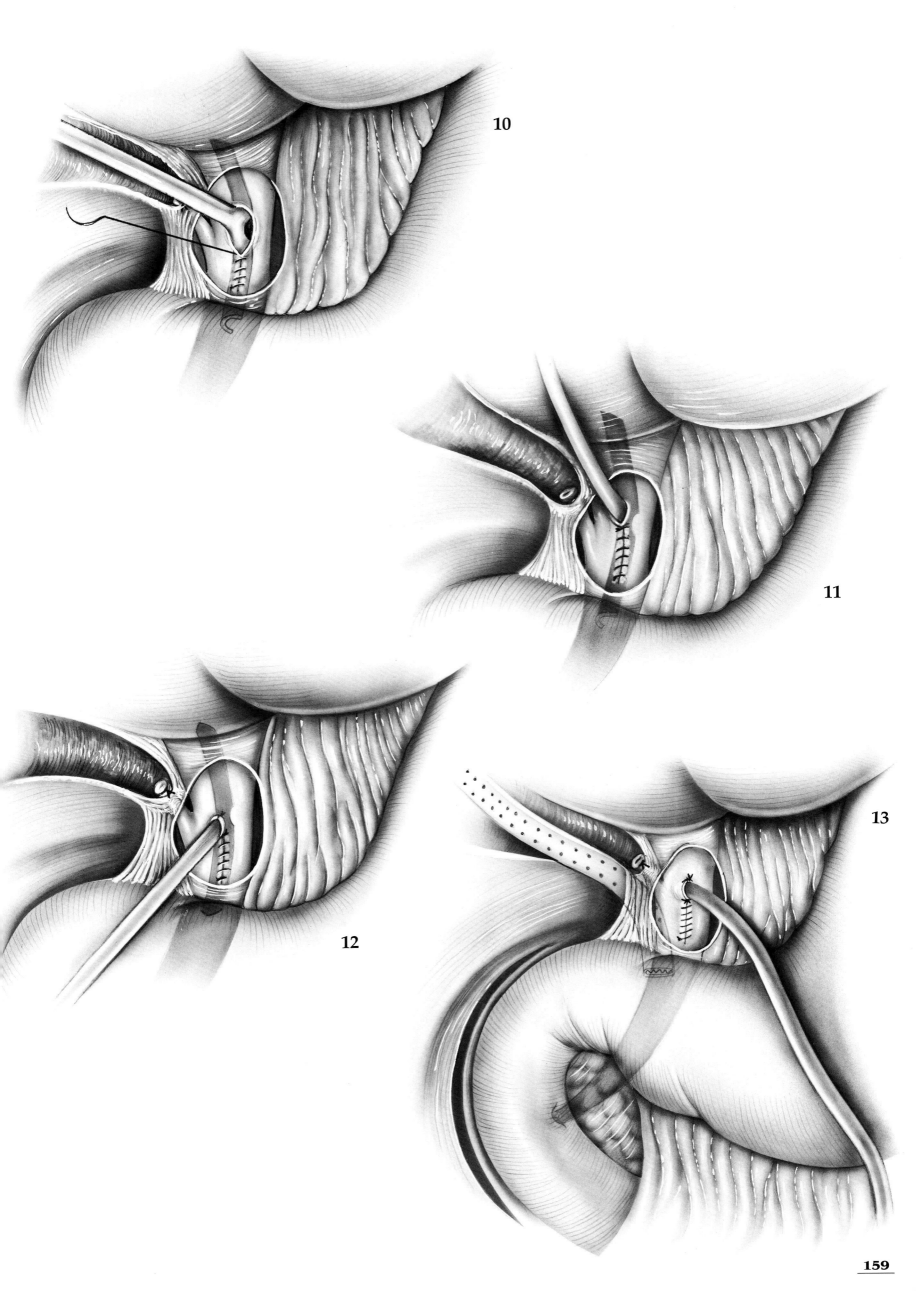

Choledochoduodenostomy

1 A choledochoduodenostomy is performed as an adjunct to, or instead of, a common bile duct exploration when the duct is dilated to a diameter greater than 14 mm. It is very useful in cases of impacted stones when preoperative pancreatitis is absent. The duodenum is mobilized by incising the peritoneum lateral to its first and second portions. The anterior wall of the common duct is dissected from its surrounding tissues. A choledochotomy is created with a #15 scalpel and then extended with an angled Pott's scissors. The choledochotomy must be at least 2.5 cm in length. A transverse duodenotomy is made on the anterosuperior border of the first portion of the duodenum. It should be centered on the choledochotomy, to facilitate the subsequent anastomosis. Though a formal duct exploration is not required with this procedure, stones that are easily accessible are removed.

2 The entire anastomosis is performed with a single layer of interrupted #000 polyglycolic acid sutures. A suture is placed from the outside in at the midportion of the medial wall of the choledochotomy, and then from the inside out at the medial corner of the duodenotomy. The ends of this suture are clamped. Similarly, the lateral wall of the choledochotomy is bisected with a stitch placed from the outside in. This suture is then brought through the lateral corner of the duodenotomy from the inside out. The remaining sutures on the posterior row of the choledochoduodenostomy are placed from within the lumen of the anastomosis by sequentially bisecting the previously placed sutures. The sutures are not tied until the posterior row is complete.

3 Once all of the stitches are placed, they are tied. Except for the two "corner" stitches, the tails of these stitches are cut.

4–6 The anterior row of sutures in the choledochoduodenostomy are placed from the outside of the anastomosis, starting with the central stitch and bisecting the previously placed stitches. The medial anterior row is placed last. The completed choledochoduodenostomy is usually bile-tight; however, closed suction drainage is commonly employed. The drain is placed behind the choledochoduodenostomy and brought out through the gallbladder bed. There is no need to perform intraoperative cholangiograms, since any residual stone will either pass through the choledochoduodenostomy or be of no clinical consequence.

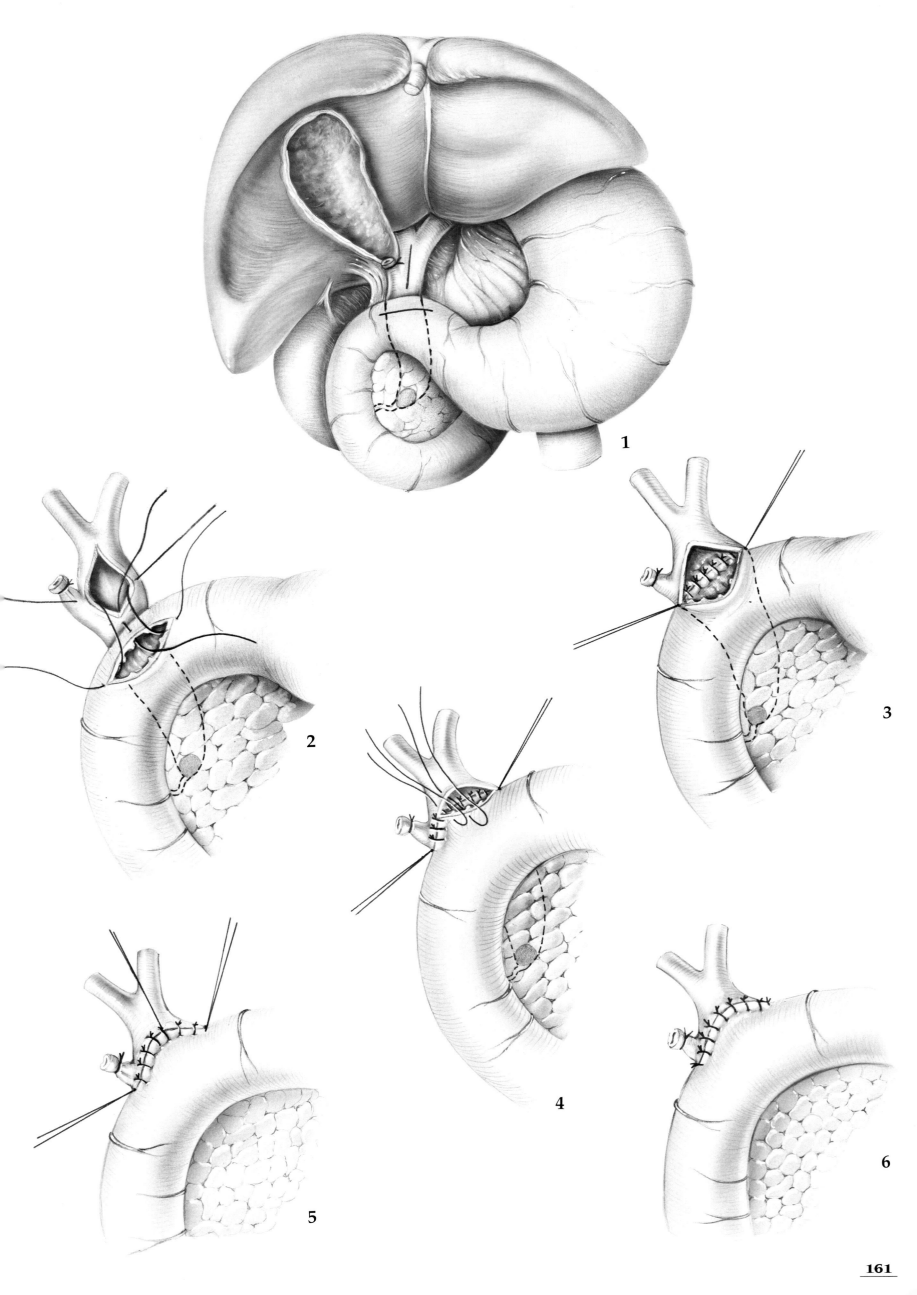

Sphincteroplasty

In cases where the common duct is too small for a choledochoduodenostomy, or where preoperative pancreatitis has resulted from a stone impacted at the ampulla which could not be removed from above during a common duct exploration, sphincteroplasty is indicated. Sphincteroplasty is also used when common duct drainage is required following surgery on a small common bile duct.

1 The duodenum is mobilized by incising the peritoneum lateral to its first and second portions. The ampulla of Vater is palpated in the medial midportion of the descending duodenum. Two #000 silk stay sutures are placed in the anteromedial and anterolateral walls of the duodenum overlying the ampulla.

2 The anterior duodenal wall is opened by electrocautery. A transverse #000 silk suture is placed below the papilla, to provide traction and to stabilize it during manipulation. A #0000 vascular silk suture is placed through the papilla at 12 o'clock.

3 Two small straight mosquito clamps are advanced into the papilla and up the distal common bile duct as traction is applied to the stitch in the papilla. The mosquito clamps should be placed between 12 and 1 o'clock, avoiding injury to the pancreatic duct. Using electrocautery, the portion of the papilla and posterior duodenal wall between these clamps is divided.

4 Three or four #0000 polyglycolic acid sutures are placed around each clamp, through both the duodenal and bile duct walls.

5 The duodenal mucosa and submucosal layer are closed with a continuous #000 polyglycolic acid suture.

6 The outer later is accomplished with an interrupted layer of #000 silk.

If there is any difficulty in identifying the papilla or placing the suture for seating the clamps in **Figs. 2** and **3**, the common duct should be opened and a fine red rubber catheter passed down the duct and through the papilla, allowing placement of the clamps between which the sphincteroplasty is performed.

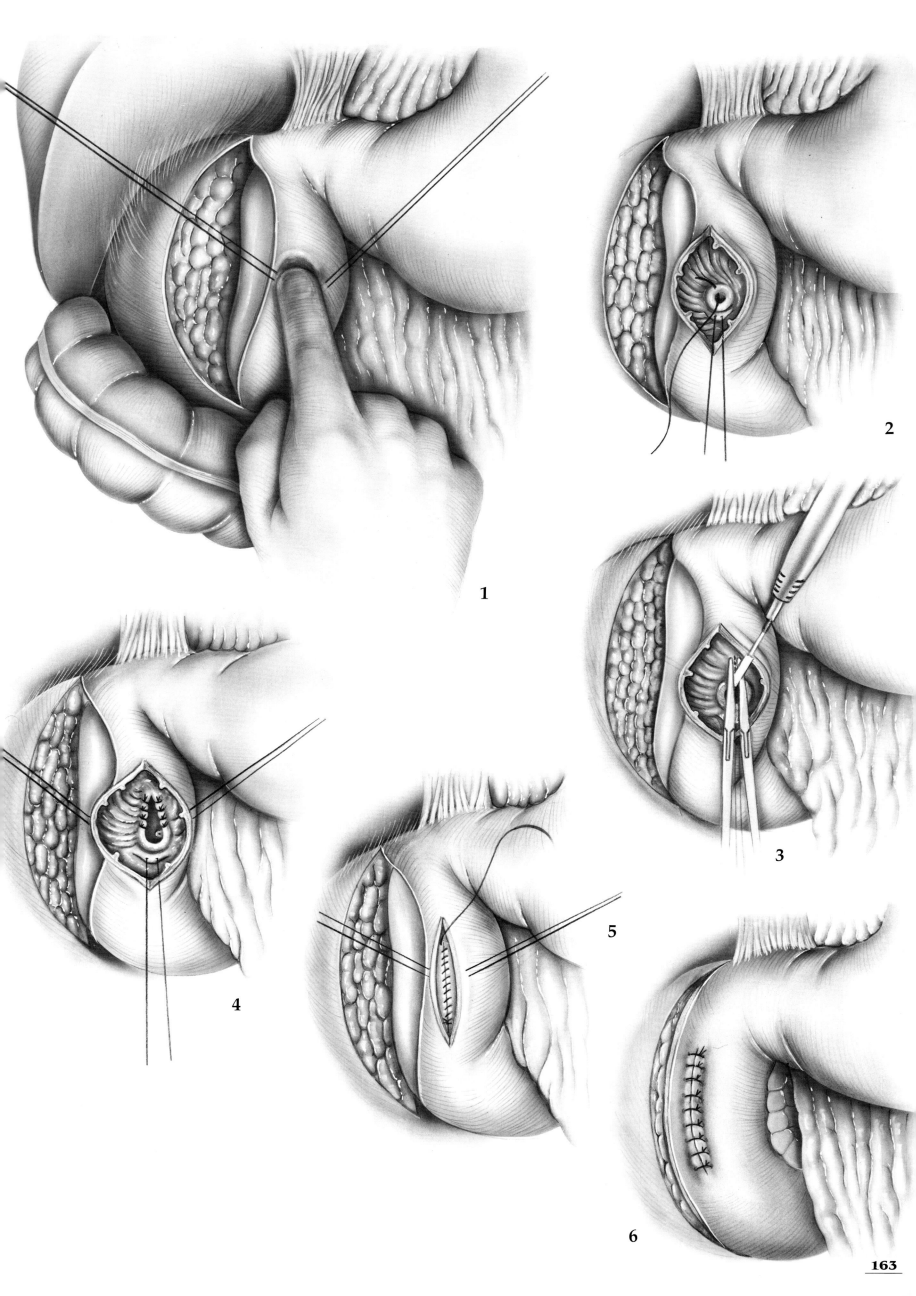

1

2

3

4

5

6

Lowering of the Hepatic Plate

1 The abdomen is explored through a bilateral subcostal incision. The round ligament of the liver is grasped with a Kelly clamp. The falciform ligament is then dissected free of the abdominal wall until the dome of the diaphragm is reached. The round ligament is traced posteriorly to where the quadrate and left lobes of the liver fuse, as indicated by the broken line.

2 This fusion plane is most often very thin, and in some cases may even be absent. When present, it is divided using electrocautery over a fine clamp.

3 While some physicians advocate elevating the round ligament, we pull it caudally as the liver is retracted cephalad. The left hepatic duct is identified by dissection in the plane indicated by the broken line.

4 There are variable veins and small hepatic arteries crossing the duct at this level. These are dissected with a fine right-angle clamp, ligated with #0000 silk, and divided. The duct can be exposed from the umbilical fissure to the hilus of the liver, permitting a wide anastomosis to be fashioned to the left hepatic duct.

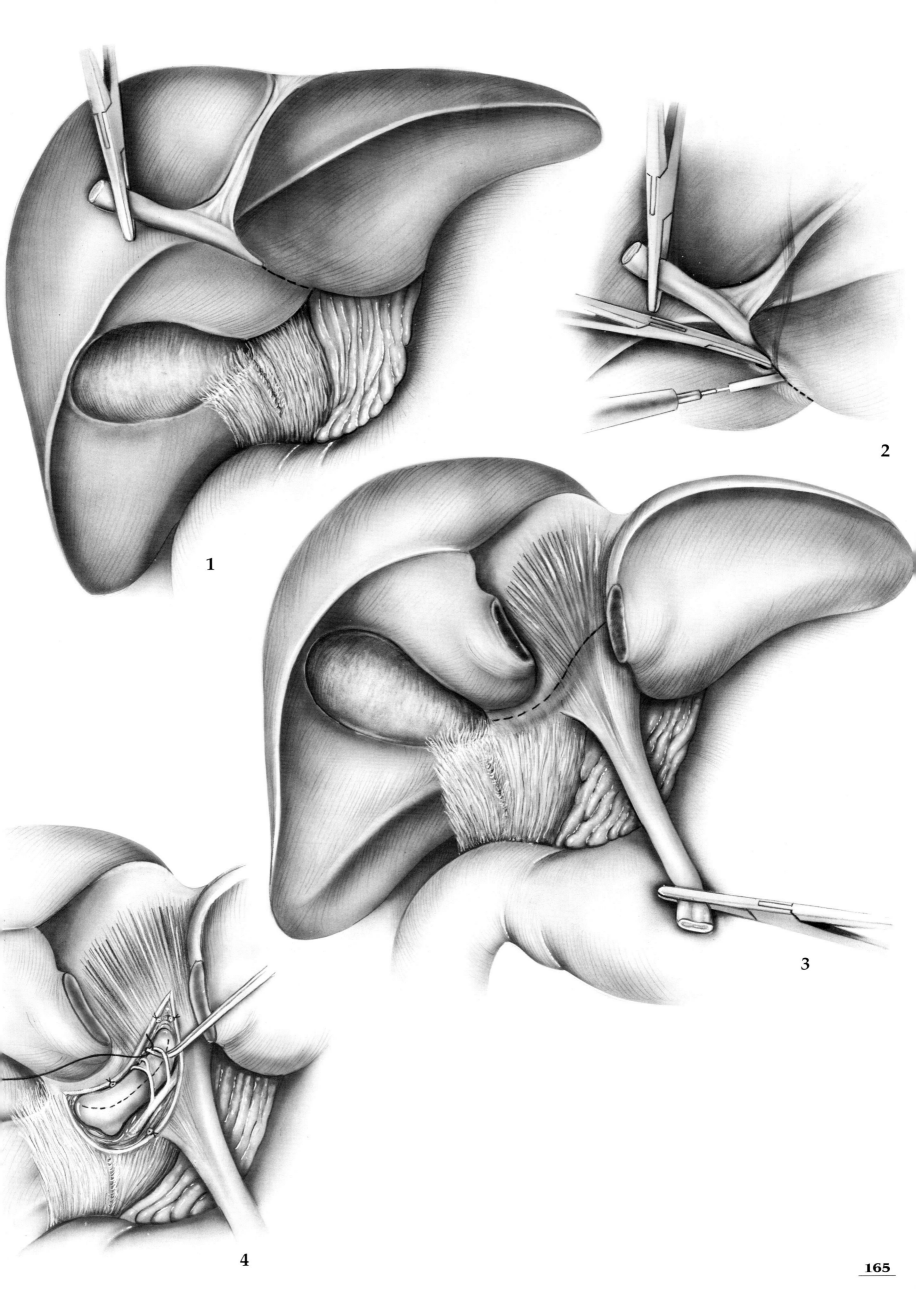

1

2

3

4

Hepaticojejunostomy (Sutured)

1 A Roux-en-Y loop (see **Plates 47–50**) is brought up for a side-to-side anastomosis between the left hepatic duct and the jejunum. The end of the jejunal limb is stapled closed. A choledochotomy and an enterotomy are made. A full-thickness posterior row of #000 polyglycolic acid sutures is placed by serially bisecting the space between previously placed sutures. A suture holder is helpful in avoiding entanglement of the untied sutures. The posterior row sutures are tied with the knots within the lumen of the anastomosis.

2 The anterior row is fashioned in a similar manner; however, the knots are tied on the outside of the anastomosis. The closure should be bile-tight.

3 The jejunum on either side of the anastomosis is sutured to the tissue around the anastomosis, to reduce the tension on the suture line created by the weight of the Roux-en-Y loop. The area is drained with closed suction catheters.

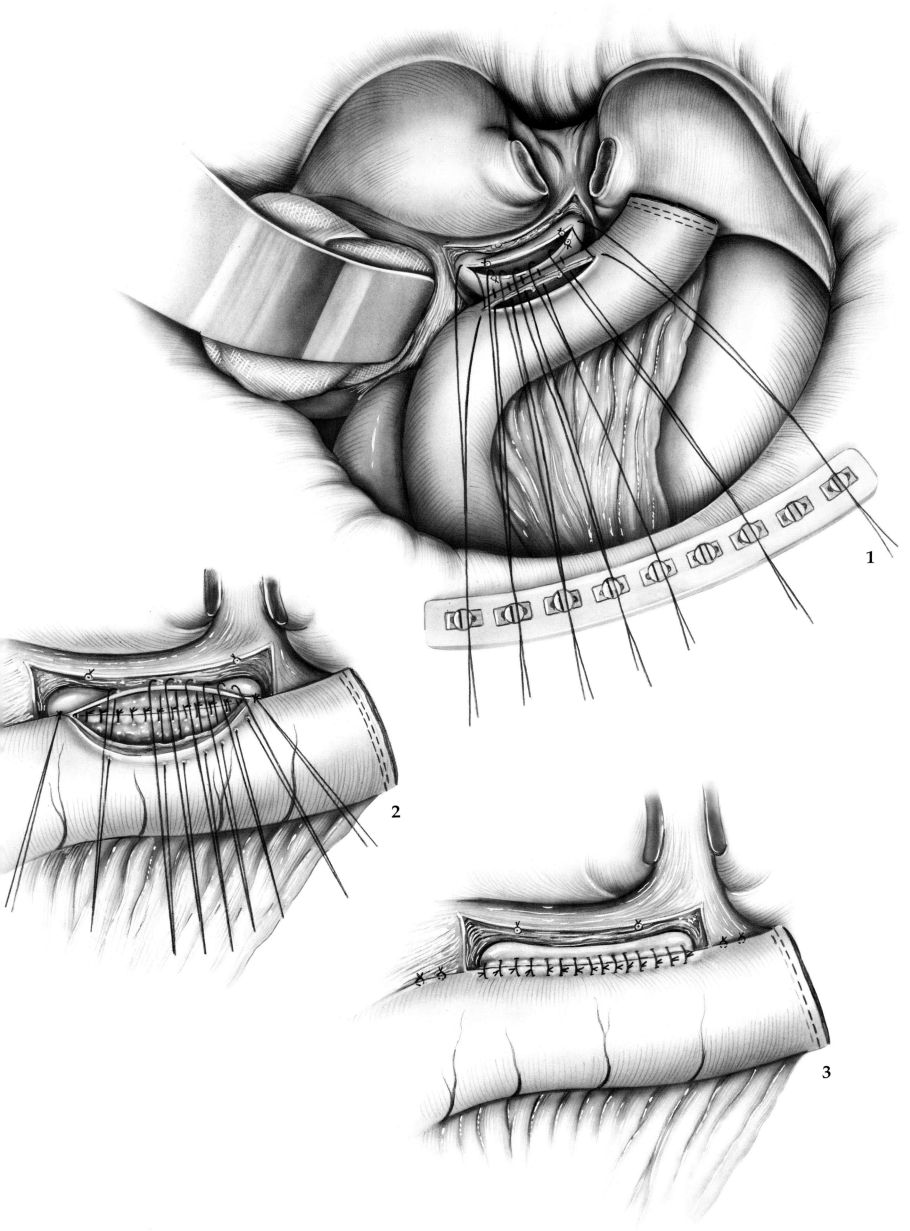

1

2

3

Hepaticojejunostomy (Mucosal Technique–Rodney Smith Procedure)

1 The abdomen is explored through a bilateral subcostal, or "hockey stick," incision. The hepatic plate is lowered as described in **Plate 82**. The falciform ligament is retracted caudally. By palpating the right and left hepatic ducts, after dropping the hepatic plate, one can better assess the most proximal extent of the tumor.

2 The hepatoduodenal ligament is incised immediately above the duodenum. The common bile duct is dissected circumferentially and a small Penrose drain is used to encircle the duct. Traction on the Penrose drain facilitates the dissection as it proceeds toward the liver.

3 The gallbladder is dissected from the liver. The cystic artery is ligated and divided with a #000 silk tie. The gallbladder may be left on the specimen or the cystic duct may be divided, thus removing the gallbladder from the operative field. The distal common bile duct, immediately above the duodenum, is divided between clamps. The lower end is suture-ligated with #00 silk. The clamp remaining on the superior cut end of the duct is used as a handle to facilitate the subsequent dissection.

4 Invasion of the portal vein underlying the bile duct tumor is often the limiting factor in this dissection. Therefore, care is taken posteriorly as the duct is separated from the portal vein. This dissection is carried as far into the liver as is necessary to get beyond the tumor in the right and left hepatic ducts. Occasionally, the duct from the medial segment of the left lobe of the liver has to be divided separately from the lateral segmental duct. In these instances, three separate hepatojejunal anastomoses are required. Similarly, the dissection is carried into the right lobe of the liver until uninvolved duct is visualized. Again, a bifurcation of the right duct may be reached. If divided separately, each duct will require an independent mucosal graft.

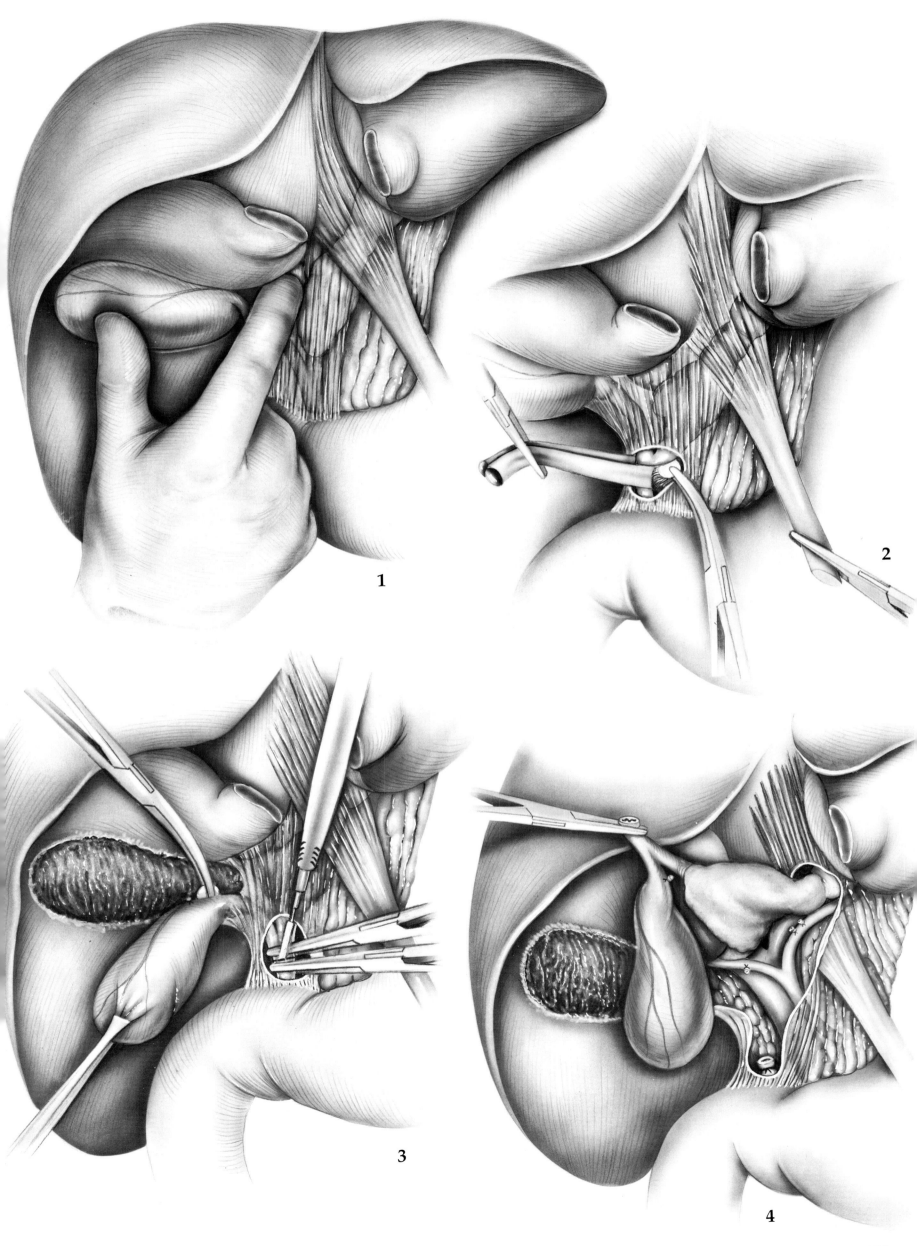

Hepaticojejunostomy (Mucosal Technique– Rodney Smith Procedure) (*cont.*)

5–6 Polyethylene intravenous tubing is used to anchor the mucosal grafts. Because this tubing is generally packaged with only the luminal surfaces sterilized, it must be gas-sterilized prior to surgery. A 3-mm Bakes dilator is passed into the right hepatic duct. A long curved clamp is applied near the handle of the Bakes dilator. This serves as an extension for the dilator, preventing it from being lost in the intrahepatic ductal system. When the Bakes dilator reaches the periphery of the ductal system, it is palpated under the liver capsule. Using electrocautery, the capsule and liver parenchyma are cauterized directly over the dilator tip. This provides hemostasis and improves the seal of the capsule and parenchyma around the tubing. After exiting the liver capsule, the dilator is bent and the sterile intravenous tubing is placed over its tip. The "olive" at the tip of the dilator will securely hold the tubing as it is withdrawn into the substance of the liver and the ductal system. The tubing is retrieved from the open end of the hepatic duct in the porta hepatis. Several small side holes are cut in the tubing for a distance of 20 cm. The left ductal system is cannulated in a similar fashion.

7 A Roux-en-Y loop of jejunum is prepared as previously described (see **Plates 47–50, Figs. 12–18**) and brought through the transverse mesocolon. A separate mucosal nipple is prepared for each duct orifice. Most often, only two nipples are required for the left and right hepatic ducts. The serosa and muscular layers of the jejunum are cauterized down to the submucosa. The distance between mucosal nipples is determined by the distance separating the cut ends of the hepatic ducts.

8 The submucosa and mucosa pout from the nipple site as pressure is applied immediately below the cauterized serosa and muscularis. A #000 polyglycolic acid purse-string suture is placed around the base of the pouting mucosa.

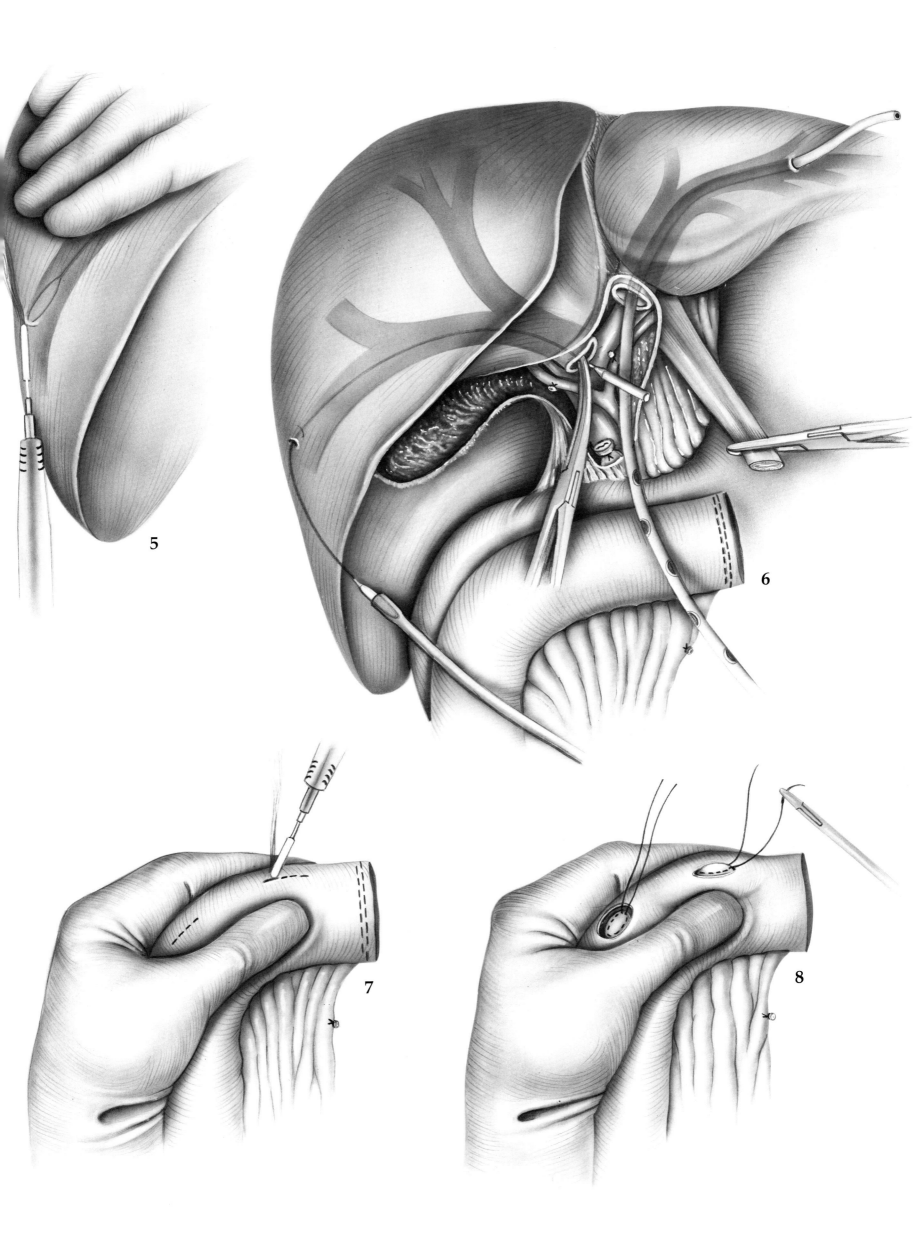

5

6

7

8

Hepaticojejunostomy (Mucosal Technique–Rodney Smith Procedure) (*cont.*)

9 A tiny enterotomy is made in the center of each purse-string and the intravenous tubing is inserted into the jejunal limb. Only 4 to 5 cm of tubing with side holes is allowed to protrude from the jejunal limb, so as to avoid pulling a side hole outside the liver as the mucosal grafts are drawn into the hepatic ducts. A second tie is placed on the pouting mucosa, fixing it more securely to the intravenous tubing.

10 With very gentle traction of the intravenous tubing, two #000 polyglycolic acid stitches are placed through the jejunal wall and through the wall of each intravenous tube in the Roux-en-Y limb. These sutures prevent the tubing from sliding out of the mucosal nipple as traction is applied to the tubing to draw the nipple into the hepatic ducts.

11 Traction is applied to the tubing as it exits the liver capsule, advancing the nipples into the hepatic ducts. The mucosal nipples enter the ducts and the jejunal serosa comes to rest against the cut ends of the ducts. The tubing exiting the liver capsule is brought out through the skin as directly as possible, in an attempt to seal the liver against the abdominal wall. The tubing is secured to the skin with #00 silk stitches. Surgical tape is wrapped around the tubing, forming a roll that further prevents the tubing from retracting into the skin. Both of these maneuvers hold the tubing in place, maintaining the traction on the mucosal nipples within the hepatic ducts.

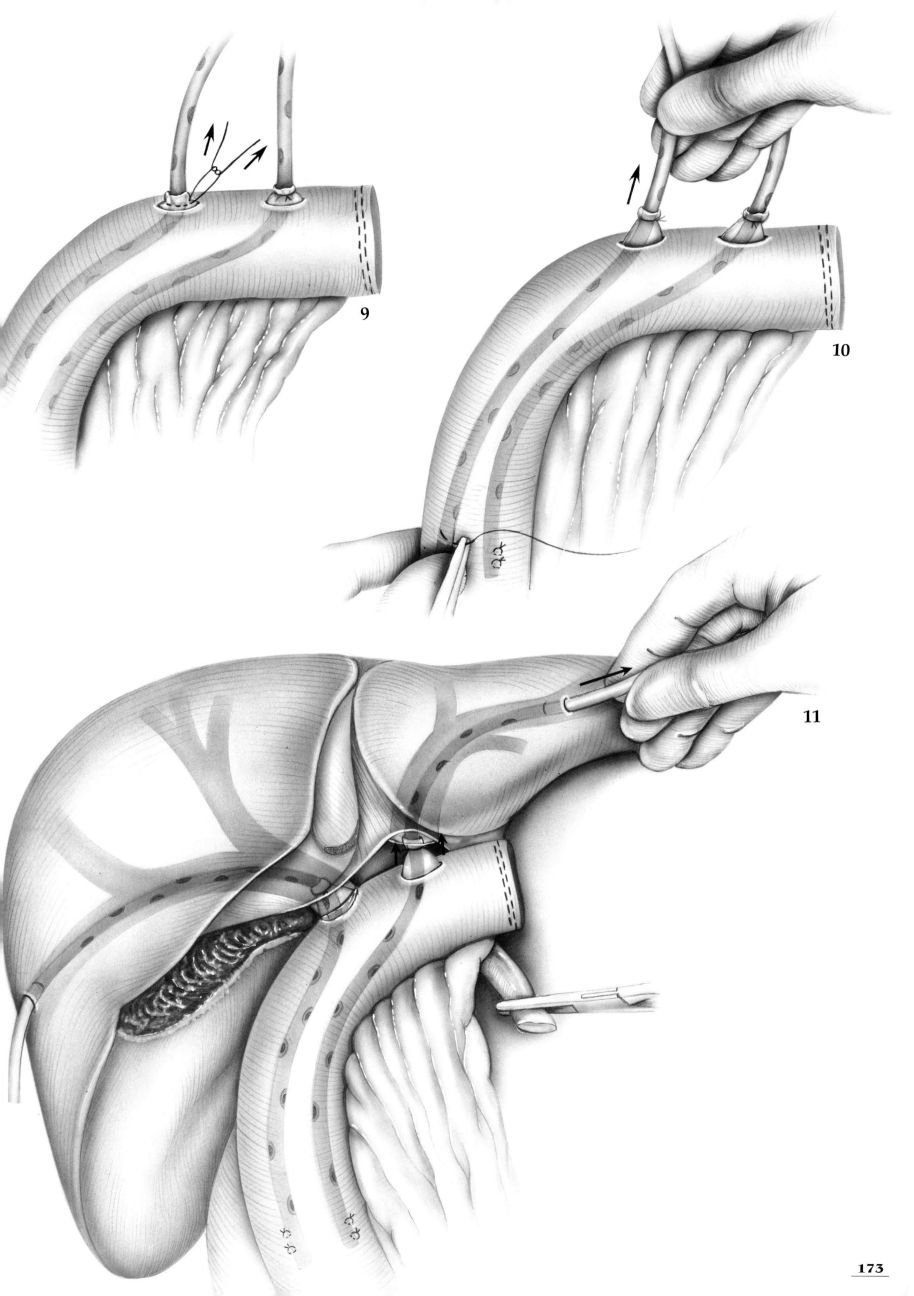

9

10

11

Hepaticojejunostomy (Mucosal Technique– Rodney Smith Procedure) (*cont.*)

12 The jejunal loop is suspended from the areolar tissue within the porta hepatis with interrupted simple #000 silk sutures. A closed suction drain is placed near the site where each tube exits the liver capsule. Two drains are placed behind the Roux-en-Y limb in the porta hepatis. These drains are removed when no further bile drainage is noted.

13 The usual exit sites of the tubing through the skin are shown. While transhepatic percutaneous biliary drainage catheters, placed prior to surgery, are most helpful during the dissection of the tumor and of the proximal hepatic ducts within the liver, it is our experience that they rarely follow the course desired for traction on the mucosal nipples. Therefore, we commonly use the percutaneous catheters to guide the dissection but remove them prior to the reconstruction. The tubes holding the mucosal nipples are removed at 6 to 8 weeks; however, no problems have been encountered when the catheters have spontaneously extruded at 4 weeks.

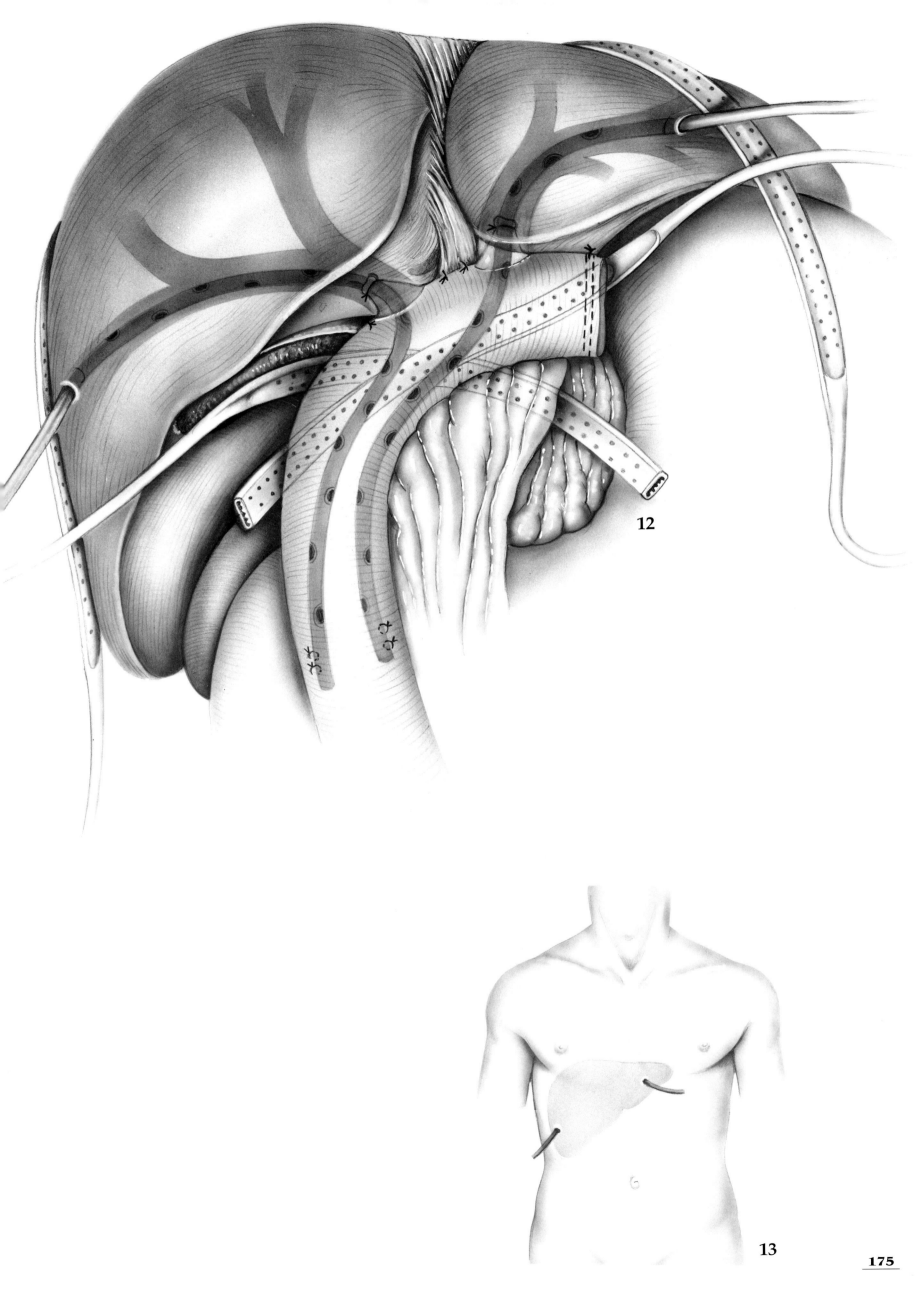

12

13

Right Hepatic Lobectomy

1 The abdomen is explored through a subcostal chevron incision extending obliquely from the right anterior axillary line to a point midway between the xiphoid and umbilicus, and then across the left rectus muscle.

2 The diaphragmatic surface of the liver is mobilized by dividing the falciform, round, and triangular ligaments.

3 The right lobe is rotated medially and the lateral attachments are cut, exposing the vena cava.

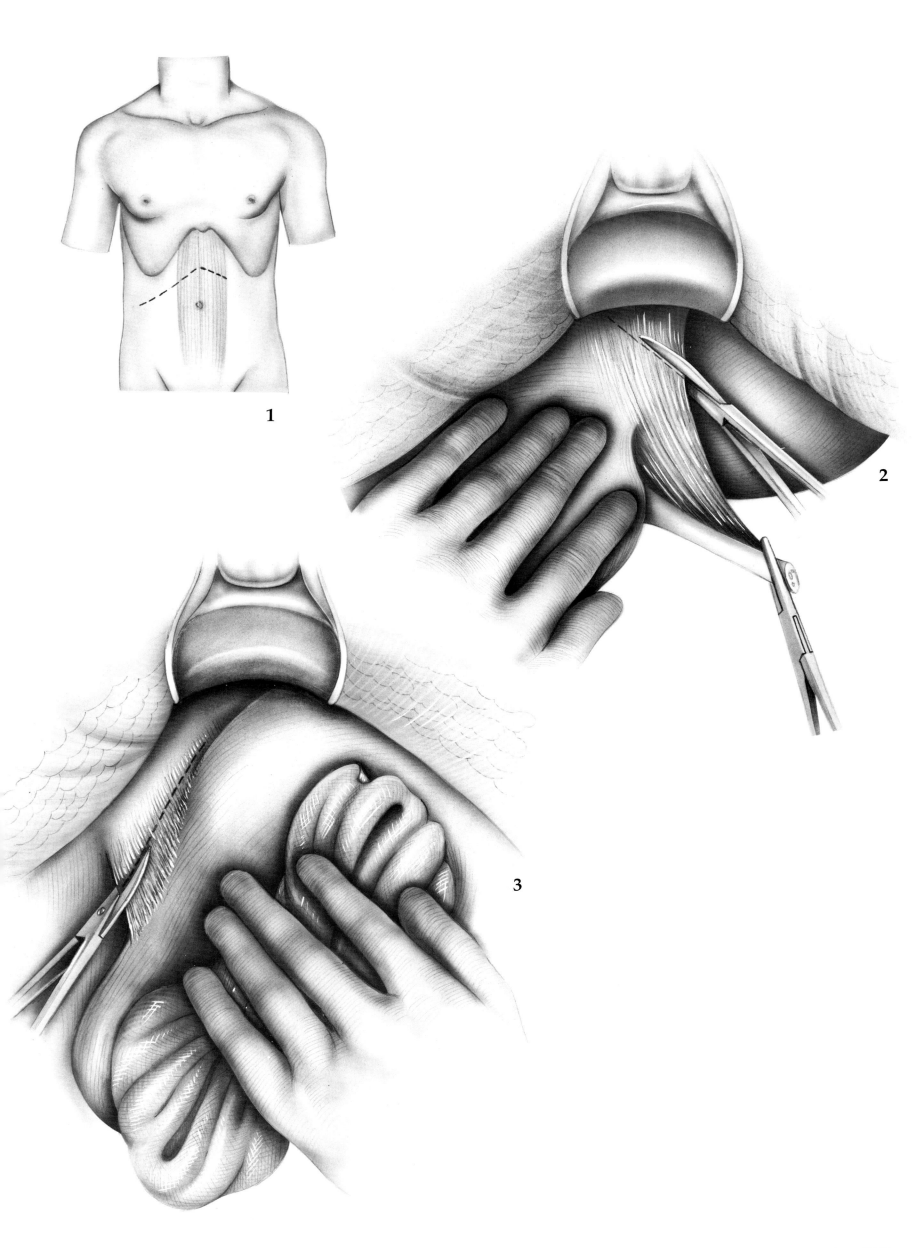

1

2

3

Right Hepatic Lobectomy (*cont.*)

4 The gallbladder is removed as previously described (see **Plates 73–75, Figs. 2–11** and **Plate 76, Figs. 1–3**).

5 The right hepatic artery and right hepatic bile duct are divided between clamps and tied.

6 The right portal vein is dissected, encircled with a #0 silk tie to separate it from other tissue, divided between clamps, tied with #000 silk, and then suture-ligated with a #000 silk stitch.

7 The technique for division and suture ligation of the portal vein is depicted.

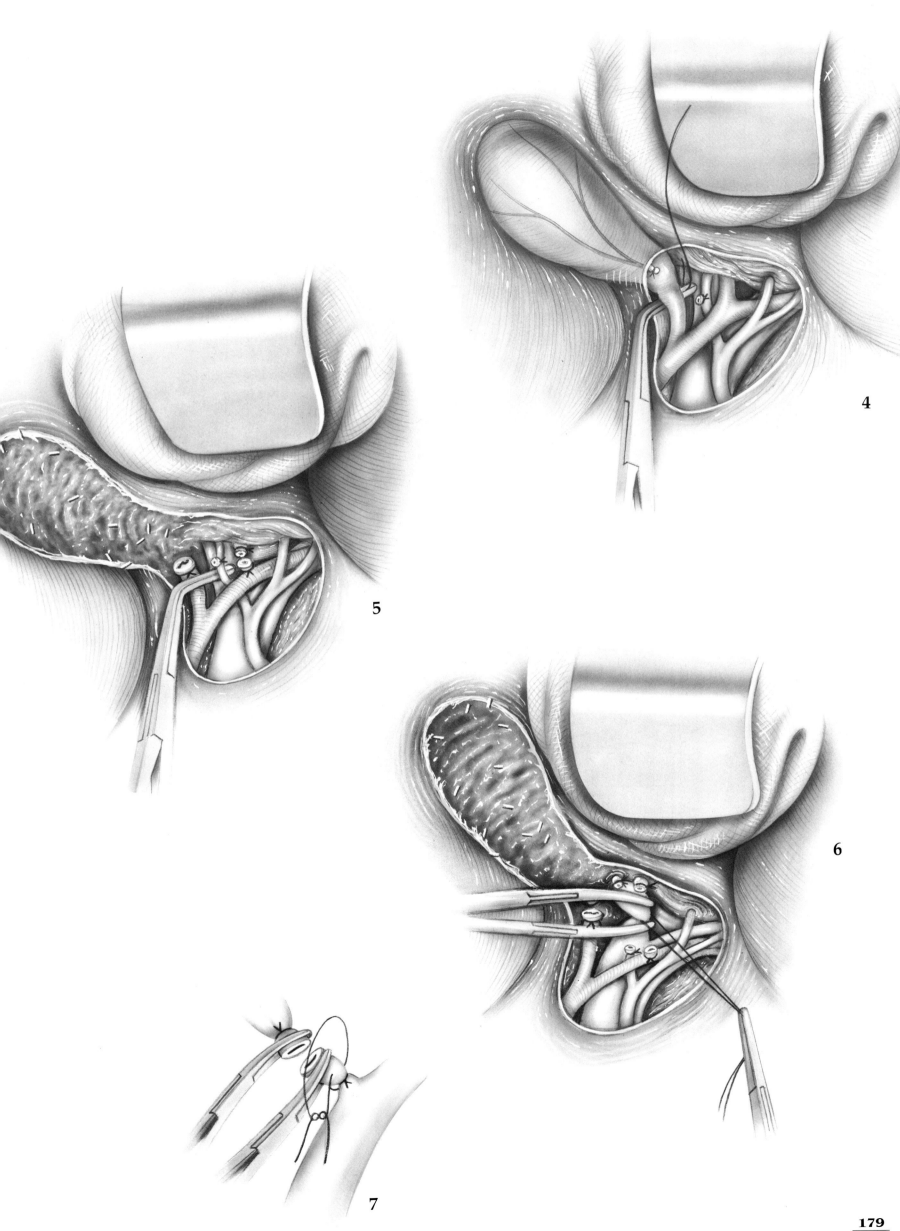

Right Hepatic Lobectomy (*cont.*)

8 Once the right lobe is devascularized, a line of demarcation becomes readily apparent. The capsule and most superficial portion of the liver parenchyma are scored with electrocautery along the demarcation.

9 The parenchyma is divided either with the "finger crushing" technique or with the back of a long scalpel handle (shown). Either technique allows one to identify small vessels and ducts within the liver parenchyma without disrupting them. Additionally, one can reduce the mass of liver tissue remaining on these vessels and ducts by aspirating over them with a strong suction.

10 Ordinarily we ligate the vessels and ducts on the side of the cleft to remain in the patient, while surgical clips are applied to the specimen side of the vessels.

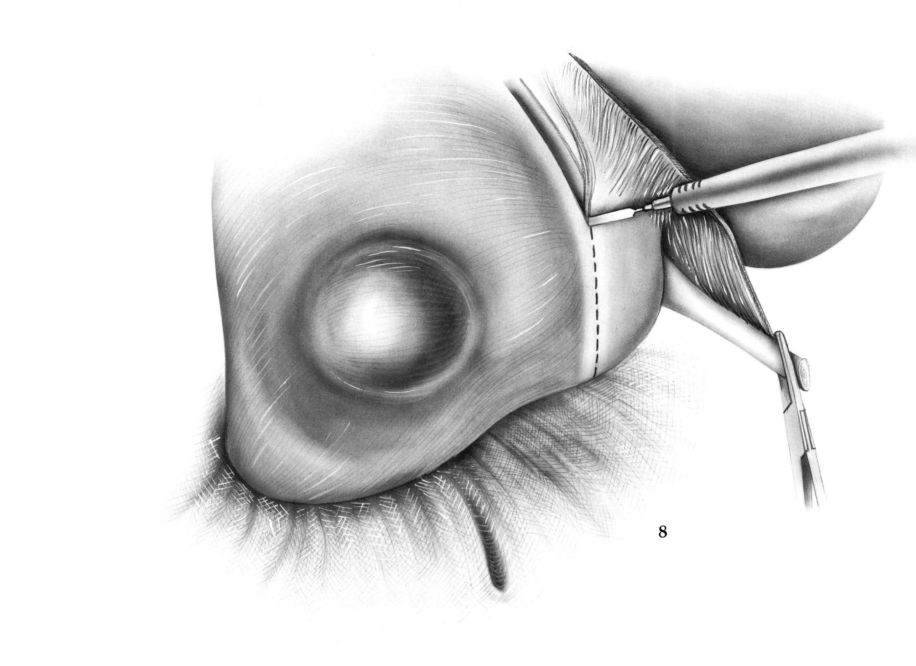

8

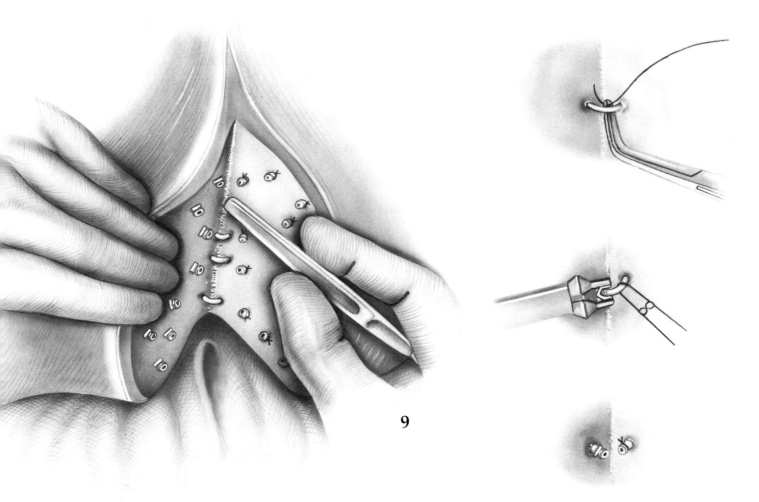

9

10

Right Hepatic Lobectomy (*cont.*)

11 While some surgeons advocate taking the major right hepatic veins via the lateral extrahepatic approach, we have found it more convenient to continue the dissection, intraparenchymally, to the hepatic vein. By dissecting the hepatic vein through the parenchyma more length can be obtained, allowing it to be tied in continuity, divided between clamps, and then suture-ligated.

12 The smaller hepatic veins draining the liver directly into the vena cava are ligated as the anterior and lateral surfaces of the vena cava are exposed by the dissection.

13 The divided liver may be examined for bile leak by injecting methylene blue through a catheter placed in the cystic duct, while the distal common bile duct is occluded manually. The methylene blue exits the liver through untied bile ducts. The cut edge is drained with a sump catheter and closed suction drains. The sump drain is removed as soon as it is apparent that postoperative bleeding is not a problem. The closed suction drains remain until no further bile is aspirated.

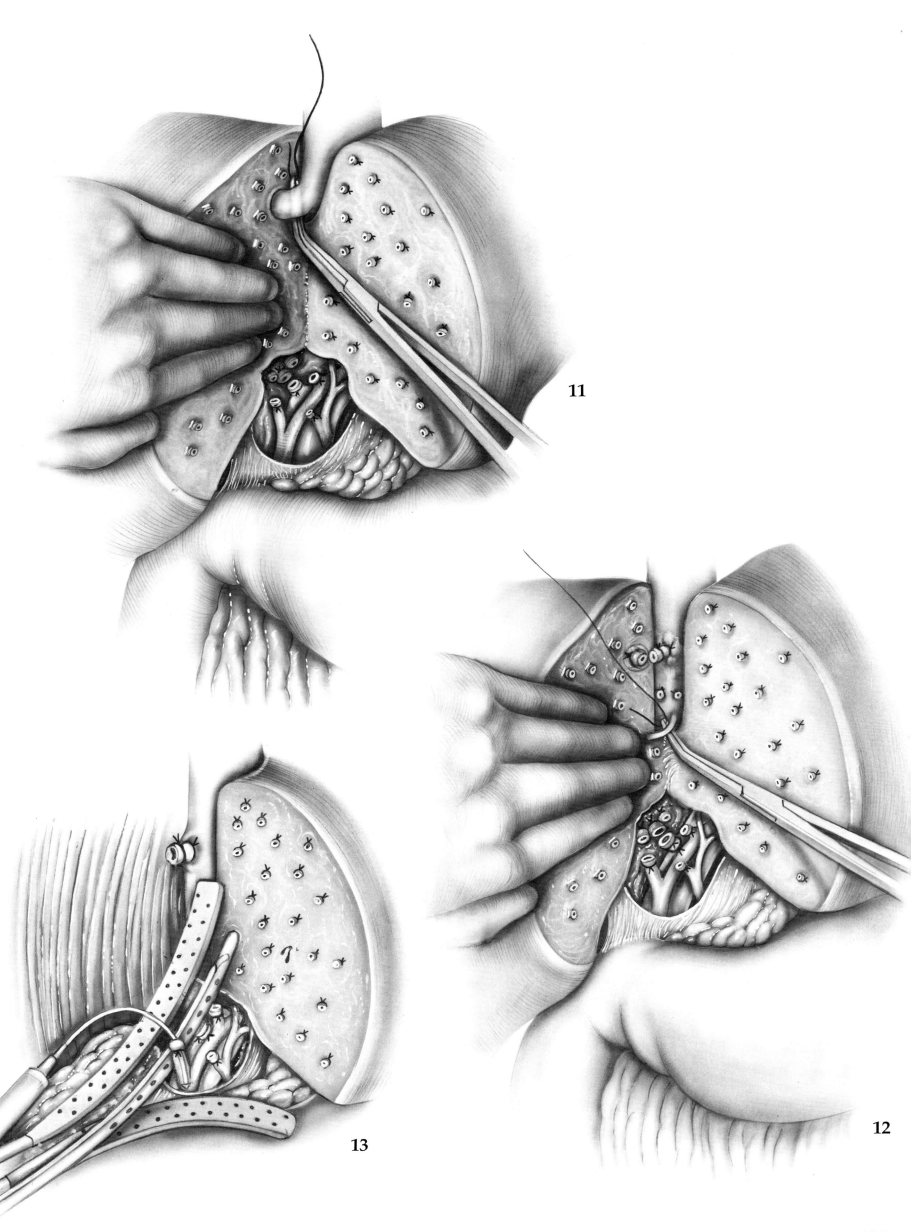

11

12

13

Left Hepatic Lobectomy

1 The abdomen is explored through a long midline incision.

2 The falciform ligament is divided along the dome of the liver.

3 The left triangular ligament is transected. As the dissection proceeds to the right, the anterior layers of the coronary ligaments are divided.

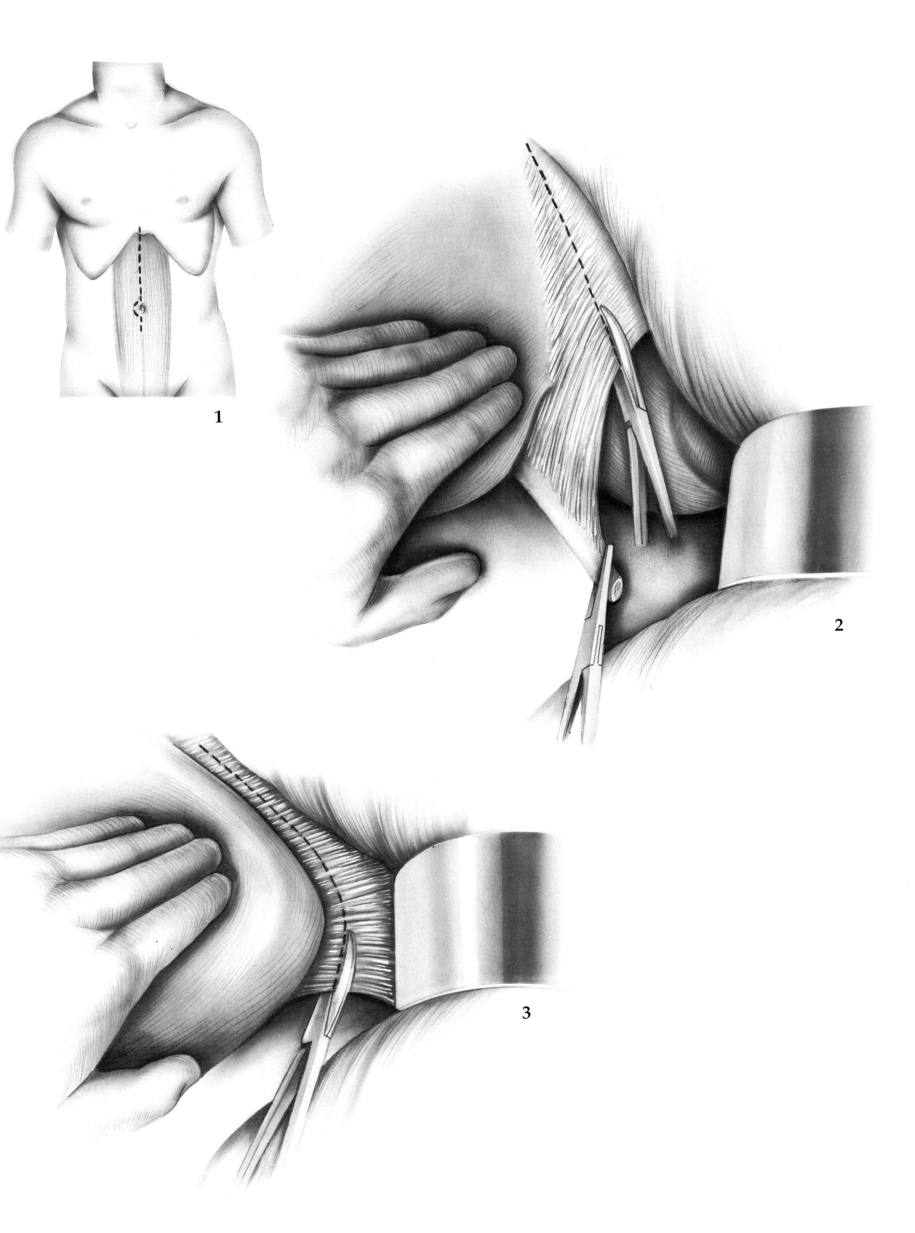

1

2

3

Left Hepatic Lobectomy (*cont.*)

4 Although it is not necessary routinely to remove the gallbladder, its removal does provide better exposure of the hilus of the liver. A long cystic-duct remnant is left so that it can be subsequently cannulated when evaluating the cut edge of the liver for residual bile leaks.

5 The hepatic artery is ligated with #000 silk ties and divided.

6 The left hepatic duct is ligated and divided.

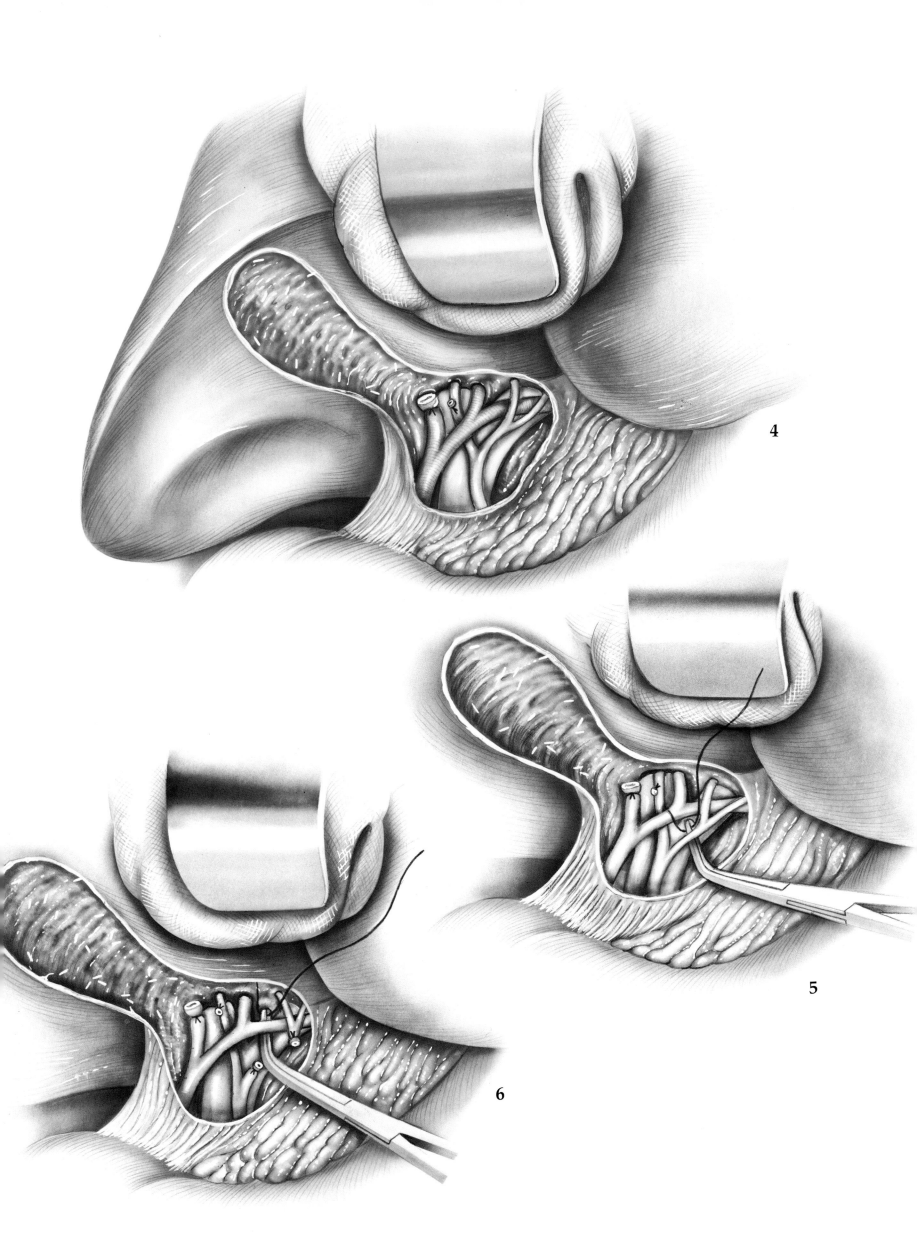

4

5

6

Left Hepatic Lobectomy (*cont.*)

7 A #00 silk tie is passed around the portal vein to separate and distract it from adjacent structures. The left portal vein is divided between clamps, tied, and then suture-ligated with a #000 silk stitch.

8 The technique for the suture ligation of the left portal vein is shown.

9 Electrocautery is used to incise Glisson's capsule and the most superficial layers of the liver parenchyma to the left of the line of demarcation caused by the devascularization of the left lobe. This demarcation always occurs well to the liver-hilus side of the falciform ligament.

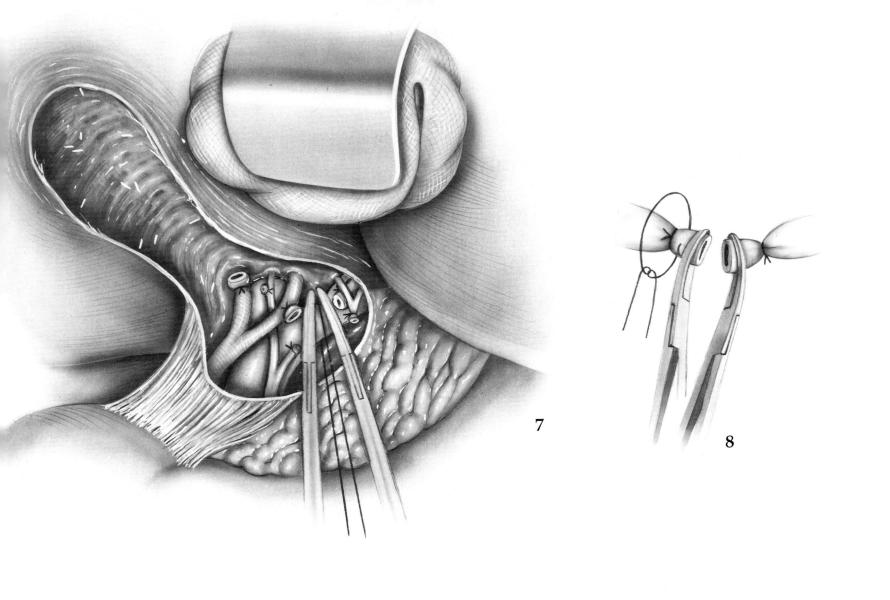

7

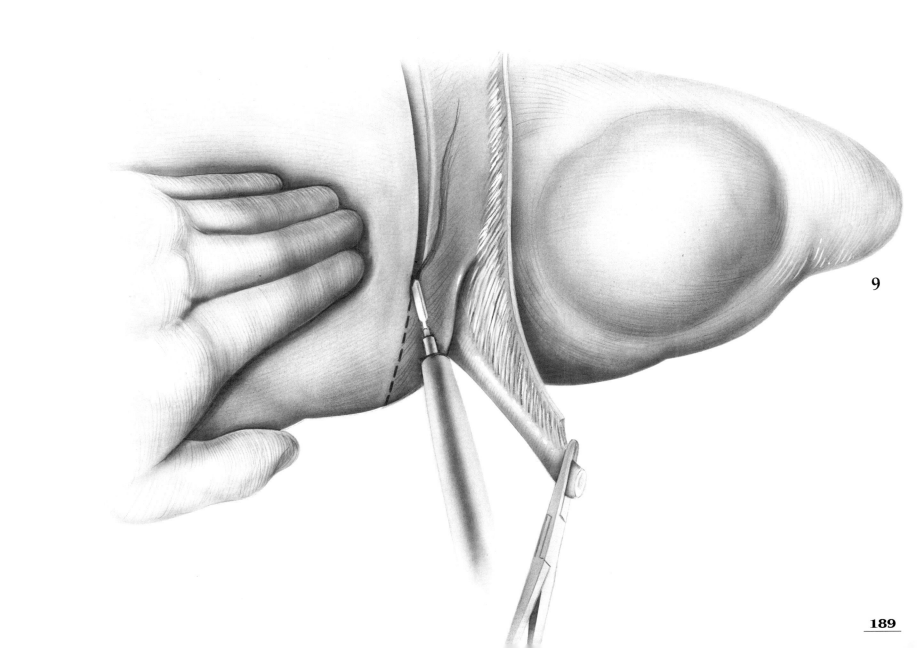

8

9

Left Hepatic Lobectomy (*cont.*)

10 Using either the "finger crushing" technique or the blunt end of a long scalpel, the liver parenchyma is divided toward the vena cava.

11 The left hepatic vein is tied in continuity within the liver parenchyma, divided between clamps, and suture-ligated with #00 silk.

12 To check for bile ducts that were not ligated during the transection of the liver, a catheter is placed into the long cystic duct and methylene blue is injected while the distal common bile duct is occluded manually. Methylene blue will leak through untied bile ducts, which are identified and ligated. The cut edge of the liver is drained with closed suction catheters and a sump catheter. The sump is removed as soon as it is determined that there is no significant postoperative bleeding, and the closed suction drain is removed when it is apparent that there is no continuing bile leak.

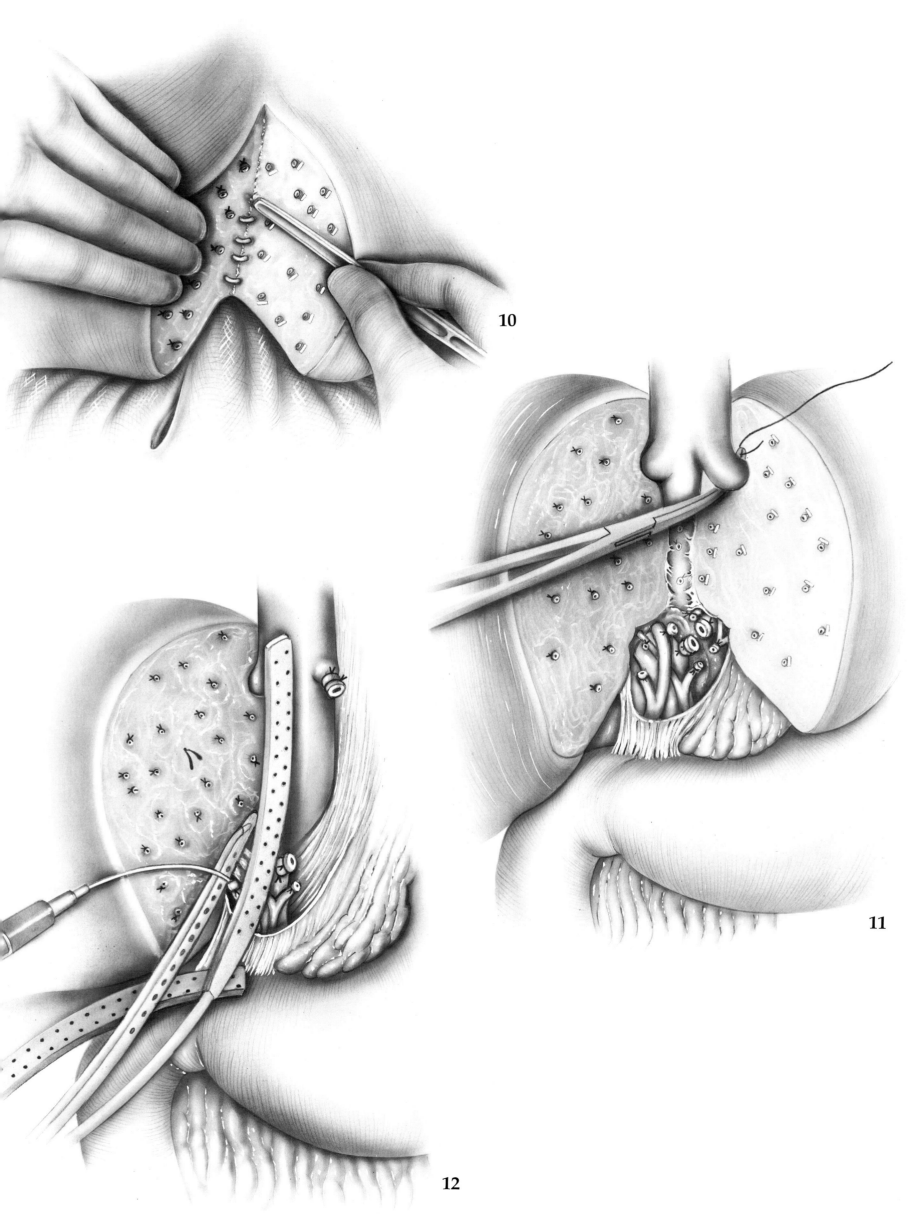

10

11

12

Drainage of Liver Abscess—Wedge Liver Biopsy

1 Depending on the location of the abscess, the abdomen is explored through either a right subcostal or an upper midline incision. It is often necessary to divide the falciform ligament to mobilize the liver. The seal between the liver and diaphragm is broken by passing the hand over the dome of the liver. A needle attached to a syringe is introduced into the presenting abscess wall, or through the hepatic parenchyma, into the abscess cavity. Deep-seated abscesses can be localized with intraoperative ultrasound. A specimen is obtained for a Gram stain and cultures.

2 The liver parenchyma overlying the abscess cavity, or the abscess wall itself, is incised with electrocautery. The abscess wall can be tented up with the aid of a bend at the end of the needle, as depicted.

3 A suction catheter is introduced through this defect into the abscess cavity and the purulent material is emptied. The suction is advanced into any satellite, or daughter, abscess. The surgeon must be certain that these satellite abscesses communicate adequately with the primary abscess cavity, thus allowing single drainage of all collections. If another abscess close to the primary abscess does not empty, it must be drained separately.

4 A portion of the abscess wall is excised for pathological examination.

5 A #20 French Pezzer catheter is prepared by removing its distal half and making several radial cuts on its surface. The Pezzer catheter is placed through the defect in the abscess wall and the cavity is irrigated. The primary and communicating abscesses should fill and collapse during the irrigation. The Pezzer catheter is brought out to the skin, secured with a heavy silk suture, and placed on low continuous suction using a closed chest suction apparatus.

WEDGE LIVER BIOPSY

6 The area on the edge of the liver to be sampled is identified and a #00 silk suture is placed through the liver at this site, approximately 2 to 4 mm from its edge. Hemostasis will be achieved in the area outlined by the broken lines with two #00 polyglycolic acid sutures placed at its margins. This allows a wedge of liver to be removed within the hemostatic sutures.

7 The stitch is passed, via the undersurface of the liver, through the apex of the wedge, and is brought out through the liver. It is then brought over the liver edge to the undersurface and passed through the liver again. The second loop of the suture is placed approximately halfway from the edge to the apex of the first bite. In addition, the second loop is placed closer to the area to be excised, preventing the longer loop from slipping off the cut edge of the liver once the wedge has been removed. The suture is tied snugly against the liver edge, causing the included tissue to blanch and indent slightly.

8 A second suture is placed to complete the wedge. Again, it is important that the second throw of the suture be within the first.

9 The wedge of liver is excised sharply about 2 mm from the hemostatic sutures, using the previously placed silk suture as a handle to manipulate, and finally remove, the specimen.

10 The ends of the hemostatic sutures may be tied together.

11 If this is done, a closed liver wound results. However, if the liver is soft, it is generally better to leave the defect open than to risk cracking the liver as these sutures are tied.

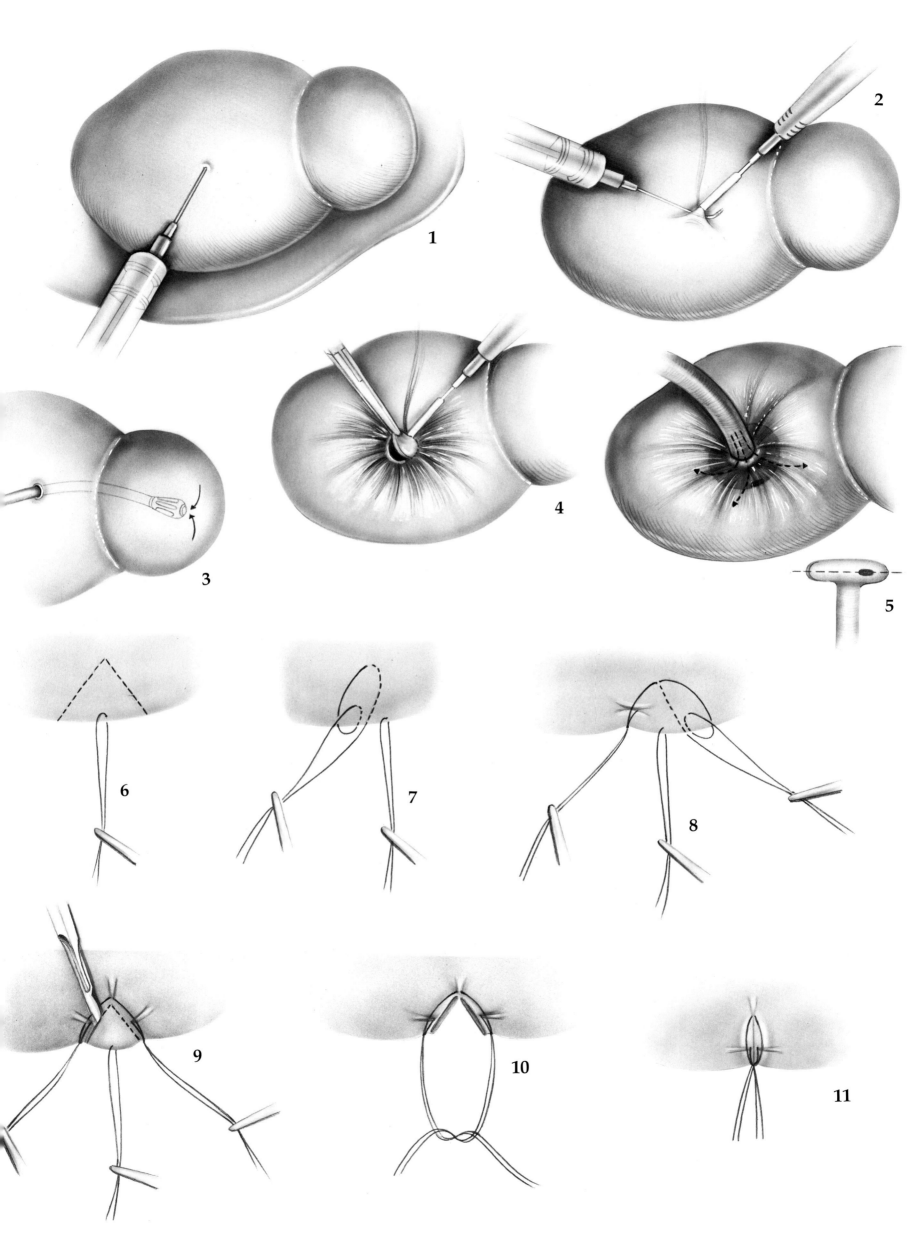

Splenectomy

Normal-Sized Spleen

1 A left subcostal incision is used for the removal of a normal-sized (or slightly enlarged) spleen.

2 The gastrosplenic ligament, containing the gastroepiploic and short gastric vessels, is divided between clamps and tied with #00 silk ligatures as shown.

3 The spleen is retracted medially and the lateral attachments are incised.

4 Once the spleen is mobilized anteriorly from the stomach and posteriorly from the retroperitoneum, it is turned anteriorly and brought up into the wound. The splenic hilar vessels, the tail of the pancreas, and accessory spleens are clearly visualized. The splenic artery is divided between clamps, tied with #00 silk, and then suture-ligated. The veins are taken subsequently, avoiding injury to the pancreas during the placement of the clamps. The veins are suture-ligated and the remaining splenic attachments divided. The spleen is then removed. The splenic bed is examined for residual bleeding. If hemostasis is complete, the wound is closed without drainage of the splenic fossa.

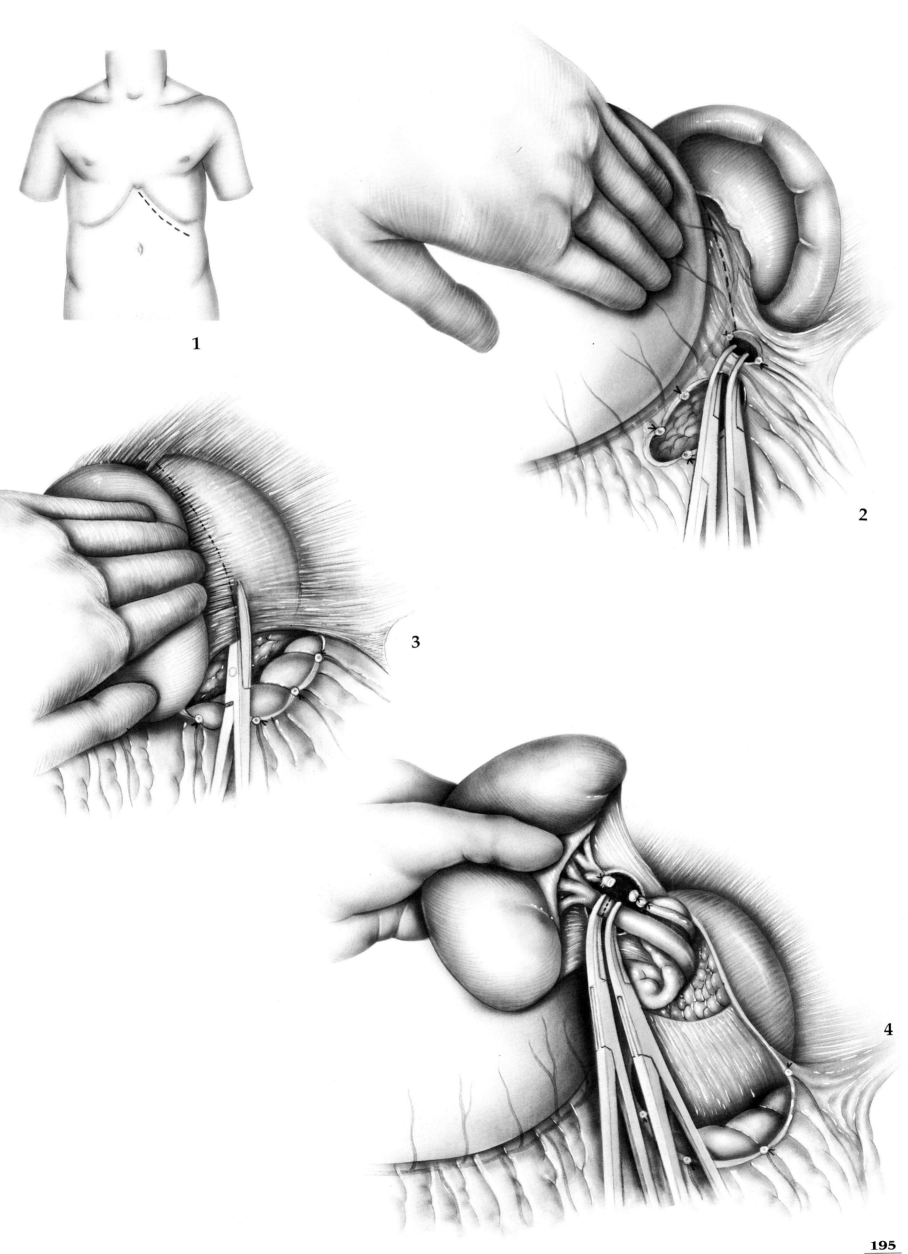

Splenectomy (*cont.*)

Enlarged Spleen

5 If the spleen is massively enlarged and extends below the costal margin, a midline incision is chosen.

6 The gastrosplenic ligament, containing the gastroepiploic and short gastric vessels, is divided—either between clamps, with ligature, or with a stapling device that applies hemostatic clips as it divides the tissue.

7 Entry is gained to the lesser sac by retracting the stomach medially. The splenic artery is palpated at the superior margin of the pancreas. It is then dissected circumferentially for a short distance near the junction of the tail and body of the pancreas, encircled with a #0 silk tie, and ligated in continuity. Early arterial ligation allows the spleen to drain partially and minimizes arterial bleeding should there be a misadventure during the dissection of the splenic hilus.

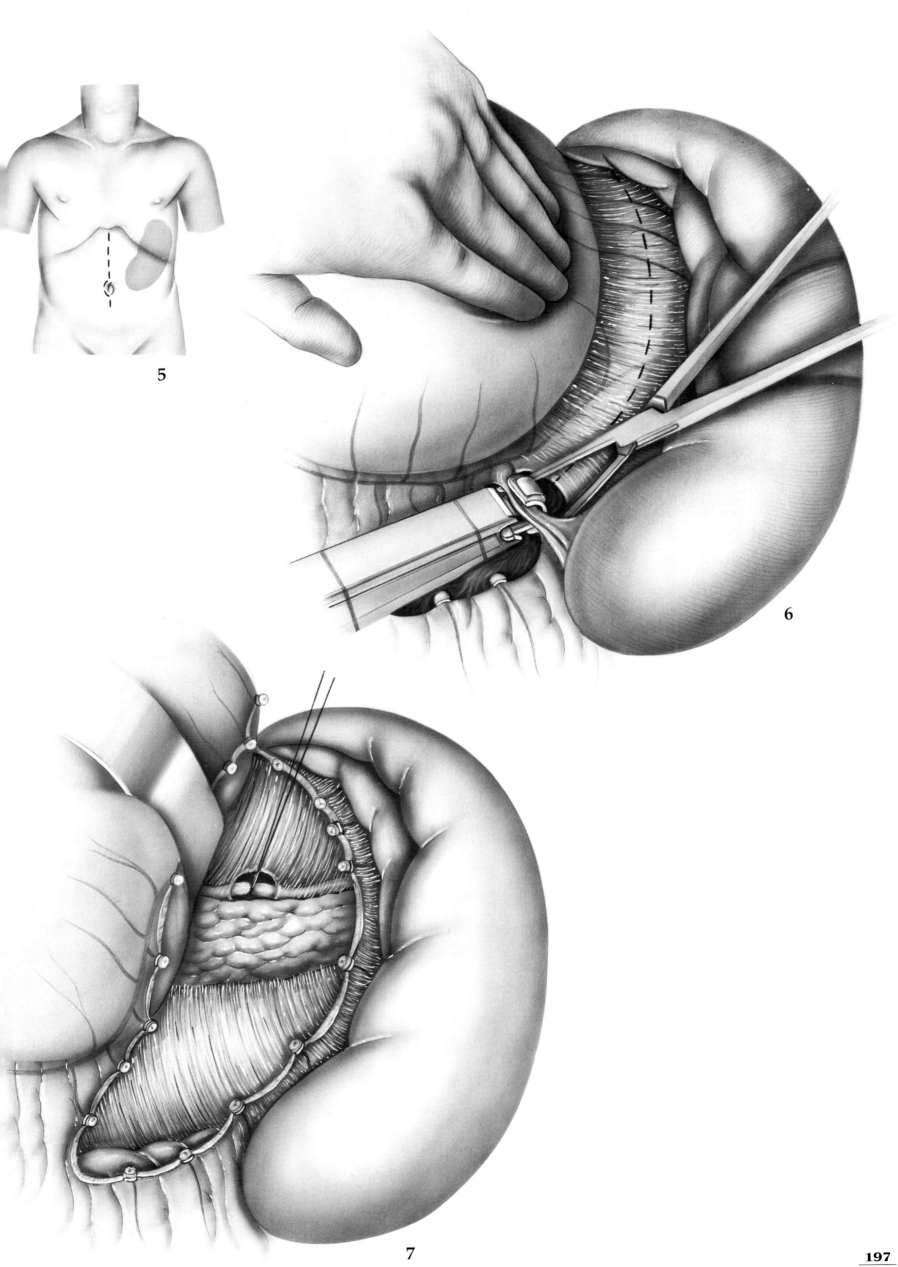

5

6

7

Splenectomy (*cont.*)

Enlarged Spleen (*cont.*)

8 The spleen is rotated medially and the lateral and superior attachments are incised.

9 With the spleen rotated medially, the splenic artery and vein are divided between clamps and doubly ligated. The residual investments of the spleen are divided and the spleen is removed. The splenic bed is examined for bleeding, which, if present, is controlled with cautery. Depending on the moistness of the splenic bed and the pancreatic manipulation, a decision to drain the area is made.

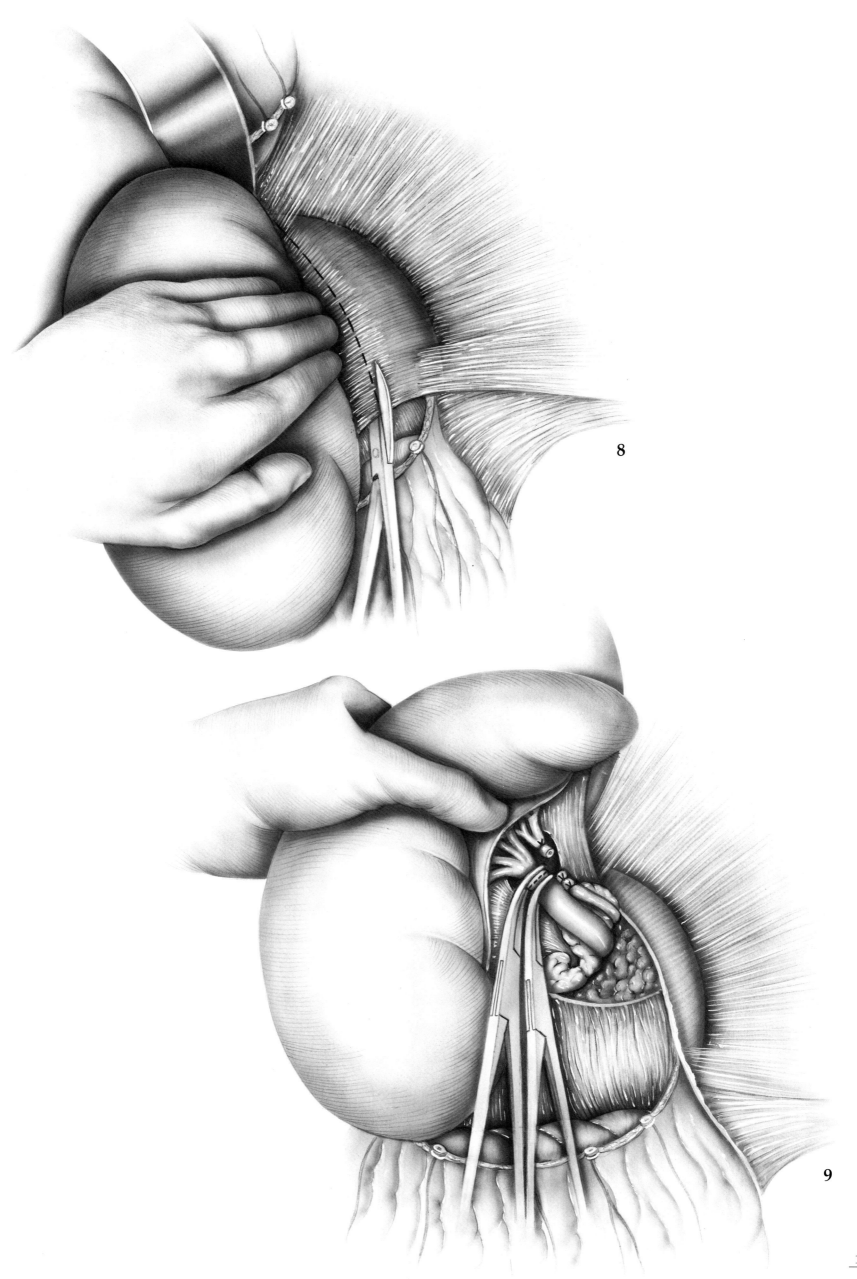

8

9

Splenectomy (*cont.*)

Shattered Spleen

10 In the situation of a shattered spleen (most commonly resulting from blunt abdominal trauma) it is essential to remove the spleen quickly. The spleen is first rotated medially, and the lateral and superior attachments are incised.

11 The splenic artery and vein are identified, divided between clamps, and doubly ligated with #0 silk ties. The gastrosplenic ligament is also divided from the posterior approach. Due to extravasation of blood into the adjacent tissues, the nearby pancreatic border is difficult to identify clearly. Further, the manipulation of the spleen prior to division of the gastrosplenic ligament may leave the stomach wall close to the hilus of the spleen where it can be injured in the clamping of the splenic vessels. Therefore, injury to the pancreas or stomach must be scrupulously avoided during the removal of the shattered spleen. The decision to drain the splenic bed is made, as described, in **Plate 99**, based on the hemostasis achieved and the apparent or potential damage to the pancreas.

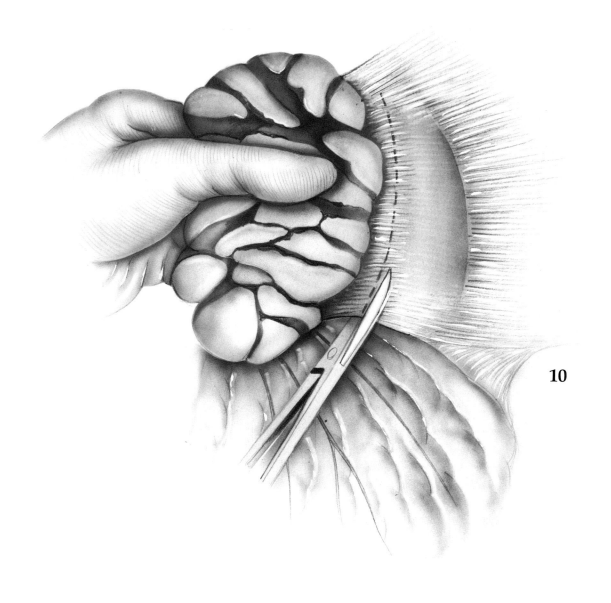

10

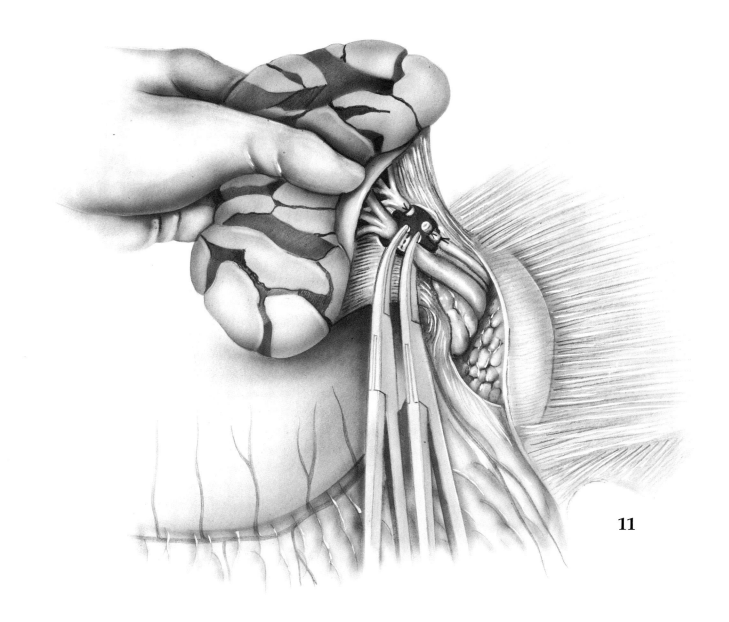

11

Splenorrhaphy

There are numerous maneuvers described for repair of splenic laceration; only two will be depicted here. The mobilization of the spleen and temporary occlusion of the splenic artery allow appropriate appraisal of the injury and careful repair.

1 In the circumstances depicted, there is a longitudinal laceration of the spleen leaving a cleft in the splenic parenchyma. The lateral attachments of the spleen are incised, exposing the vessels at the splenic hilus.

2 The splenic artery is temporarily occluded with a bulldog clamp.

3 A tongue of omentum is placed into the cleft and secured with a row of interrupted #0 polyglycolic acid sutures, thus compressing the spleen about the omental tongue. The arterial clamp is removed and the spleen is examined for residual bleeding.

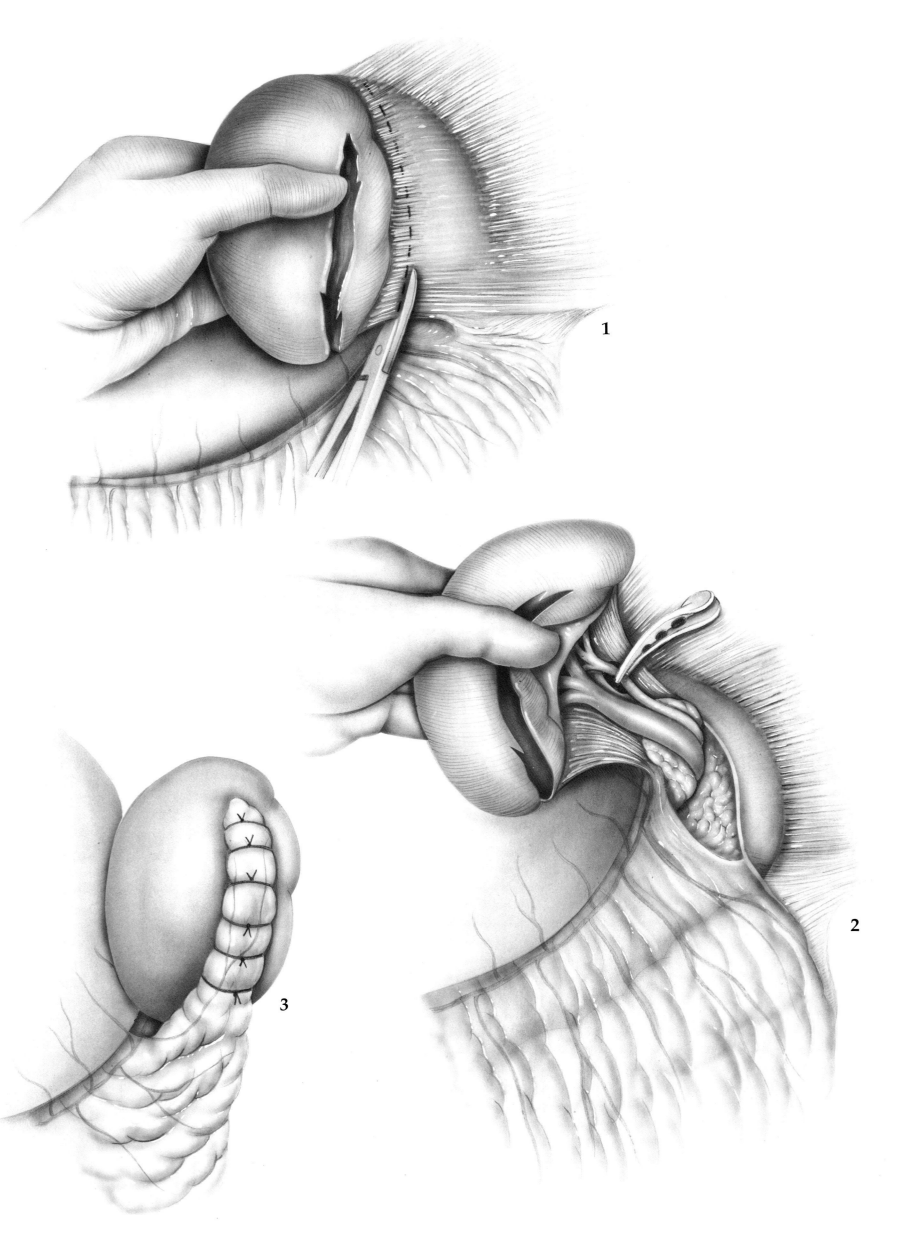

Splenorrhaphy (*cont.*)

4 In the case of a transverse laceration or partial avulsion of the spleen, another technique is applicable. The inferior pole of the spleen, shown here, is partially transected. Entry to the lesser sac is gained through the divided gastrosplenic ligament. The splenic artery is identified at the superior border of the pancreas and temporarily occluded. The segmental vessels to the injured portion of the spleen are taken between clamps and tied. These vessels may be found within the parenchyma of the injured spleen.

5 The splenic transection is completed with electrocautery.

6 The cut edge of the spleen is closed with mattress sutures buttressed with Teflon pledgets, which prevent the sutures from cutting through the splenic parenchyma. These compressive sutures will ordinarily control the bleeding, but additional sutures approximating the oozing portion of the parenchyma between the mattress sutures may be necessary. The spleen must be observed long enough after the release of the splenic artery clamp to make sure that hemostasis has been achieved. When the spleen has been repaired, the wound should be drained with a sump suction catheter. This drain allows the surgeon to monitor the patient for postoperative bleeding.

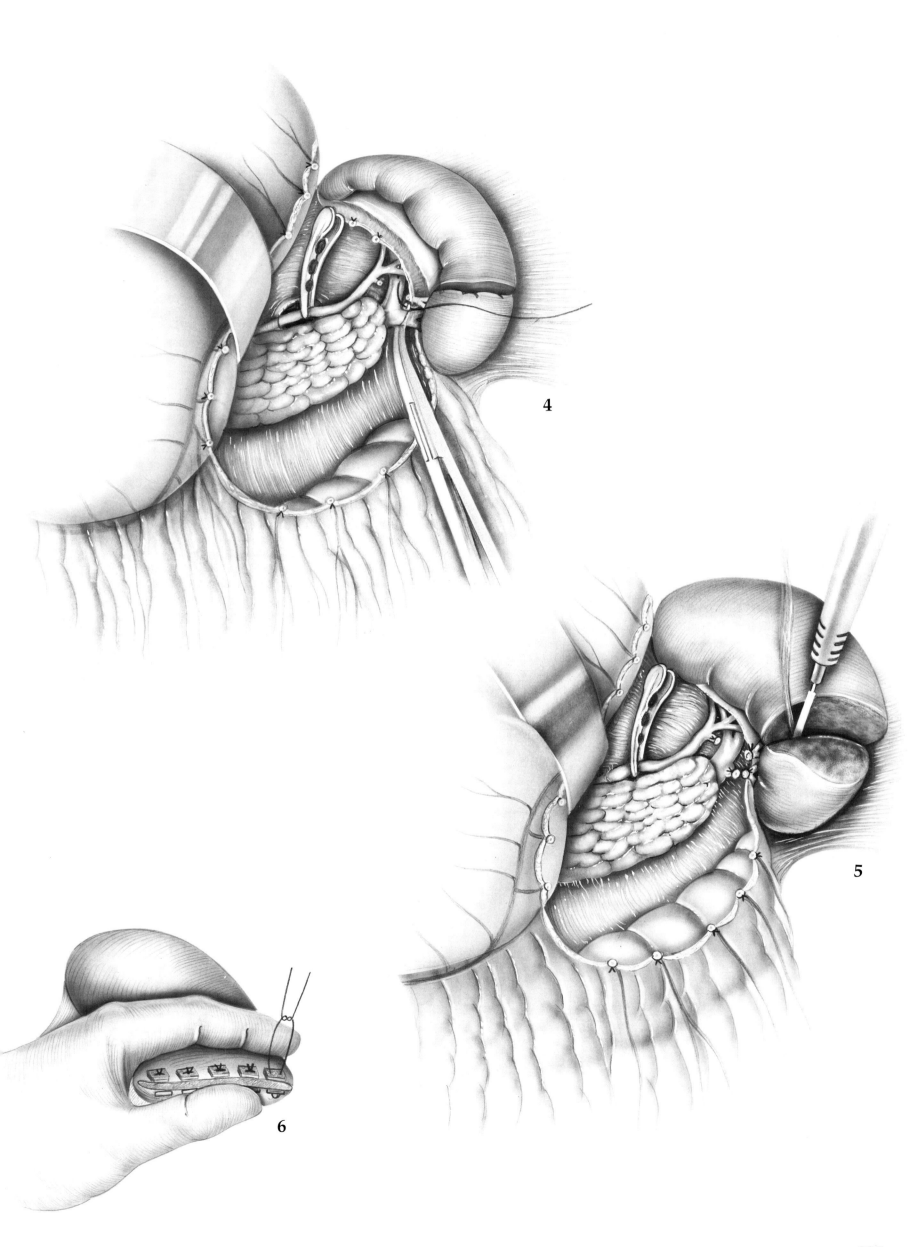

4

5

6

Portacaval Shunt

1 The patient is positioned supine on the operating table, with the right arm extended and the kidney support elevated. The abdomen is explored through a right subcostal incision.

2 The liver is retracted cephalad, the stomach medially, and the transverse colon caudally, exposing the hepatoduodenal ligament. The hepatoduodenal ligament is incised. The portal vein is identified and dissected free of the common bile duct. It must be freed circumferentially at this level. The duodenum is mobilized by dividing the peritoneum laterally and superiorly, as indicated by the line.

3 The duodenum is retracted medially along with the pancreas, exposing a greater length of the portal vein as well as the vena cava. Enough of the anterior, medial, and lateral surfaces of the vena cava is dissected free to allow the placement of a partially occluding Satinsky vascular clamp.

4 Two Satinsky clamps are placed on the portal vein, at the superior and inferior limits of the dissection. The portal vein is divided immediately below the upper clamp. The hepatic end of the portal vein is closed with a continuous #0000 polypropylene suture sewn back and forth across the stump of the vein and tied at its point of origin.

5 An additional Satinsky clamp is placed on the vena cava, but only partially occludes the lumen. An ellipse of the anterior wall of the vena cava is excised to match the luminal size of the portal vein. The lower portion of the portal vein is rotated to approximate it to the vena cava. Two 5-0 polypropylene corner stitches are placed and tied.

6 A 5-0 vascular stitch is placed in the lateral side of the vena cava venotomy and is used to distract this wall as the medial row is sewn. The needle on the inferior corner stitch is passed into the lumen of the anastomosis through the outer medial wall of the vena cava, adjacent to the corner stitch. The medial suture line is run inside the lumen of the anastomosis from below upward. When the medial row is completed, the suture is passed through the medial wall of the portal vein and tied to the free end of the superior corner stitch.

7 The suture that was used to distract the lateral wall of the vena cava is removed and the lateral row of the anastomosis is run from above downward, on the outside of the anastomosis. At the completion of this row, this suture is tied to the free end of the lower corner stitch.

8 The vascular clamps are removed and the anastomosis is inspected for hemostasis. Any defect in the anastomosis is repaired with a simple 6-0 vascular silk or polypropylene stitch.

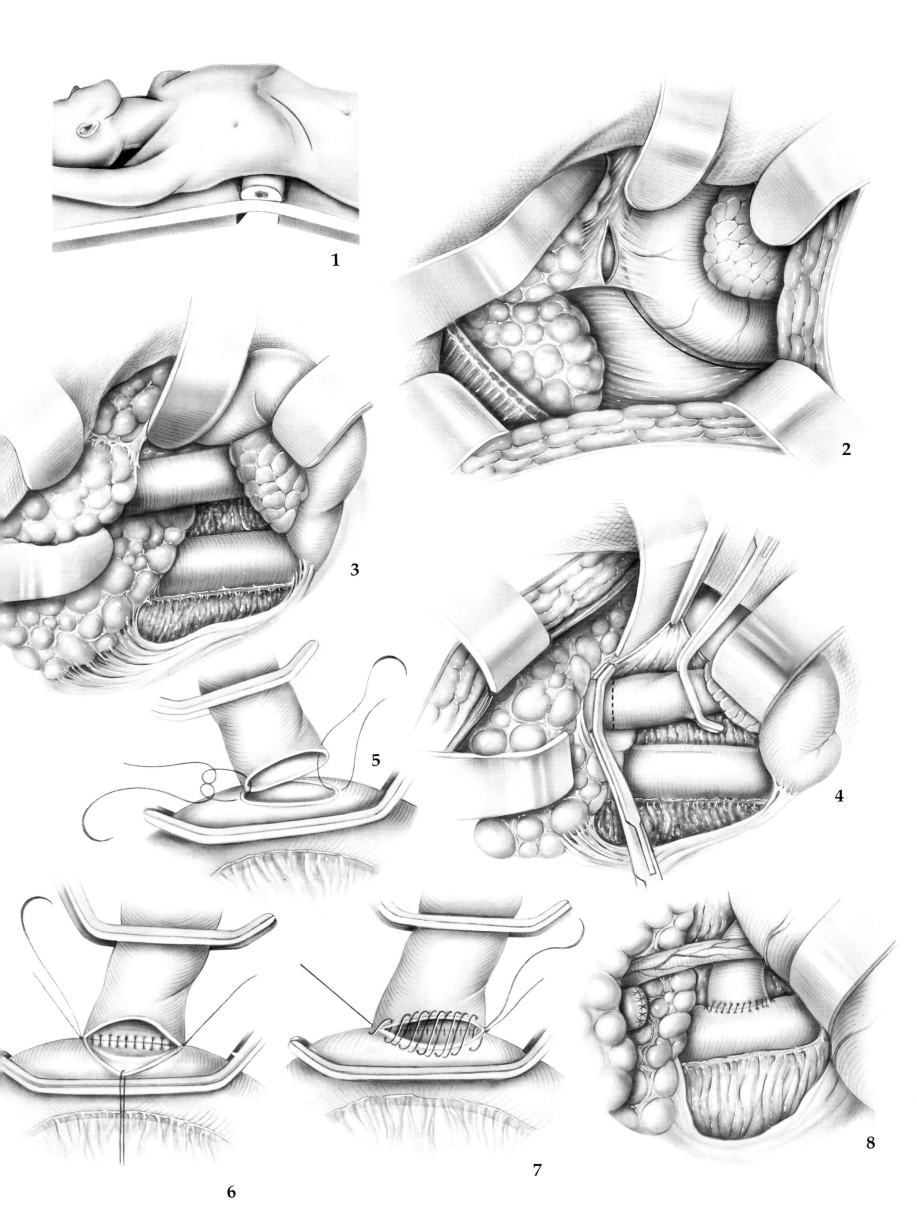

Mesocaval Shunt

Both the classic Marion-Clatworthy J-type and the H-graft mesocaval shunt are described.

1 A midline incision is made, extending from approximately 8 to 10 cm below the umbilicus to approximately two-thirds the way to the xiphoid.

2 The transverse colon is retracted cephalad, exposing the root of the mesocolon. The peritoneum at the base of the mesocolon is incised transversely, exposing the superior mesenteric vein. The superior mesenteric vein usually lies to the right of the lateral border of the vertebral body palpated posteriorly; it is somewhat more lateral to the superior mesenteric artery than is commonly thought. The superior mesenteric vein is freed from the level of the middle colic vein, which enters it on the anterior surface just below the inferior border of the pancreas, to below the junction of the ileocolic and ileal tributaries. Tributaries entering the lateral border of the superior mesenteric vein between the middle and ileocolic veins are carefully dissected, divided between clamps, and tied with fine silk, thereby clearing an adequate length of superior mesenteric vein for the caval or prosthetic graft anastomosis. The length of vein dissected should be great enough to allow the vascular anastomosis to be performed above the confluence of the ileocolic and superior mesenteric vein proper. It is permissible to extend the anastomosis onto the ileocolic vein and still achieve a functional decompression of the portal system; however, the major portion of the anastomosis must be to the superior mesenteric vein.

The classic Marion-Clatworthy shunt requires circumferential dissection of the superior mesenteric vein, to afford greater mobility of this vessel and to allow a tension-free anastomosis to the divided inferior vena cava. In contradistinction, only the anterior, right lateral, and part of the posterior walls of the superior mesenteric vein are dissected for the H-graft mesocaval shunt.

The J-Shunt (Marion-Clatworthy Shunt)

3 The right colon is reflected medially to a point where it is turned like a page of a book hinged on the superior mesenteric vein. The descending and transverse portions of the duodenum are mobilized by incising the peritoneum investing the duodenum, starting behind the superior mesenteric vein and ending at the first part of duodenum. The patient with portal hypertension has many collateral vessels within these investments which should be divided between surgical clips for hemostasis. This dissection commonly opens the ligament of Treitz behind the superior mesenteric vein.

4 The inferior vena cava is cleared from the common iliac veins below and the renal veins above. All tributaries between these sites are divided between clamps and tied securely. The lumbar veins are divided between surgical clips, which expedite the posterior dissection of the cava. The tissue between the duodenum and cava is divided to prevent subsequent sharp angulation of the upturned vena cava after it is sewn to the superior mesenteric vein. Once the cava has been mobilized circumferentially, it is divided between two Satinsky clamps placed at the confluence of the right and left common iliac veins. In order to place the Satinsky clamps, it is usually necessary to mobilize and retract the right iliac artery to the left as it crosses the inferior vena cava.

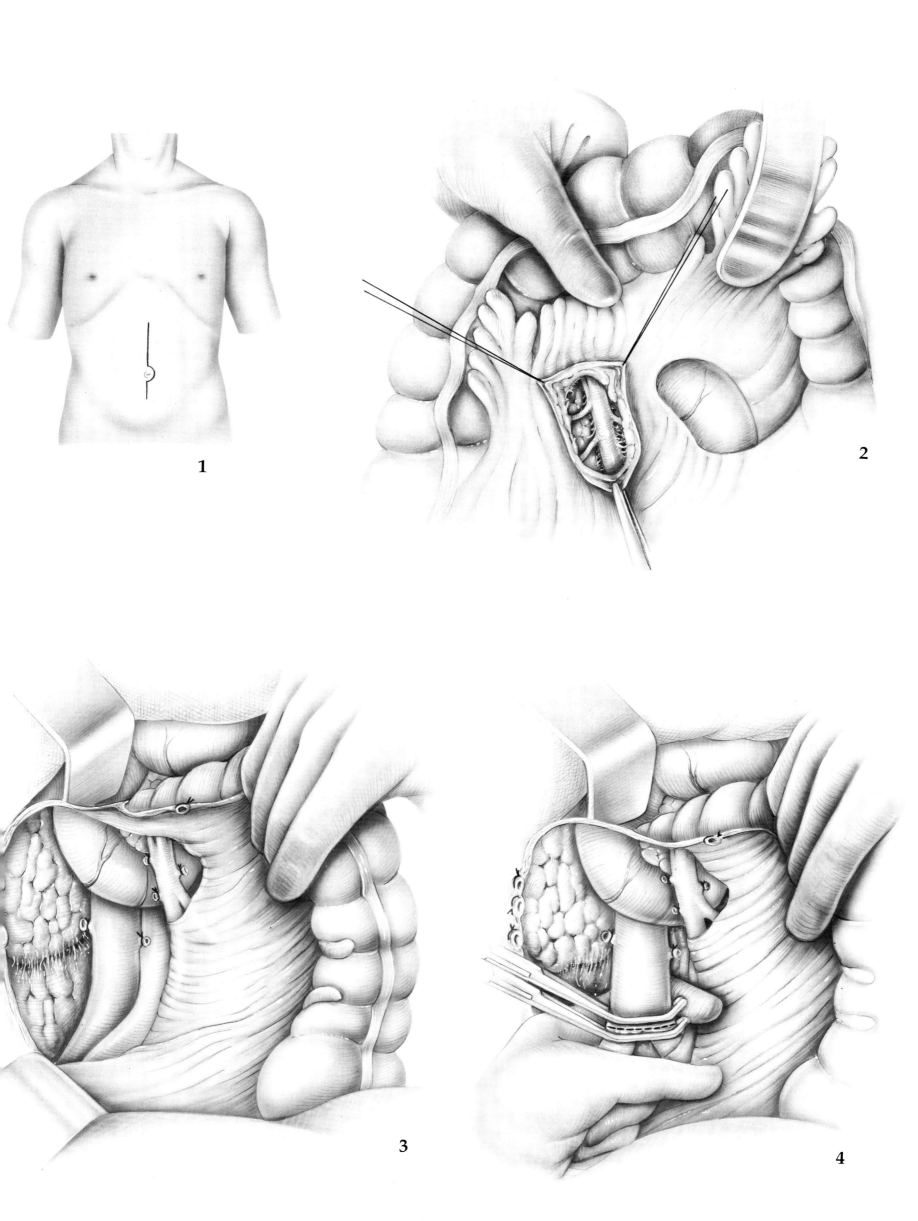

Mesocaval Shunt (*cont.*)

The J-Shunt (Marion-Clatworthy Shunt) (*cont.*)

5–6 The distal stump of the cava is closed with a continuous over-and-over #000 polypropylene suture run from right to left and then back to the right.

7 The proximal stump of the vena cava is turned medially, approximating it to the lateral border of the superior mesenteric vein so that the right side of the cava becomes the caudal end of the anastomosis. A #000 vascular silk suture is placed through the lateral wall of the superior mesenteric vein near a previously ligated branch. The superior mesenteric vein is tented up, allowing the placement of a Satinsky clamp with its jaws pointing cephalad. All tributaries to the superior mesenteric vein must be occluded with this clamp, and the superior mesenteric vein must bow between the toe and heel of the clamp. A venotomy is created by excising a small portion of the superior mesenteric vein, as indicated by the broken line.

8–10 Using vascular 5-0 polypropylene sutures, corner stitches are placed with the knots tied on the outside of the anastomosis. The needle on the lower corner is passed through the wall of the cava posterior to the knot. This maneuver allows the right-handed surgeon to run the posterior row from below upward, in a forehand fashion, from within the lumen of the anastomosis. At the completion of the posterior row this suture is brought out through the wall of the superior mesenteric vein and tied to the free end of the superior corner stitch on the outside of the anastomosis. The anterior row is run from above downward, in a forehand fashion, starting the needle on the superior corner stitch. Care is taken to avoid catching the posterior wall in the anterior suture line. At the conclusion of the anterior wall suture line, this stitch is tied to the free end of the lower corner stitch.

11 The Satinsky clamps are removed. The effectiveness of the shunt is immediately apparent—the superior mesenteric vein narrows as the pressure within it falls. With adequate mobilization of the duodenum, inferior vena cava, and superior mesenteric vein, there is little tension of the anastomosis and there is no constriction of the duodenum or inferior vena cava.

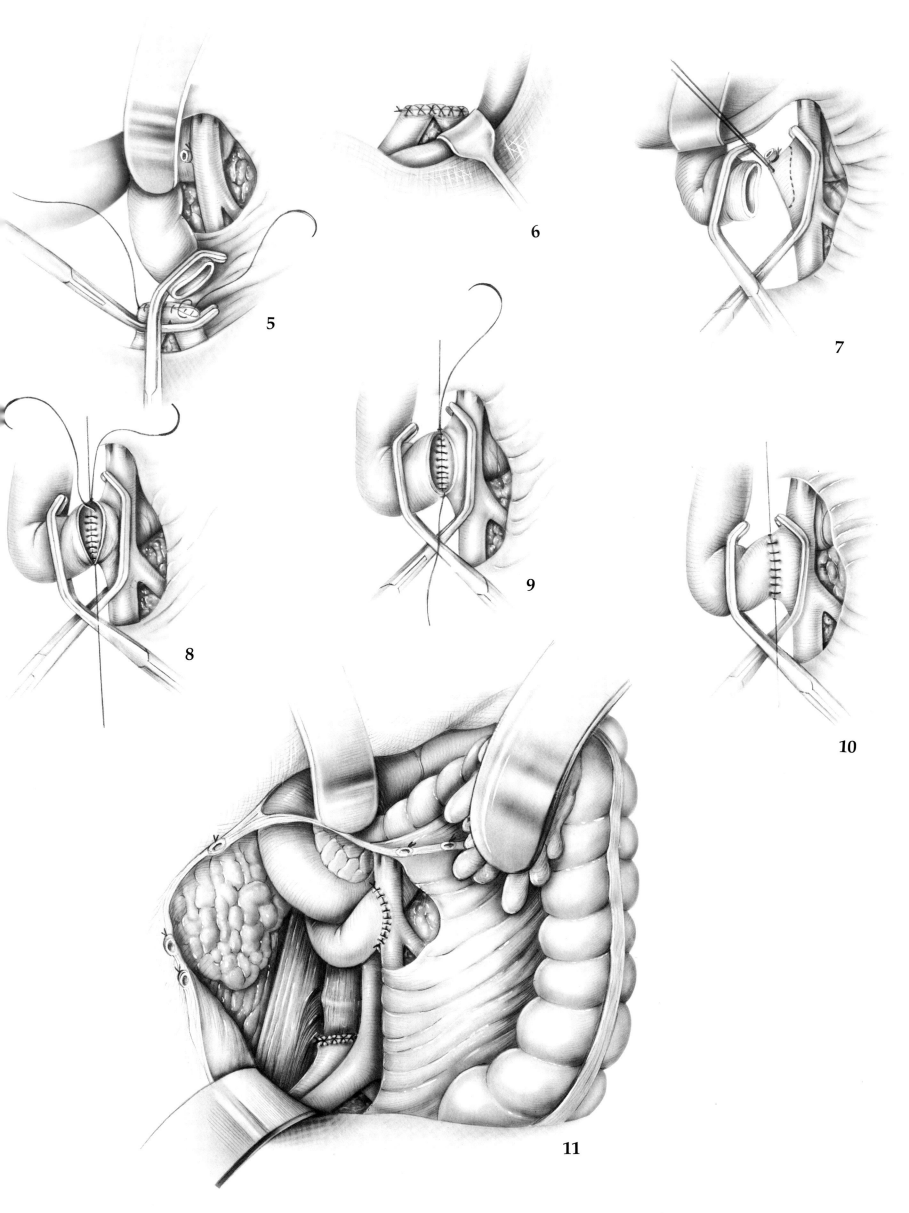

5

6

7

8

9

10

11

Mesocaval Shunt (*cont.*)

Mesocaval H-Graft

The procedure for the mesocaval H-graft, using a woven Dacron or "ringed" PTFE graft connecting the superior mesenteric vein to the inferior cava, is quite similar to the procedure described above. In contrast to the Marion-Clatworthy J-shunt, extensive mobilization of the superior mesenteric vein and inferior vena cava to provide an adequate length of vein for a tension-free anastomosis is unnecessary because these vessels do not have to be approximated. The minimal retroperitoneal dissection required for the H-graft shunt is a considerable advantage in the patient with portal hypertension. Division of the retroperitoneal portal to systemic collateral vessels can result in significant blood loss prior to the decompression of the portal circulation.

12 The inferior vena cava is exposed directly through the posterior retroperitoneum just lateral to the superior mesenteric vein, without mobilizing the colon. Frequently, the ileocolic artery is encountered coursing anterior to the cava during this dissection. It is divided between clamps and tied as close as possible to its origin from the superior mesenteric artery. Bowel viability is not compromised by the division of this artery; an arterial pulsation can be palpated in the distal stump. The retroperitoneal investments of the descending and transverse duodenum are divided between surgical clips as described for the J-shunt. The duodenum is elevated, exposing the vena cava. The tissue enveloping the vena cava in the retroduodenal region is the thinnest, making exposure relatively easy. The areolar tissue investing the inferior vena cava is dissected in a single layer from enough of the anterior, lateral, and medial walls of the vena cava to allow placement of a Satinsky vascular clamp. The lumbar tributaries are not divided.

13 The anastomosis of the graft to the vena cava must be performed prior to that between the superior mesenteric vein and the graft. By performing the caval anastomosis first, the portal circulation is occluded for a shorter period of time. In addition, during the period of superior mesenteric vein occlusion the portal pressure increases, with a commensurate increase in retroperitoneal bleeding. The increased retroperitoneal bleeding would make the caval anastomosis much more difficult if it were done second.

A #000 vascular silk suture is placed in the anterior wall of the vena cava with the entry and exit sites separated by 4 mm. The inferior vena cava is tented upward with this suture, and a large Satinsky clamp is placed so that it partially occludes the lumen of the cava. However, the heel and toe of the vascular clamp must completely occlude the isolated portion of the cava so as to prevent bleeding during the anastomosis.

14 The suture used to tent the cava is removed, and a venotomy is made with a #15 blade. This venotomy is extended proximally and distally with an angled Pott's scissors. Some surgeons remove a small ellipse of the anterior wall of the vena cava, but this is unnecessary. The stiffness of the graft material, in combination with the wide bites taken on the cava during the anastomosis, will make the lumen of the anastomosis gape widely at its completion.

15 Usually a 14- to 18-mm Dacron or reinforced PTFE graft is used. It is beveled slightly on the vena cava side of the anastomosis. Two reinforcing rings are removed from the vena cava end of the graft in those instances where reinforced PTFE is employed, thus making the placement of the stitches easier. Corner sutures are placed, using either #0000 polypropylene or #00 PTFE sutures, and tied on the outside of the anastomosis. Both suture lines are done from the outside. The Satinsky clamp and graft are rotated, allowing the surgeon to look down on the line of the anastomosis.

16 Because the area of the caval anastomosis is dependent, blood and lymph tend to collect there, obscuring the surgeon's view of the field. It is recommended that the retractors be replaced at this point, so that the duodenum is elevated adequately and the other viscera are packed away from the operative field. A second assistant aspirates all fluid collecting at the anastomotic site. A stay suture may be placed in the medial wall of the vena cava to distract the medial wall during the completion of the lateral suture line. The lateral suture line is begun,

running the inferior corner suture superiorly in a continuous fashion. This suture is tied to the free end of the superior corner stitch.

17 After the completion of the lateral suture line the Satinsky clamp is rotated. This suture line is inspected from within the lumen of the anastomosis, using a nerve hook to retract the unsutured medial side of the cava. The medial suture line is accomplished using the superior corner stitch, running it from above downward. Care must be taken to avoid catching the lateral portion of the anastomosis in the medial suture line. Once completed, this suture is tied to the free end of the inferior corner stitch.

18 The entire anastomosis is examined through the lumen of the graft with the aid of a flexible flashlight. On occasion a small gap is noted in the suture line. Any such gap should be repaired with a 5-0 vascular suture. As the graft is held vertically, the Satinsky clamp is partially removed and the suture line examined for bleeding.

19 The Satinsky clamp is then replaced on the graft immediately above the suture line, thus restoring full flow within the vena cava. Gentle traction is applied to the graft, which is cut to an appropriate length to reach the superior mesenteric vein. While there is considerable elasticity in the Dacron graft, the reinforced PTFE is inelastic; therefore the length of the graft required must be carefully measured prior to transection. Usually 4 to 5 cm of graft is needed, although in an obese patient it may be as much as 7 cm.

In a fashion similar to the caval anastomosis, a vascular suture is used to tent the portion of the superior mesenteric vein overlying the duodenum for the placement of the Satinsky clamp. The Satinsky clamp must occlude the entire lumen of the superior mesenteric vein. No ellipse of vein is excised. A venotomy is created on the anterolateral surface of the superior mesenteric vein with a #15 blade. The venotomy is enlarged with an angled Pott's scissors. However, when a large lateral tributary of the superior mesenteric vein has been ligated, the venotomy should be created by excising this stump.

Because the superior mesenteric vein is delicate and additional length is difficult to obtain if the corner sutures tear out, 5-0 polypropylene sutures are placed transversely across the vein at the upper and lower margins of the venotomy. These are used to anchor the corner sutures.

20–21 5-0 polypropylene corner sutures are placed and tied outside. The Satinsky clamp on the graft is replaced with a straight vascular clamp. This clamp is elevated to reduce tension on the suture line until the posterior row is completed. The needle of the lower corner stitch is passed through the graft wall, from the outside inward, immediately posterior to the lower corner stitch. This permits the right-handed surgeon to run the posterior row from within the lumen of the anastomosis in a forehand fashion. By applying traction to the suture the surgeon can "follow himself," thus facilitating the anastomosis. The last few sutures of the posterior row tend to be difficult to place. It is most useful to pass the needle through the back wall of the superior mesenteric vein, retrieve it between the graft and vein, and then bring it back into the lumen through the back wall of the graft. At the completion of this row, the suture is passed through the posterior wall of the vein and tied to the free end of the upper corner stitch.

22 The anterior row is run outside the lumen from above downward, using the needle on the superior corner stitch. By rotating the Satinsky clamp on the vein toward the right, the vein and graft are more closely approximated, facilitating the anastomosis. A nerve hook is used to expose the edges to be approximated and prevents the surgeon from catching the posterior wall in the suture line.

23 The completed graft is almost straight from the cava to the superior mesenteric vein. The effect of the graft is immediately apparent upon removal of the clamps, with the collapse of the superior mesenteric vein. A distinct thrill is commonly felt when the graft is palpated between the thumb and forefinger. The peritoneum overlying the superior mesenteric vein and the area opened for the dissection of the cava is closed loosely with interrupted absorbable sutures, allowing egress of retroperitoneal fluid.

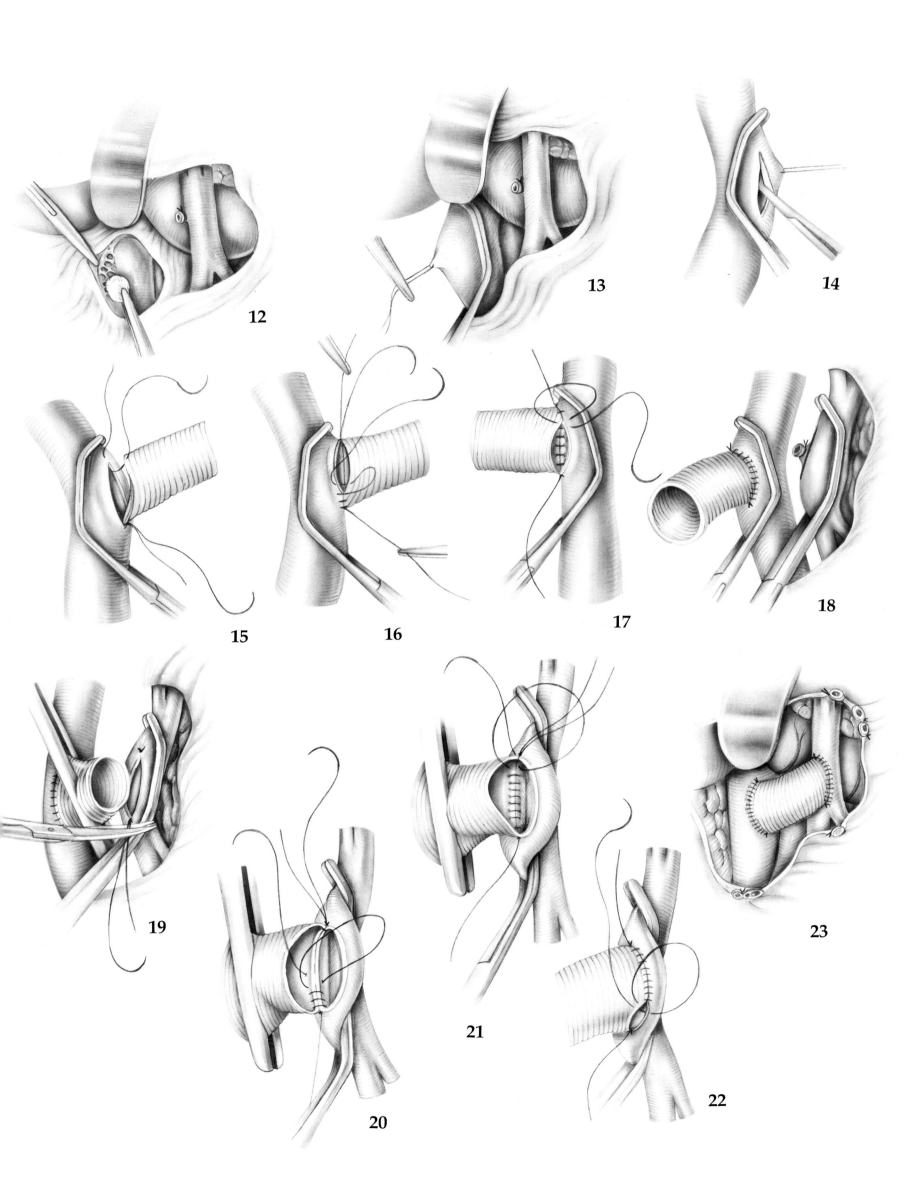

Splenorenal Shunts

1 The abdomen is explored through a midline incision extending from 6 cm below the xiphoid to 6 to 8 cm below the umbilicus.

2 The small intestine is either removed from the abdominal cavity or retracted to the right behind laparotomy pads. The transverse colon is retracted cephalad, the peritoneum at the base of the mesocolon is incised parallel to the inferior border of the pancreas, freeing the ligament of Treitz as indicated by the broken line.

3 The inferior mesenteric vein, left renal vein, and lower margin of the pancreas are exposed by this incision. The inferior mesenteric vein is dissected cephalad until its confluence with the splenic vein is identified.

4 Retraction of the pancreas cephalad and dissection on its posterior surface allows mobilization of a portion of the splenic vein proximal and distal to the entrance of the inferior mesenteric vein. This segment of vein, in contradistinction to those portions beneath the tail of the pancreas or splenic hilus, is almost completely free of pancreatic tributaries. However, if present, any tributaries to the splenic vein must be ligated between clamps and divided. Immediately inferior and deep to this area of dissection, the left renal vein is identified and cleared of its investing tissues. The genital and adrenal tributaries can be divided, allowing more length for a tension-free anastomosis.

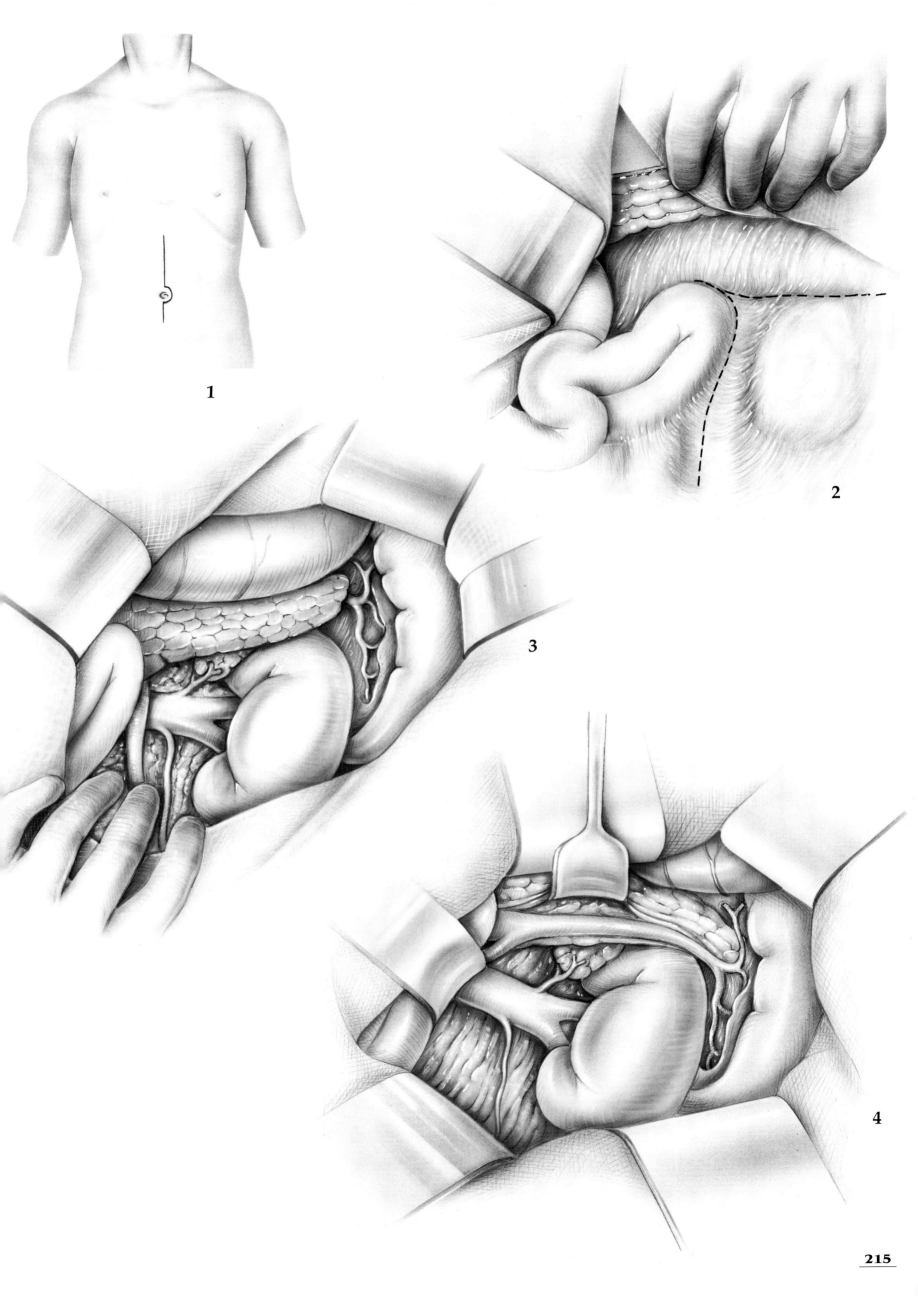

Splenorenal Shunts (*cont.*)

Central

5–6 If the splenic artery is easily accessible, a proximal tie is placed around it prior to dividing the splenic vein to prevent splenic congestion. The splenic vein is divided between Satinsky clamps. The proximal splenic vein (closest to the spleen) is oversewn with a #0000 vascular polypropylene suture run to and fro across the stump and tied at its point of origin. The distal stump of the splenic vein is rotated, approximating it to the superior and anterior surface of the left renal vein. If greater length of splenic vein is required, the inferior mesenteric vein may be divided and ligated. A Satinsky vascular clamp is placed so as to partially occlude the lumen of the renal vein. A venotomy is created in the renal vein and two 5-0 polypropylene corner sutures are placed. The posterior row of the anastomosis is performed from within the lumen in a fashion similar to that described for the end-to-side portacaval shunt.

7 The anterior row of the anastomosis is run from the right to the left outside the lumen, ensuring that the posterior row of the anastomosis is not caught in this suture line. The vascular clamps are removed. The coronary vein, found in the lesser omentum, is then ligated betewen clamps; alternatively, a linear stapler may be used to ligate all vessels in the lesser omentum without extensive dissection, thus selectively decompressing the stomach.

Splenectomy is then performed by serially clamping, dividing, and tying the vessels at the splenic hilus after division of the short gastric vessels (see **Plates 98–99, Figs. 6–9**).

Reverse or Distal

8–9 The splenic vein is approached in a fashion similar to that used for the central splenorenal shunt. The splenic vein, once circumferentially dissected and freed of all pancreatic tributaries, is divided between Satinsky vascular clamps medially. As with the central splenorenal shunt, if a greater length of splenic vein is required, the inferior mesenteric vein may be divided and tied. The medial stump of the splenic vein is oversewn with a 5-0 vascular polypropylene suture run to and fro across the stump of this vessel and tied at its point of origin. The peripheral portion of the splenic vein is sewn to the anterosuperior surface of the renal vein after creation of a venotomy in the same fashion described for the central splenorenal shunt. The spleen is not removed. Again, either the coronary vein is divided directly or a stapling device is used to divide the vessels in the lesser omentum.

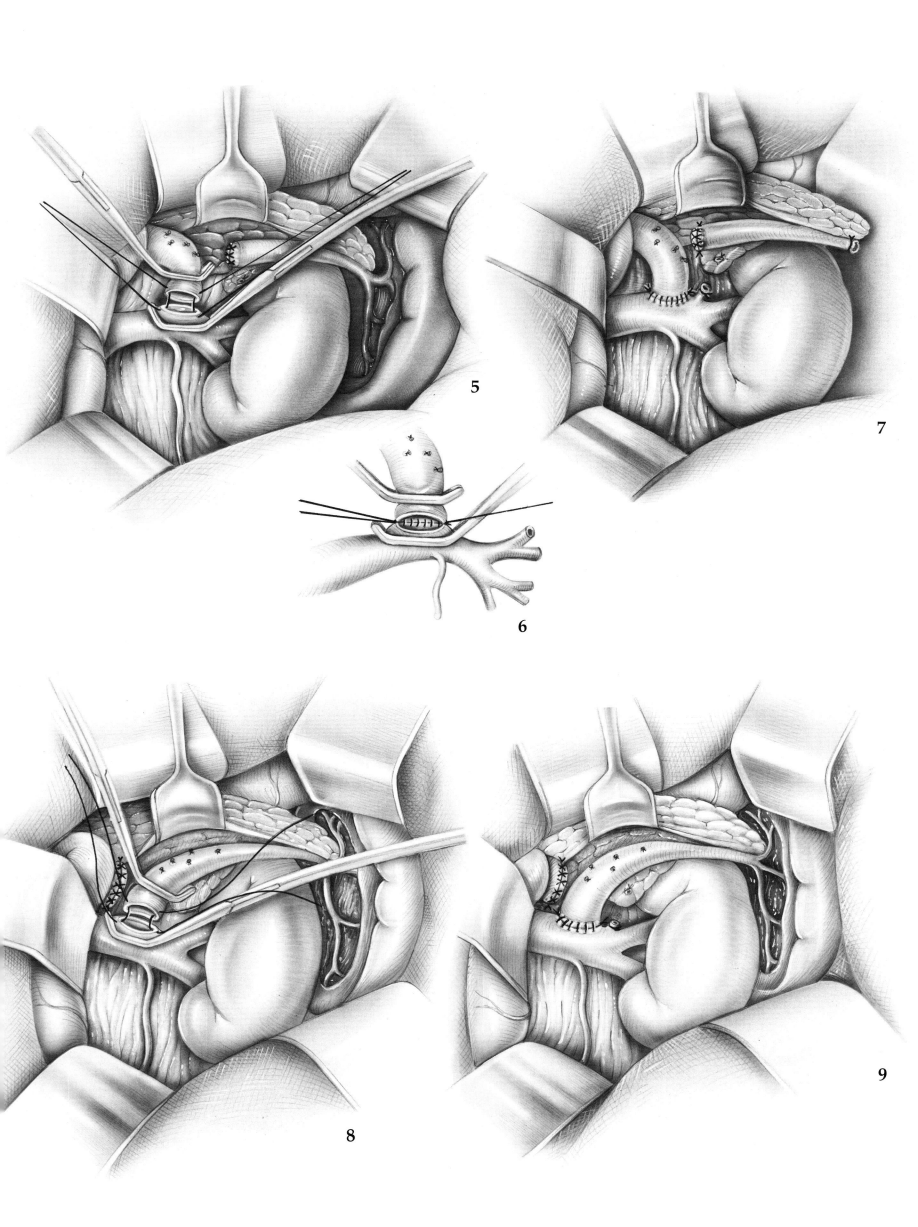

5

6

7

8

9

Drainage of a Pancreatic Pseudocyst

Cystogastrostomy

1 The abdomen is explored through an upper midline incision. The pseudocyst is palpated deep to the stomach, and the anterior wall of the stomach, overlying the pseudocyst, is opened with electrocautery. Some surgeons prefer to open the stomach with a stapling device; however, the staples create artifacts on CT scans used to follow the patient's progress.

2 A needle, bent at its distal centimeter and attached to a syringe, is inserted into the pseudocyst through the posterior wall of the stomach. A sample of the cyst fluid is aspirated and sent for culture, Gram stain, and biochemical analysis.

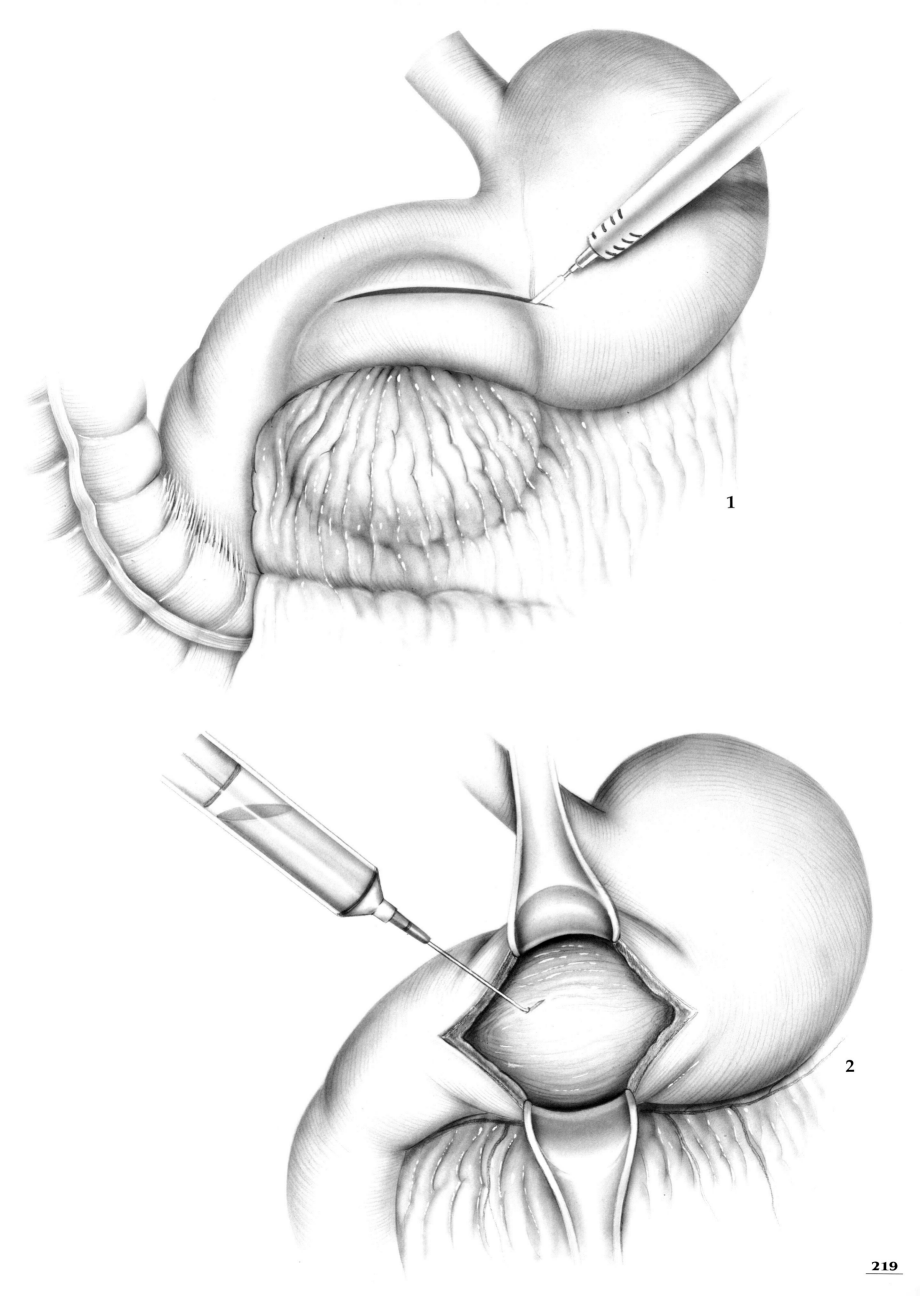

Drainage of a Pancreatic Pseudocyst (*cont.*)

Cystogastrostomy (*cont.*)

3 Using the bent needle to tent up the posterior wall of the stomach, the cyst is entered. A circular area of the posterior stomach that makes up the anterior cyst wall is mapped for excision, as indicated by the broken line.

4 Upon opening the cyst cavity, suction is used to empty its contents. Over the open jaws of a right angle clamp, a circular defect is created in the posterior gastric and anterior cyst walls with electrocautery.

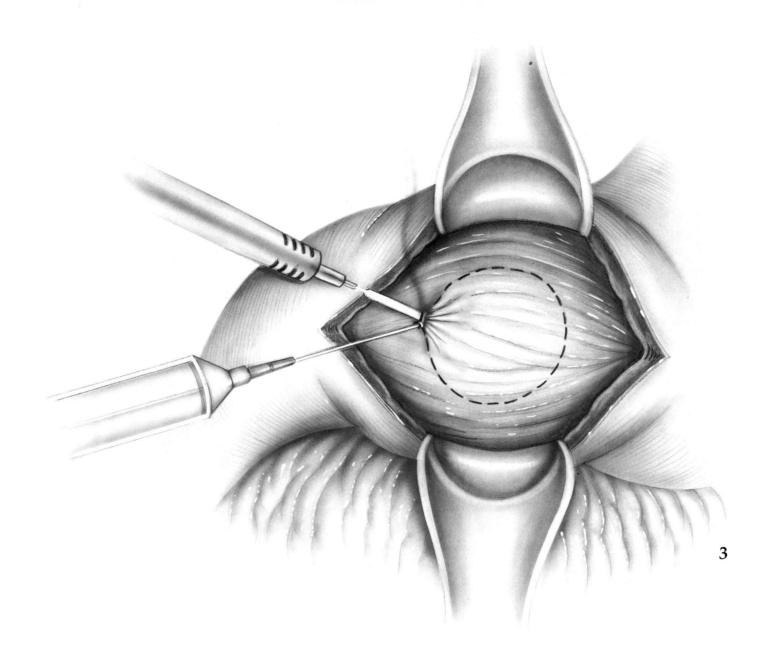

3

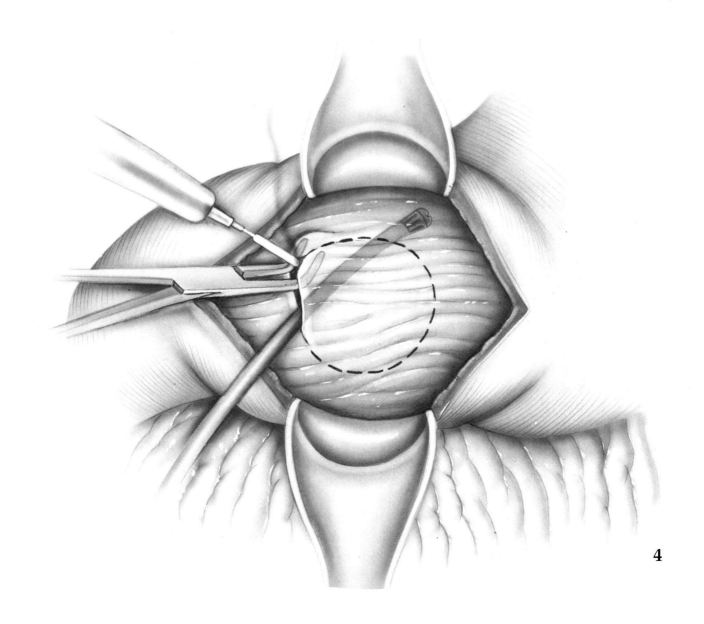

4

Drainage of a Pancreatic Pseudocyst (*cont.*)

Cystogastrostomy (*cont.*)

5 The usual defect is about 2½ cm in diameter. Searing the gastric surface to map out the area to be excised is helpful.

6–7 The cystogastrostomy is performed with a continuous #00 polyglycolic acid suture carried around the circumference of the opening twice, to "X" the cut edges. The running suture establishes the anastomosis and provides complete hemostasis.

8 The tip of the sump nasogastric tube is placed into the pseudocyst, and the anterior wall of the stomach is closed with an inner layer of continuous #00 polyglycolic acid sutures and an outer layer of interrupted seromuscular #000 silk sutures. Again, staples may be used to close the gastrotomy; but for reasons mentioned above (see page 218, paragraph 1), this is not recommended.

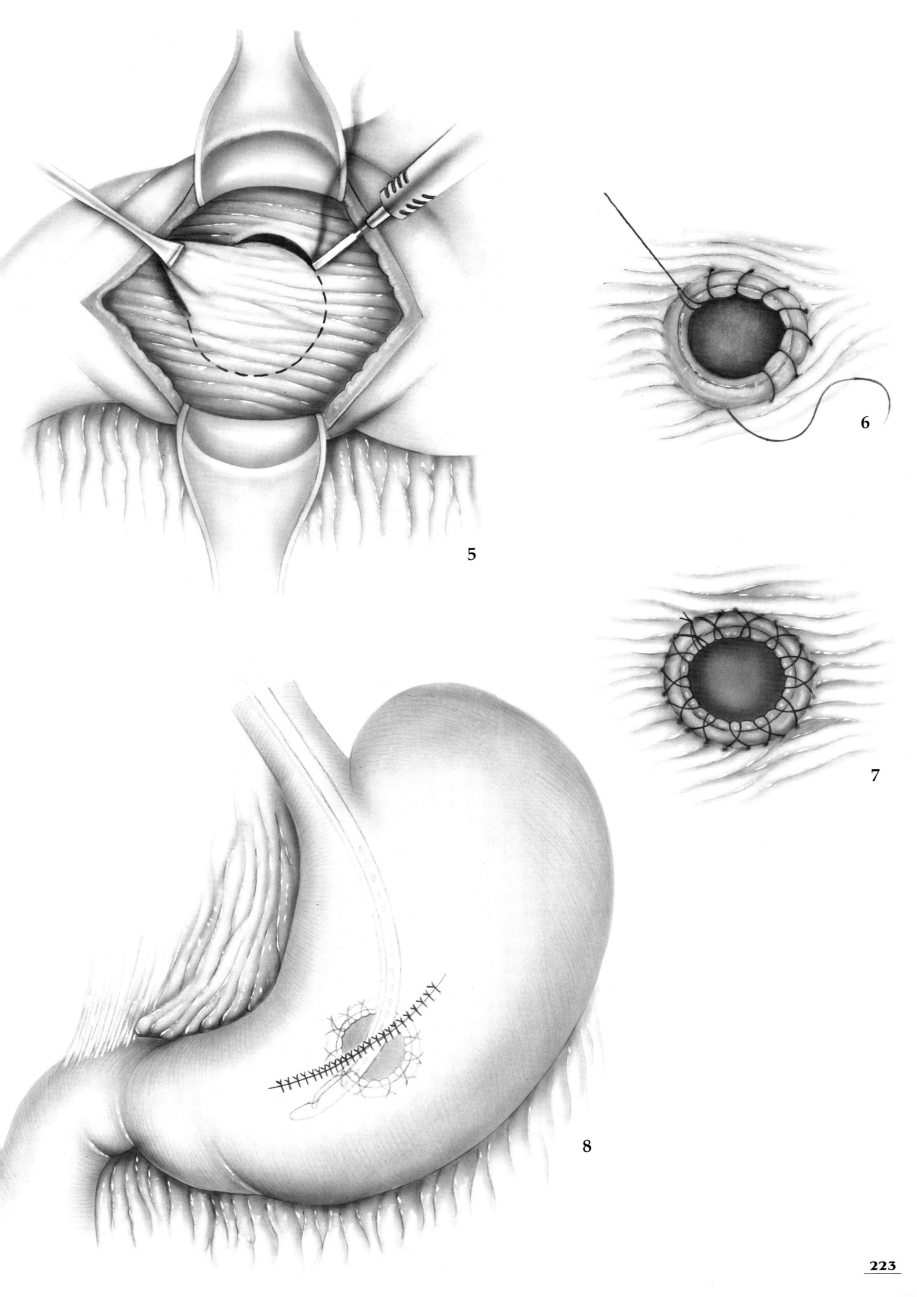

5

6

7

8

Drainage of a Pancreatic Pseudocyst (*cont.*)

Cystoduodenostomy

9 Cystoduodenostomy is a convenient way to drain a pancreatic pseudocyst located in the head of the pancreas or abutting the curve of the duodenum. The cyst is palpated through the duodenal wall. The duodenum is opened opposite the wall that directly abuts the cyst.

10 A needle attached to a syringe is inserted into the cyst through the lumen of the duodenum. A sample of the cyst fluid is sent for culture, Gram stain, and biochemical analysis.

11 A bend fashioned at the distal end of the needle allows it to be used as a hook to tent up the duodenal wall. The duodenal and cyst walls are incised over the needle tip with electrocautery. The cyst contents are aspirated. A circular portion of the abutting duodenal and cyst walls is excised with electrocautery over the open jaws of a right-angle clamp.

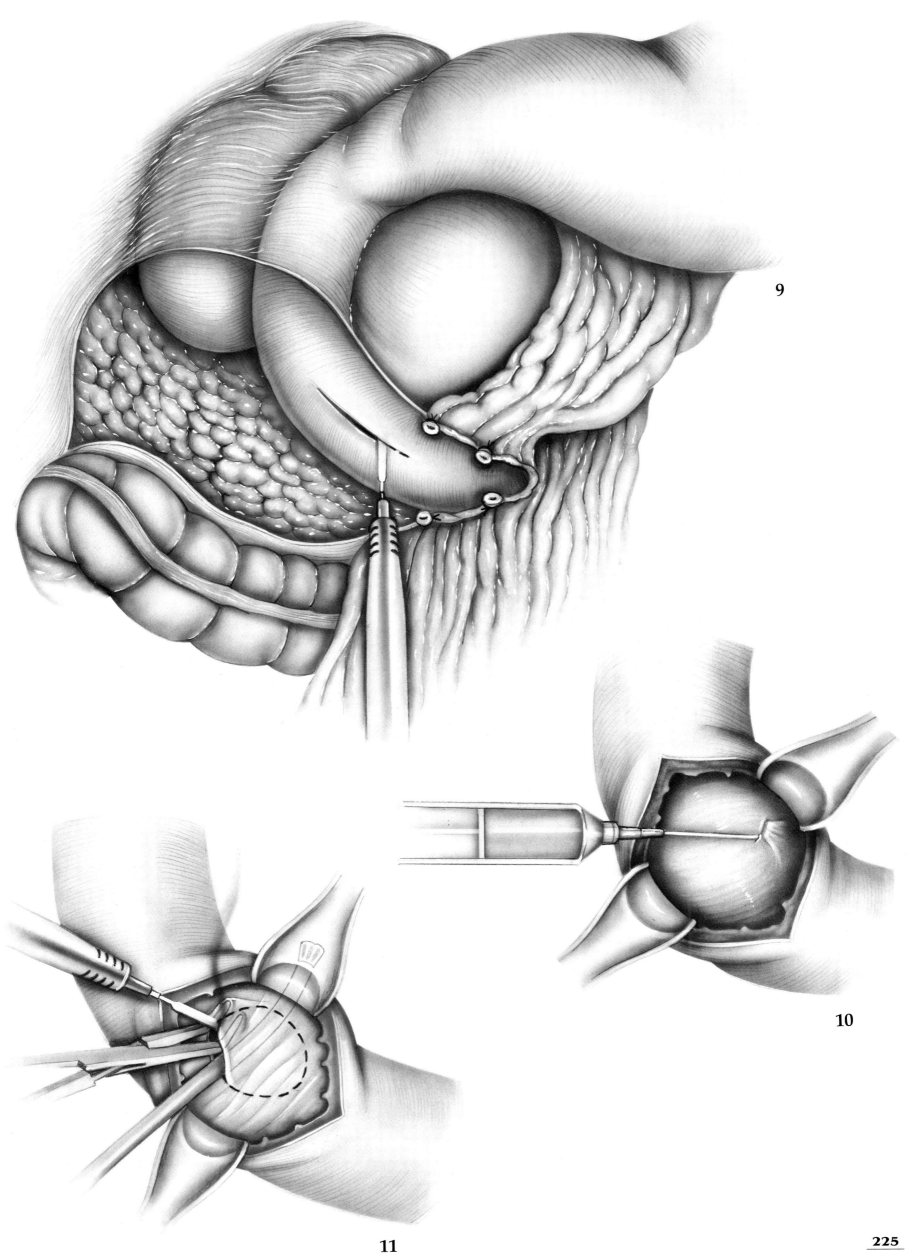

9

10

11

Drainage of a Pancreatic Pseudocyst (*cont.*)

Cystoduodenostomy (*cont.*)

12 On occasion, vigorous bleeding will occur from branches of the inferior and superior pancreaticoduodenal arteries during the excision of the duodenal and cyst walls. These are oversewn with interrupted silk sutures. In addition a larger vessel may be identified in the cyst wall, or the common bile duct may be seen within the pseudocyst cavity.

13–15 The anastomosis between the cyst and duodenum, as well as hemostasis, is achieved with a circumferential #00 polyglycolic acid suture line run around the defect twice so as to "X" the cut edges.

16 A Pezzar catheter may be inserted into the gallbladder and used as a cholecystostomy if there is any suspicion of bile leakage into the pseudocyst or transient ampullary obstruction resulting from local injury. The end of the Pezzar catheter is bisected, forming a flat surface, and four radial cuts are made to allow easy removal of the catheter.

17 The Pezzar catheter is introduced into the gallbladder and held in place with a #000 polyglycolic acid purse-string suture. It is brought out to the skin through a separate incision and placed on low continuous suction. The duodenum is closed longitudinally in layers, with a continuous #000 polyglycolic acid suture on the inner layer. Interrupted #000 silk sutures are used for the seromuscular outer layer. When indicated, the area lateral to the duodenum is drained with a closed suction catheter.

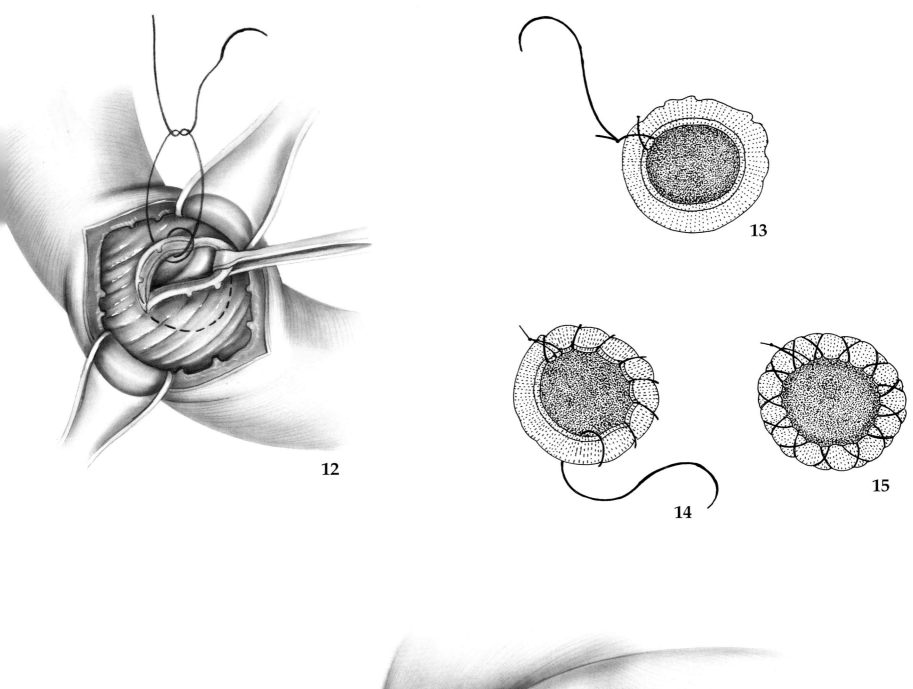

12

13

14

15

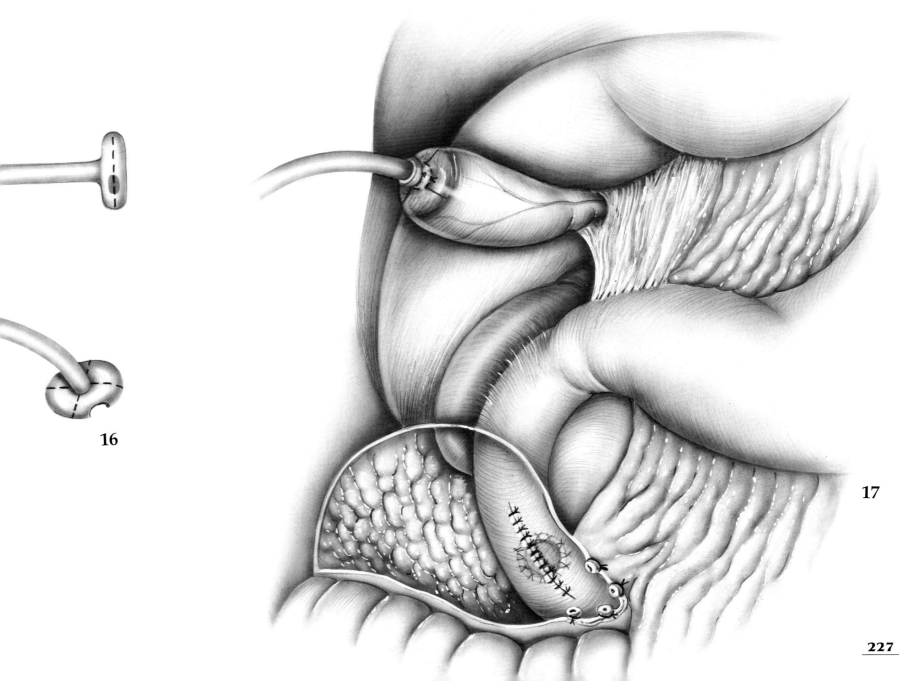

16

17

Drainage of a Pancreatic Pseudocyst (*cont.*)

Roux-en-Y Limb

18 When the pancreatic pseudocyst presents in a position that is not convenient for gastric or duodenal drainage, a Roux-en-Y limb is used to drain the cyst. Commonly this occurs when the pseudocyst presents inferiorly through the transverse mesocolon.

19 The transverse colon is retracted superiorly. The cyst is palpated and, through the bare area of the transverse mesocolon posterior to the vascular arcades, aspirated with a needle attached to a syringe. An opening into the pseudocyst is facilitated by tenting up the transverse mesocolon and cyst wall with a needle bent at the tip. The mesocolon and cyst wall are incised on the needle tip using electrocautery.

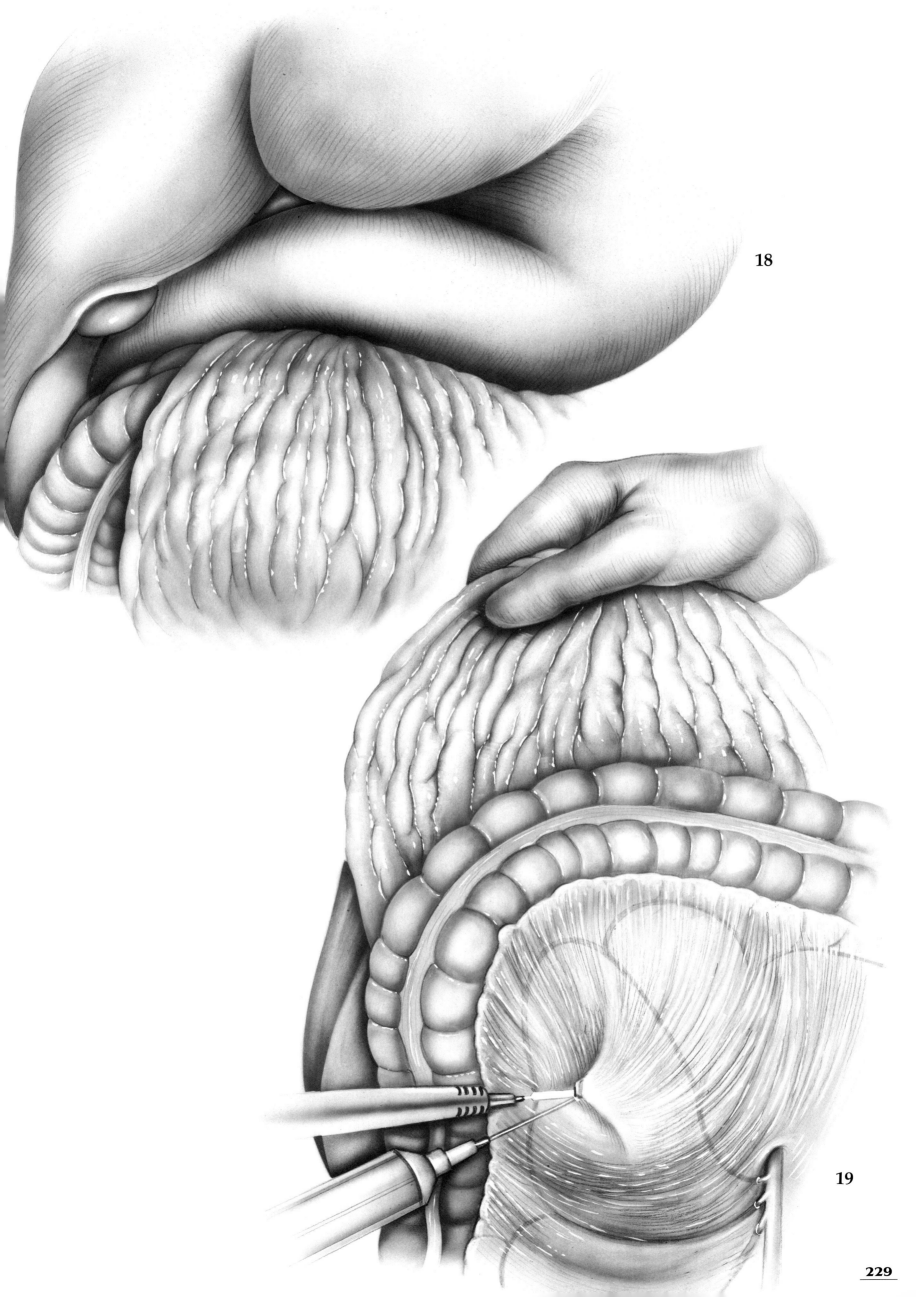

18

19

Drainage of a Pancreatic Pseudocyst (*cont.*)

Roux-en-Y Limb (*cont.*)

20 A suction catheter is placed into the cyst cavity through this defect in the mesocolon and cyst wall. A portion of the mesocolon and cyst wall is excised, using electrocautery over the open jaws of a right-angle clamp.

21 A Roux-en-Y limb is constructed (**Plates 47–49, Figs. 12–17**). The orifice of the open end of the jejunal limb is enlarged by incising the antimesenteric border, as shown by the broken line.

22 The open end of the Roux-en-Y limb is sutured to the mesocolon and cyst wall with interrupted #000 or #00 polyglycolic acid sutures.

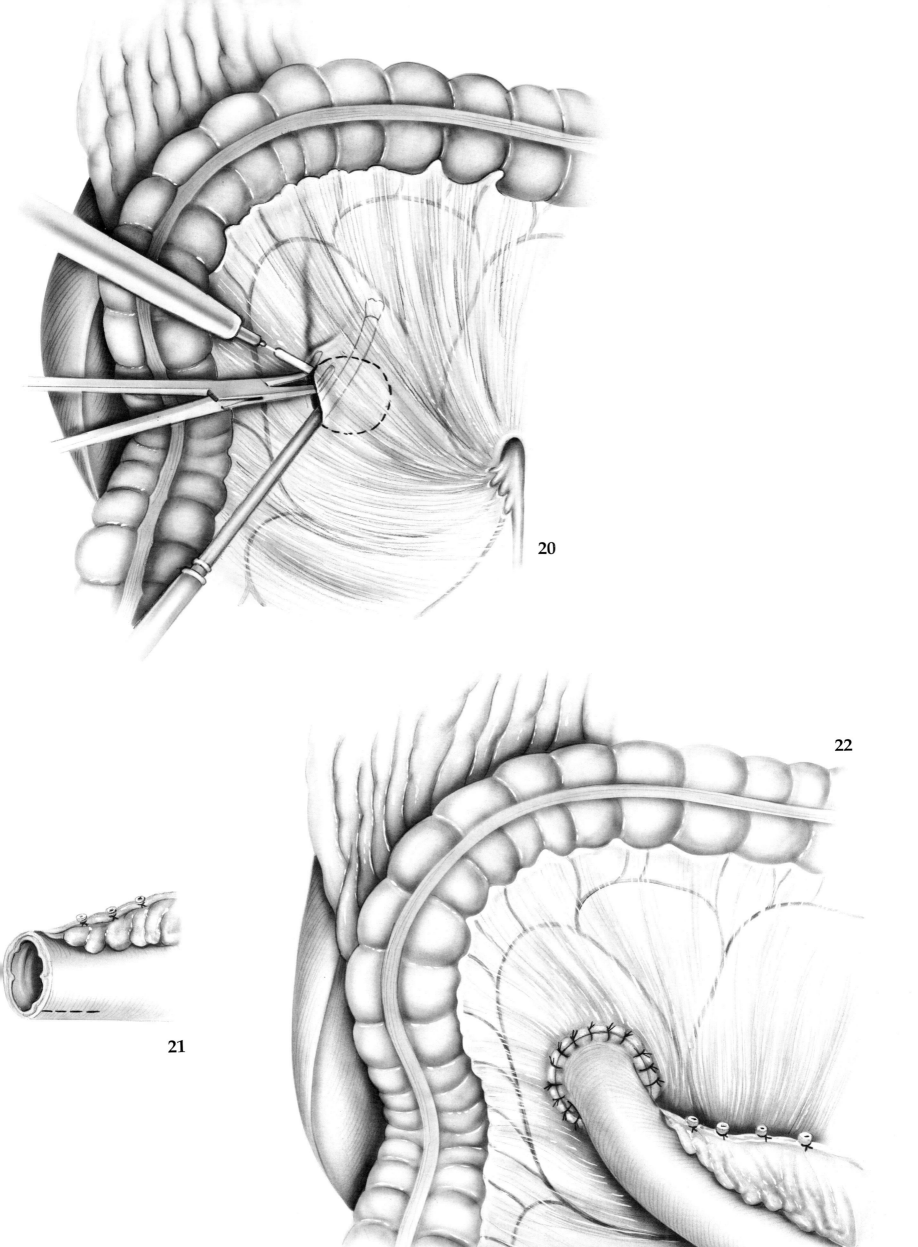

20

21

22

Pancreaticojejunostomy (Puestow Procedure)

1 The abdomen is explored through a long midline incision. The gastrocolic ligament is divided and the lesser sac is entered. The stomach is retracted cephalad, exposing the pancreas. The pancreatic duct is palpated in the substance of the pancreas. A needle with a bend at its tip is inserted into the pancreatic duct, fluid is aspirated for culture, Gram stain, and biochemical analysis, and the duct is opened with a #15 scalpel over the needle in the duct.

2 An angled Pott's scissors is used to extend the opening in the duct medially and laterally.

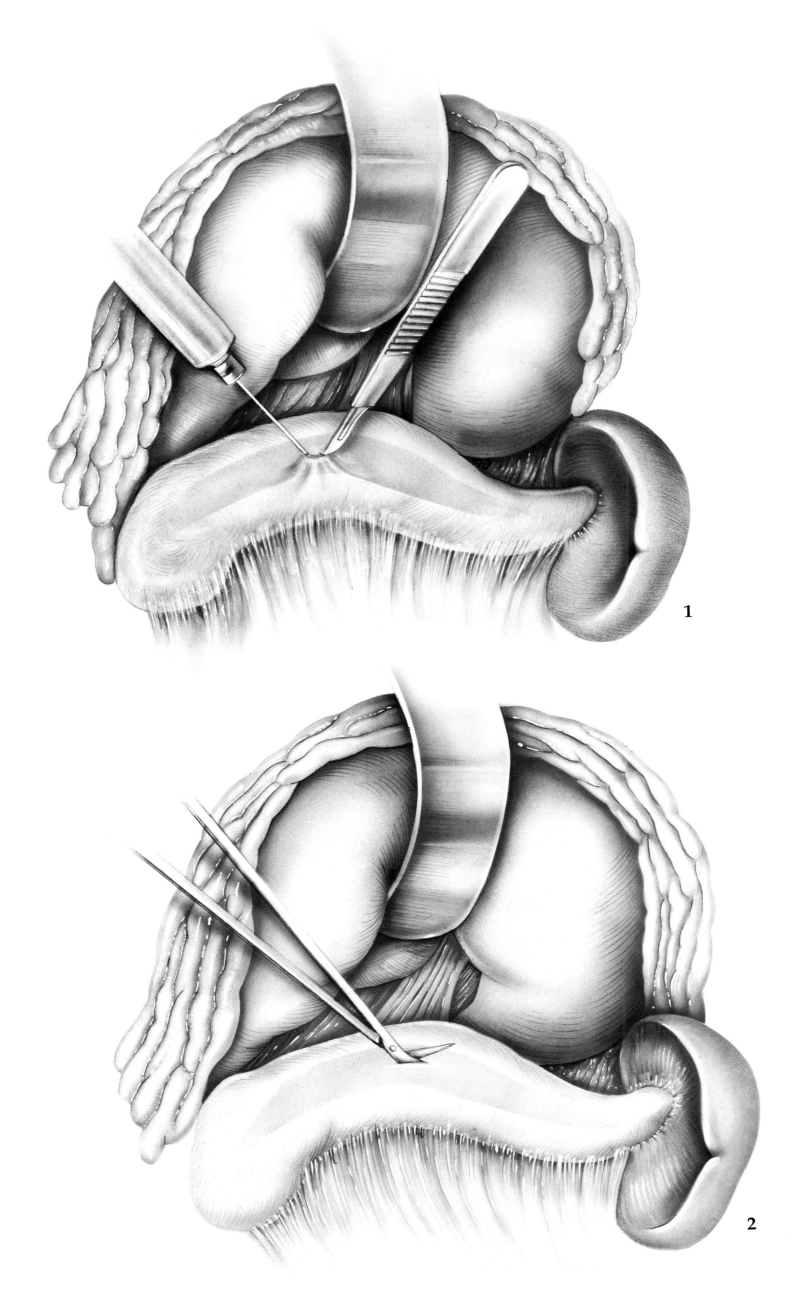

Pancreaticojejunostomy (Puestow Procedure) (*cont.*)

3 Concretions, calculi, and septa within the dilated ductal system are removed.

4 A Roux-en-Y jejunal limb is constructed (**Plates 47–49, Figs. 12–17**) and brought through the mesocolon into the lesser sac.

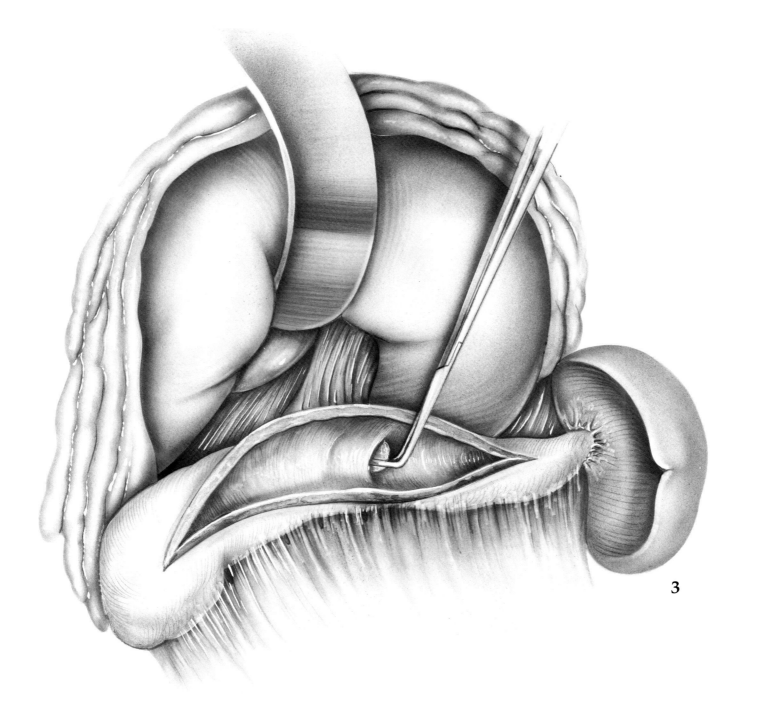

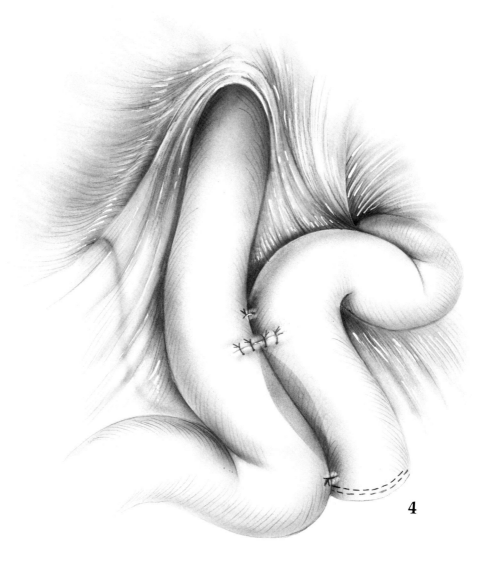

3

4

Pancreaticojejunostomy
(Puestow Procedure) (*cont.*)

5 The antimesenteric border of the jejunal limb is opened for a length equal to the opening in the pancreatic duct.

6 Full-thickness interrupted #000 polyglycolic acid sutures are placed at 4- to 7-mm intervals through the inferior duct wall and then through the superior wall of the opened jejunum. The sutures are clamped until this row is completed.

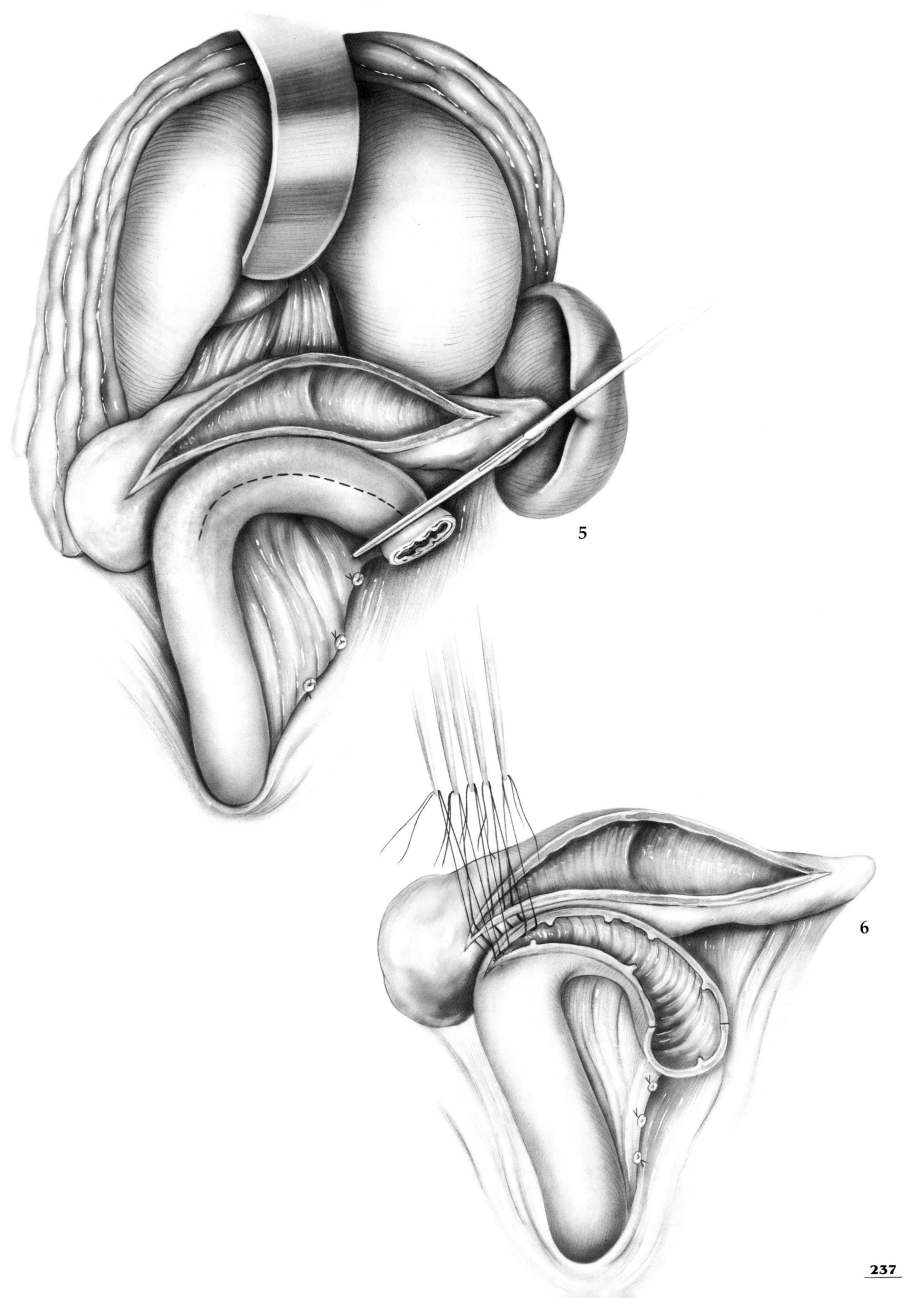

5

6

PLATE
1 1 9

Pancreaticojejunostomy
(Puestow Procedure) (*cont.*)

7 It is convenient to line the clamps up on an empty sponge stick holder as the stitches are placed. The end of the Roux loop is tailored as indicated by the broken line.

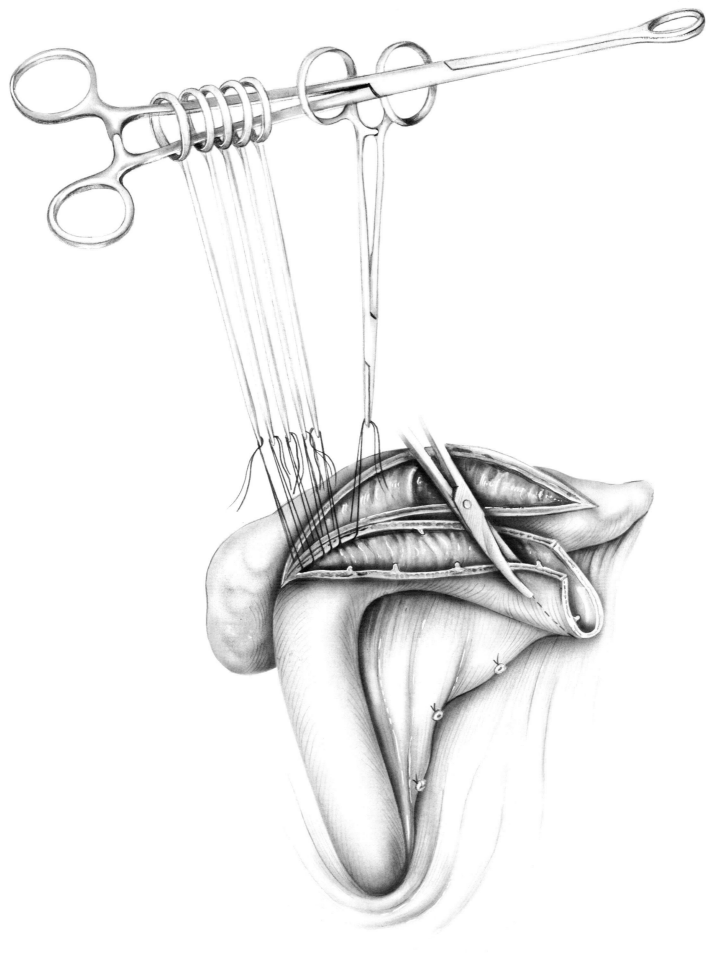

7

Pancreaticojejunostomy
(Puestow Procedure) (*cont.*)

8 The inferior row is tied and the ends of the stitches are cut.

9 Similarly, the superior cut edge of the pancreatic duct is sewn to the jejunum with interrupted full-thickness #000 polyglycolic acid sutures.

10 Usually there is a "dog's ear" of jejunum that is closed with interrupted #000 silk seromuscular stitches, as depicted. The Roux-en-Y is secured to the defect in the mesocolon with interrupted #000 silk sutures. A closed suction drain is placed at the anterior inferior border of the pancreas, behind the jejunal limb, and brought out to the skin through separate incisions.

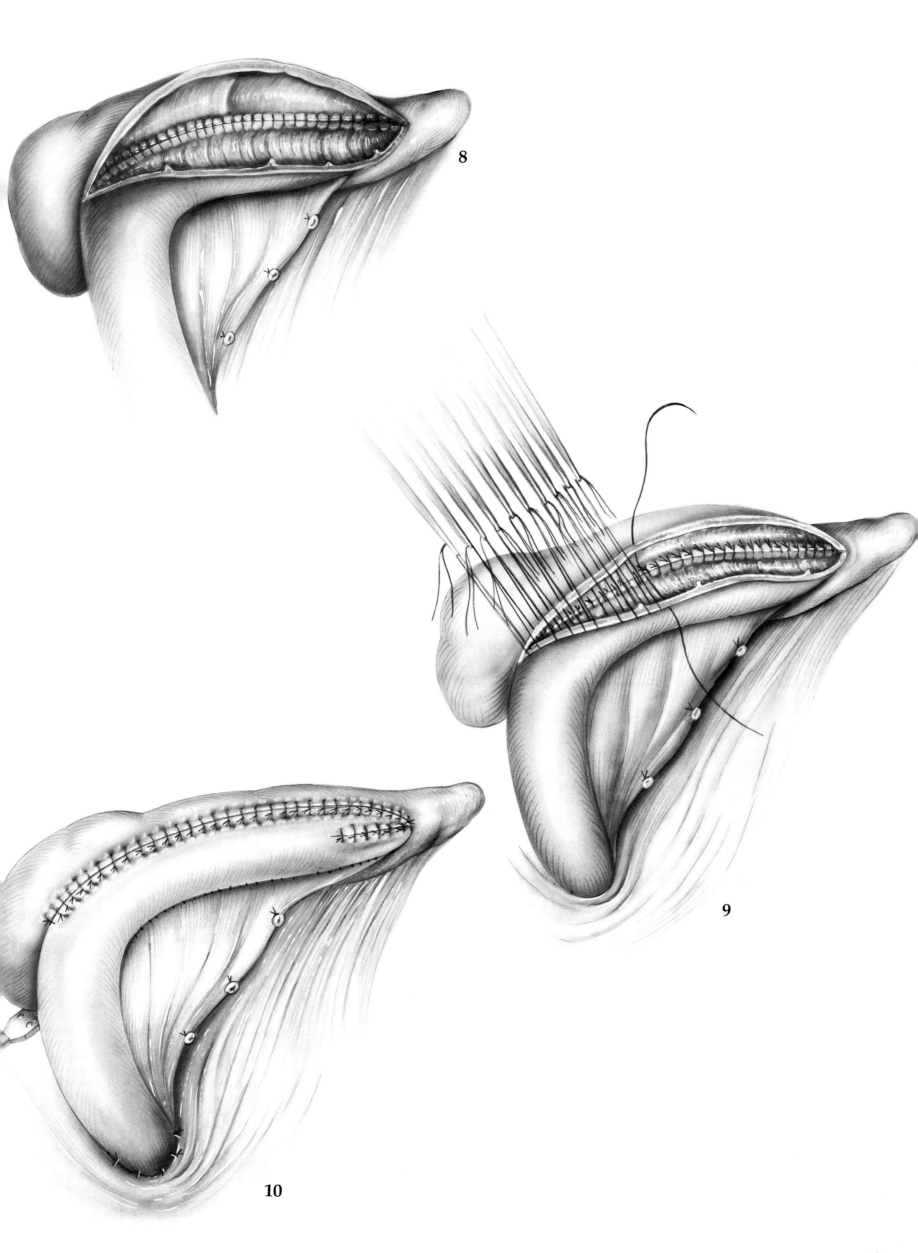

8

9

10

Marsupialization of the Lesser Sac for Pancreatic Abscess or Necrosis

1 The abdomen is explored through either a transverse or a midline incision. The location and extent of the pancreatic phlegmon will determine which incision is best suited to the case at hand.

2 The contents of the lesser sac usually push the gastrohepatic ligament anteriorly, almost to the abdominal wall. The gastrocolic ligament is palpated and the area of greatest swelling and/or fluctuance is identified, shown here by the dashed line.

3 Using a syringe, a sample of the fluid in the lesser sac is aspirated for culture, Gram stain, and biochemical analysis.

4 An area of the gastrocolic ligament is cauterized; then a right-angle clamp is introduced into the lesser sac. The contents of the lesser sac are aspirated with a large suction catheter. The gastrocolic ligament is then opened transversely with electrocautery.

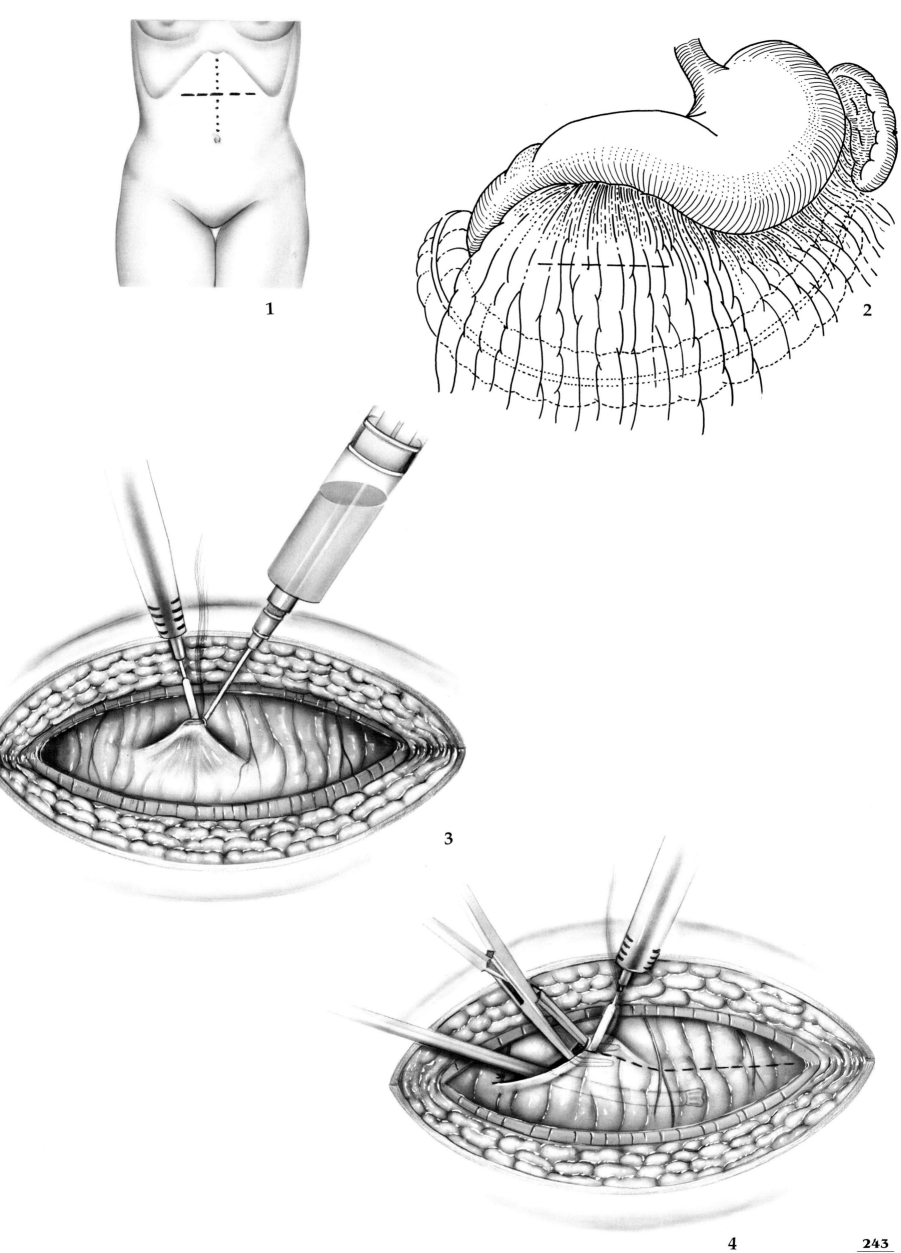

Marsupialization of the Lesser Sac for Pancreatic Abscess or Necrosis (*cont.*)

5 Necrotic fat and pancreas are bluntly debrided with a stick sponge and gentle finger dissection. The lesser sac is then irrigated with copious amounts of warm saline solution.

6 Wide Penrose drains or rubber dams are placed into the lesser sac inferiorly, superiorly, and in each corner. The lesser sac is packed fairly tightly with vaginal gauze. These packs will also elevate the stomach, transverse colon, and omentum to the abdominal wall, facilitating the subsequent fixation of omentum to the wound.

   Each of the packs is identified with sutures—e.g., one suture for the first, two sutures for the second, and so on, allowing the packs to be removed in reverse order of placement. (That is, the last pack placed is the first pack removed.)

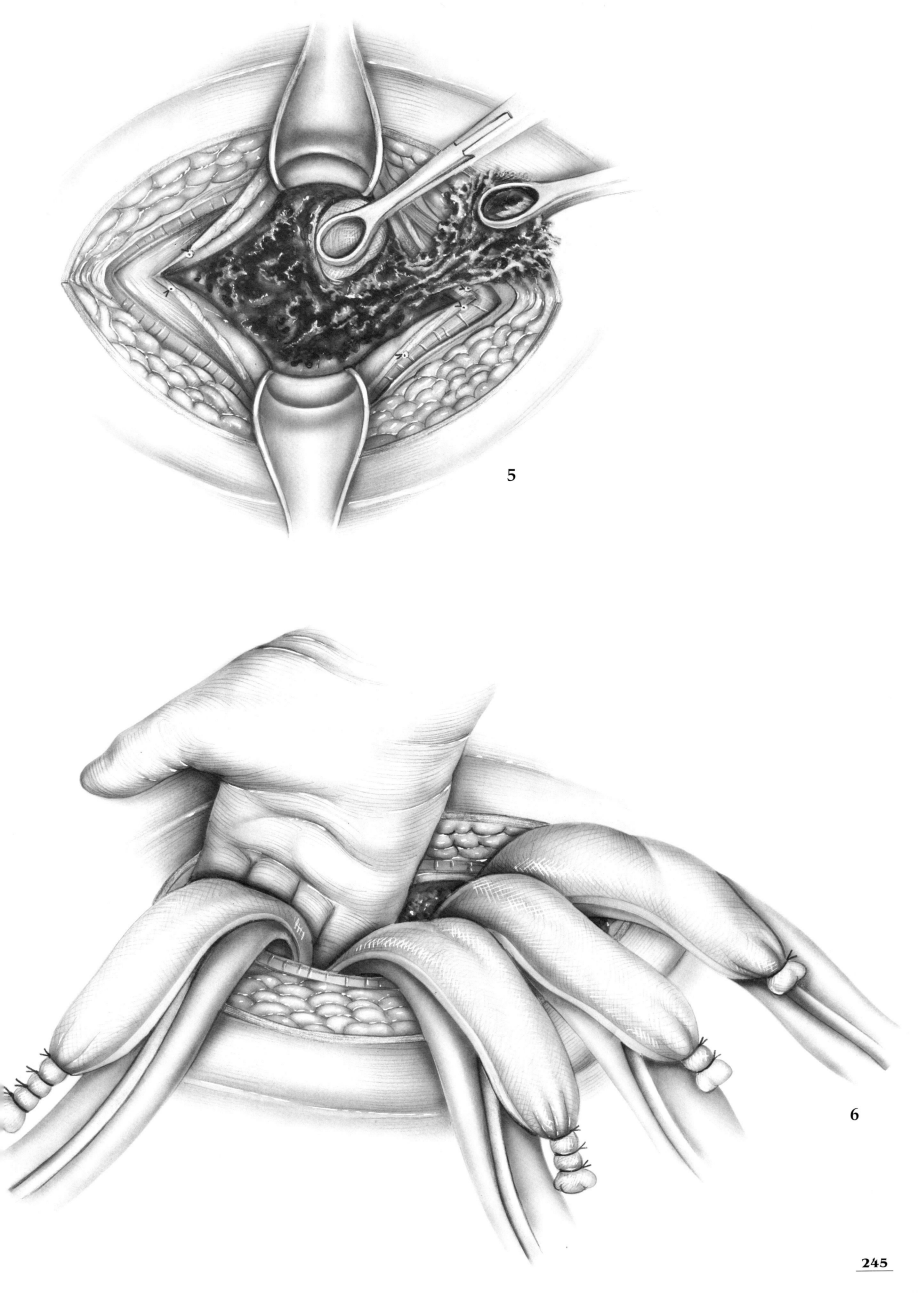

5

6

Marsupialization of the Lesser Sac for Pancreatic Abscess or Necrosis (*cont.*)

7 A wedge of subcutaneous fat is removed, allowing the skin to be sutured to the fascia and muscle with interrupted #000 polyglycolic acid sutures.

8 The skin is sutured to the fascia and muscle circumferentially around the wound to prevent the pancreatic ferments from coming into contact with the subcutaneous fat—which might cause further necrosis or infection in this layer.

9 The margins of the defect in the gastrocolic ligament are sutured to the abdominal wound with #00 polyglycolic acid sutures. In the corners, where the incision may extend beyond the defect in the gastrocolic ligament, portions of the abdominal wall are closed with interrupted #1 polyglycolic acid sutures. Corner stitches including the omentum are used to separate the area marsupialized from the partial abdominal wall closure. This maneuver seals the remainder of the abdominal cavity but permits easy access to the lesser sac and its contents.

10 After the completion of the marsupialization the lesser sac and its packing are readily accessible through the anterior abdominal defect. If the patient's clinical course is benign, the first pack is removed on the fifth postoperative day. In the septic patient the packs are removed after three days. Early removal may provoke bleeding from the pancreatic tissues and adherent omentum. By the fifth postoperative day, the packs generally separate from the pancreatic bed and the walls of the lesser sac. The packs are removed, over two days, at the patient's bedside with the assistance of mild sedation. The cavity is irrigated twice daily with saline to wash out any residual pancreatic fragments. The wound opening will remain large enough to permit removal of the necrotic tissues. Once the packs are removed, the wound will close fairly rapidly without a ventral hernia. The wound is cultured intermittently.

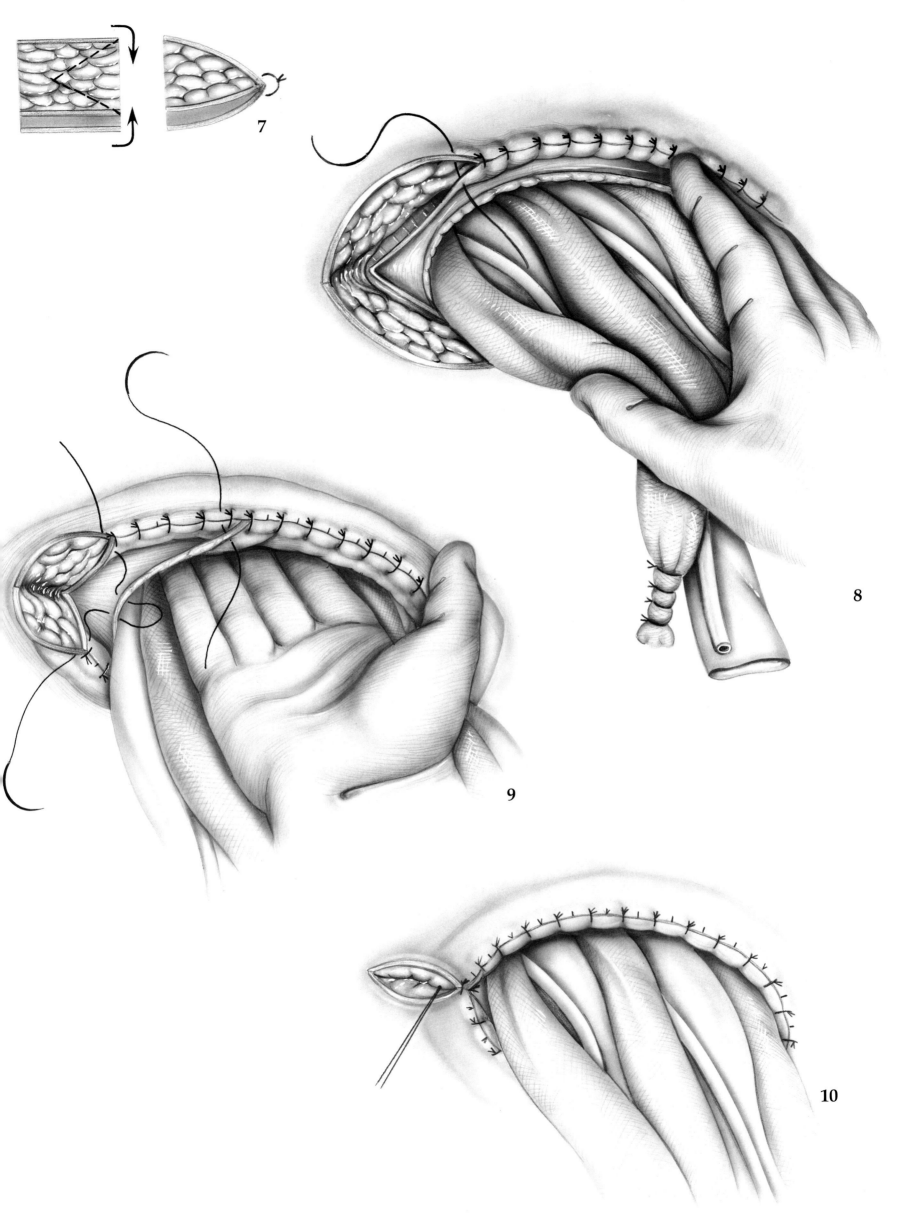

7

8

9

10

Radical Pancreaticoduodenectomy (Whipple Procedure)

1 The abdomen is explored through a hockey stick–shaped incision extending from the right anterior axillary line obliquely across the abdomen to a point in the midline halfway between the xiphoid and umbilicus, and then across the left rectus muscle. It is essential to evaluate the liver, peritoneal surfaces, and abdominal viscera for evidence of metastases before proceeding with this operation.

2 Access to the lesser sac is gained through the gastrocolic ligament, which is divided between clamps and tied. The stomach is retracted cephalad, exposing the anterior surface of the pancreas. Again the potential for resection is assessed.

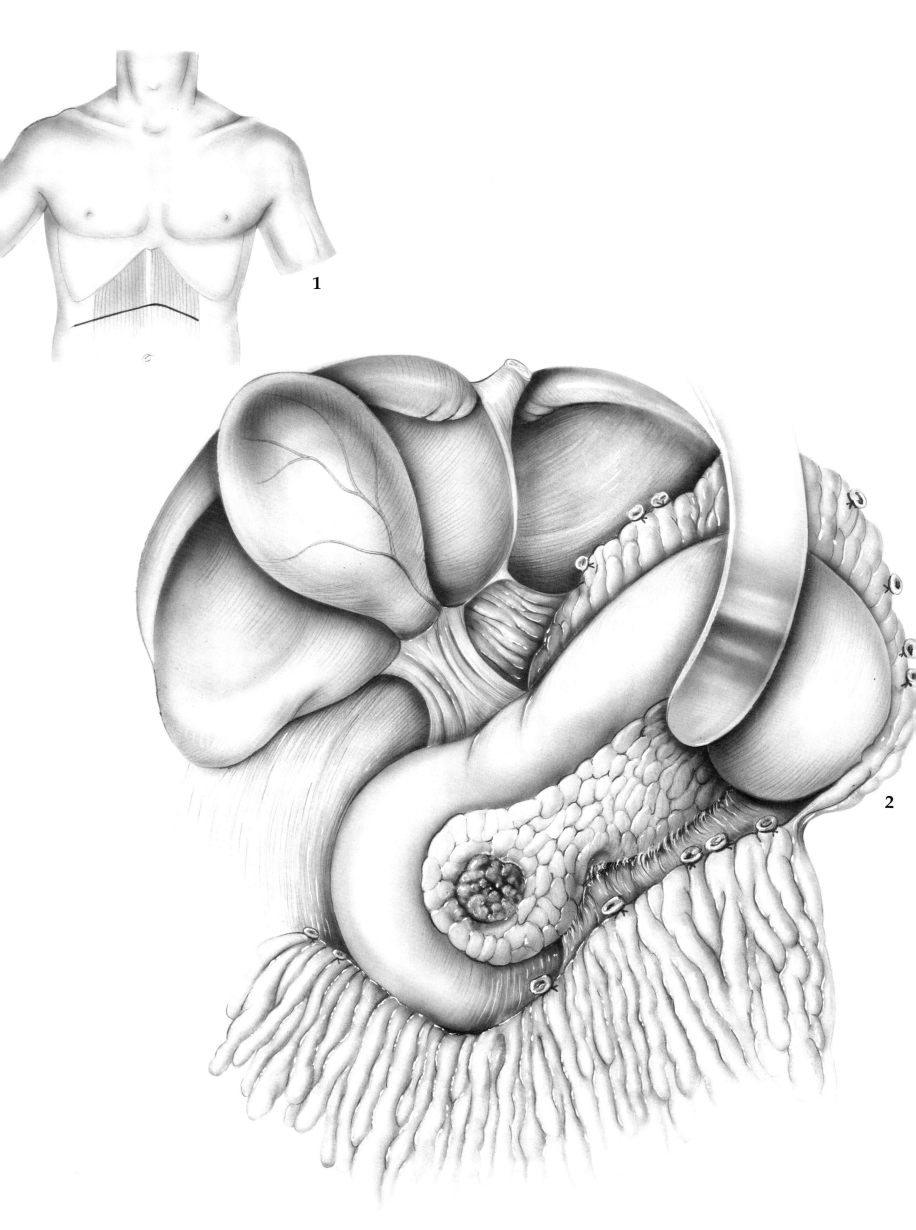

Radical Pancreaticoduodenectomy (Whipple Procedure) (*cont.*)

3 The duodenum is mobilized by incising the peritoneal investment lateral to its first, second, and third portions. This dissection is continued across the peritoneum covering the lower margin of the hepatoduodenal ligament, carefully exposing the underlying common bile duct and hepatic artery.

4 The duodenum and tumor are mobilized from the retroperitoneal location with blunt finger dissection behind the pancreas, common bile duct, and transverse duodenum. The dissection is carried medially to the portal vein.

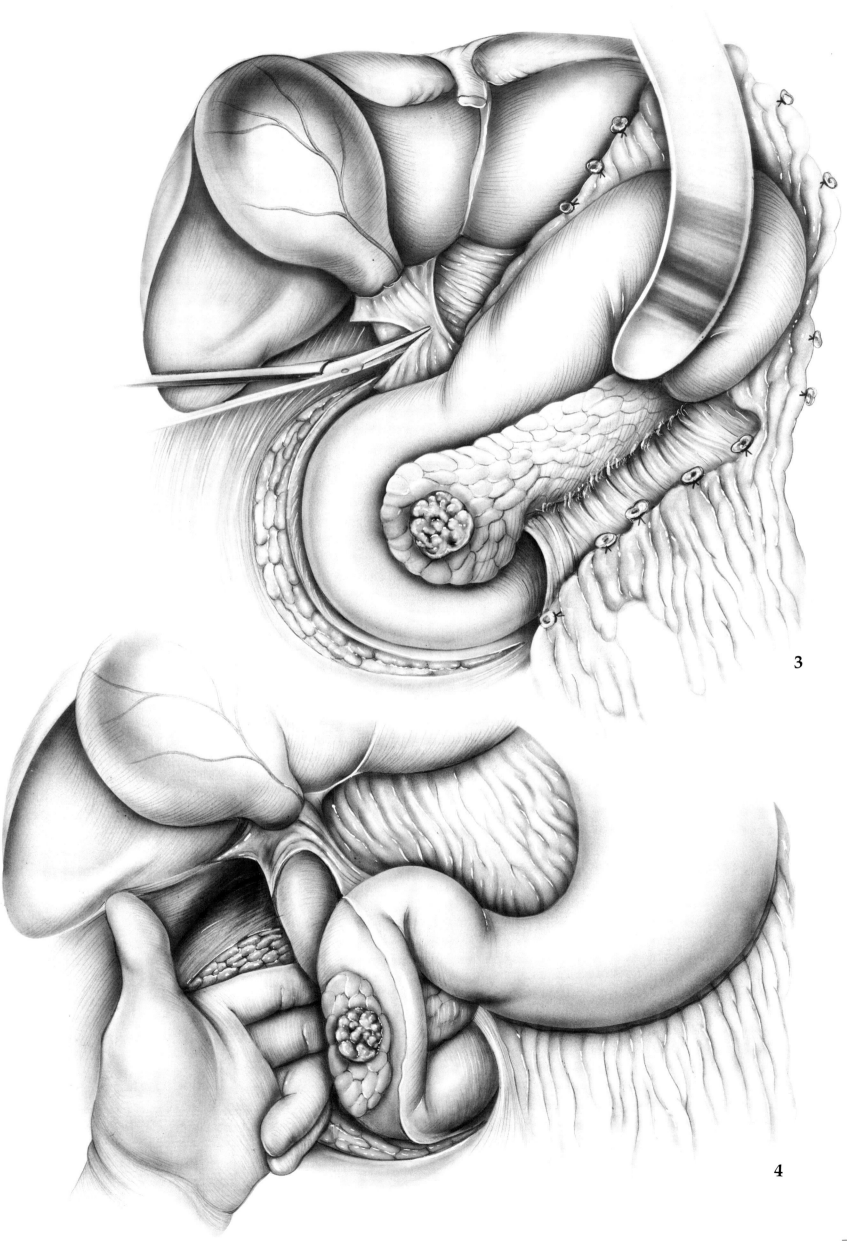

3

4

Radical Pancreaticoduodenectomy (Whipple Procedure) (*cont.*)

5 The common bile duct is bluntly dissected, medially to laterally, with a gauze pledget held at the tip of a right-angle clamp. Placing a finger behind the common bile duct through the foramen of Winslow, to provide direction and an opposing surface, facilitates this maneuver.

6 The common bile duct is encircled with a Penrose drain and retracted to the right, exposing the common hepatic, gastroduodenal, and right gastric arteries. The gastroduodenal artery is divided between clamps and tied with #00 silk ligatures.

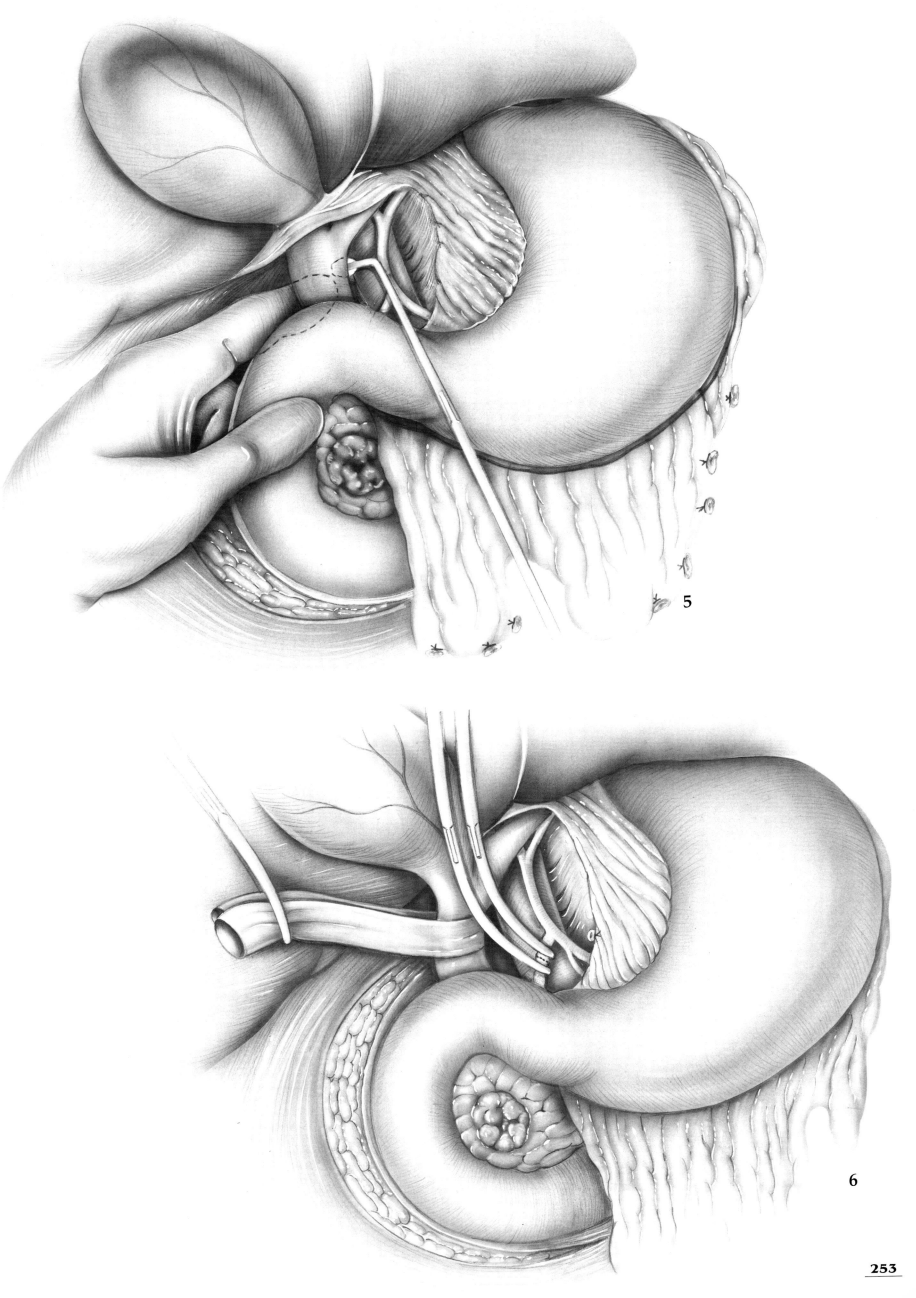

5

6

Radical Pancreaticoduodenectomy (Whipple Procedure) (cont.)

7 Similarly, the right gastric artery is divided between clamps and tied close to its origin from the hepatic artery. The common bile duct is retracted laterally, exposing the underlying portal vein.

8 From above the duodenum, a finger is insinuated between the portal vein and the posterior duodenal wall and neck of the pancreas. The areolar tissue anterior to the superior mesenteric vein and at the inferior border of the pancreas is bluntly dissected against the finger. Because there are several pancreatic venous tributaries entering the lateral wall of the portal vein at the neck of the pancreas, it is essential that the finger not stray from the anterior surface of the portal vein.

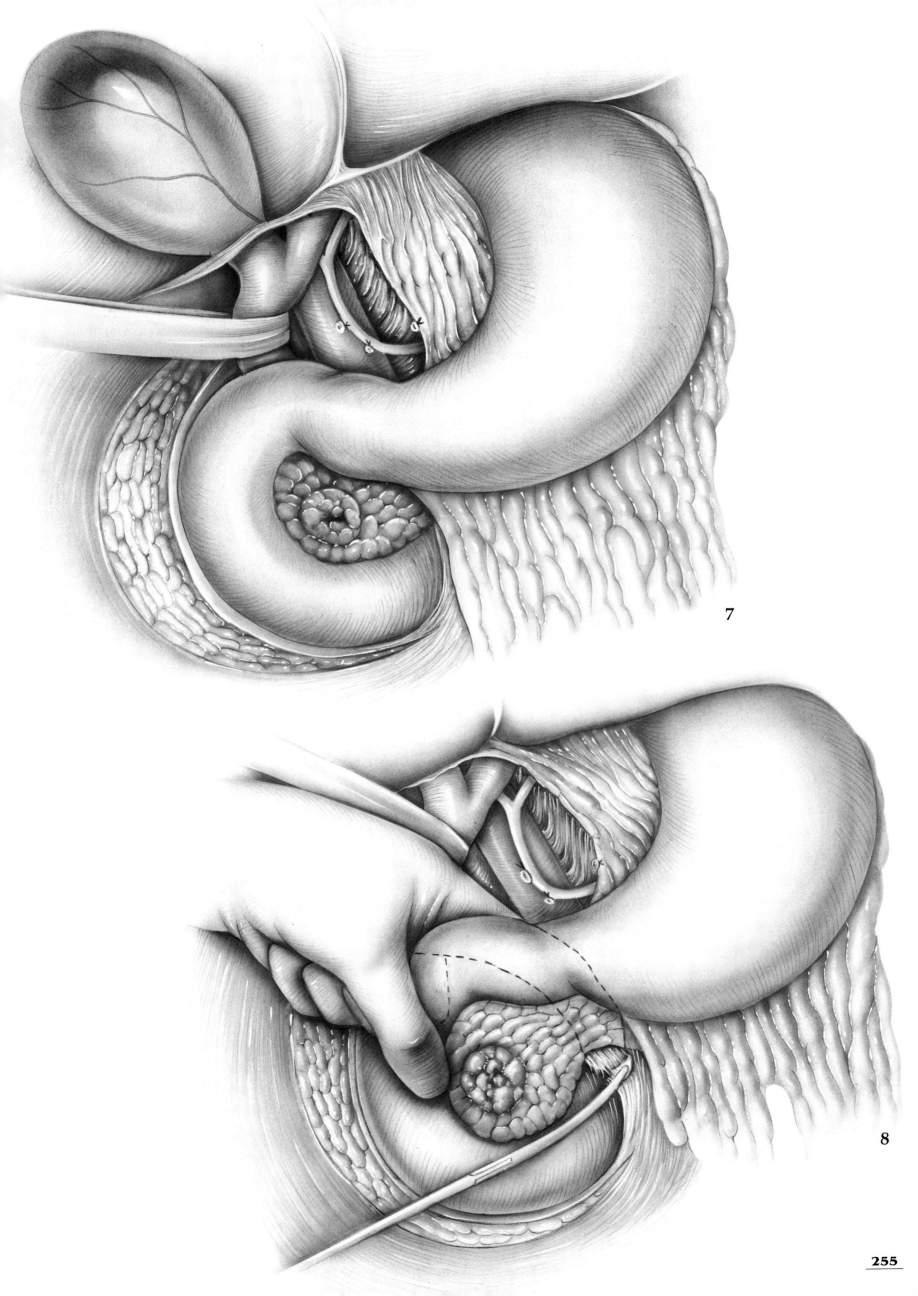

7

8

Radical Pancreaticoduodenectomy (Whipple Procedure) (*cont.*)

9–10 A long curved clamp is passed through this tunnel, clamped to the tip of the surgeon's gloved finger.

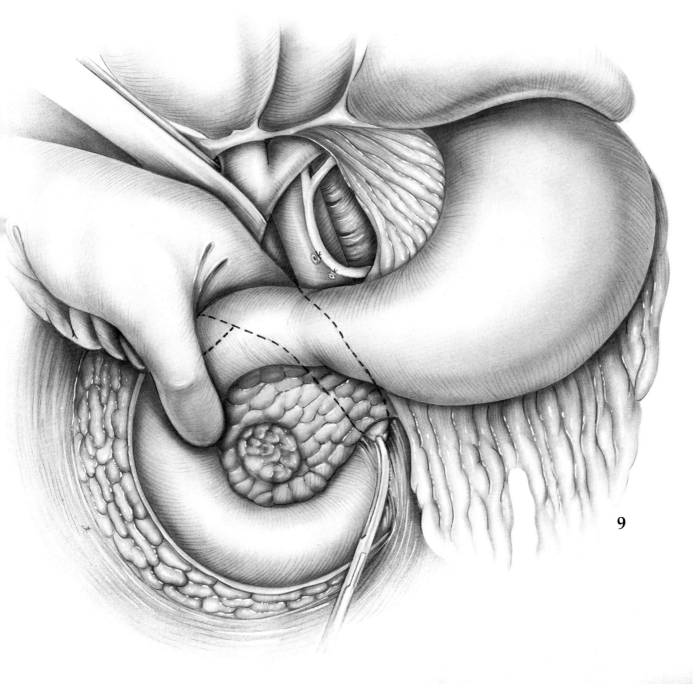

9

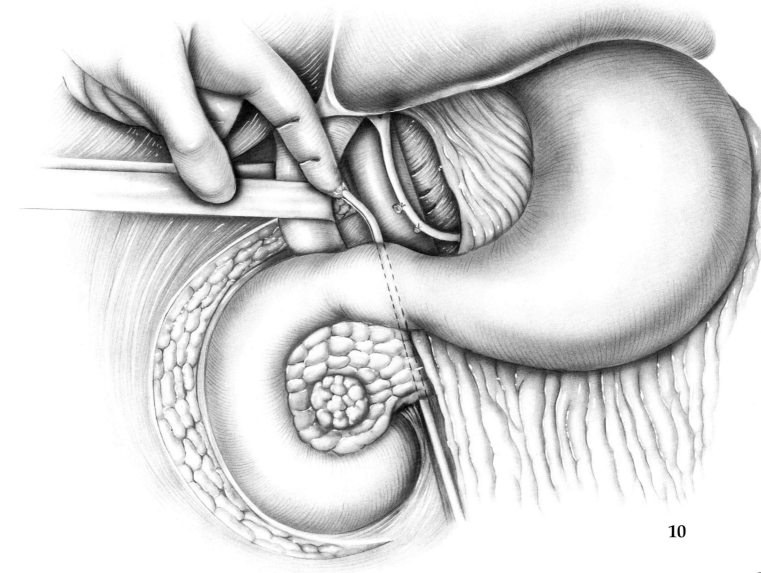

10

Radical Pancreaticoduodenectomy (Whipple Procedure) (*cont.*)

11 A Penrose drain is then brought through the plane anterior to the portal vein and posterior to the pancreas and duodenum.

12 Resectability of the tumor is reasonably assured at this point in the dissection.

13 The gallbladder is removed and the cystic duct is tied. The supraduodenal portion of the common bile duct is divided between a vascular clamp above and a crushing clamp below. The distal segment is ligated with a #00 silk tie.

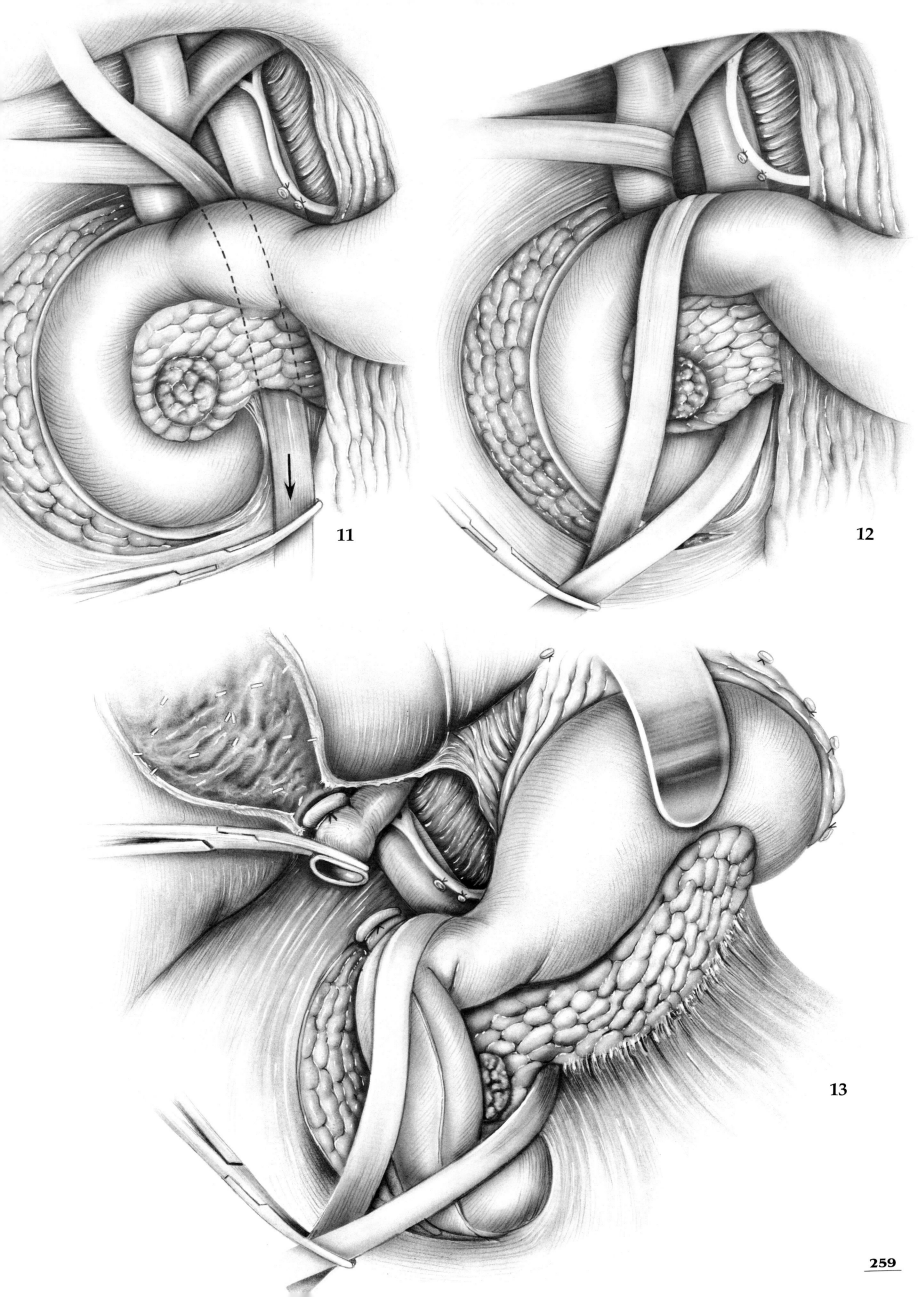

11

12

13

Radical Pancreaticoduodenectomy (Whipple Procedure) (*cont.*)

14 A Payr clamp is placed across the stomach at the level of the incisura. A linear stapling device is placed parallel and distal to the Payr clamp, and discharged. The stomach is transected between the stapler and Payr clamp with electrocautery. The stomach and proximal duodenum are then turned to the patient's right, exposing the neck of the pancreas.

15 Retraction of the neck of the pancreas with the Penrose drain permits a linear stapling device to be placed across the pancreas from below. The stapler is discharged. The pancreas is divided with electrocautery to the left of the superior mesenteric vein. Small vessels on the cut edge of the pancreas are controlled with #000 polyglycolic acid stitches.

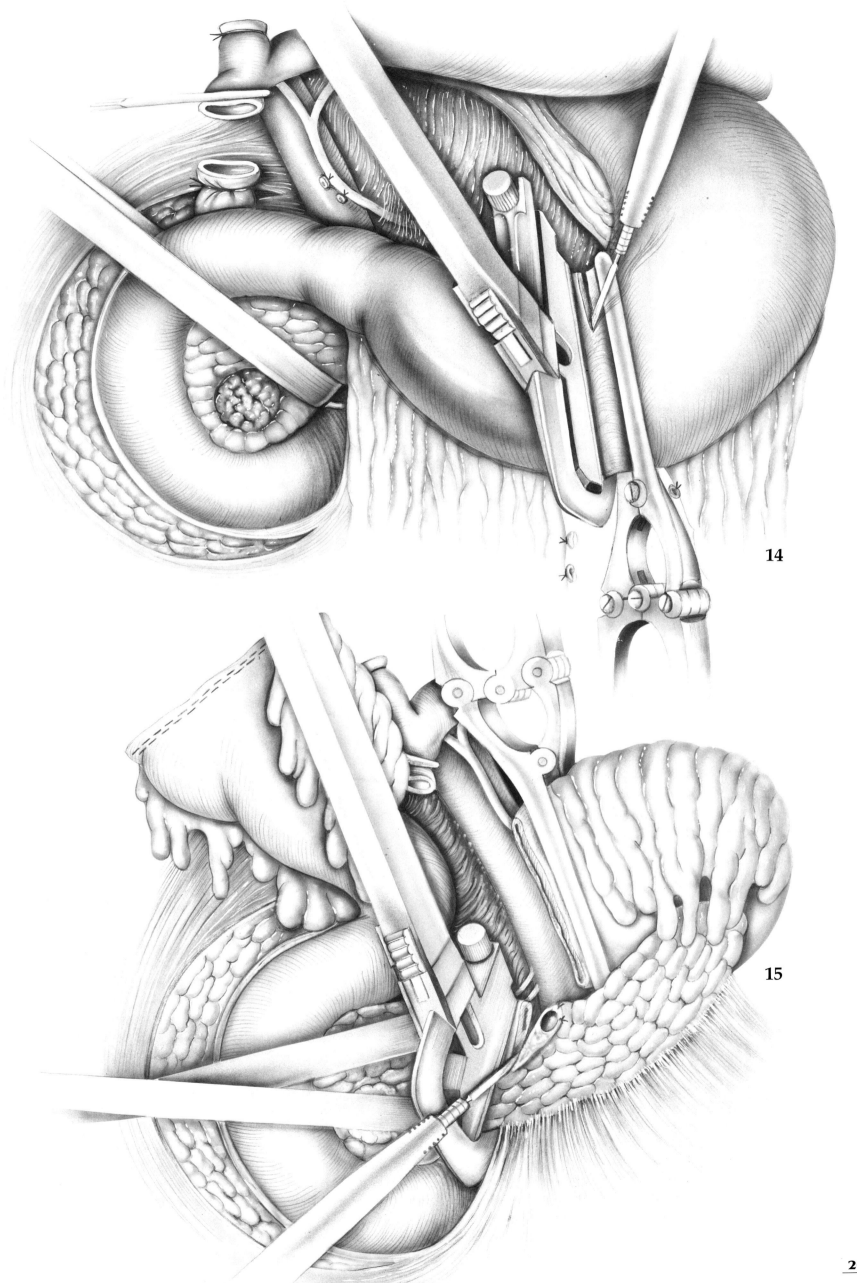

14

15

Radical Pancreaticoduodenectomy (Whipple Procedure) (*cont.*)

16 The transverse colon is retracted cephalad and the ligament of Treitz is taken down, as indicated by the broken line.

17 The jejunum, close to the ligament of Treitz, is divided with electrocautery between a linear stapling device proximally and a non-crushing bowel clamp distally. The proximal stump is then tied with an umbilical tape. The proximal jejunal mesentery is divided between clamps and tied, preserving adequate blood supply to the distal segment.

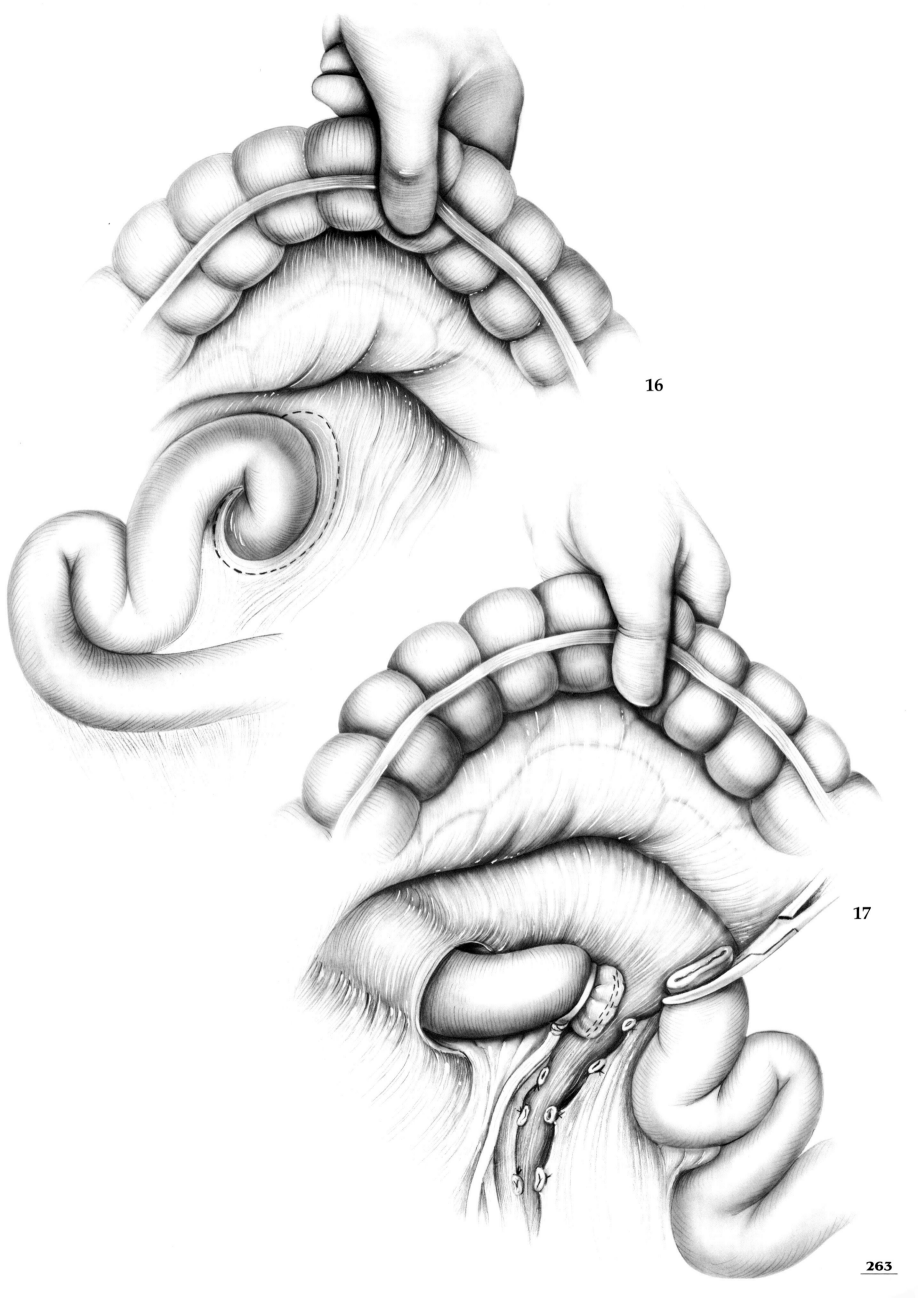

16

17

Radical Pancreaticoduodenectomy (Whipple Procedure) (*cont.*)

18 The umbilical tape is twisted around the forefinger and advanced into the lesser sac behind the most proximal jejunum, the fourth portion of the duodenum, and the superior mesenteric vessels.

19 The umbilical tape is retrieved in the lesser sac, pulling the proximal jejunum and the transverse duodenum behind it. At this point the entire specimen to be resected lies to the right of the portal and superior mesenteric veins.

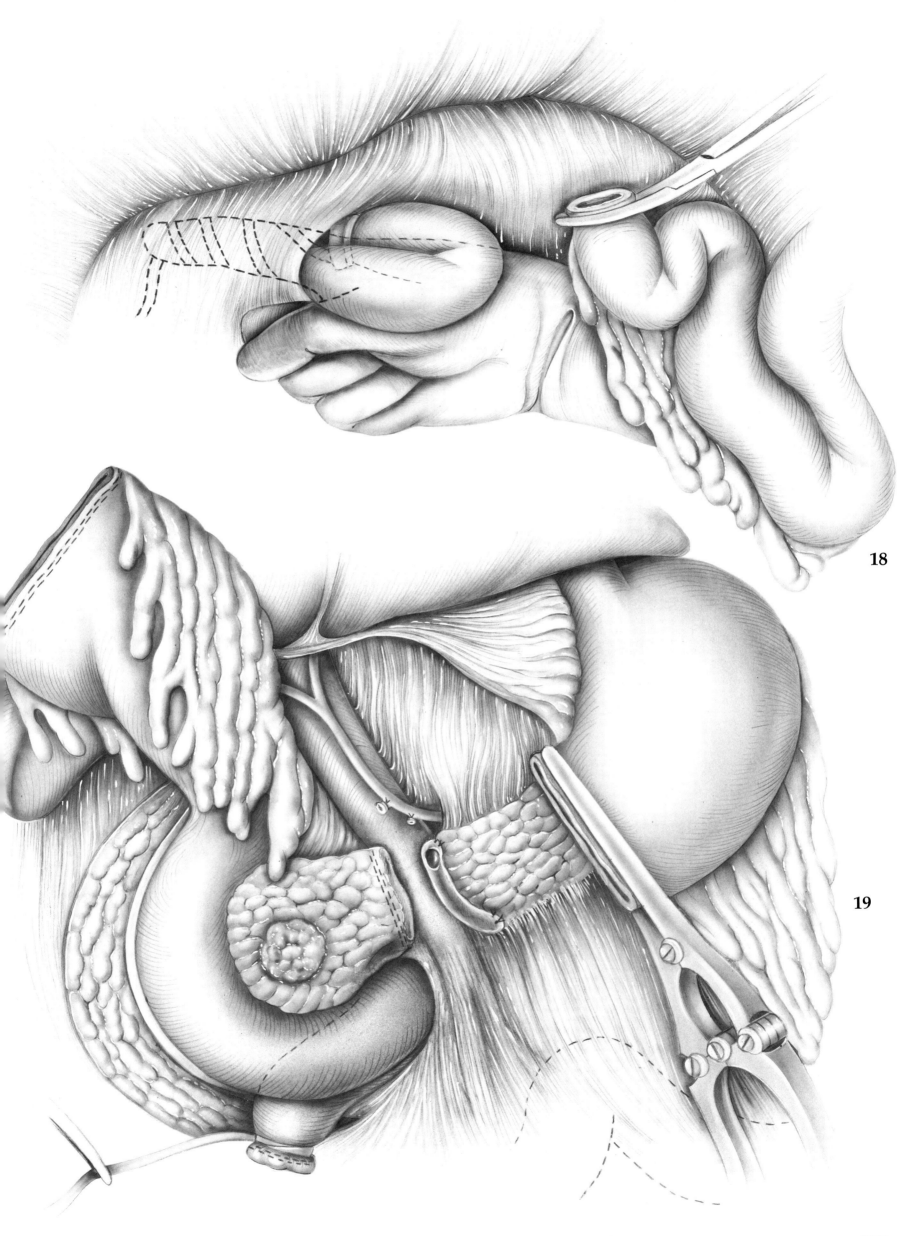

18

19

Radical Pancreaticoduodenectomy
(Whipple Procedure) (*cont.*)

20 Small communicating branches of the superior mesenteric artery and portal vein are divided on the right side of the portal vein. The portal vein may be retracted medially with the aid of a vein retractor or the open jaws of a right-angle clamp. Because the vessels to the right of the portal vein are small and avulsion can result in significant bleeding, dissection of these vessels should be minimized. This can be facilitated by passing swaged sutures under these veins, blunt end first, with the needle reversed on the needle holder. The remaining vessels to the proximal jejunum from the superior mesenteric artery and vein are divided between clamps and tied. The specimen is then removed from the operative field for pathological examination.

21 The distal jejunum is brought under the superior mesenteric vessels with the aid of a long non-crushing clamp passed from the lesser sac.

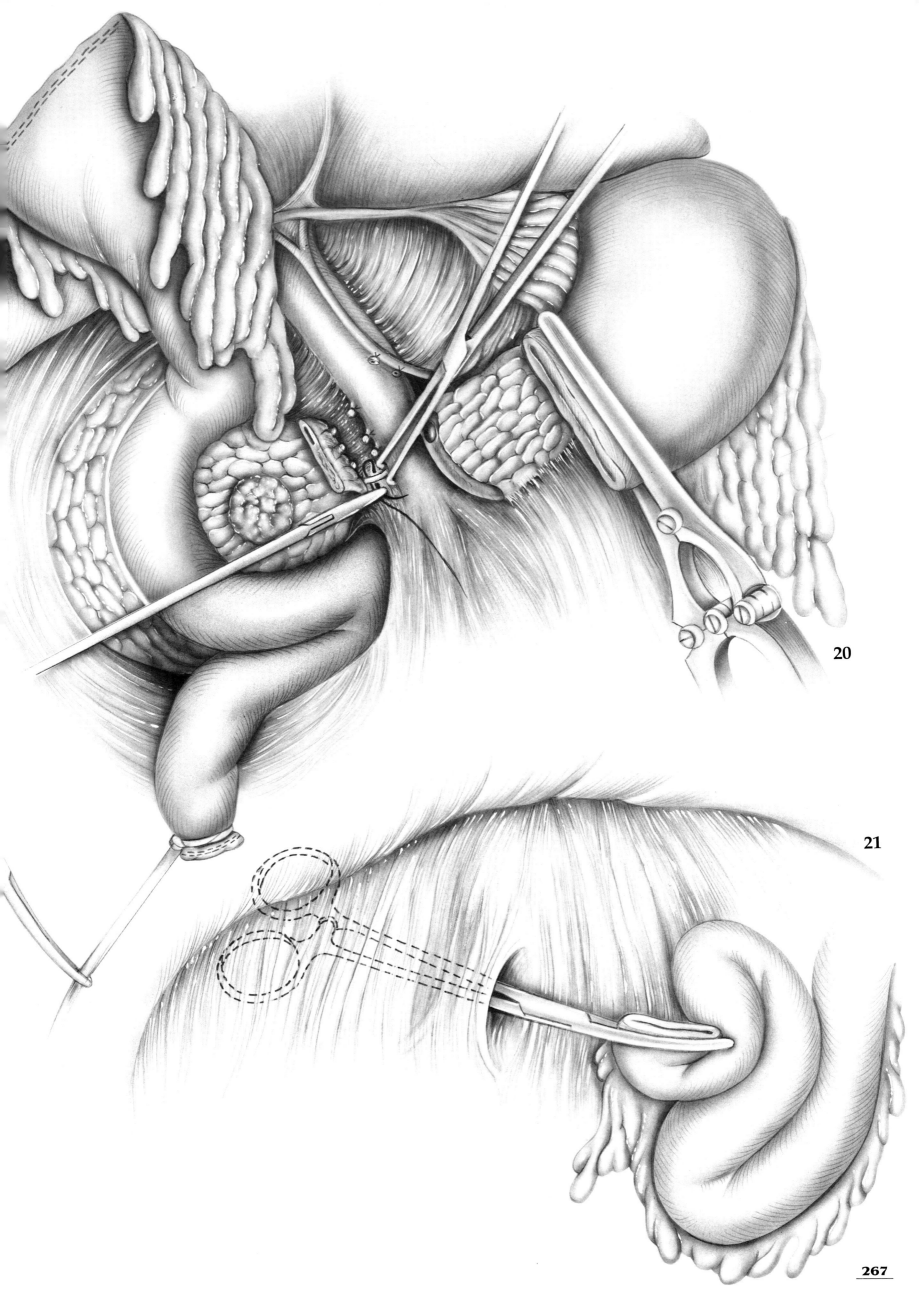

20

21

Radical Pancreaticoduodenectomy
(Whipple Procedure) (*cont.*)

22 A sufficient length of jejunum is advanced into the lesser sac for construction of the pancreaticojejunostomy, choledochojejunostomy, and gastroenterostomy.

23 A 15- to 20-cm length of Silastic tubing with side holes is introduced into the pancreatic duct.

24 A sufficient length of tubing is required to divert the pancreatic flow beyond the proposed choledochojejunostomy. The Silastic tube is held in place with two #000 polyglycolic acid sutures placed in the duct wall, into the pancreatic parenchyma, and around the catheter (**Fig. 28**).

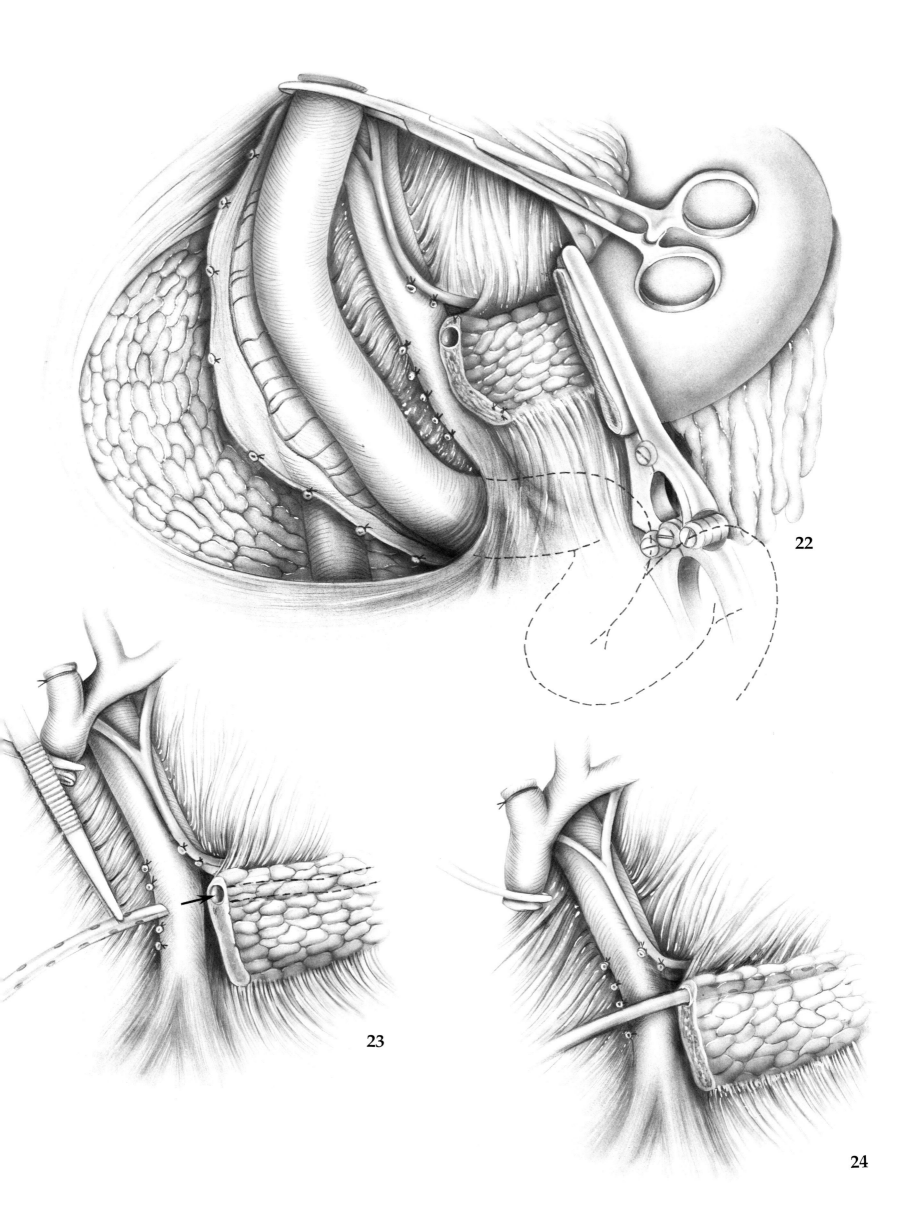

22

23

24

Radical Pancreaticoduodenectomy
(Whipple Procedure) (*cont.*)

25–30 The pancreaticojejunostomy is constructed so as to place the proximal 2 cm of pancreas within the lumen of the jejunum, similar to a hand in a glove. The perforated catheter in the pancreatic duct is passed down the lumen of the jejunum. The pancreaticojejunostomy is accomplished by everting the mucosa and submucosa of the distal 3 cm of jejunum. Two or three Allis clamps are placed into the jejunal lumen (**Fig. 25**), grasping the mucosa and submucosa, thus permitting the bowel to be folded back upon itself (**Fig. 26**). On cross section, this exposes the full thickness of the bowel at the everted edge (**Fig. 27**). The cut edge of the pancreas is sewn to the everted jejunal wall. This suture line is performed circumferentially with interrupted #000 polyglycolic acid stitches which include the mucosa, submucosa, and muscular coats of the jejunum (**Fig. 28**). The jejunum is then turned right-side-out, ducking the pancreatic stump into the lumen of the jejunum. A second layer of interrupted #000 polyglycolic acid sutures secures the pancreatic capsule to the cut end of the jejunal limb both posteriorly and then anteriorly (**Figs. 29–30**). This technique places the transected pancreas completely and securely within the lumen of the jejunum, without tension. If the pancreas is too wide to allow inversion, the anterior muscular coat of the jejunum may be incised to increase the luminal diameter.

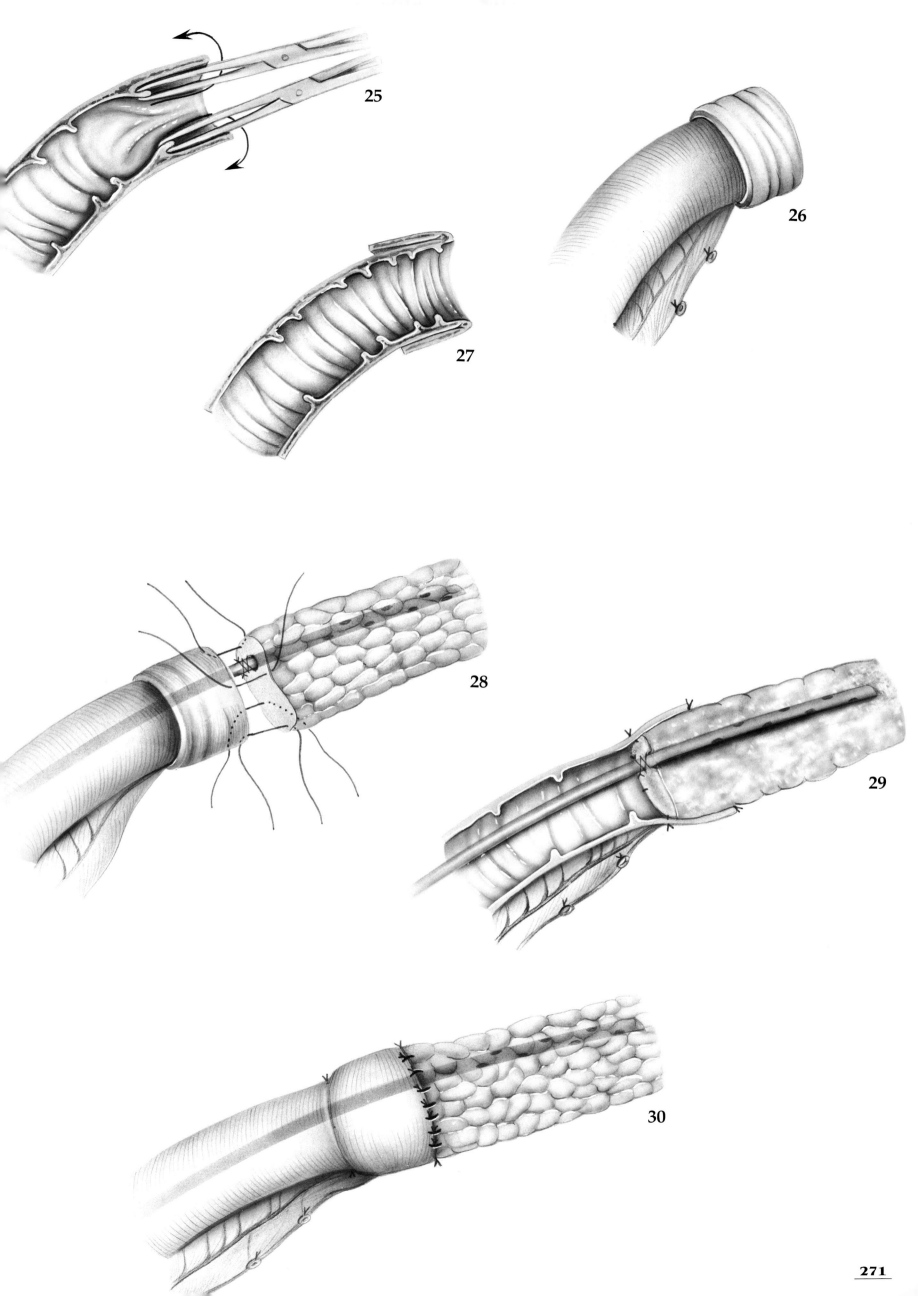

Radical Pancreaticoduodenectomy (Whipple Procedure) (*cont.*)

31 The choledochojejunostomy is constructed at a point where the cut end of the common bile duct rests against the jejunum. This usually occurs 7 to 10 cm distal to the pancreatico-jejunostomy. An antimesenteric jejunal enterotomy is made, matching the diameter of the common bile duct.

32 Two full-thickness #000 polyglycolic acid corner sutures are placed. The posterior suture line is accomplished in an interrupted fashion with #000 polyglycolic acid stitches from within the lumen of the anastomosis.

33 The interrupted anterior layer completes the anastomosis between the common bile duct and the jejunum.

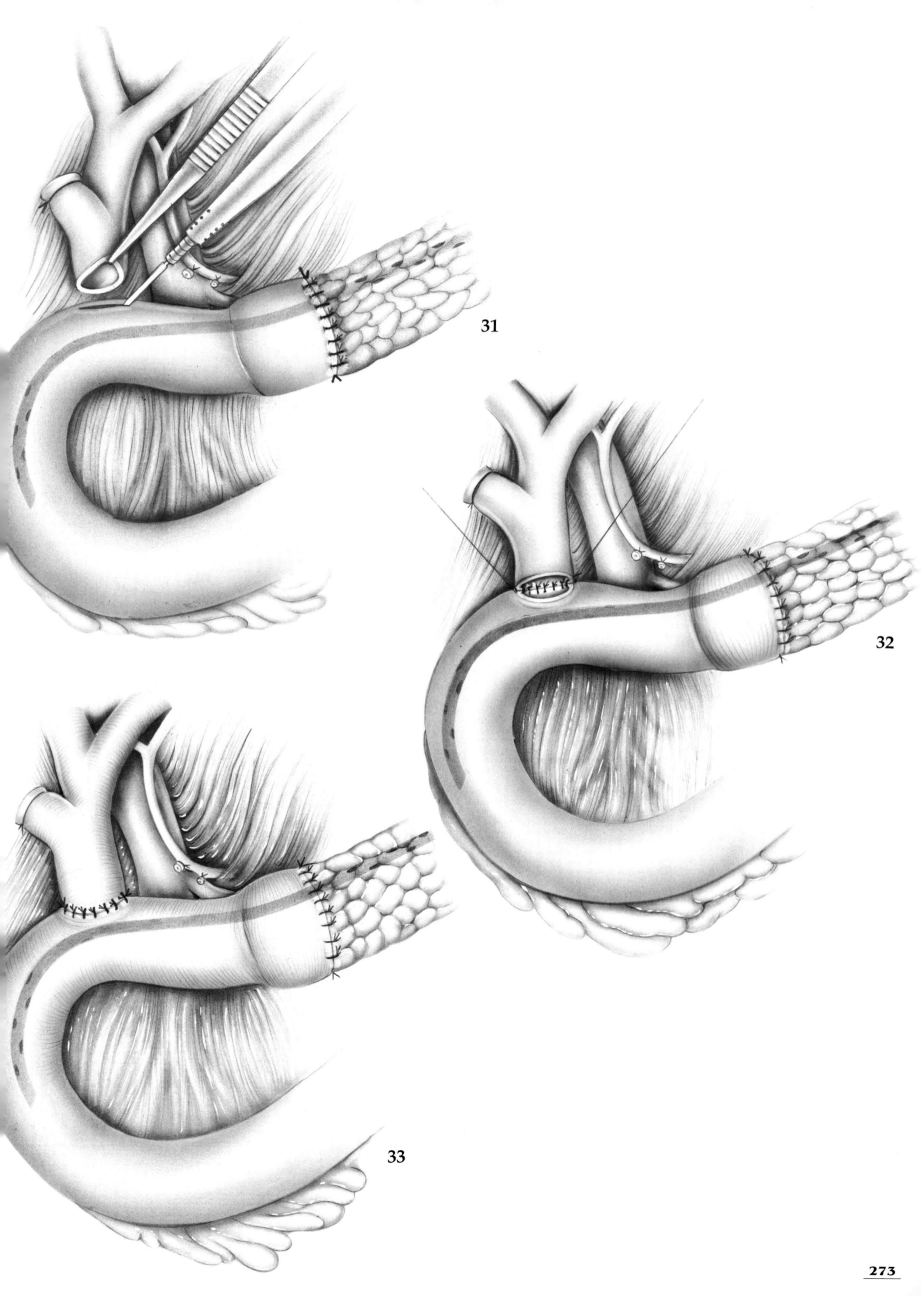

31

32

33

Radical Pancreaticoduodenectomy
(Whipple Procedure) (*cont.*)

34 The gastrojejunostomy is constructed at least 45 cm from the choledochojejunostomy. The full width of the gastric lumen is used for the anastomosis. The two-suture gastrojejunostomy may be used here (see **Plates 20–22, Figs. 4–11**). A posterior, seromuscular, running #00 polyglycolic acid suture line is created between the closed jejunum and the gastric remnant prior to removal of the Payr clamp. This suture is set aside, and a jejunal enterotomy is made opposite the cut edge of the stomach.

35 A full-thickness continuous #00 polyglycolic acid layer is run circumferentially from the posterior and the anterior inner suture lines.

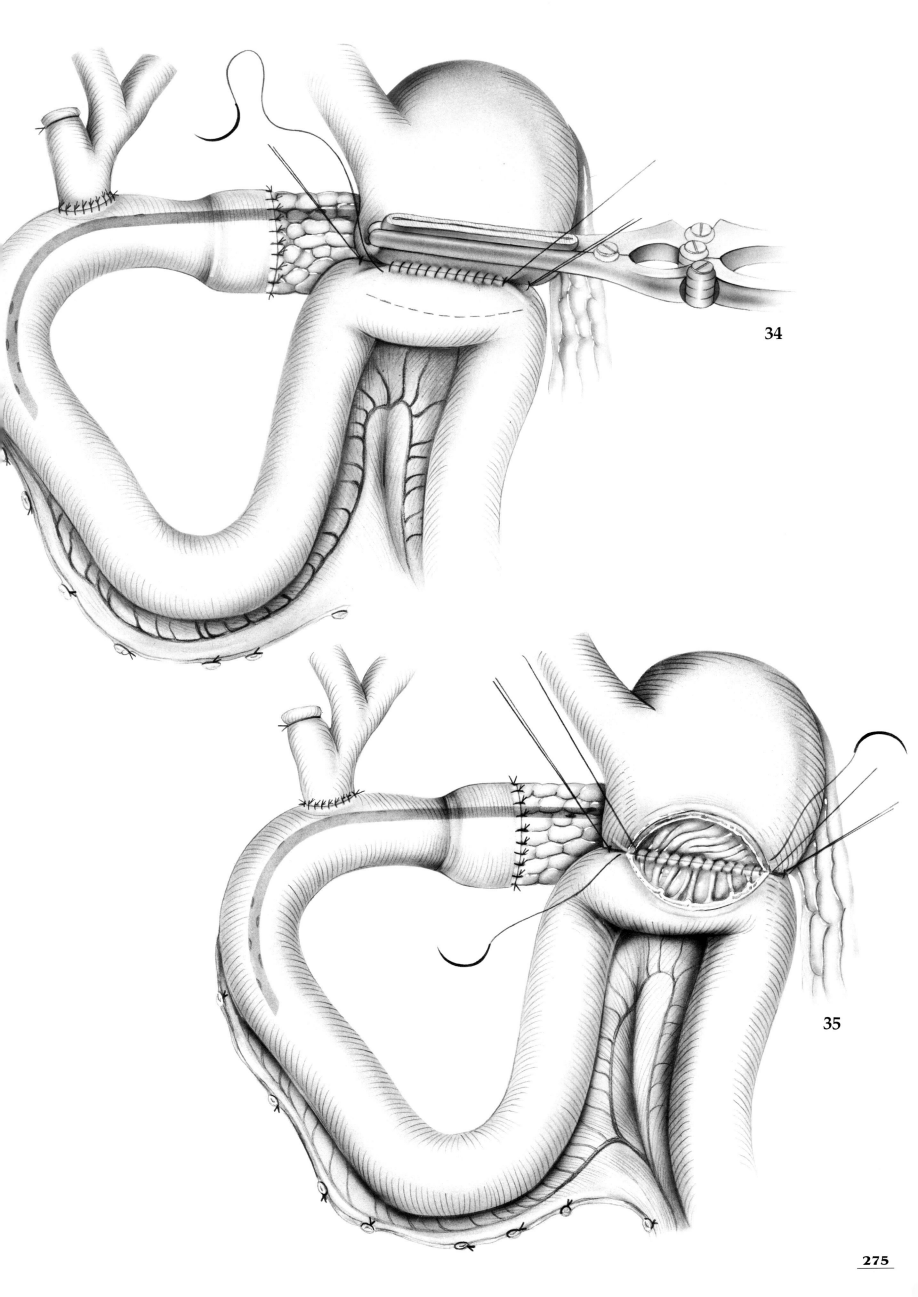

34

35

Radical Pancreaticoduodenectomy (Whipple Procedure) (*cont.*)

36 The inner suture line is completed by tying the stitch to the tail of the suture at the starting point.

37 The original suture is retrieved and the anterior, outer, seromuscular suture line is accomplished, completing the gastrojejunostomy.

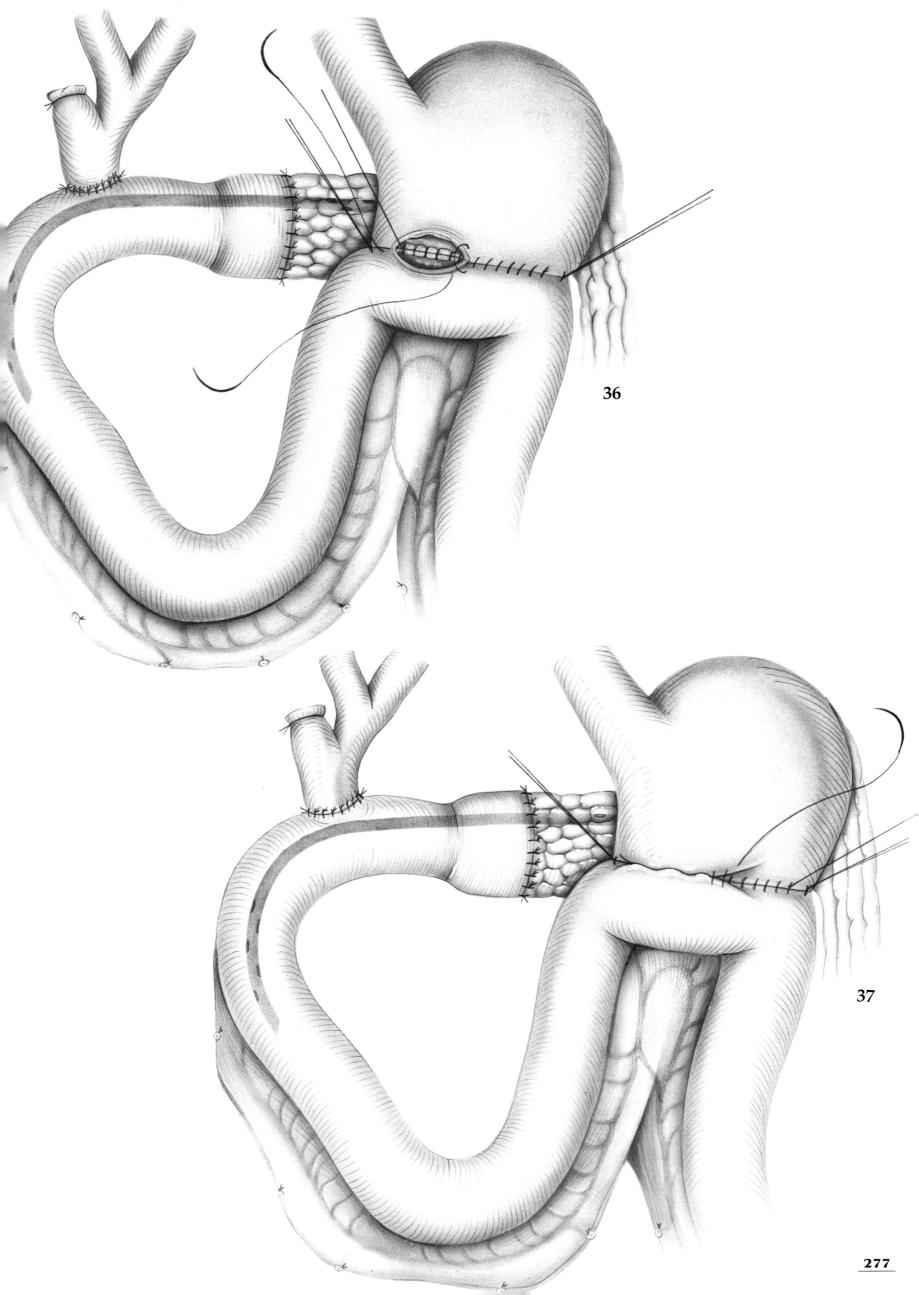

36

37

Radical Pancreaticoduodenectomy
(Whipple Procedure) (*cont.*)

38 A sump nasogastric tube is advanced through the gastrojejunostomy. Several #000 poly-glycolic acid sutures are used to tack the jejunum in place as it passes under the superior mesenteric vessels. These sutures are placed from either above or below the transverse mesocolon, whichever is more convenient.

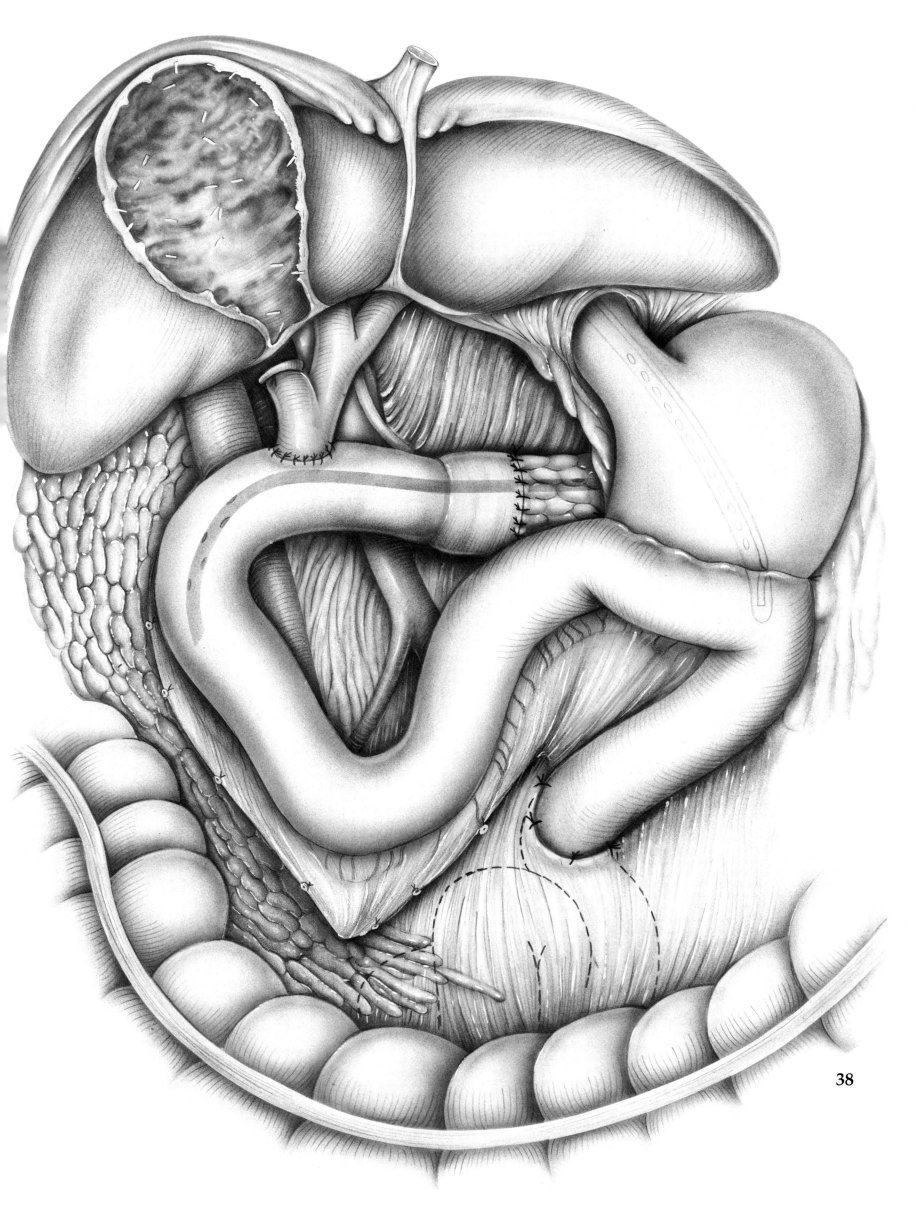

38

Distal Pancreatectomy

1 The abdomen is explored through an upper midline or left subcostal incision. The lesser sac is entered by dividing the gastrocolic ligament between clamps, or with a ligating and dividing stapling device.

2 With the stomach retracted cephalad, the splenic artery is identified at the superior border of the pancreas near its origin at the celiac axis. The artery is then dissected free, divided, and tied with #00 silk ligatures.

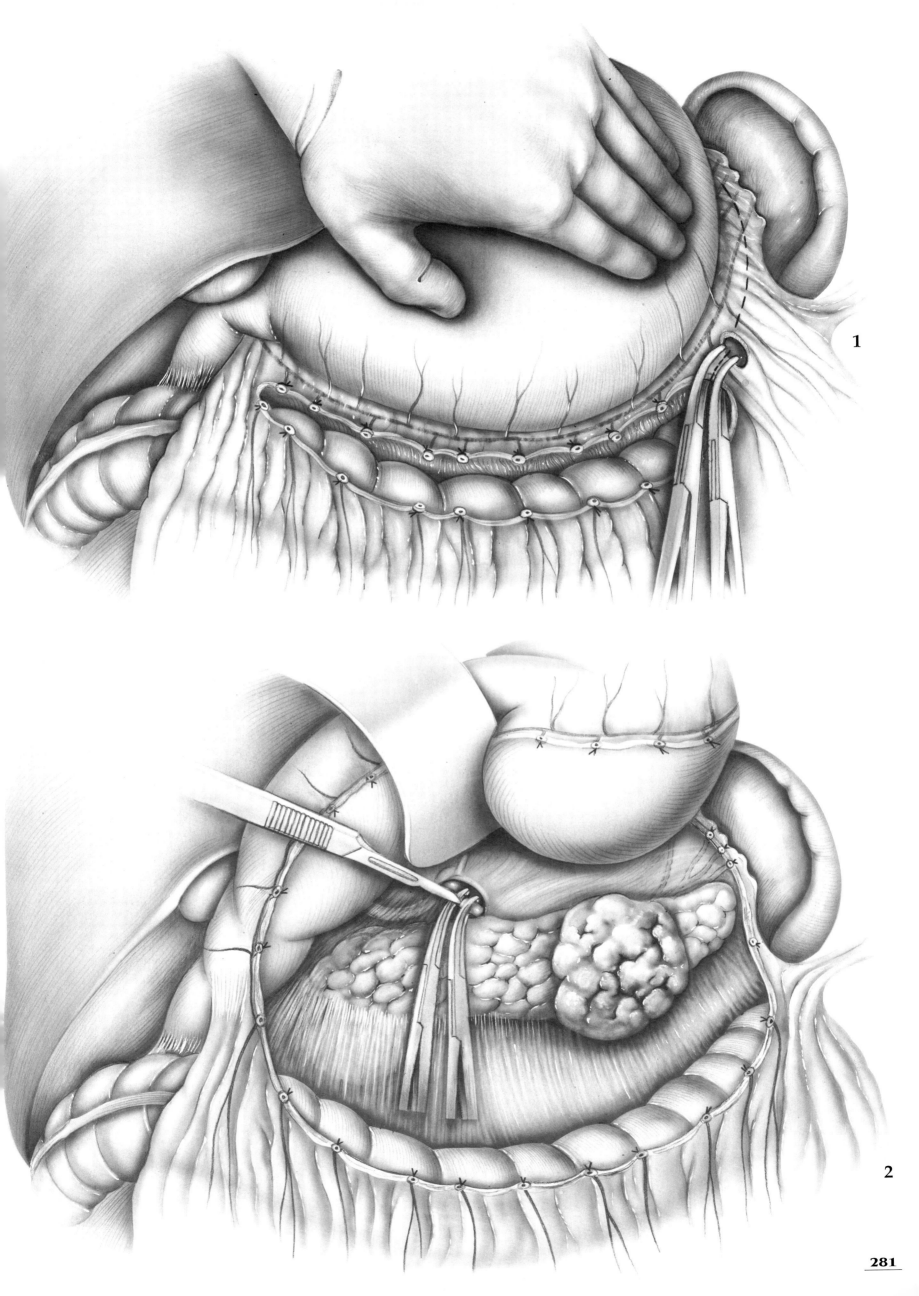

Distal Pancreatectomy (*cont.*)

3 The retroperitoneal investments of the pancreas are incised both superiorly and inferiorly with electrocautery over the open jaws of a right-angle clamp. The inferior mesenteric vein is identified, dissected free, clamped, divided, and securely tied.

4 A finger is insinuated beneath the pancreas from below and tunneled toward the hepatic artery. The finger commonly passes between the pancreas and the splenic vein.

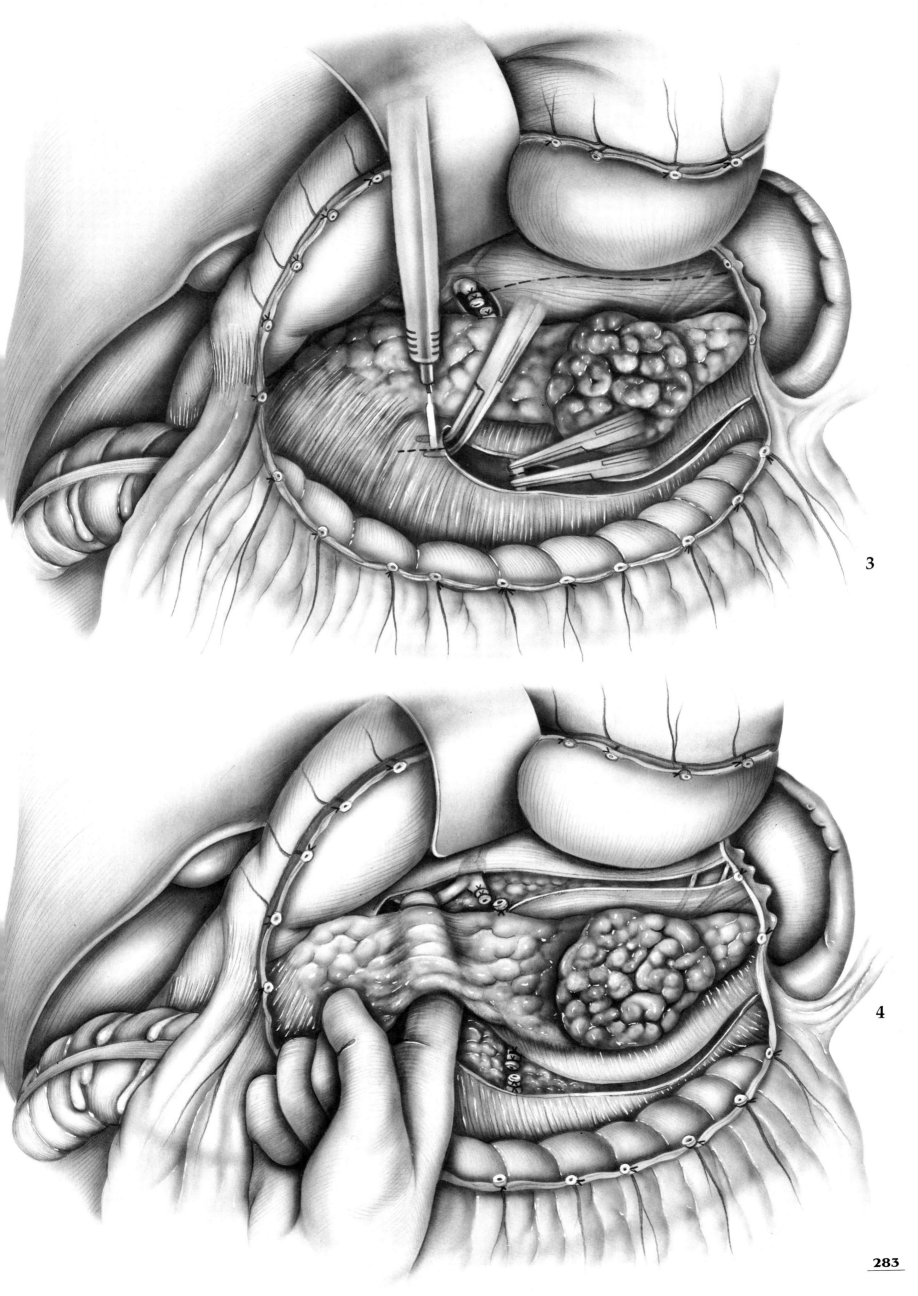

3

4

Distal Pancreatectomy (*cont.*)

5 The body of the pancreas is encircled with a Penrose drain. The Penrose drain is retracted to the patient's left, and a linear stapling device is fired across the neck of the pancreas. The pancreas is then divided with electrocautery, carefully avoiding injury to the underlying splenic vein, which may or may not be included in the staple line.

6 The splenic vein either has been included in the staple line or is visible beneath the divided pancreas, as shown. If it has been stapled shut, an additional ligature is placed toward the side of the portal and superior mesenteric veins by passing a clamp around the vein beyond the staple line. More commonly the intact vessel is seen in the retroperitoneum behind the pancreas. In these cases it is divided between clamps and ligated. Alternatively, it may be left intact at this time and divided after the spleen is mobilized, as in **Fig. 8.**

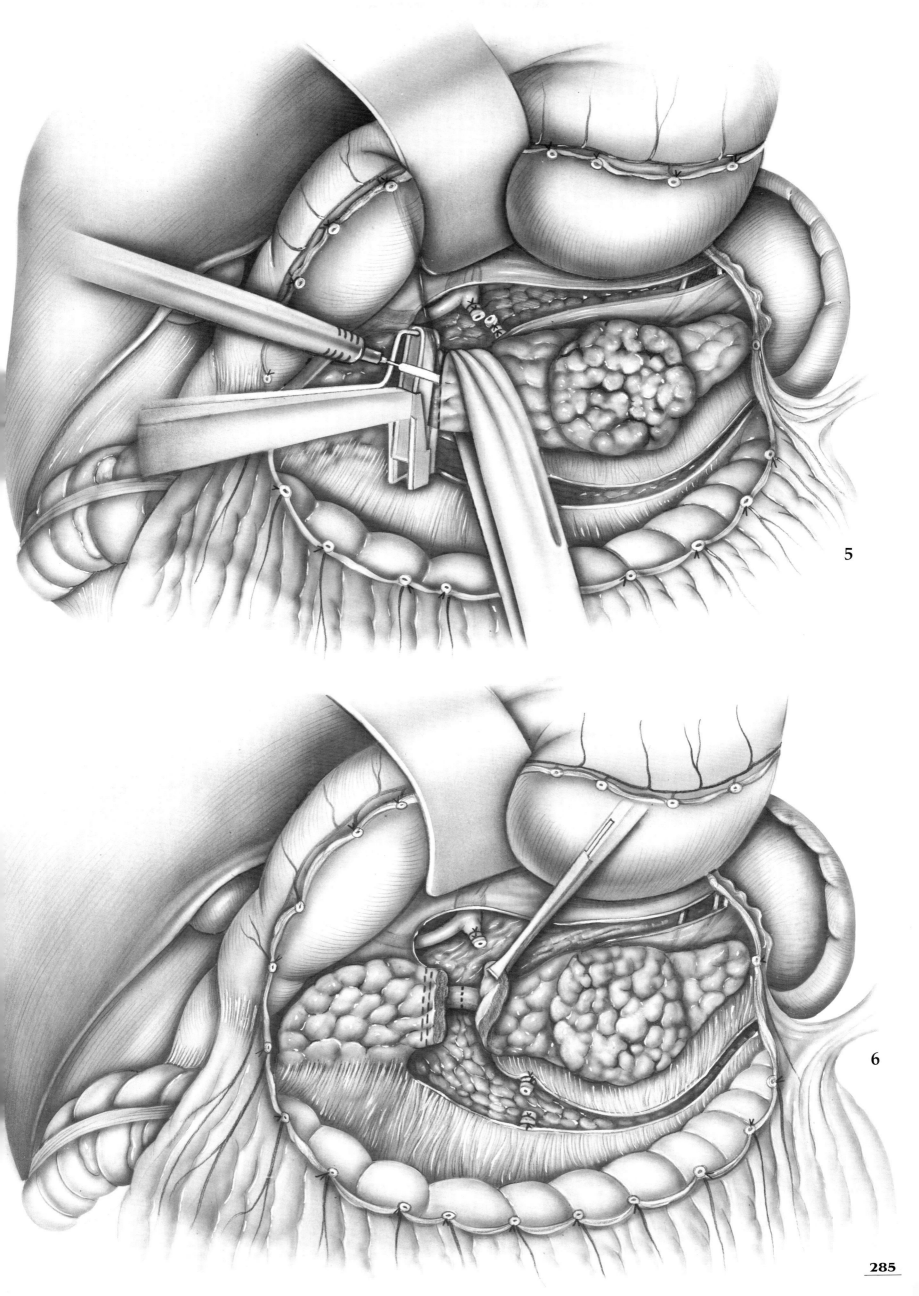

5

6

Distal Pancreatectomy (*cont.*)

7 The lateral splenic attachments are freed.

8 The spleen and pancreas are bluntly dissected from the retroperitoneum and rotated medially. If the splenic vein remains intact it is clamped, divided, and ligated. The specimen, including the tail of the pancreas and spleen, is removed.

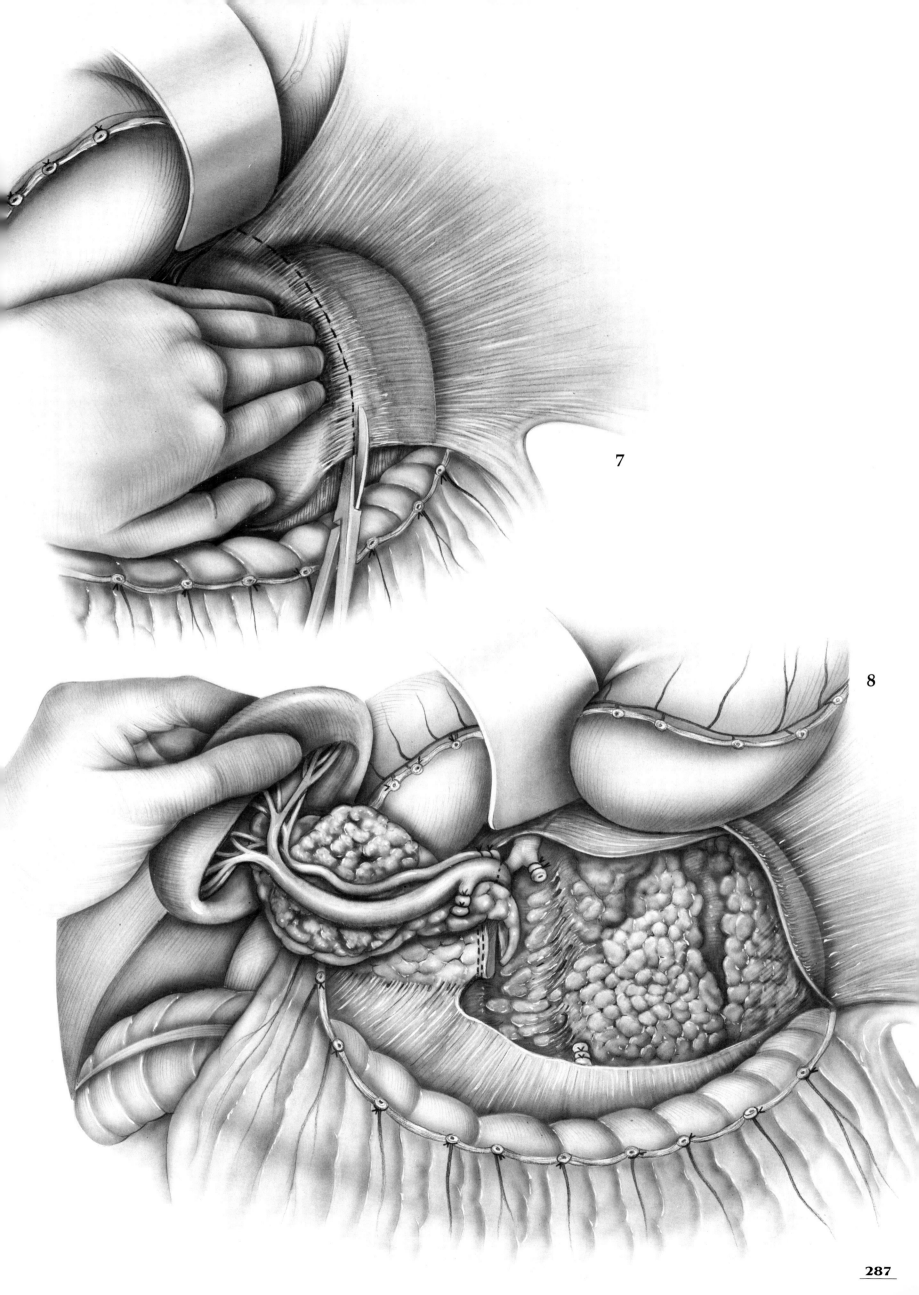

7

8

Distal Pancreatectomy (*cont.*)

9 A tongue of omentum is brought up and sutured with #000 polyglycolic acid stitches over the stapled neck of the pancreas. Two closed suction drains are placed in the pancreatic and splenic bed and brought out to the skin through separate incisions. They are secured to the skin with heavy silk sutures.

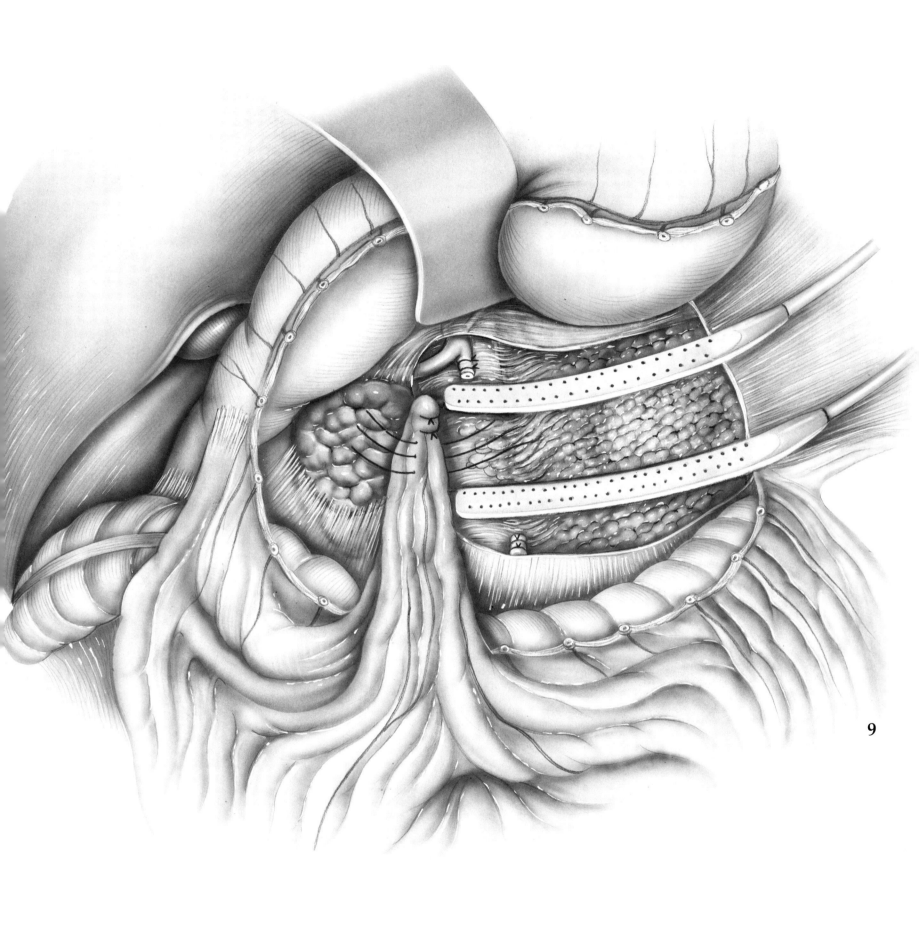

9

Choledochogastrostomy for Palliative Biliary Bypass

1 Most other techniques of biliary and duodenal bypass performed for unresectable pancreatic cancer drain the bile distal to the gastrojejunostomy. Because the pancreatic duct is obstructed by the malignancy in the head of the pancreas and the bile is diverted beyond the gastrojejunostomy, the stomach acid remains unbuffered by either the pancreatic bicarbonate or the diverted bile—putting the patient at risk for marginal ulceration of the gastrojejunostomy. The choledochogastrostomy bypasses the obstructed biliary system into the stomach, which serves to buffer the gastric acid, thus protecting the gastrojejunal anastomosis from marginal ulceration. In addition, the patency of this bypass can easily be assessed either by aspiration of the gastric lumen—looking for bile—or by visualization of the biliary tree with a soluble-contrast upper gastrointestinal series.

   If the pancreatic tumor is locally unresectable or the patient is not a candidate for radical resection, a choledochogastrostomy is performed along with a gastrojejunostomy for palliative bypass of both the duodenum and the biliary system.

   Cholecystectomy is not necessary. By not performing it, one avoids dissection of the soft, friable livers of these patients. The gallbladder shrinks within 1 month to a small diverticulum off the common bile duct.

2 The common duct is freed circumferentially immediately above the duodenum.

3 The common bile duct is encircled with a Penrose drain.

4 Retraction on the Penrose drain facilitates further dissection of the common bile duct.

5 The distal common bile duct is clamped, and transected above the clamp.

6 The distal stump of the common bile duct is closed with a #00 polyglycolic acid suture ligature.

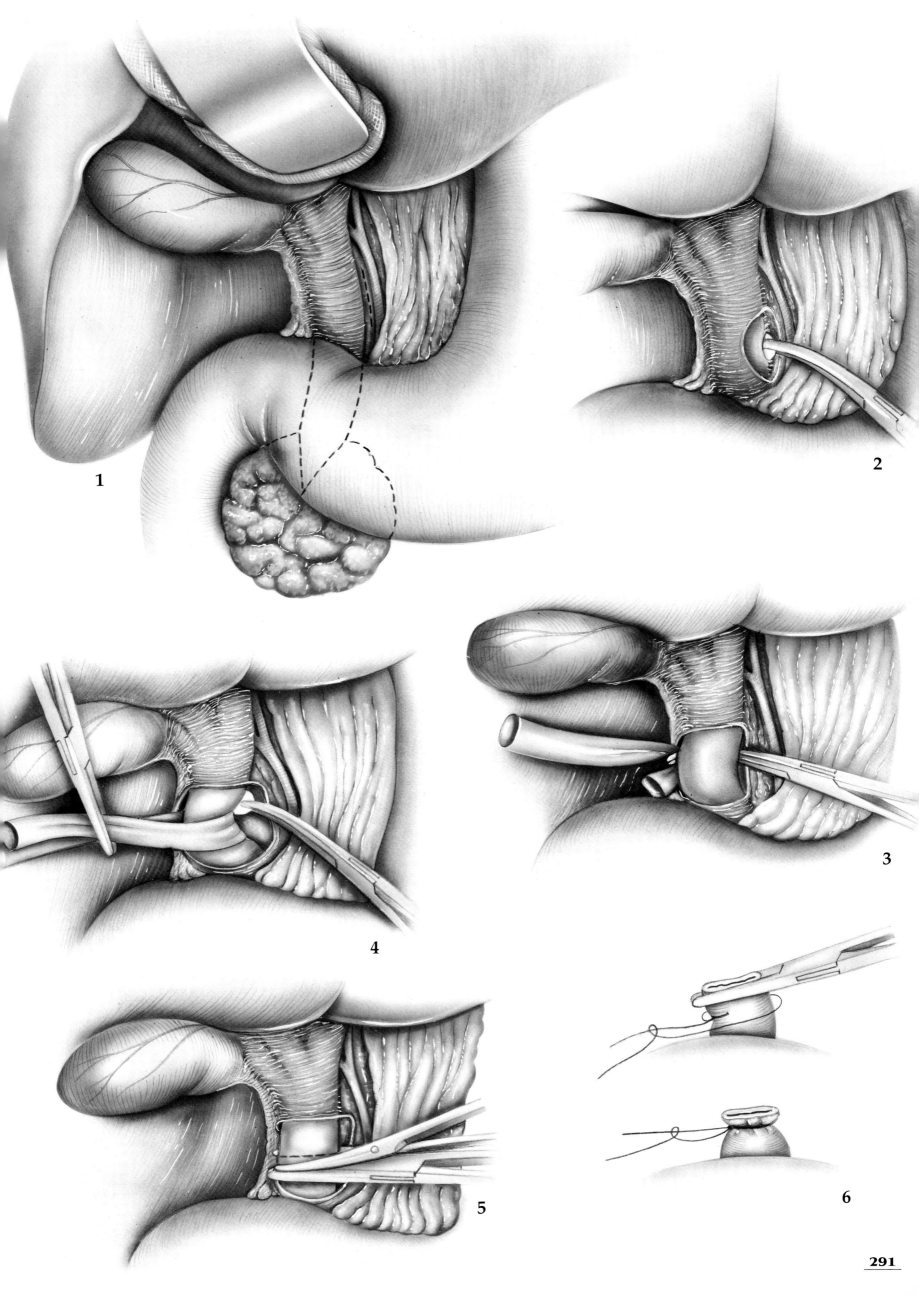

Choledochogastrostomy for Palliative Biliary Bypass (*cont.*)

7 A single-layer end-to-side choledochogastrostomy is fashioned between the proximal common bile duct stump and the distal antrum. The distal stomach can always be brought high into the hilus of the liver without dissection. A gastrotomy is made with electrocautery at the site of the proposed anastomosis. Two #000 polyglycolic acid corner stitches are placed.

8–9 Occasionally the cystic duct is transected and presents in the wall of the posterior suture line. To avoid obstructing the cystic duct lumen with the suture, a stitch is placed on the common wall of the cystic duct and common duct. A triangular segment of this wall is excised so that the gallbladder will continue to drain after the completion of the anastomosis.

10 The posterior row is accomplished from within the lumen of the anastomosis with interrupted #000 polyglycolic acid sutures. These sutures are not tied until the posterior row is complete. The knots are tied inside the lumen.

11–12 Interrupted #000 polyglycolic acid sutures are placed to complete the anterior row of the anastomosis. A gastrojejunostomy is then carried out as previously described (**Plates 20–22**). A closed suction drain is placed posterior to the anastomosis and brought out through a separate incision.

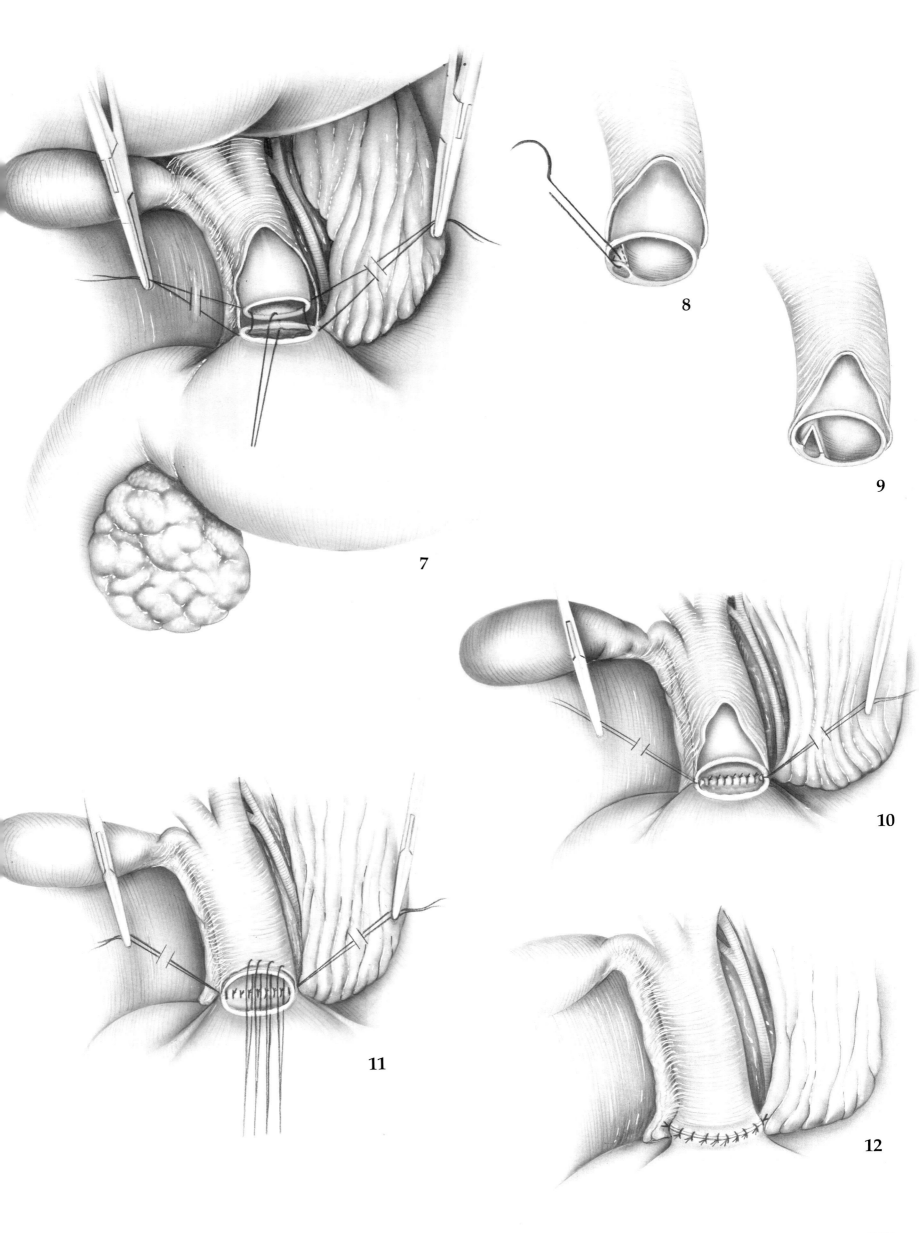

7

8

9

10

11

12

Adrenalectomy (Abdominal Approach)

1 The abdomen is explored through a bilateral subcostal incision.

2 There are two anterior approaches to the left adrenal, either through the lesser sac or via the base of the mesocolon. When approaching the adrenal through the mesocolon, the retroperitoneum behind the pancreas is exposed as for the splenorenal shunts (**Plate 107, Figs. 2–4**). The procedure performed through the lesser sac is illustrated. The gastrocolic ligament is divided between clamps, and the lesser sac is entered.

3 The peritoneum at the lower border of the pancreas is incised and the inferior mesenteric vein exposed, clamped, divided, and tied with #00 silk ligatures.

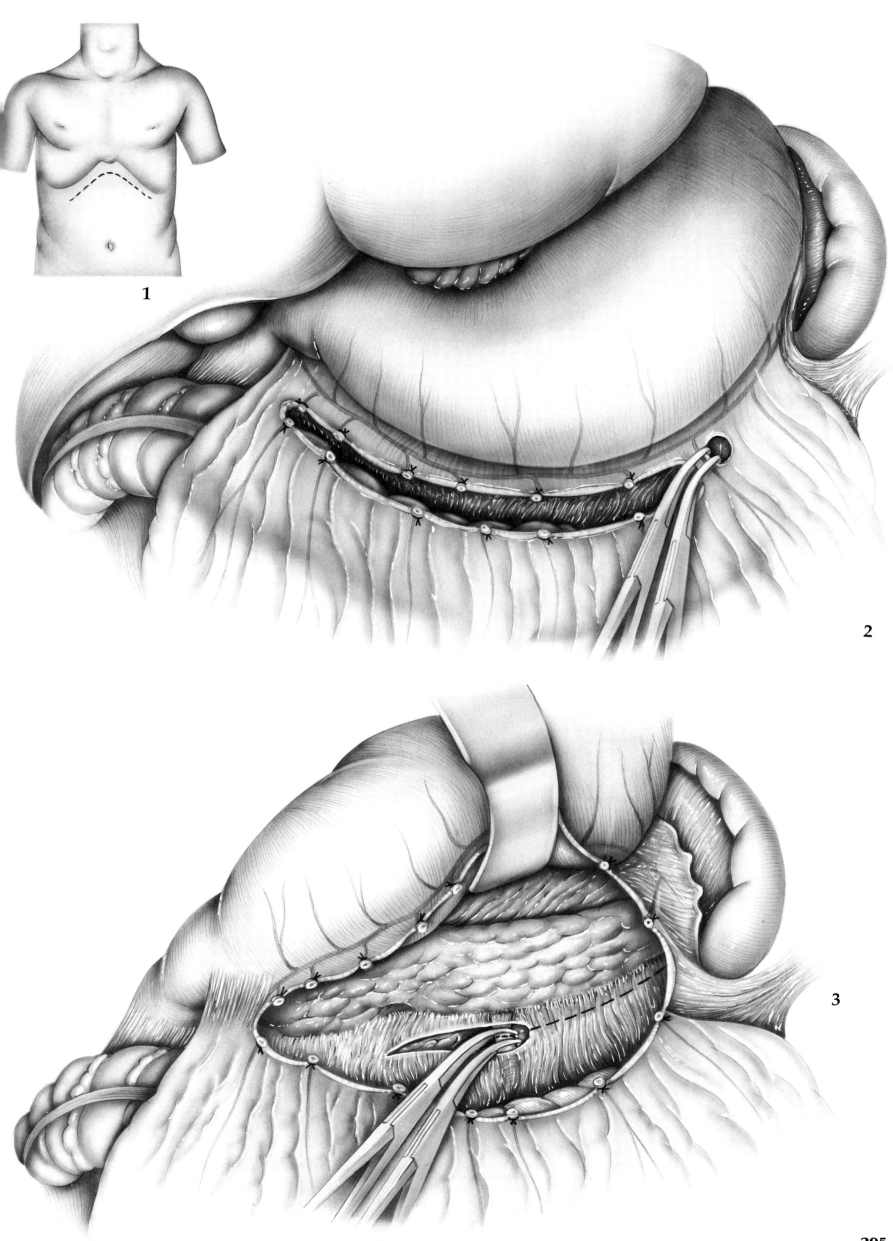

Adrenalectomy (Abdominal Approach) (*cont.*)

4 Gentle retraction of the pancreas cephalad, and blunt dissection in the plane deep to the pancreas, exposes the left adrenal medial to the superior pole of the kidney. The left adrenal vein is dissected from its entrance into the left renal vein. It is safest to divide and ligate this vein first, thus preventing continued catecholamine flow from a pheochromocytoma. In addition, a clamp on the adrenal side of this vein provides a handle for the subsequent dissection of the adrenal.

5 Traction on the proximal adrenal vein stump exposes small arteries and veins arising from the retroperitoneum and kidney capsule. These vessels are divided between surgical clips. Once these vessels are divided, the adrenal can be manipulated and freed from its attachments. Because the adrenal is manipulated on the stump of the adrenal vein and because the vessels are ligated with clips, compression of the gland is minimized along with the potential for release of vasoactive mediators.

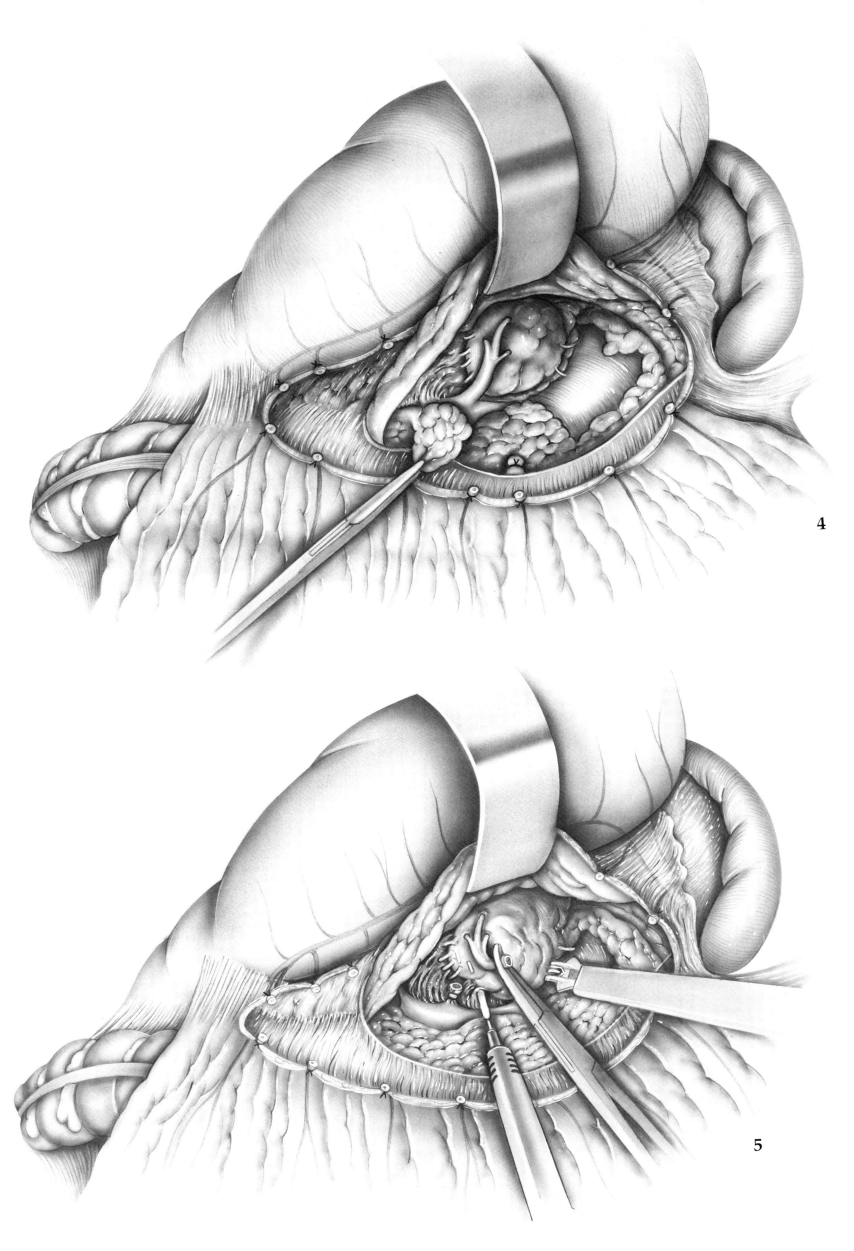

4

5

Adrenalectomy (Abdominal Approach) (*cont.*)

6 The right adrenal is exposed by incising the peritoneum lateral to the duodenum (Kocher incision). A superior extension of this incision is made toward the junction of the posterior retroperitoneum and the posterior attachments of the liver, as indicated by the broken line.

7 The right adrenal is palpated on the vena cava, medial to the superior pole of the right kidney, after retraction of the liver superiorly and the duodenum medially. The right adrenal may extend well behind the vena cava and superiorly beneath the liver. It is easiest to start the dissection at the inferior pole of the adrenal. A segment of the renal capsule is incised with the electrocautery. The edge of the capsule is grasped; with a tonsil clamp with which the adrenal is manipulated as it is bluntly dissected from its retroperitoneal attachments.

8 Medial retraction of a vascular silk suture placed through the anterior wall of the vena cava, adjacent to the adrenal, is one technique for approaching the short, and commonly retrocaval, right adrenal vein. This maneuver exposes a longer length of the adrenal vein, which is tied in continuity and then divided.

9 Alternatively a vein retractor can be used to distract the vena cava from the adrenal, exposing the adrenal vein. A tonsil clamp is used to dissect the adrenal vein. Again, the adrenal vein is ligated in continuity prior to division.

10 Using the clamp on the proximal adrenal vein, a finger can be used to tease the adrenal from its retroperitoneal bed. Surgical clips are applied to the small arteries and veins that fix the adrenal to the retroperitoneum and to the renal capsule.

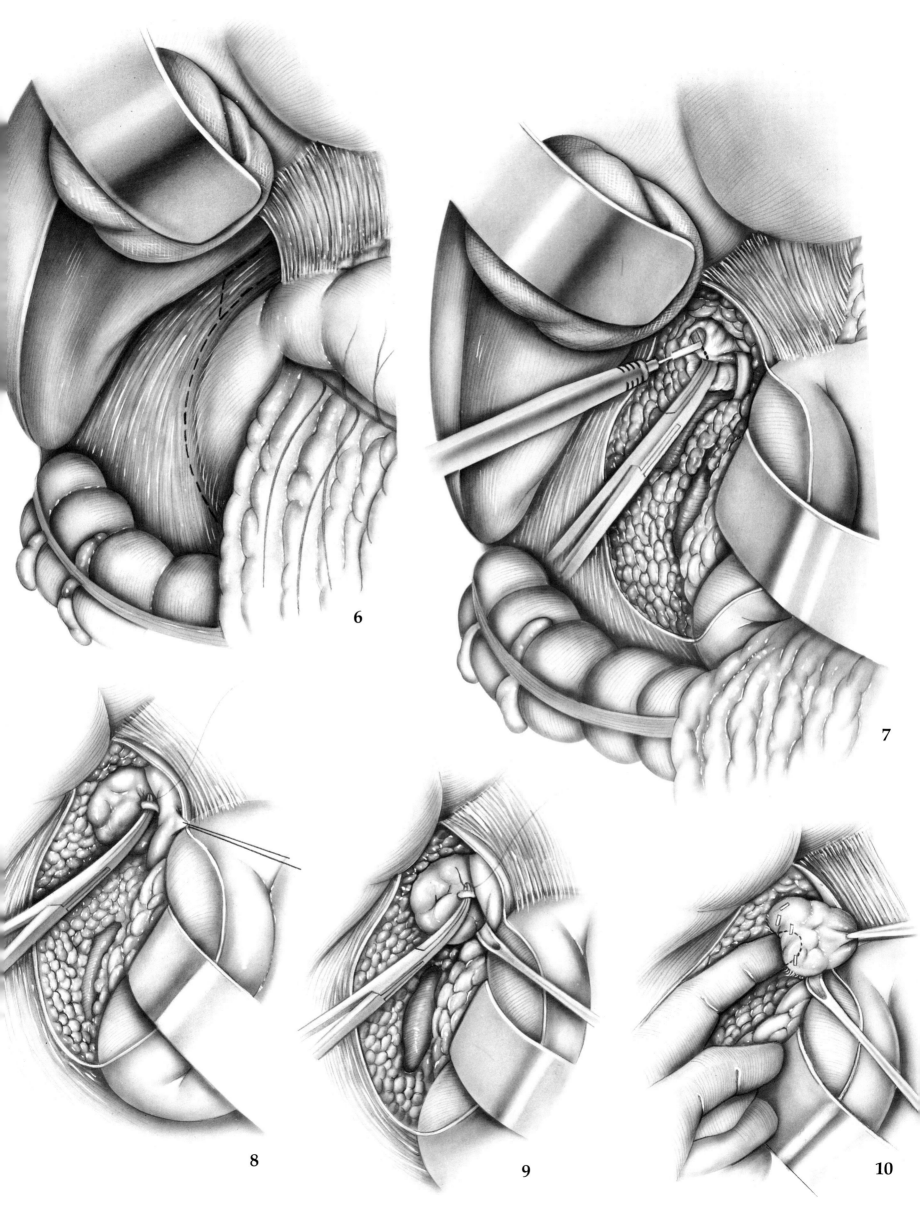

6

7

8

9

10

Superior Mesenteric Artery Embolectomy

1 The patient with an embolus lodged in the superior mesenteric artery (SMA) as demonstrated on a preoperative angiogram is explored through a long midline incision. Care must be taken, in positioning the patient, not to dislodge the angiogram catheter which has been placed into the superior mesenteric artery to be used for intraarterial infusion of papaverine in the immediate preoperative and postoperative period. The superior mesenteric artery is identified at the base of the transverse mesocolon, which is retracted cephalad.

2 With emboli lodged peripherally in the SMA, the proximal SMA pulsations can be palpated. In cases where the embolus is proximal, the middle colic artery is dissected proximally to its origin at the SMA. The peritoneum overlying the SMA is incised sharply, exposing the anterior surface of the vessel.

3 The artery is dissected circumferentially, and vessel loops are placed around the vessel and its branches. Alternatively, a small vascular clamp can be placed on the proximal artery. A longitudinal anterior arteriotomy is created. The arteriotomy is enlarged with an angled Pott's scissors. The embolus is removed. The artery is allowed to back-bleed; this should flush out all residual small clots, but a Fogarty catheter may be used to clear the vessel of any residual debris. The proximal clamp is released momentarily to flush any residual clot from the proximal vessel.

4 The arteriotomy is closed, usually without a vein patch, using a running 5-0 polypropylene vascular suture. Bowel viability is then determined.

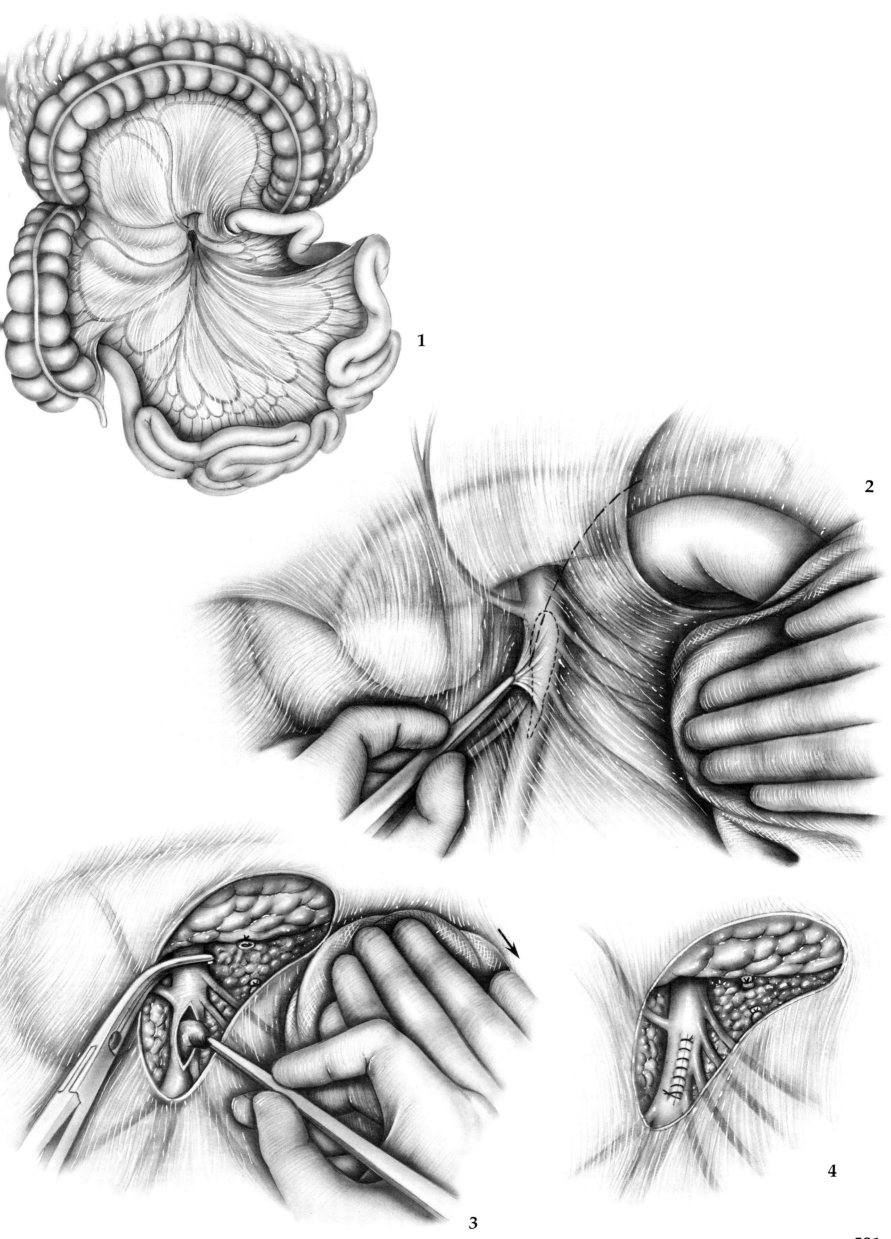

1

2

3

4

Nonocclusive Mesenteric Ischemia: Operative Technique and Placement of Intraarterial Infusion Catheter

1 In nonocclusive mesenteric ischemia or superior mesenteric artery embolism, there is a significant component of vasospasm of the mesenteric circulation as demonstrated on a preoperative angiogram. It has been shown that a papaverine infusion can salvage compromised small intestine; however, excision is often a necessary component of the therapy. The compromised segment is indicated between the broken lines.

2 The bowel is reapproximated with a closed single-layer anastomosis as described in **Plate 27, Figs. 22–25.**

3 If a preoperative angiogram was not performed, or if a catheter could not be placed into the superior mesenteric artery for postoperative infusion of papaverine, a 2- to 3-mm catheter can be introduced into a small artery in the peripheral small bowel mesentery. The catheter is advanced into the proximal superior mesenteric artery and secured in place with elastic yarn tied around the catheter proximal to the arteriotomy. The catheter is brought out to the skin through a separate incision in the abdominal wall, and a papaverine infusion is begun. The catheter can be used to perform a postoperative angiogram to reassess the mesenteric circulation for persistent vasospasm. It is usually removed within 2 days, by simple withdrawal. The elastic yarn on the proximal arteriotomy occludes the arterial lumen.

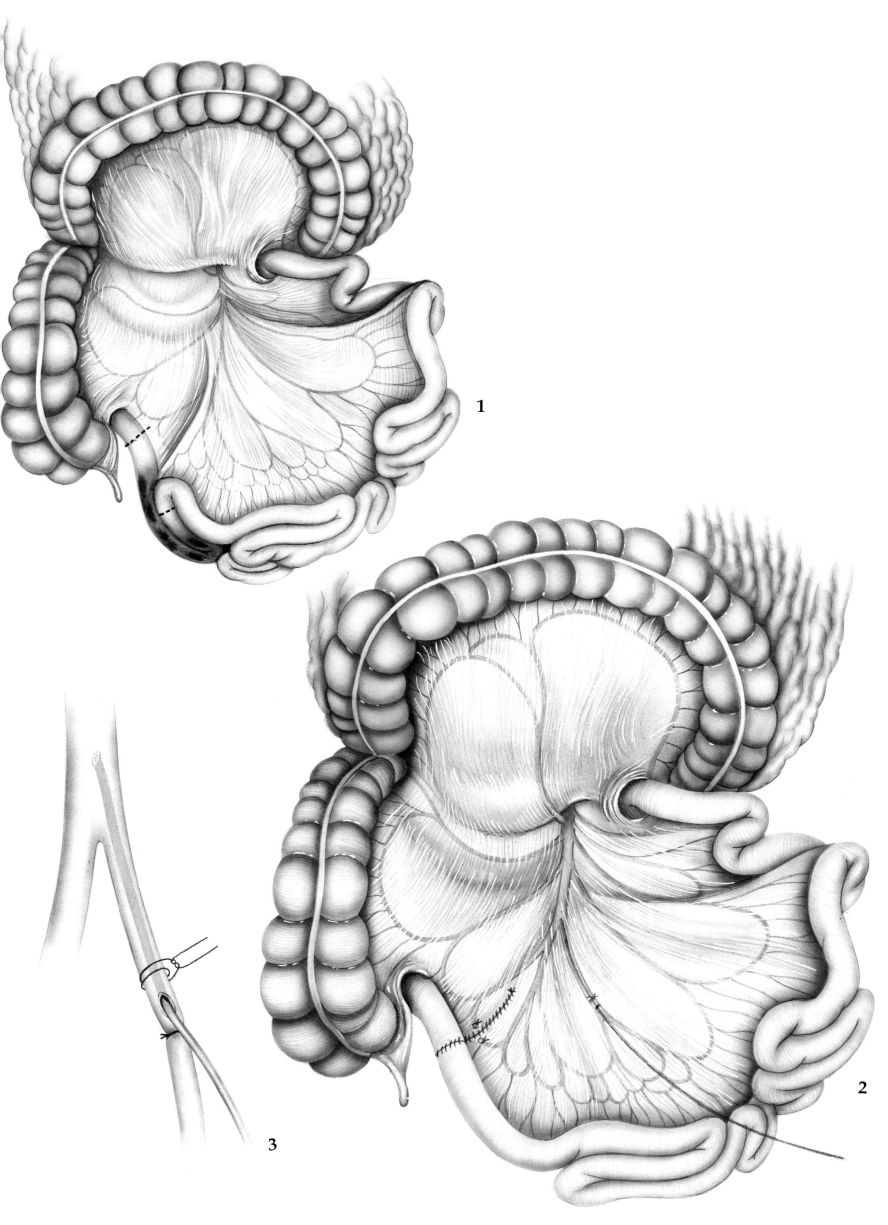

1

2

3

Nonocclusive Mesenteric Ischemia: Operative Technique and Placement of Intraarterial Infusion Catheter (*cont.*)

4 In cases of catastrophic and irretrievable massive ischemia, where there is only little viable proximal and distal small bowel, some surgeons have recommended a very proximal jejunostomy and a distal ileostomy. We disagree. We have found that restoring the continuity of the bowel, however short, is better tolerated by the patient. Unfortunately, the proximal and distal ends often are not long enough for a tension-free anastomosis.

5 The lateral gutter of the right colon and the hepatic flexure are freed as indicated by the broken line. The right colon is then reflected medially, allowing the proximal jejunum to be reapproximated to the distal ileum.

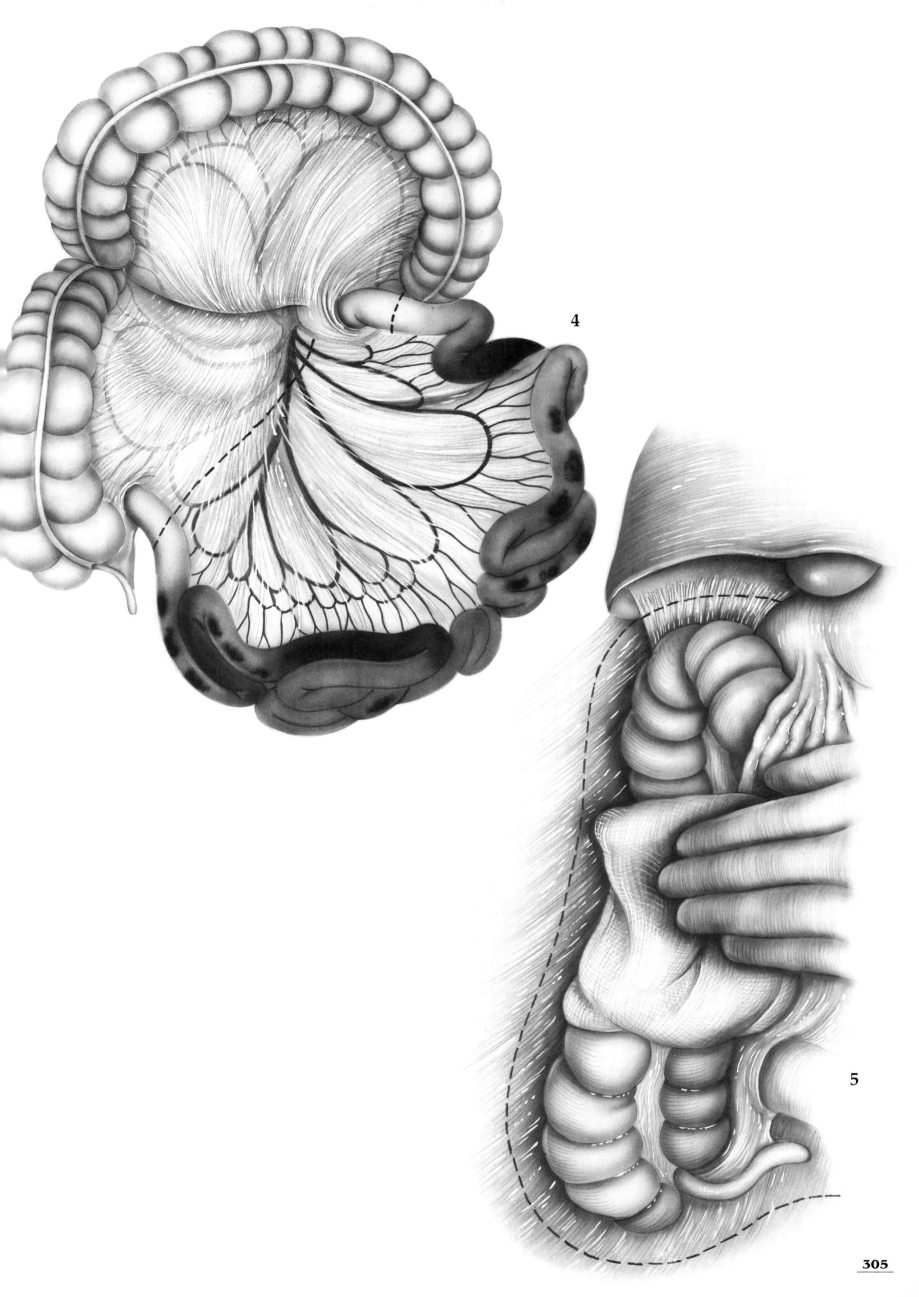

Nonocclusive Mesenteric Ischemia: Operative Technique and Placement of Intraarterial Infusion Catheter (*cont.*)

6 The colon is fixed to the retroperitoneum with #000 polyglycolic acid sutures, thus avoiding tension on the anastomosis. In this case, the patient will require long-term parenteral nutrition.

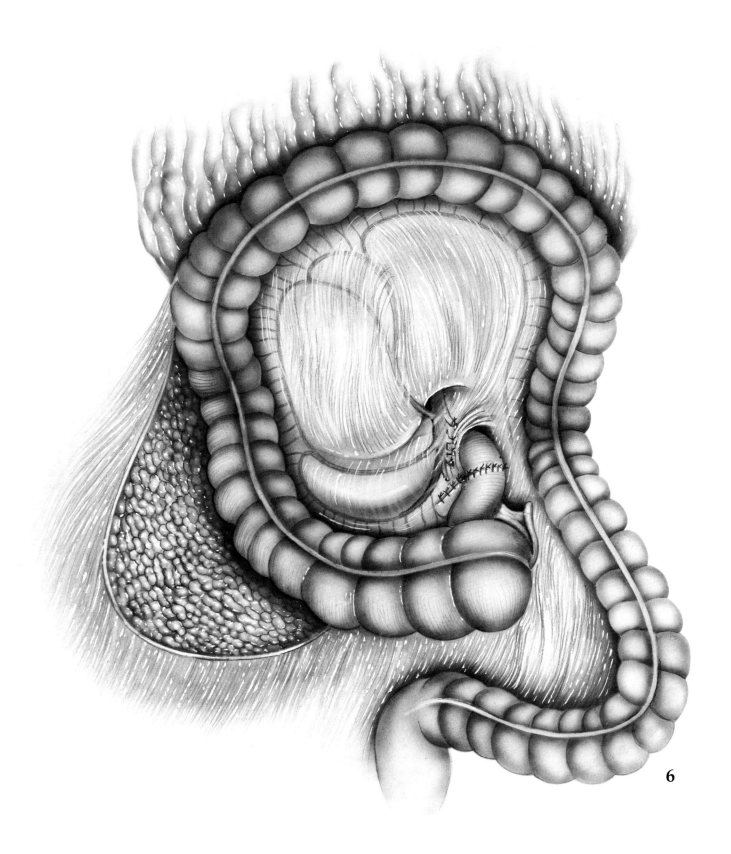

6

Appendectomy

McBurney Incision (Muscle-Splitting)

1 Numerous incisions have been recommended for the removal of the inflamed appendix. Each has its ardent advocates. The most popular incision is the muscle-splitting approach, with either an oblique (*a*) or a transverse (*b*) skin incision. The incision should be performed over the point of maximum tenderness.

2 Following the skin incision, the aponeurosis of the external oblique muscle is incised in the axis of its fibers for approximately 6 to 7 cm.

3 A Kelly clamp is inserted into the substance of the external oblique muscle and then opened, splitting the muscle's fibers. Similarly, the substance of the internal oblique is split and retracted.

4 The transversalis muscle is split in the axis of its fibers, exposing the transversalis fascia and peritoneum.

5 With the tip of the surgeon's finger, the peritoneum and transversalis fascia are bluntly dissected free of the overlying musculature. The peritoneum and transversalis fascia will then pout into the wound. These layers are opened transversely, as indicated by the broken line, allowing entry into the peritoneal cavity.

6 The closure of the peritoneum and transversalis fascia is accomplished with a continuous #000 polyglycolic acid suture.

7 The split internal and external oblique muscles are closed with several interrupted #000 polyglycolic acid sutures.

8 The aponeurosis of the external oblique is closed with interrupted #000 polyglycolic acid sutures. The wound is irrigated and the skin is closed.

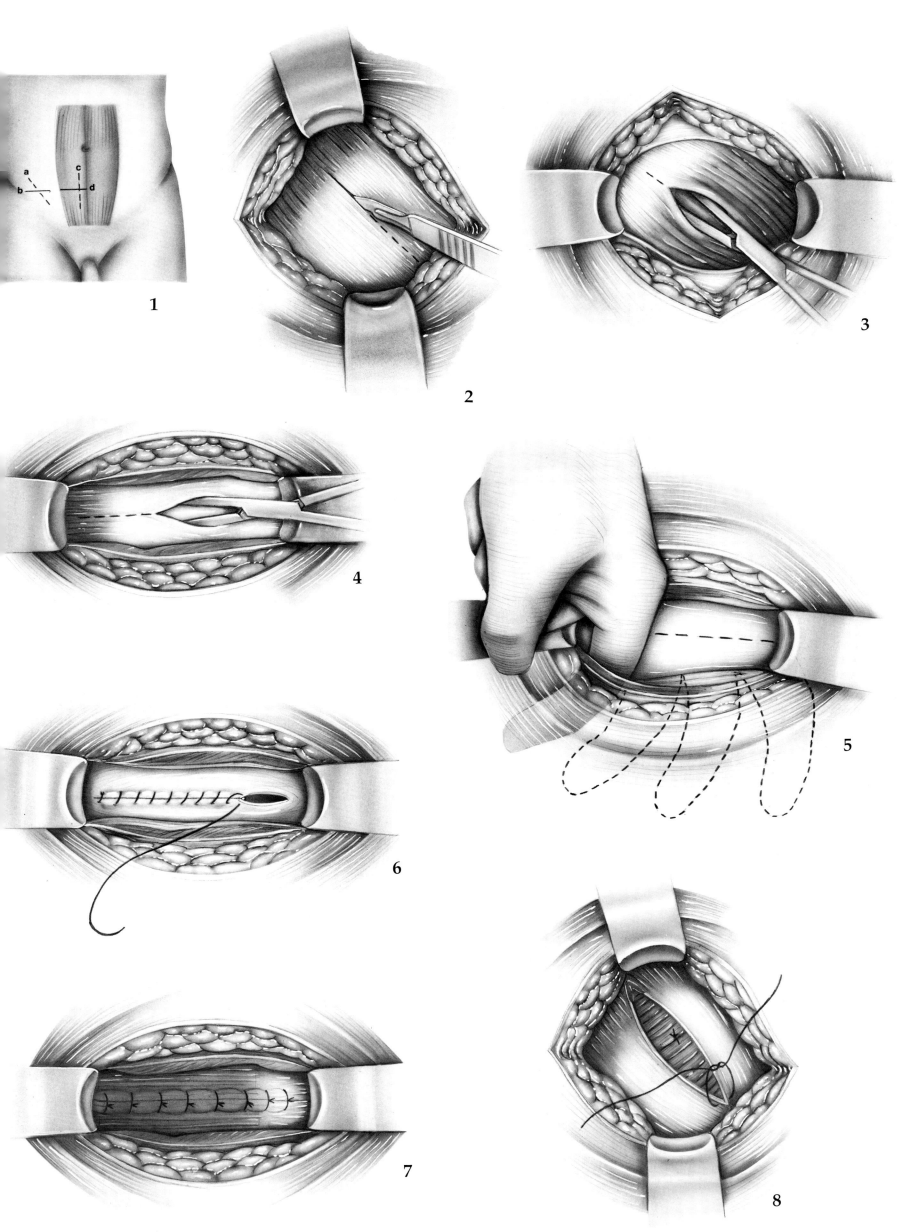

Appendectomy (*cont.*)

Transverse Rectus Retracting Incision

9 The transverse incision over the rectus at the area of maximal tenderness is our preferred incision. This incision allows greater flexibility should the pathology be other than acute appendicitis. This incision can be extended laterally, or across the left rectus, should the need arise.

10 The incision is brought down to the anterior rectus fascia. This fascia is opened transversely. If greater exposure is required, the insertion of the oblique fascia on the rectus may be incised.

11 The rectus is undermined and retracted medially. The inferior epigastric artery is clamped, divided, and ligated. The peritoneum is bluntly dissected circumferentially, allowing it to pout into the wound. Entry into the peritoneal cavity is achieved by transversely incising the peritoneum, as indicated by the broken line. This incision permits the cecum and appendix to be easily elevated into the wound and allows excellent exposure of the fallopian tubes and ovaries.

Appendectomy

12 It is essential to have clear visualization of the terminal ileum, cecum, and appendiceal mesentery prior to removal of the appendix.

13 The appendiceal mesentery is dissected, divided between clamps, and tied with #000 silk ligatures.

14 The appendiceal base is divided between clamps with the electrocautery.

15 A #000 silk purse-string suture is placed around the clamped appendiceal stump. A #0 silk tie is placed through a loop in the purse-string opposite its point of origin, to be used for countertraction when the stump is inverted.

16 The appendiceal stump is inverted into the cecal wall as countertraction is applied to the ends of the purse-string suture and the heavy silk. This traction at two points allows the cecal wall to be brought around the clamp holding the appendiceal stump. The clamp on the appendiceal stump is opened and the purse-string suture tied. The heavy silk is removed.

17 A #000 silk "Z" stitch is placed to further invert the purse-string and appendiceal stump, thus securing the closure.

18 A second "Z" stitch is placed at right angles to the first, completely burying the purse-string suture. The peritoneum is then closed with a running #000 polyglycolic acid suture.

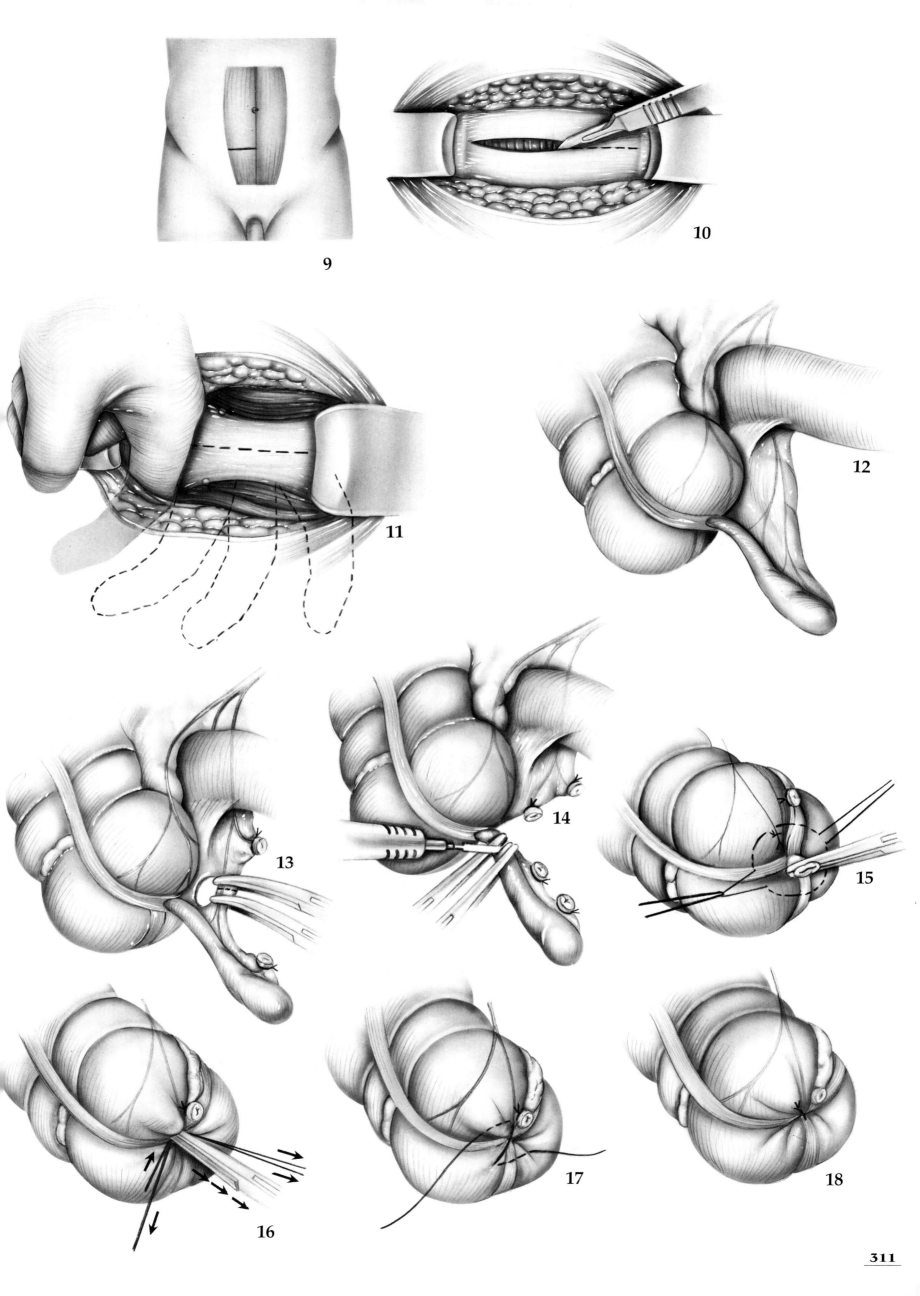

Appendectomy (*cont.*)—Appendicostomy

APPENDECTOMY (*cont.*)

19 The anterior rectus sheath is closed with interrupted #000 polyglycolic acid sutures. The wound is irrigated and the skin is closed.

APPENDICOSTOMY

20 An appendicostomy is useful for the decompression of the atonic colon distended with gas, or as an adjunct to a distal anastomosis in the transverse colon. The mesentery of the appendix is divided between clamps and tied with #000 silk ligatures.

21 The appendix is partially transected approximately 1.5 cm from its base.

22 A #16 French catheter is introduced into the cecum through the cut appendix and secured in place with two #00 polyglycolic acid ties. The distal end of the appendix is excised.

23 The appendix and the catheter are brought into the lateral abdominal wall, with the catheter exiting through a separate incision made in the skin. The cecum is fixed to the lateral peritoneum with #000 polyglycolic acid sutures. The catheter will remove gas from the cecum and right colon as long as it is irrigated frequently. It may be removed after 1 week; the tract will close spontaneously.

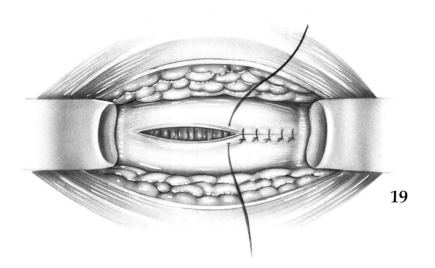

19

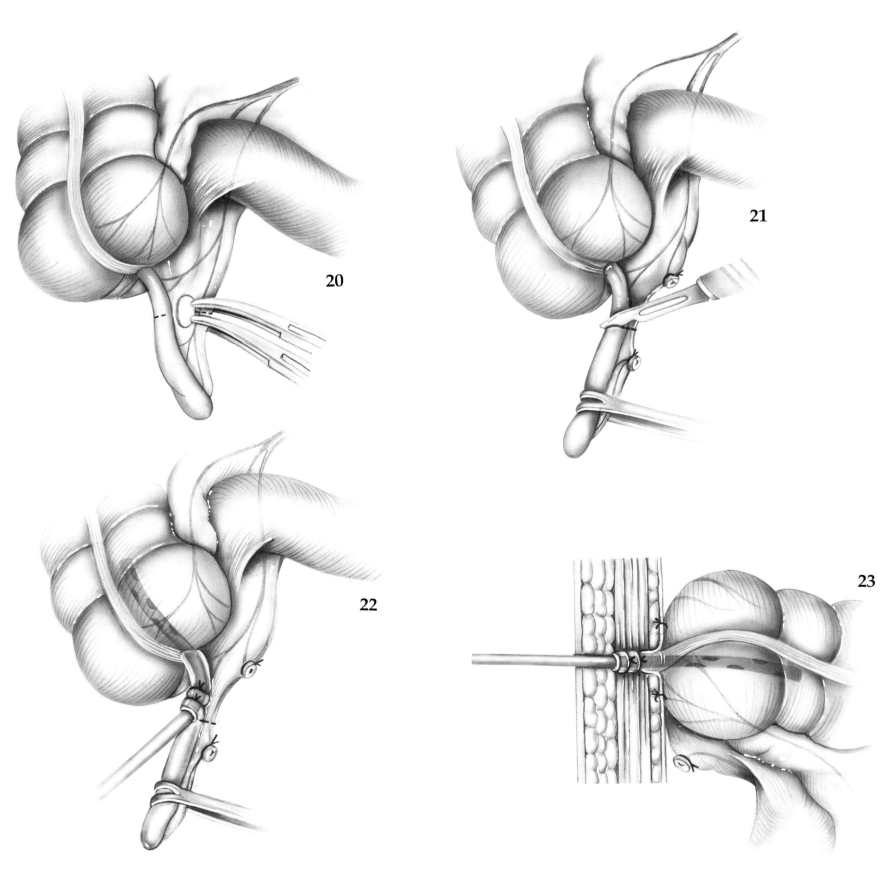

20

21

22

23

Loop Colostomy—Closure of Loop Colostomy

LOOP COLOSTOMY

314

1 A transverse loop colostomy may be used if the patient has a significant obstruction proximal to a lesion in the descending or sigmoid colon and/or is not a candidate for a resection at the time of presentation. The transverse loop colostomy will decompress the colon and allow appropriate preparation for elective resection. A right upper quadrant transverse incision is used for the approach to the proximal transverse colon.

2 The right side of the transverse colon is retracted into the wound, allowing the greater omentum to drape backward toward the liver. This will make dissection of the overlying omentum unnecessary. Two glass or plastic rods, attached to short segments of plastic or rubber tubing, are placed through the transverse mesocolon and used to secure the colon above the abdominal wall. Gas in the distended colon is evacuated with the aid of a 19-gauge needle inserted into the open end of a #24 French red Robinson catheter attached to a tonsil suction.

3 The needle point is inserted into the muscular wall of the colon, tunneled for approximately 1 cm within the muscle, and then passed into the bowel lumen. With bowel collapsed, the formal opening of the colostomy may be delayed for 24 to 48 hours, after which a firm seal has formed around the colostomy, isolating it from the peritoneal cavity.

4 Only one supporting rod is used if the colostomy is matured immediately. A transverse colotomy is made along the taenia with the electrocautery. The colostomy is matured with #000 polyglycolic acid stitches taken through the full thickness of the bowel at the edge of the colotomy, then again through the colon at the level of the skin in a seromuscular fashion, and finally through the skin.

5 As these sutures are tied the mucosa everts, creating the stoma. The glass rod may be removed after 5 days.

CLOSURE OF LOOP COLOSTOMY

6 Closure of the mature colostomy is accomplished by incising the skin close to the mucocutaneous junction.

7 The bowel is freed from the subcutaneous tissues down to the abdominal fascia. The skin remaining on the colostomy is grasped with Allis clamps.

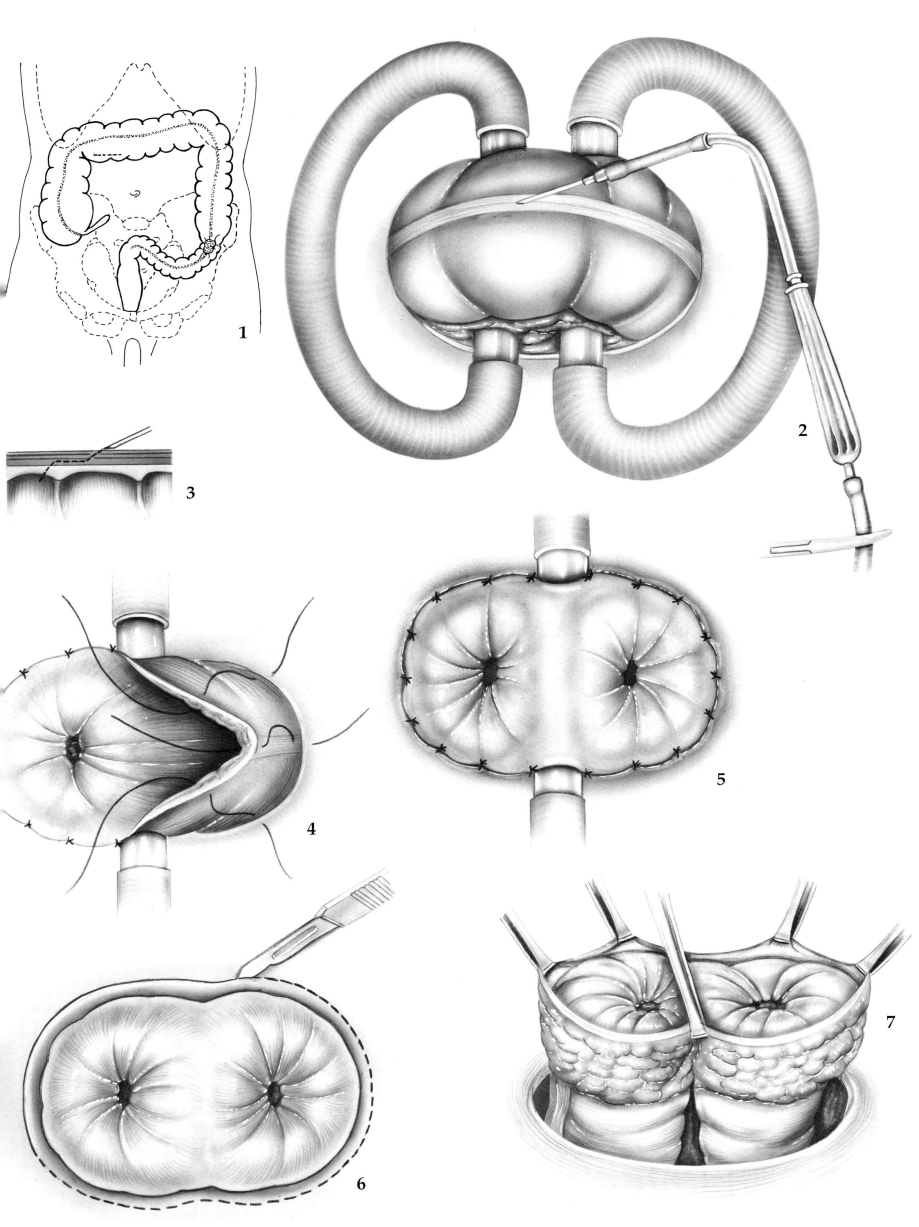

Closure of Loop Colostomy (*cont.*)— Cecal Decompression

CLOSURE OF LOOP COLOSTOMY (*cont.*)

8 The skin is peeled from the bowel wall using sharp and blunt dissection. The pouting and raw mucosa at the edges of the colostomy is excised.

9 The bowel is closed transversely with either an interrupted or a continuous layer of #000 polyglycolic acid sutures.

10 This layer is inverted with an additional row of interrupted #000 silk Lembert stitches.

11 The abdominal wall is closed with simple #1 polyglycolic acid sutures.

12 According to the surgeon's preference, the skin may be either loosely approximated or left open for a delayed closure.

CECAL DECOMPRESSION

13 If the patient has presented with a massively distended cecum and right colon resulting from proximal transverse or ascending colon lesions, it is important to avoid manipulation of the cecum. The thinned and distended cecum disrupts easily, causing fecal contamination of the peritoneum. Insertion of a catheter into the cecum through an enterotomy in the distal terminal ileum is a useful technique for cecal decompression.

14 A #000 silk purse-string suture is placed in the terminal ileum approximately 5 cm proximal to the ileocecal valve. A heavy silk tie (to be used for countertraction when the catheter is inserted) is placed under a loop of the purse-string.

15 A small enterotomy is created in the center of the purse-string. A catheter is advanced through the enterotomy and into the cecum. The contents of the cecum and ascending colon are aspirated through this catheter without manipulation of the cecum.

16 Once the colon is decompressed, the catheter is removed and the purse-string tied. A #000 silk "Z" stitch is placed over the tied purse-string, further securing the closure of the enterotomy.

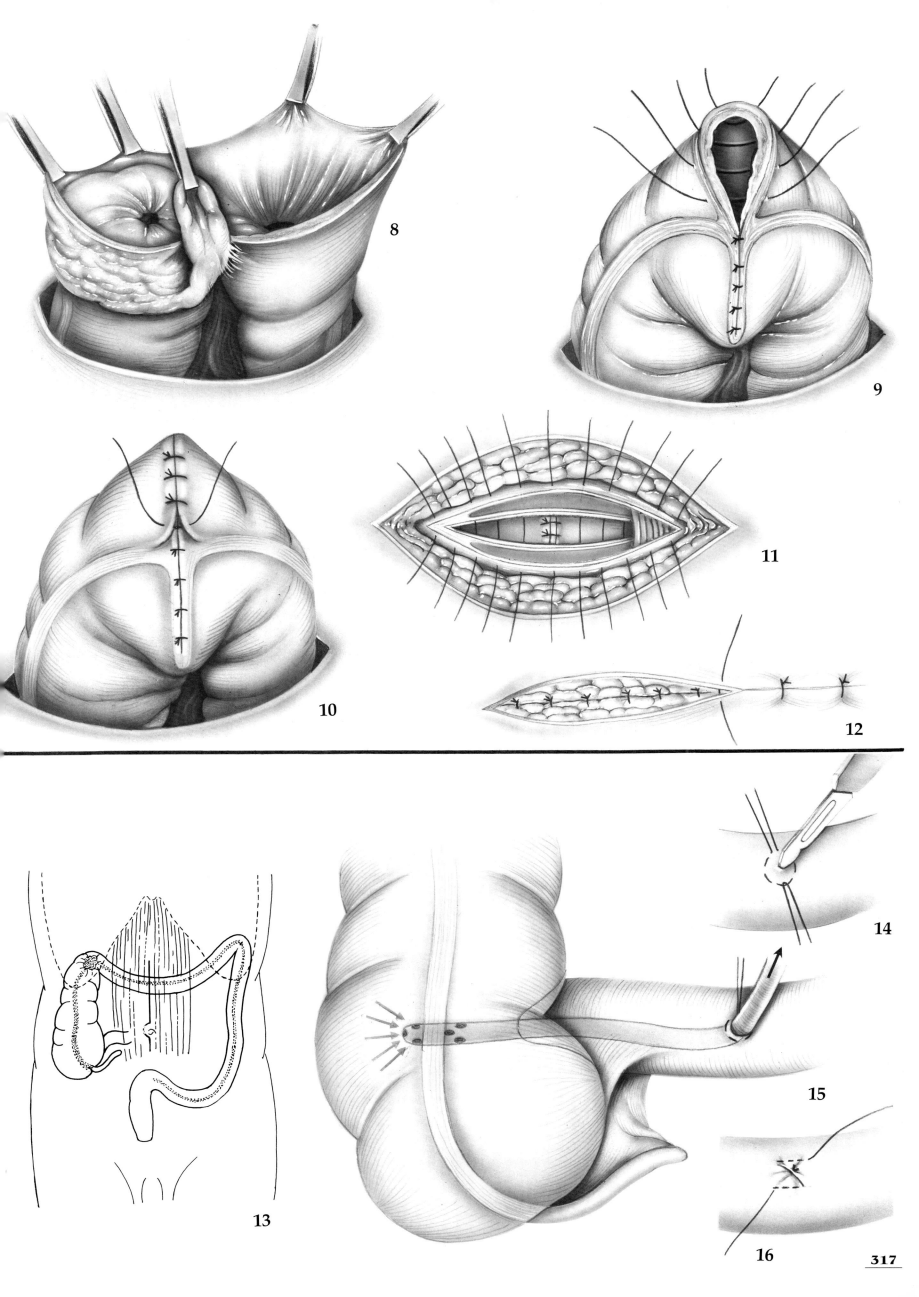

8

9

10

11

12

13

14

15

16

End Colostomy (Matured)

1 The skin in the area of the proposed colostomy is tented up with two Allis clamps. An ellipse of skin is excised. The natural skin tension converts this ellipse into a circular defect. The subcutaneous tissues are divided until the aponeurosis of the external oblique muscle is identified.

2 The aponeurosis of the external oblique is incised transversely with the electrocautery.

3 A vertical incision is made in the aponeurosis of the external oblique with the electrocautery. The cruciate incision in the aponeurosis guarantees that there will be no compression of the bowel that traverses this fascia.

4 The underlying muscles are split along their fibers.

5 Two fingers push the peritoneum through the defect in the skin and fascia from within the peritoneal cavity. The peritoneum is widely incised with electrocautery or scissors.

6 The segment of bowel is brought through the defect in the abdominal wall.

7 A full-thickness #000 or #0000 polyglycolic acid stitch through the stump of the colon is taken.

8 The stitch passes through the serosa and muscularis of the colon at the level of the skin . . .

9 . . . and is then passed through the skin.

10–12 This is repeated around the stoma, in the order shown in **Fig. 12**. The sequence of suture placement is generally appropriate for complete eversion and fixation of the stoma. The stoma should protrude 1 to 2 cm from the surface of the skin. Additional #000 silk sutures are placed in the peritoneum and posterior abdominal wall fascia and then into the bowel in a seromuscular fashion, further fixing the colostomy in place.

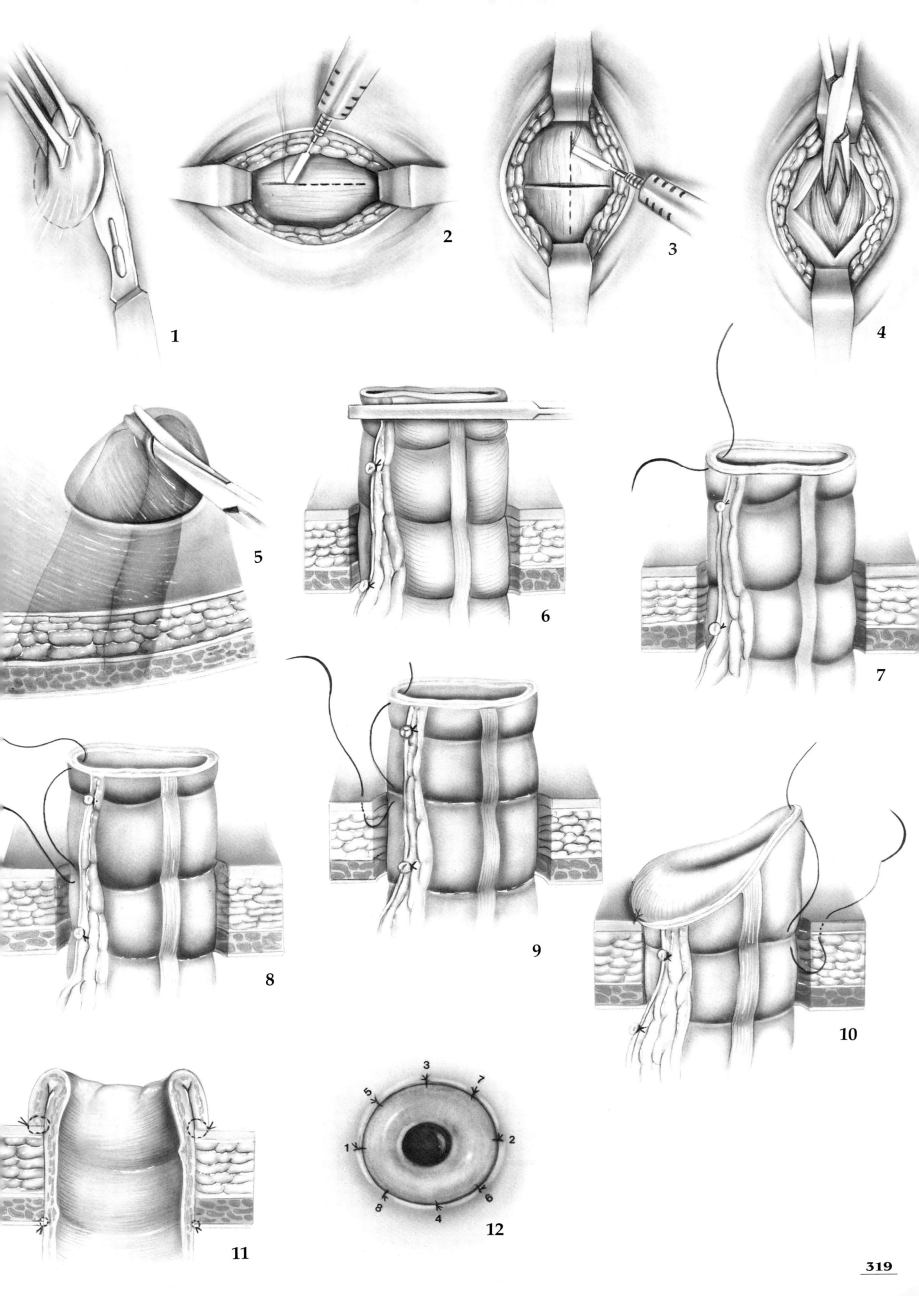

Right Hemicolectomy (Stapled Ileotransverse Colostomy)

1 The abdomen is explored through a transverse incision located either above or below the umbilicus, depending on the location of the cecum and transverse colon as seen on the preoperative barium enema or abdominal plain x-ray.

2 The boundaries of the right hemicolectomy performed for carcinoma of the colon are depicted by the broken line. The small intestinal mesentery and the transverse mesocolon are divided on a line paralleling the superior mesenteric and middle colic arteries. Much of the greater omentum is included in the resection specimen.

3 The tumor is covered with a laparotomy pad if it extends to the serosa. The right colon is then retracted medially, exposing its lateral peritoneal investments, which are incised as indicated by the broken line.

4 The hepatic flexure is divided, either sharply or with the electrocautery.

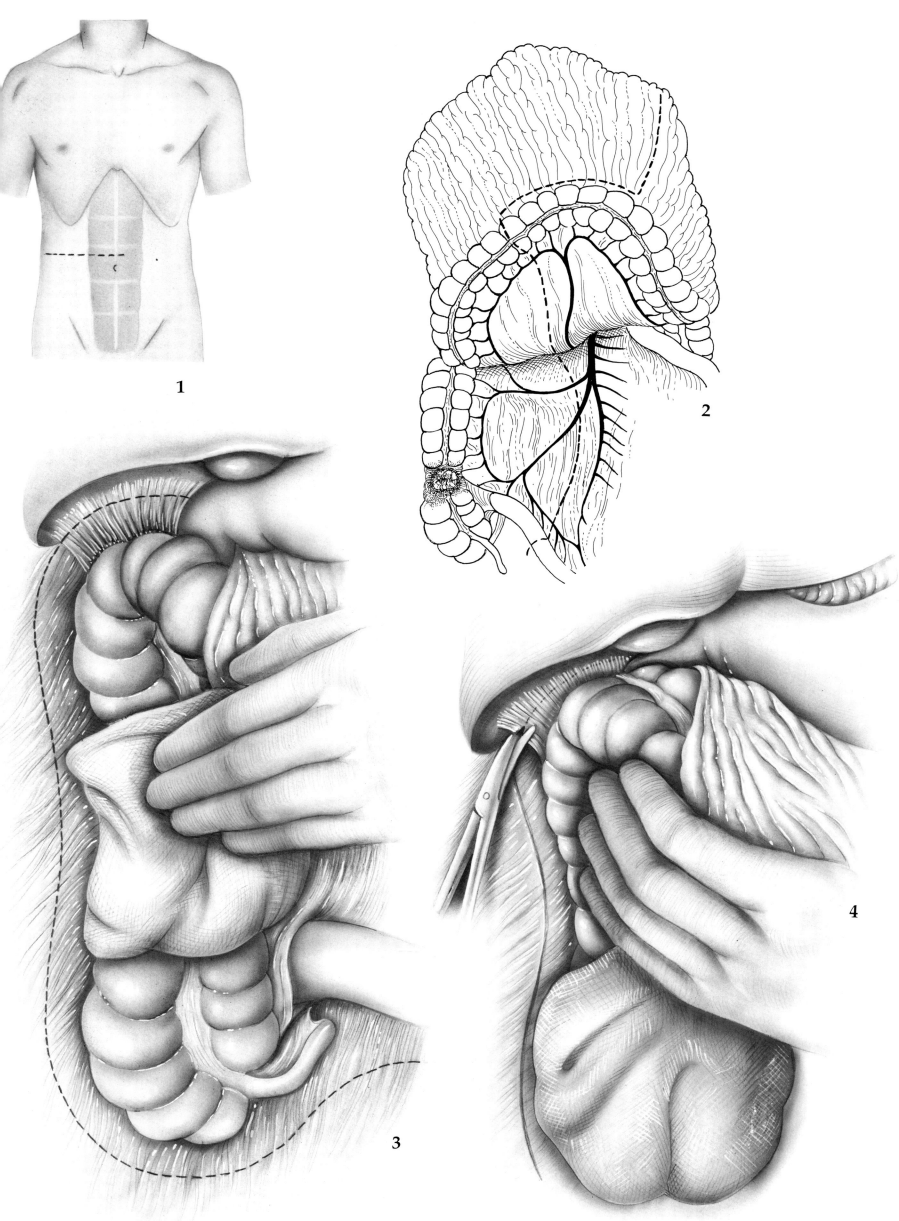

Right Hemicolectomy (Stapled Ileotransverse Colostomy) (*cont.*)

5 The right colon is retracted medially as it is bluntly dissected from the retroperitoneum. It is freed superiorly from the underlying duodenum and pancreas. The right ureter is identified and carefully preserved.

6 The gastrocolic ligament is divided between clamps, preserving the gastroepiploic arcades, so that most of the greater omentum can be removed with the specimen.

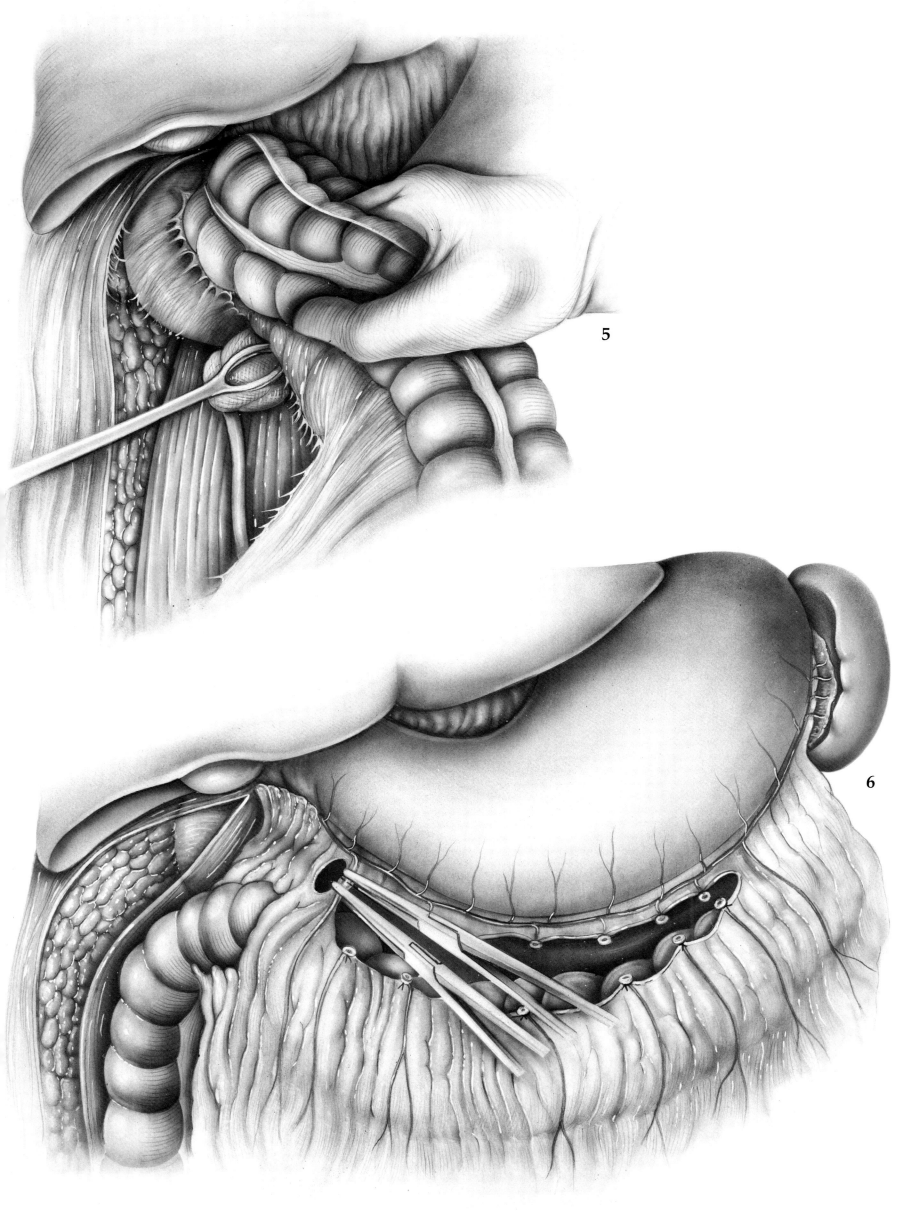

5

6

Right Hemicolectomy (Stapled Ileotransverse Colostomy) (*cont.*)

7 The right half of the greater omentum is divided as indicated by the broken line. A 15-cm portion of the transverse colon, which will be used for the subsequent ileotransverse colostomy, is dissected free of the greater omentum.

8 The peritoneum overlying the mesentery of the right and proximal transverse colon is incised over the open jaws of a right-angle clamp. The vessels within the mesentery of the colon are divided between clamps and tied with #000 silk ligatures.

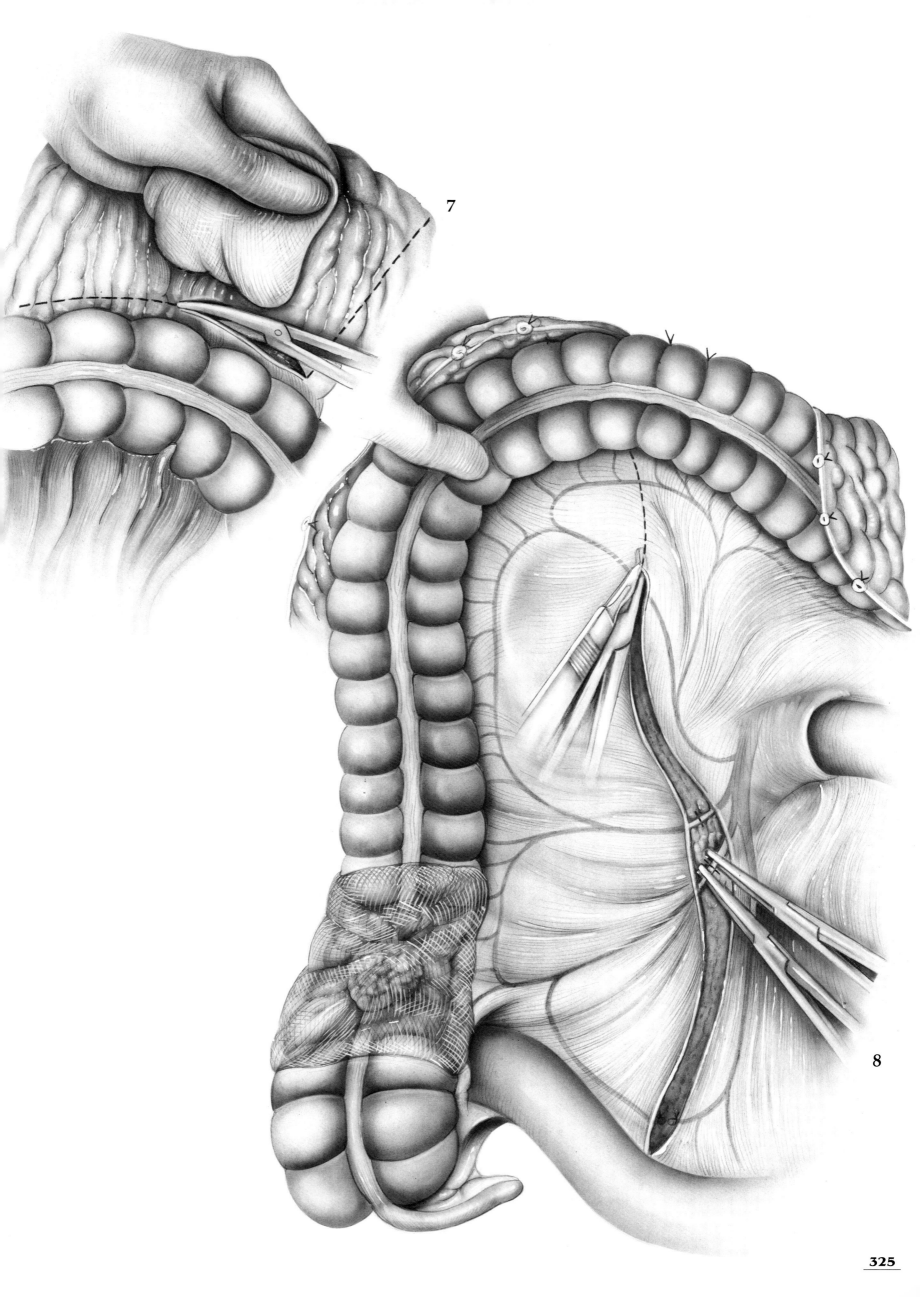

7

8

Right Hemicolectomy (Stapled Ileotransverse Colostomy) (*cont.*)

9 The terminal ileum is divided with electrocautery, 7 to 8 cm proximal to the ileocecal valve, between a Kocher clamp and a linear stapling device.

10 Similarly, the transverse colon is divided between a clamp and a linear stapling device.

11 The transverse colon and distal ileum are approximated in an isoperistaltic fashion with two #000 seromuscular silk stay sutures placed 8 to 10 cm apart. Enterotomies are created on the taenia of the colon and the antimesenteric side of the ileum. A gastrointestinal anastomotic stapler is inserted into the bowel lumen through the two enterotomies and fired, thus establishing the side-to-side anastomosis. The remaining enterotomy is closed with interrupted #000 silk sutures after the luminal surface of the anastomosis is inspected for bleeding. The benefit of the side-to-side stapled ileocolostomy is that it permits the narrow ileum to be conveniently anastomosed to the wide transverse colon. In addition, the ileum, proximal to the anastomosis, comes to lie comfortably in the area of the right gutter previously occupied by the ascending colon. The defect between the mesenteries of the transverse colon and ileum is closed with interrupted #000 silk sutures.

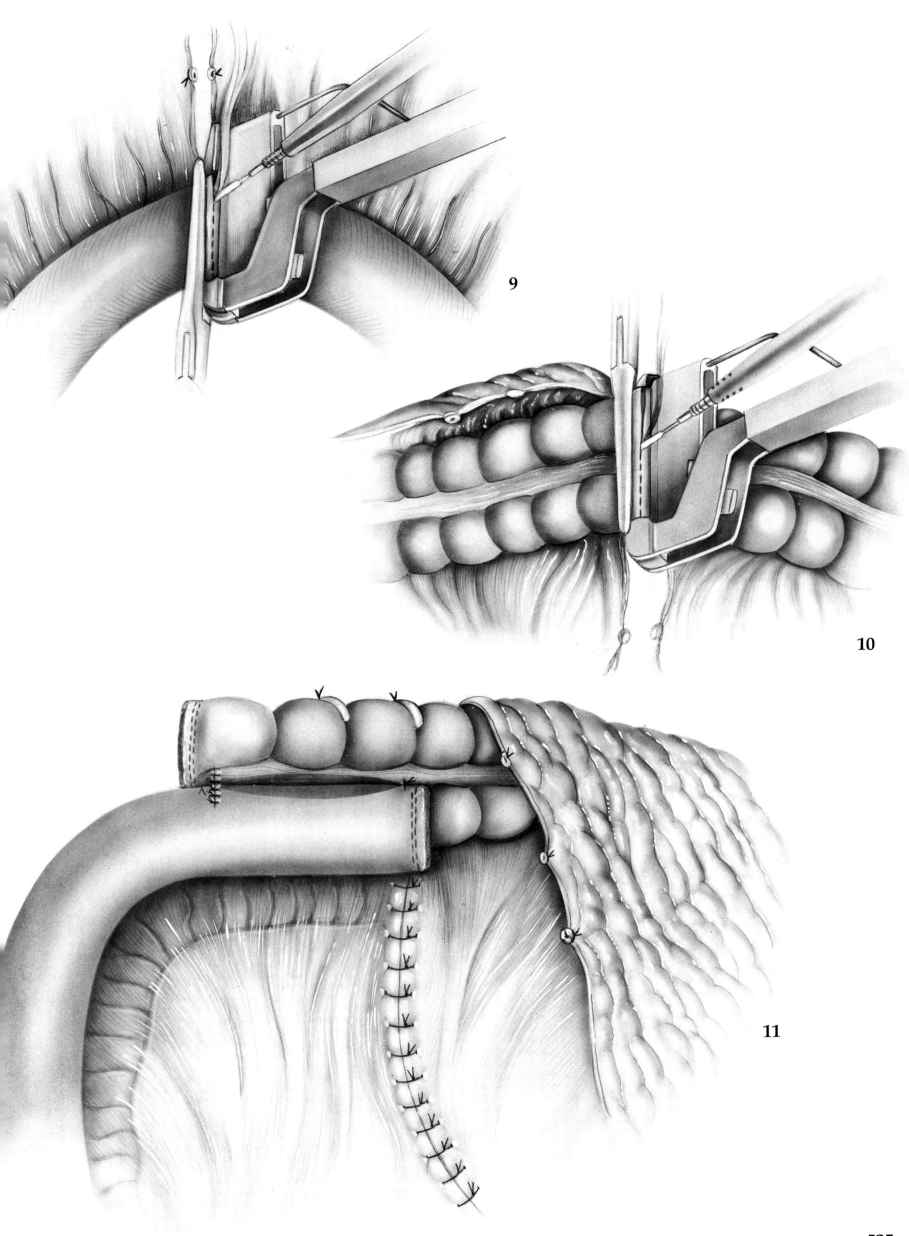

9

10

11

Left Hemicolectomy (Anastomosis with Intestinal Anastomosis Clamps)

1 The boundaries for the resection of a malignant lesion of the descending colon are indicated by the broken line. A radical excision extends from the middle of the sigmoid colon to the transverse colon near the origin of the left branch of the middle colic artery, and includes a large portion of the greater omentum and all of the colonic mesentery supplying the resected bowel.

2 The abdomen is explored through a generous midline incision. The viscera are examined to determine the presence of metastatic disease. The lesion in the colon is identified; if it extends to the serosa it is covered with a laparotomy pad during the subsequent dissection. The left colon is retracted medially, and the lateral peritoneal investments are incised.

3 The gastrocolic ligament is divided between clamps within the gastroepiploic arcades.

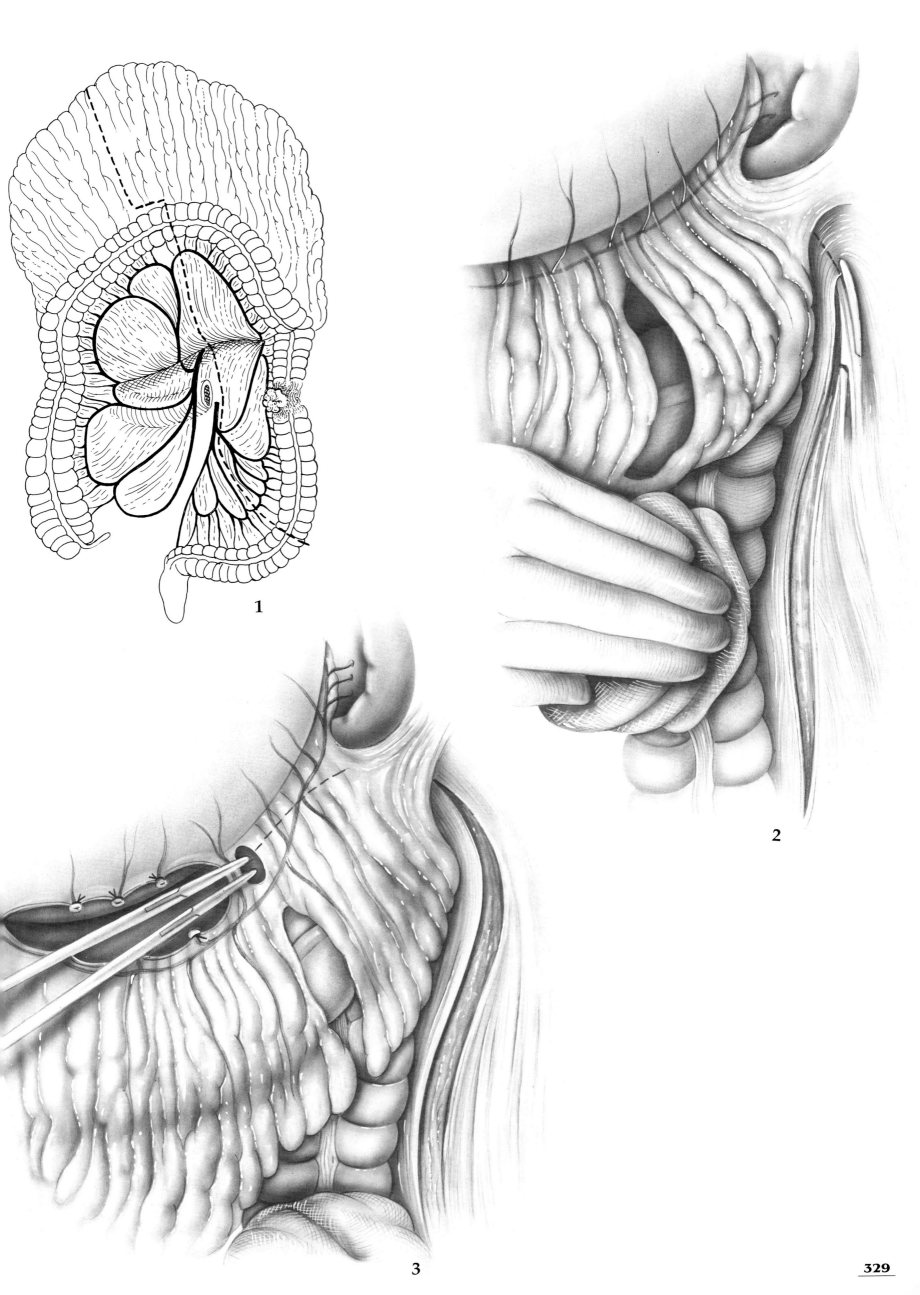

Left Hemicolectomy (Anastomosis with Intestinal Anastomosis Clamps) (*cont.*)

4 Both the transverse and descending colon should be freed prior to the division of the lieno-colic ligament. This allows easier mobilization of the splenic flexure, which is divided with either cautery or sharp dissection.

5 The descending colon is retracted medially and bluntly dissected from the retroperitoneum. The left ureter is identified and carefully preserved.

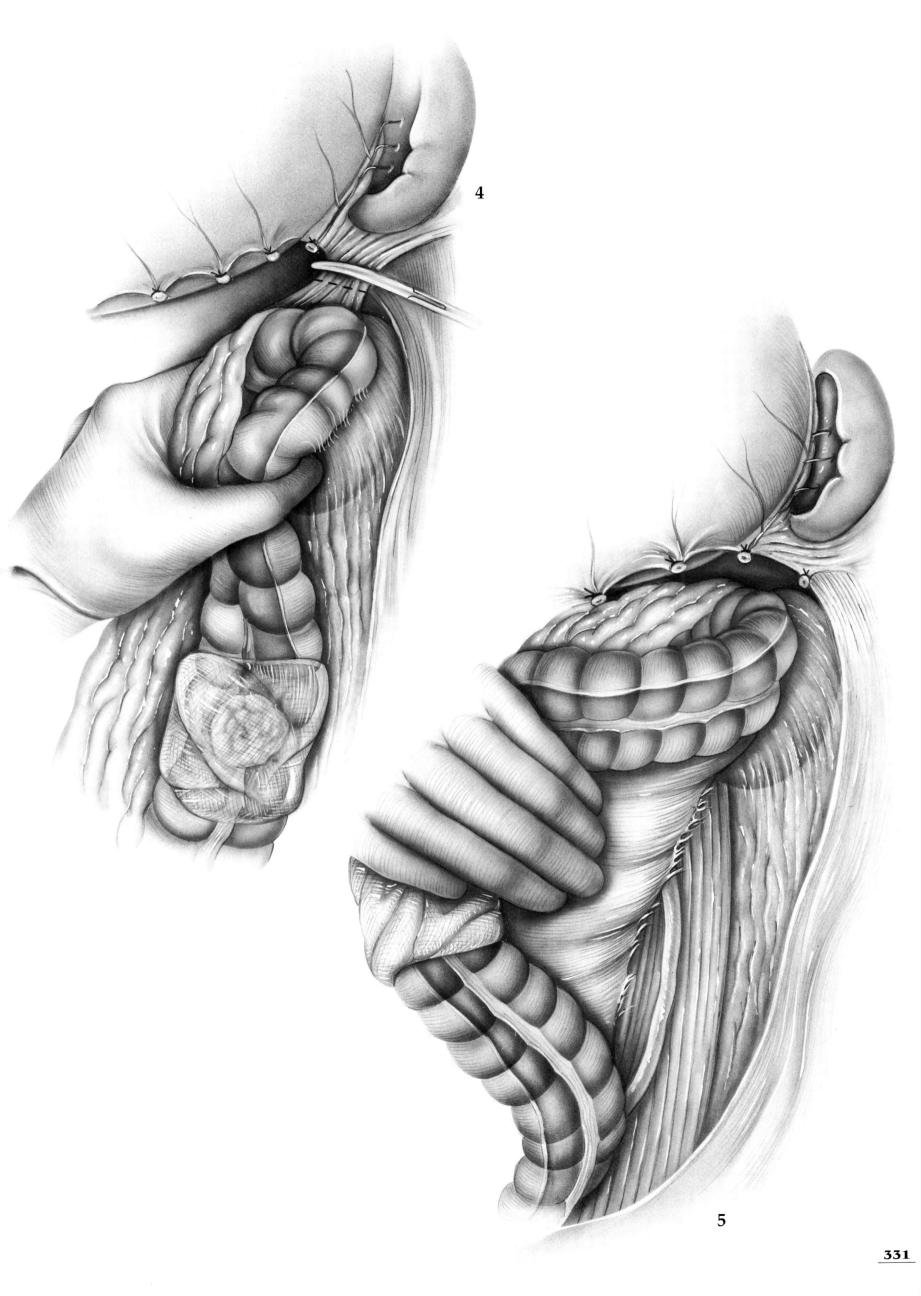

4

5

Left Hemicolectomy (Anastomosis with Intestinal Anastomosis Clamps) (*cont.*)

6 The peritoneum overlying the vessels supplying the portion of the colon to be resected is incised as shown. The vessels are dissected free, divided between clamps, and tied with #000 silk. Dennis intestinal anastomosis clamps are placed on the proximal and distal lines of resection, and Kocher clamps are placed on the specimen side of the bowel to be resected. Using electrocautery, the colon is divided between the Dennis and Kocher clamps both proximally and distally. The intestinal anastomosis clamps are placed so that a clockwise rotation of the transverse colon will put the handles of both clamps to the patient's left, allowing the assistant to manipulate them during the anastomosis.

7 The right colon is mobilized as previously described (**Plates 160–161, Figs. 3–6**) and the hepatic flexure is taken down. The right portion of the gastrocolic ligament is divided outside the gastroepiploic arcades, freeing the right side of the transverse colon.

8 The mobilization of the right and transverse colon permits a clockwise rotation of the residual transverse colon toward the distal portion of the sigmoid colon. A closed sewn anastomosis is carried out with interrupted #000 silk sutures placed in a seromuscular fashion. The posterior layer is placed initially and then tied. The anterior row is placed over the intestinal anastomosis clamps, held up in the air as the clamps are removed, and tied (see **Plate 27, Figs. 22–25**). The seal between the anterior and posterior walls of the colon is broken by palpating the anastomosis between the thumb and forefinger. The mesentery is closed with interrupted #000 silk sutures. This closure skirts, and partially reconstructs, the ligament of Treitz.

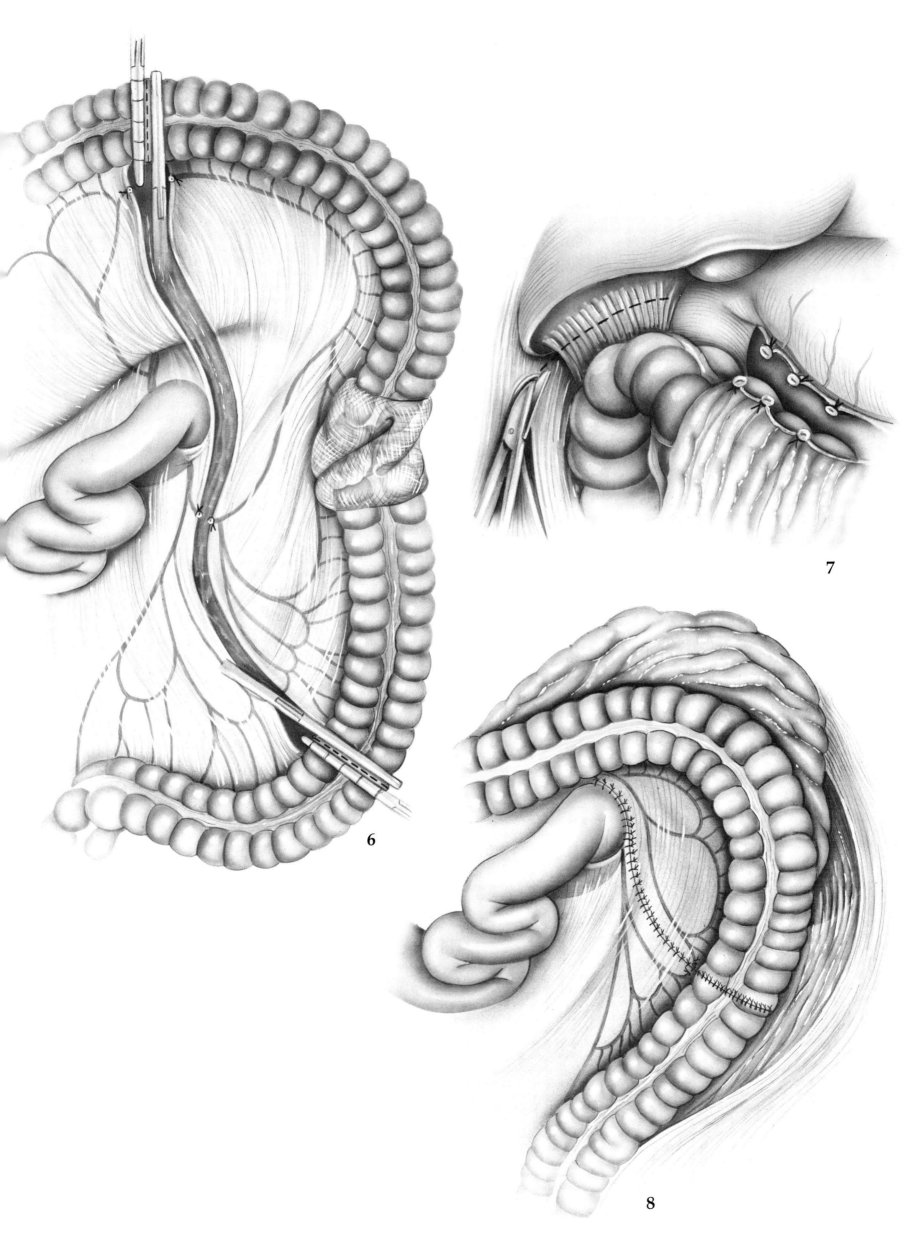

6

7

8

PLATE

1 6 7

Sigmoid Resection (Anastomosis with Intestinal Anastomosis Clamps)

1 For carcinoma located in the sigmoid colon, the sigmoid and its mesocolon are resected as indicated by the broken line. This requires that the inferior mesenteric artery be divided close to its origin at the aorta.

2 The abdomen is explored through a lower midline incision. The abdominal viscera are inspected for metastases. The peritoneum lateral to the sigmoid colon is incised, allowing the sigmoid to be retracted medially. This dissection is extended to the level of the proximal rectum. The sigmoid is bluntly dissected from the retroperitoneum. The ureter is identified and carefully preserved.

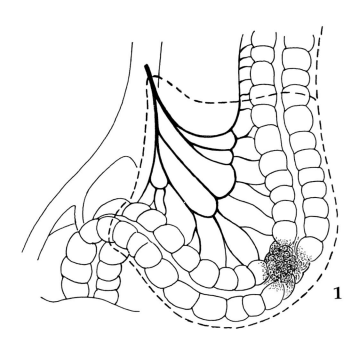

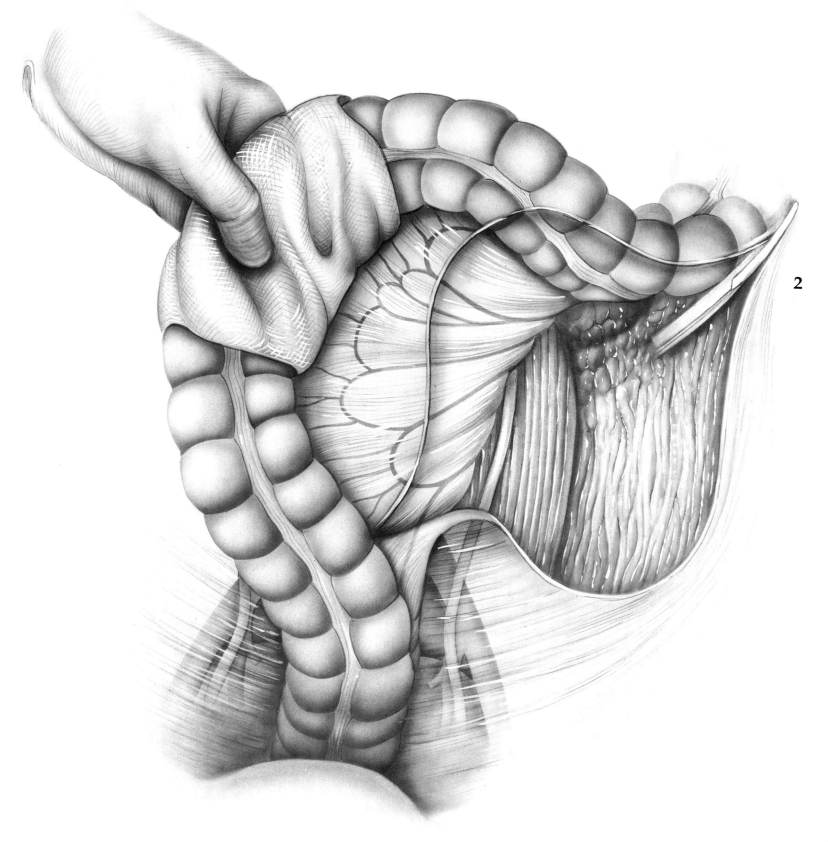

Sigmoid Resection (Anastomosis with Intestinal Anastomosis Clamps) (*cont.*)

3 The mesentery of the sigmoid colon is incised, allowing the vessels supplying this portion of colon to be divided between clamps and tied with #000 silk. The inferior mesenteric artery is divided near its origin from the aorta. Subsequently, the inferior mesenteric vein is identified coursing parallel to the aorta. It is divided and tied as it approaches the proximal jejunum and ligament of Treitz. The marginal artery is divided between clamps and tied at the site of the proposed transection, near the junction of the descending and sigmoid colon.

4 Intestinal anastomosis clamps are placed across the bowel distal to the sigmoid colon and across the proximal margin in the descending colon. These clamps are positioned so that their handles will be available to the assistant for manipulation during the anastomosis. Kocher clamps are placed proximally and distally on the specimen, and the colon is divided between the Kocher and anastomosis clamps with electrocautery.

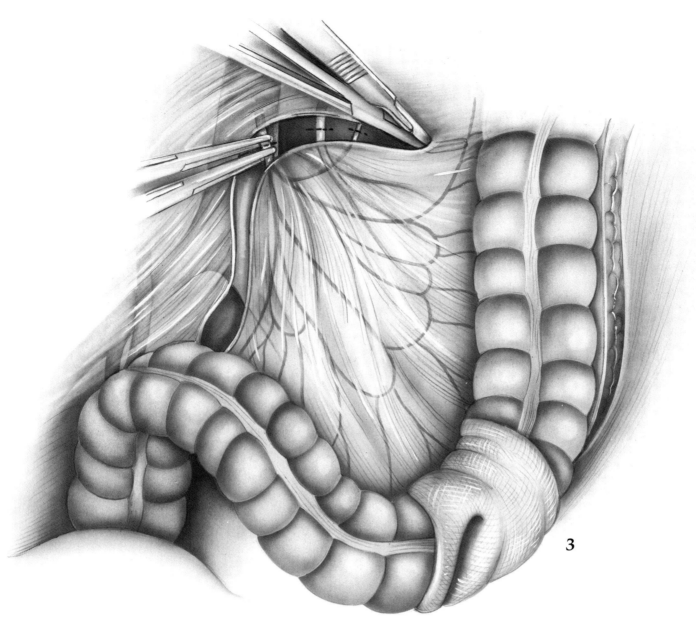

3

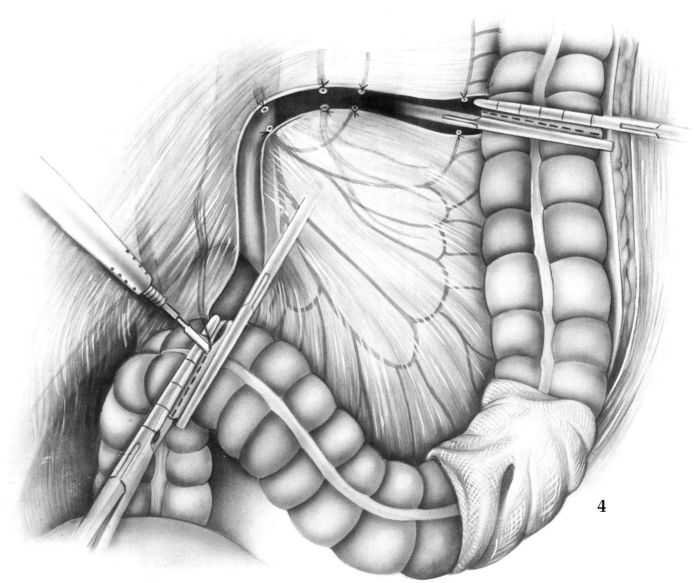

4

Sigmoid Resection (Anastomosis with Intestinal Anastomosis Clamps) (*cont.*)

5 Before freeing the splenic flexure, the retroperitoneum overlying the left kidney is bluntly dissected with the surgeon's hand. This maneuver often provides sufficient mobility to the descending colon, obviating the need to mobilize the splenic flexure.

6 If the descending colon does not reach the proximal rectum comfortably and without tension, the splenic flexure is mobilized as previously described (**Plates 164–165, Figs. 2–4**).

7 A closed single-layer anastomosis is fashioned as previously described (see **Plate 27, Figs. 22–25** and page 332, paragraph 8). The defect in the mesentery is closed with interrupted #000 silk sutures.

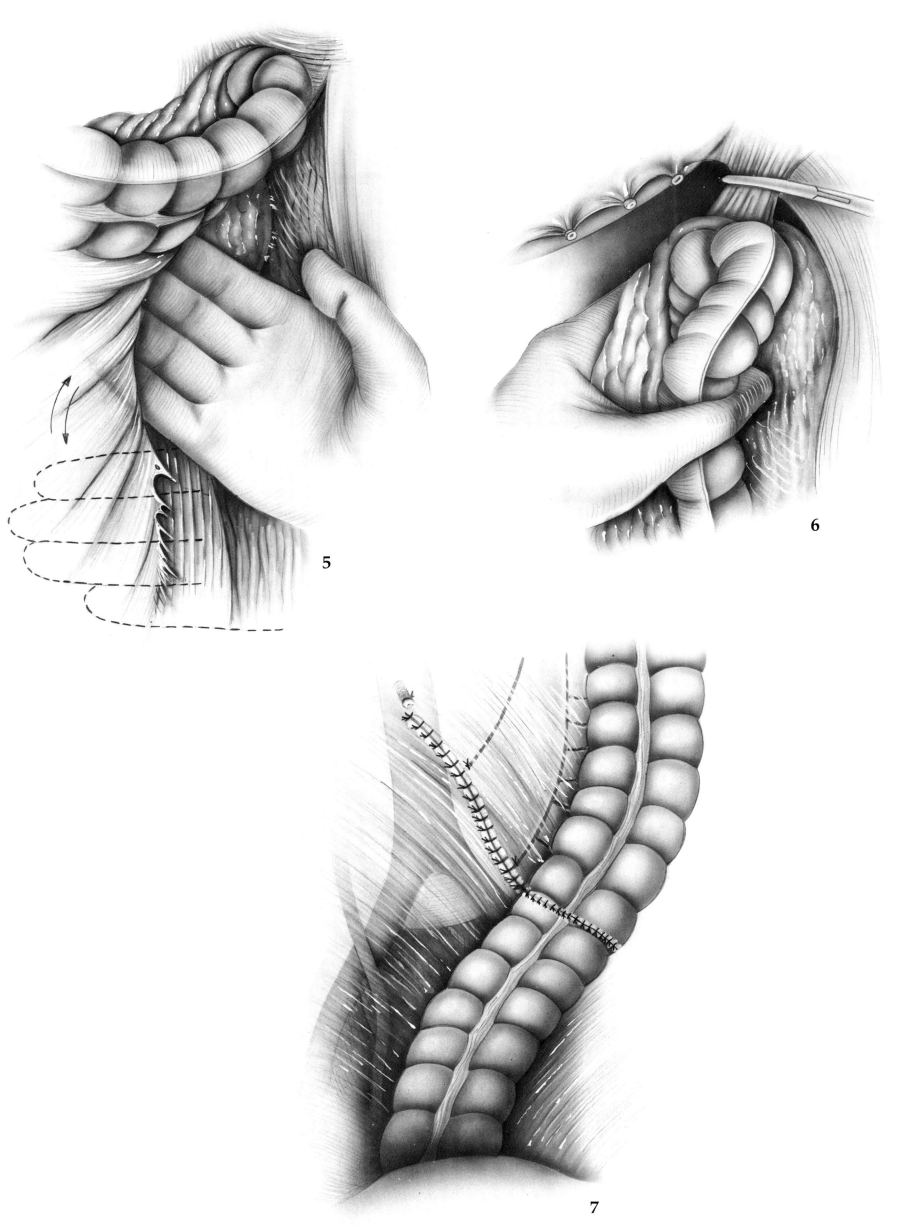

Anterior Resection

1 The patient is placed on an operating table equipped with shoulder braces. Initially the table is flat; during the pelvic dissection it is tilted into a deep Trendelenburg position, with the knees flexed parallel to the floor. A urinary catheter is placed and the abdomen is explored through a midline incision extending from above the umbilicus to the pubis.

2 The boundary of the resection for this mid-rectal lesion is illustrated by the broken line. The specimen should include the portion of the colon from the middle of the sigmoid to 5 cm below the distal margin of the tumor. The inferior mesenteric artery is divided immediately distal to the branch to the proximal sigmoid colon.

3 The left lateral peritoneum is incised and the sigmoid retracted medially, exposing the left ureter coursing through the retroperitoneum. This incision is carried anteriorly and medially, between the bladder and the rectum.

4 The right side of the sigmoid mesocolon is opened immediately to the left of the midline, allowing palpation of the descending branch of the inferior mesenteric artery. The right ureter is identified and preserved. The sigmoid mesocolon is then dissected from its retroperitoneal position, freeing the sigmoid colon between the medial and lateral peritoneal incisions. The peritoneum overlying the vessels in the mesocolon is incised from the descending branch of the inferior mesenteric artery to the proximal margin of resection. The descending branch of the inferior mesenteric artery is divided between clamps and tied with #00 silk ligatures. Two intestinal anastomosis clamps are placed across the midsigmoid colon, and the bowel is divided with electrocautery.

5 The distal sigmoid colon is retracted anteriorly and the plane between the rectum and the presacral fascia is developed manually. The presacral space can be opened to, or below, the level of the prostate with blunt dissection.

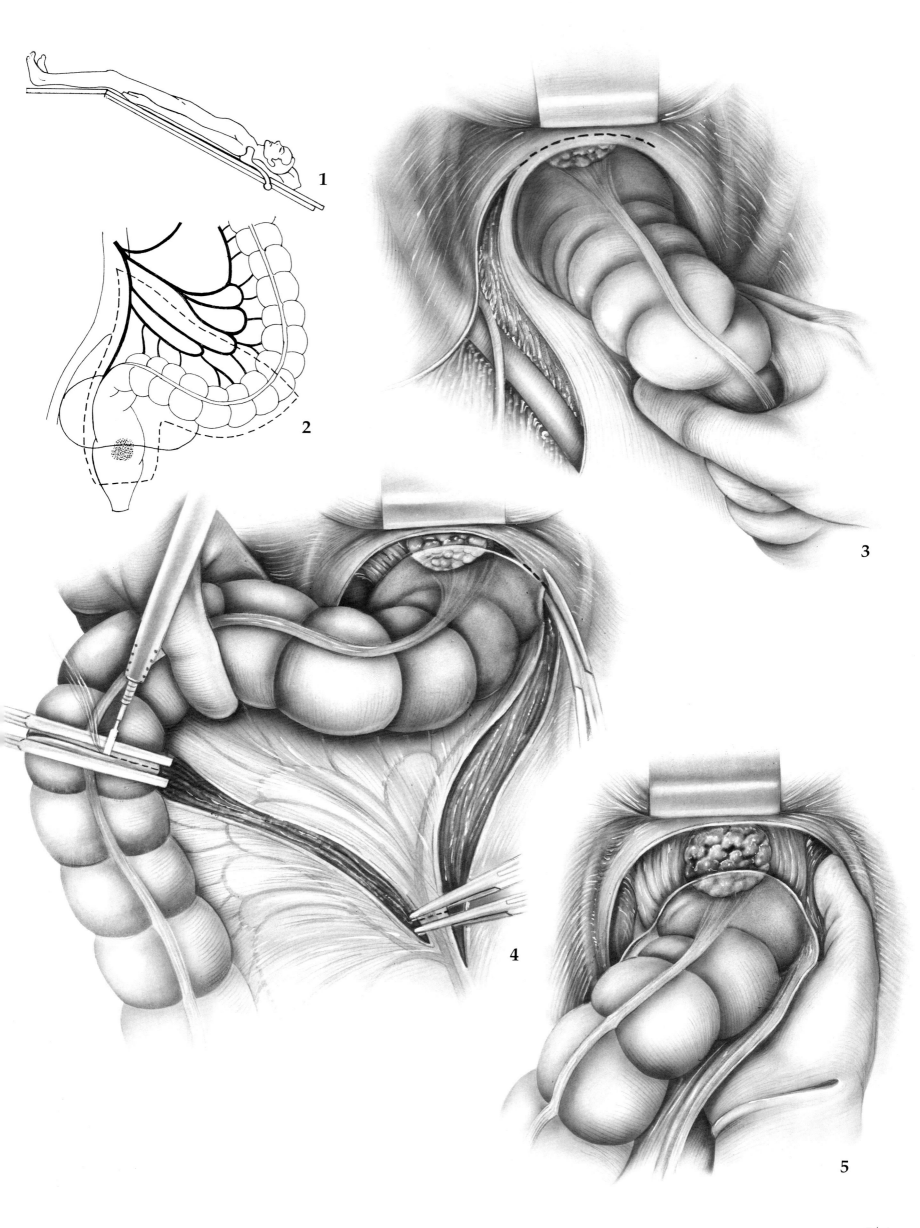

Anterior Resection (*cont.*)

6 The anterior rectum, in the rectovesical space, is dissected bluntly with the aid of a sponge stick. Sharp dissection is required to free the fascial attachments of the rectum to the prostate and the bladder. Exposure of this area is aided by manipulation of the divided distal sigmoid.

7 The lateral rectal stalks carrying the blood supply to the rectum and fixing it to the lateral pelvic sidewalls are divided as far laterally as possible. This is facilitated by retracting the free sigmoid stump to the side opposite the dissection. The lateral stalks are divided medial to a right-angle clamp placed across them.

8 The lateral stalks are suture-ligated, as shown, with #00 silk ligatures.

9 Continued blunt and sharp dissection, with the ligation of the lateral rectal attachments, allows the rectal valves to unfold, providing surprising length below the rectal tumor. A large right-angle bowel clamp is placed across the rectum immediately proximal to the distal margin of resection. The rectum is divided distal to the bowel clamp using the electrocautery, as indicated by the broken line.

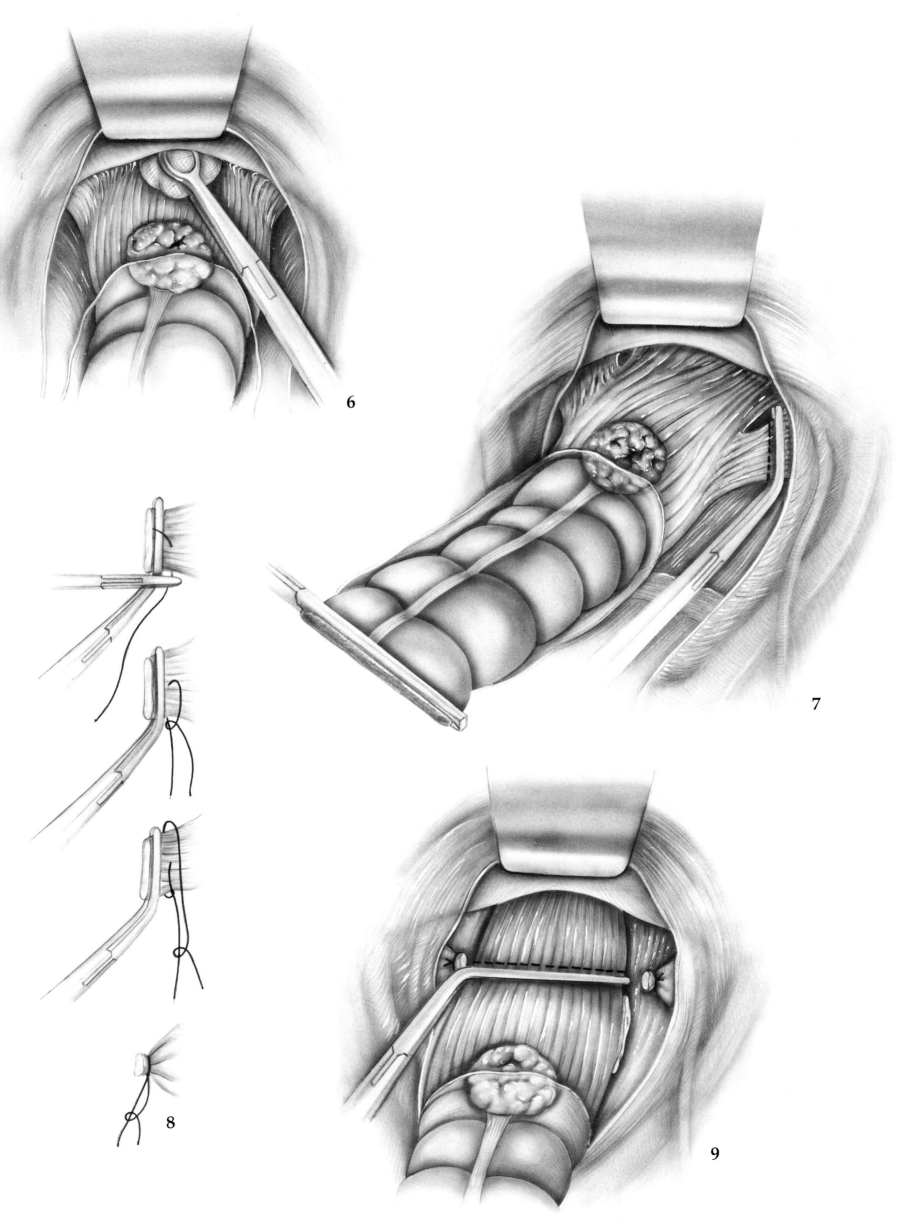

6

7

8

9

Anterior Resection (*cont.*)

Stapled, Side-to-End from Within the Abdomen

Our preferred technique for restoration of bowel continuity is the side-to-end anastomosis fashioned with the circular stapling instrument.

10 A continuous #0 polypropylene suture is placed around the open rectal stump. Each stitch should be taken through the full thickness of the rectal wall approximately 4 mm from the cut end. The stitches should be placed about 1 cm apart. This suture must start and end on the anterior rectum.

11 Sizing instruments that dilate the bowel and determine the largest-sized stapler that can be used for the anastomosis are introduced into the proximal sigmoid. During this procedure the cut edge of the sigmoid colon is stabilized with two Allis clamps.

12 A circular stapling device, with its stalk fully extended, is introduced into the lumen of the proximal sigmoid colon. The tip of the stalk is pressed against the antimesenteric wall of the colon approximately 7 to 10 cm from the cut end. A small enterotomy is created, using the electrocautery over the tip of the stapler, and the stalk is then passed through this enterotomy. The anvil is replaced on the extended stalk and tightened firmly and squarely onto the post.

13 The anvil is introduced into the open rectal lumen and the polypropylene suture is tied tightly about the stalk, and the free ends are cut 5 mm from the knot.

14 The anvil and body of the stapler are tightened together and the stapler is fired, creating the colorectal anastomosis. The stapler is opened, and then removed through the open end of the sigmoid colon. The anvil is unscrewed and removed, and the excised rings of bowel wall are inspected. An incomplete tissue ring certainly means that there is a defect in the staple line between the colon and the rectum. Even with complete rings, however, the anastomosis should be inspected and tested.

15 A flexible flashlight is introduced into the anastomosis through the open end of the sigmoid colon. This allows transillumination and direct inspection of the suture line. If a defect is identified, it is easily closed with interrupted #000 silk sutures.

16 A soft rubber catheter is introduced into the rectum through the cut end of the sigmoid colon, and saline solution is instilled to fill the distal segment. The water column should not fall if the anastomosis is free of defects.

17 After the inspection and testing of the anastomosis and the repair or reinforcement of the suture line, the cut end of the sigmoid colon is closed with a linear stapling device approximately 2.5 cm from the end-to-side stapled coloproctostomy.

18 The stapled end of the sigmoid is fixed to the lateral pelvic sidewall with interrupted #000 polyglycolic acid sutures. If it is considered necessary, a transverse colostomy is carried out in conjunction with this procedure.

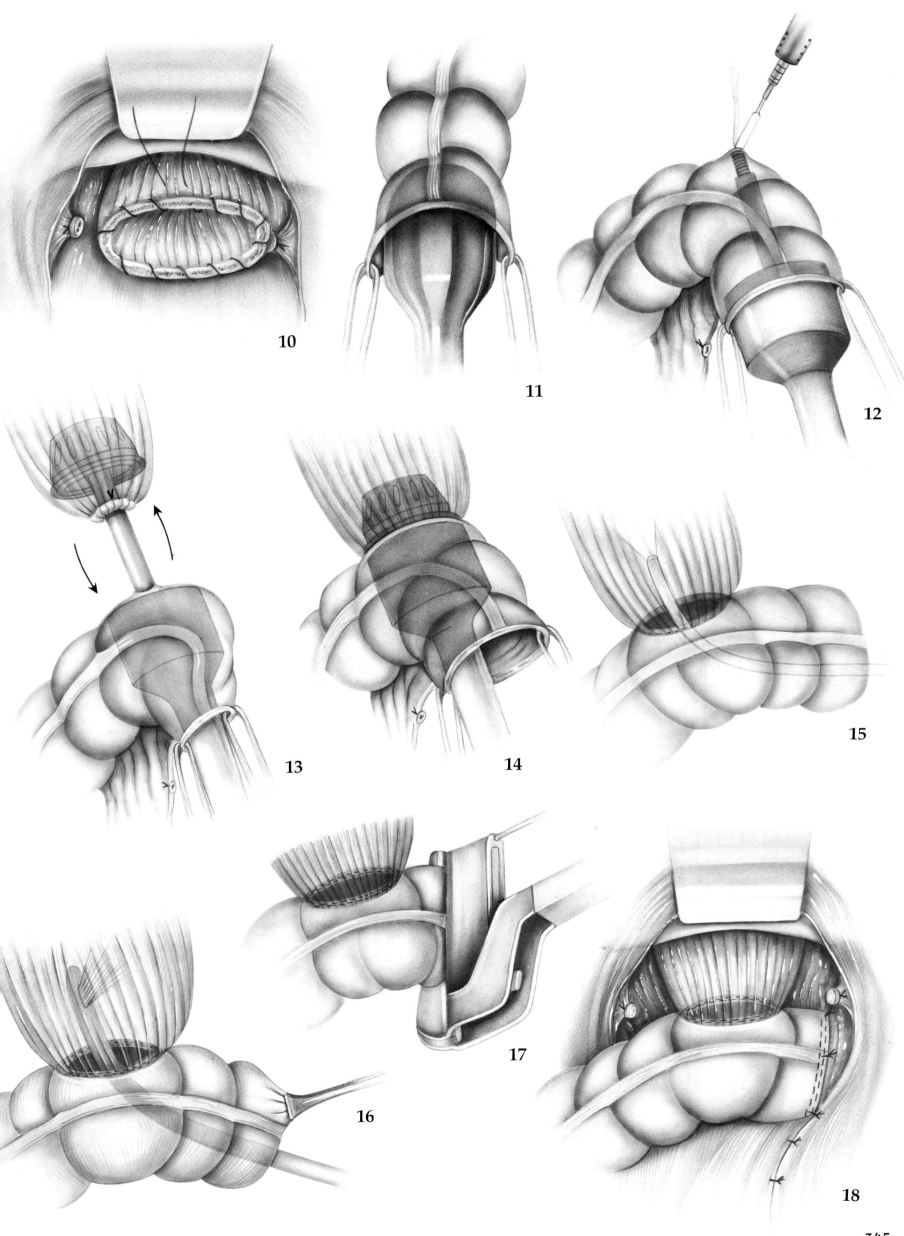

10

11

12

13

14

15

16

17

18

Anterior Resection (*cont.*)

Stapled, End-to-End Through the Rectum

An alternate method of fashioning the stapled coloproctostomy is depicted here. In this technique the stapler, with its stalk extended and the anvil attached, is introduced into the rectum through the anus. This procedure requires that the patient be prepared and draped in the lithotomy position, which significantly limits the surgeon's ability to perform a deep pelvic dissection.

19 A purse-string suture is placed around the rectal stump, as described in **Plate 172, Fig. 10**.

20 A similar purse-string is placed around the cut end of the sigmoid colon. Four #00 silk stay sutures are placed at 2, 5, 7, and 10 o'clock at the end of the bowel to aid the introduction of the anvil into the distal sigmoid segment. Traction is applied to the posterior stay sutures, and the anvil is partially advanced into the bowel lumen.

21 Further traction of the anterior stay sutures pulls the sigmoid over the anvil.

22 The purse-string sutures are tied tightly around the stalk of the stapler, and the ends of the sutures are cut. The silk stay sutures are removed. The body and anvil of the stapler are brought into apposition.

23 The stapler is fired, completing the coloproctostomy.

24 The stapler is withdrawn through the anastomosis and out of the rectum. The tissue rings are inspected. The suture line is inspected by passing a flexible light through the anus into the rectum to transilluminate the bowel. Saline solution is introduced through a catheter placed into the distal rectum from below to further test the anastomosis.

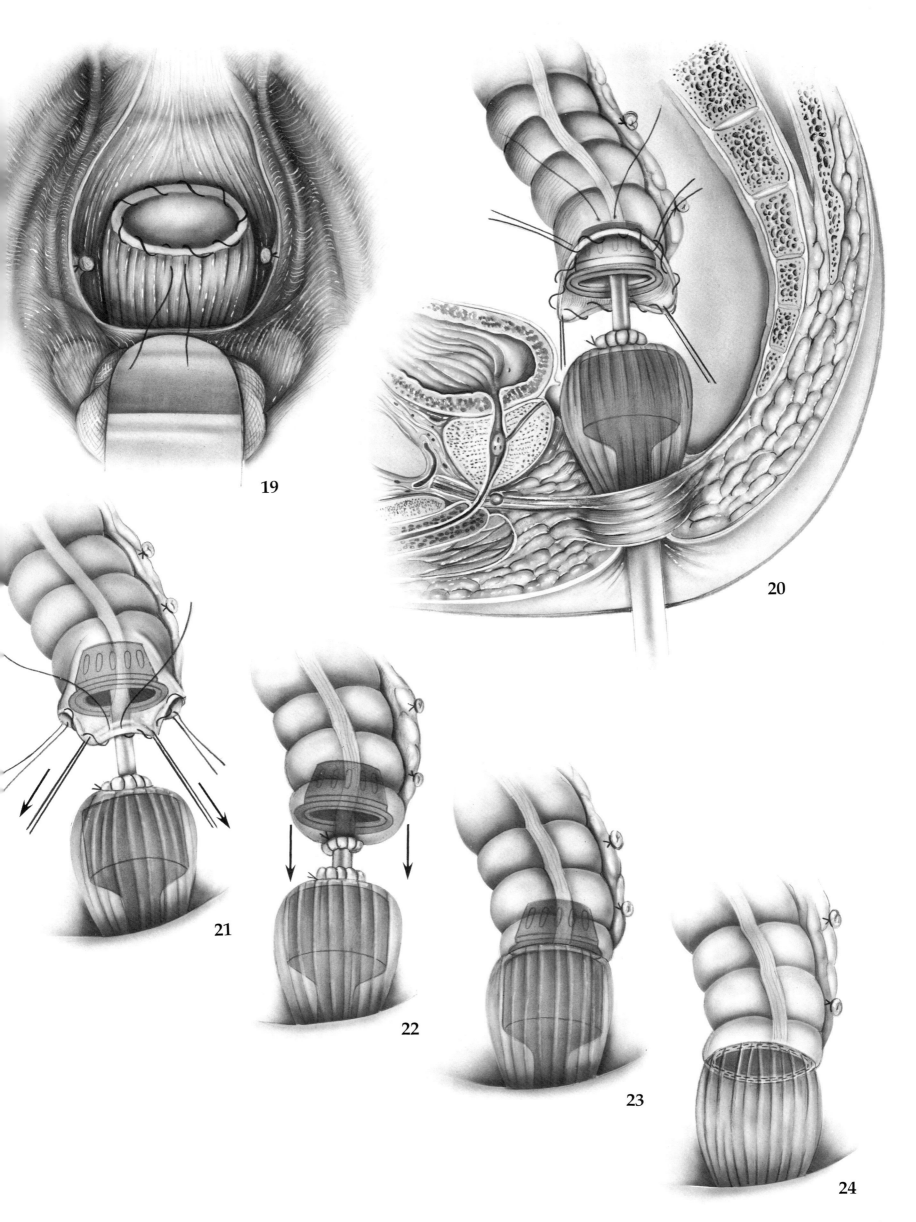

19

20

21

22

23

24

Anterior Resection (*cont.*)

Sutured, Side-to-End

The sutured side-to-end technique is used most commonly when the staple line has failed as a result of the stapler misfiring, or when there is a large defect in the staple line as evidenced by two incomplete rings of tissue upon inspection following a stapled anastomosis.

25 The end of the sigmoid colon is stapled closed. A single-layer anastomsosis using interrupted full-thickness #00 silk sutures is employed. The #00 silk sutures are used rather than #000 silk stitches because they are longer, have a sturdier needle, and present less risk of breaking while tying. Due to the large rectal circumference, the anastomosis between the side of the sigmoid stump and the rectum is accomplished by placing two corner stay sutures and then serially bisecting the remainder of the posterior bowel wall. This is facilitated by the use of a suture holder placed at the superior margin of the incision. These suture holders, commonly used for cardiac valve replacement surgery, are available in most operating rooms. Once the entire row is placed, all sutures except the corner stitches are tied with the knots within the lumen of the anastomosis. The free ends of the tied sutures are cut.

26 The anterior row is placed in a similar fashion.

27 The anterior sutures are tied with the knots outside the anastomosis, completing the coloproctostomy. If appropriate, a transverse colostomy is carried out in conjunction with the resection and anastomosis.

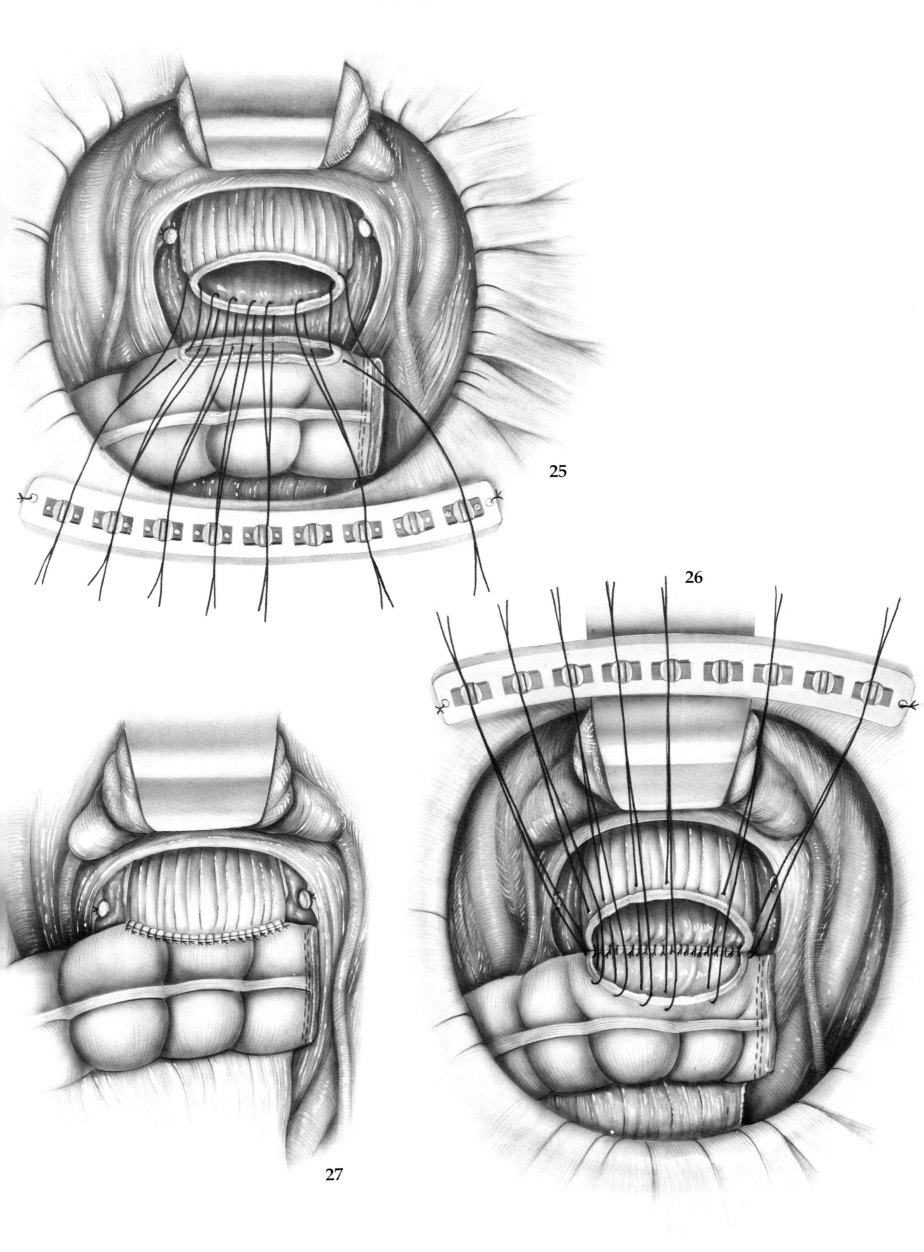

25

26

27

Abdominoperineal Resection

1 The patient is placed on an operating table equipped with shoulder braces. The abdomen is explored through a lower midline incision that extends above the umbilicus. Initially the table is flat; during the pelvic dissection it is tilted into a deep Trendelenburg position. A urinary catheter is required for this procedure. The proximal boundary of the resection for a tumor in the lower portion of the rectum is the middle of the sigmoid colon. The distal sigmoid and rectum, including the anus, is excised. As in the anterior resection (**Plate 170, Fig. 4**), the descending branch of the inferior mesenteric artery is the point where the blood supply to this portion of the colon is transected, as indicated here by the broken line.

2 The lateral peritoneal investments of the sigmoid colon are incised as the sigmoid is retracted medially. This dissection is continued anteriorly and medially between the posterior wall of the bladder and the anterior surface of the rectum. The mesentery of the sigmoid colon is bluntly dissected from the retroperitoneum. The left ureter is identified and carefully preserved. The peritoneum is incised just to the right of midline, and the right ureter is identified and preserved. With the sigmoid colon elevated, the descending branch of the inferior mesenteric artery is identified, divided between clamps, and tied with #00 silk. The remainder of the sigmoid mesentery is then divided between clamps and tied. Three DeMartel clamps are applied to the colon at the proximal line of resection. The middle DeMartel clamp is removed, and the bowel is divided with electrocautery between the two remaining DeMartel clamps.

3 The ureters are followed into the pelvis lateral to the area of dissection. Once adequate visualization of the ureters is achieved, Denonvilliers' fascia, between the rectum and the bladder, is sharply and bluntly dissected.

4 The dissection posterior to the rectum is done bluntly, anterior to the presacral fascia. The lateral stalks are then divided close to the pelvic sidewall, as for the anterior resection (**Plate 171, Figs. 7–9**). This dissection is carried as deep into the pelvis as possible. The profound Trendelenburg position improves the exposure for the pelvic dissection. It is not unusual to visualize the pelvic floor during this dissection.

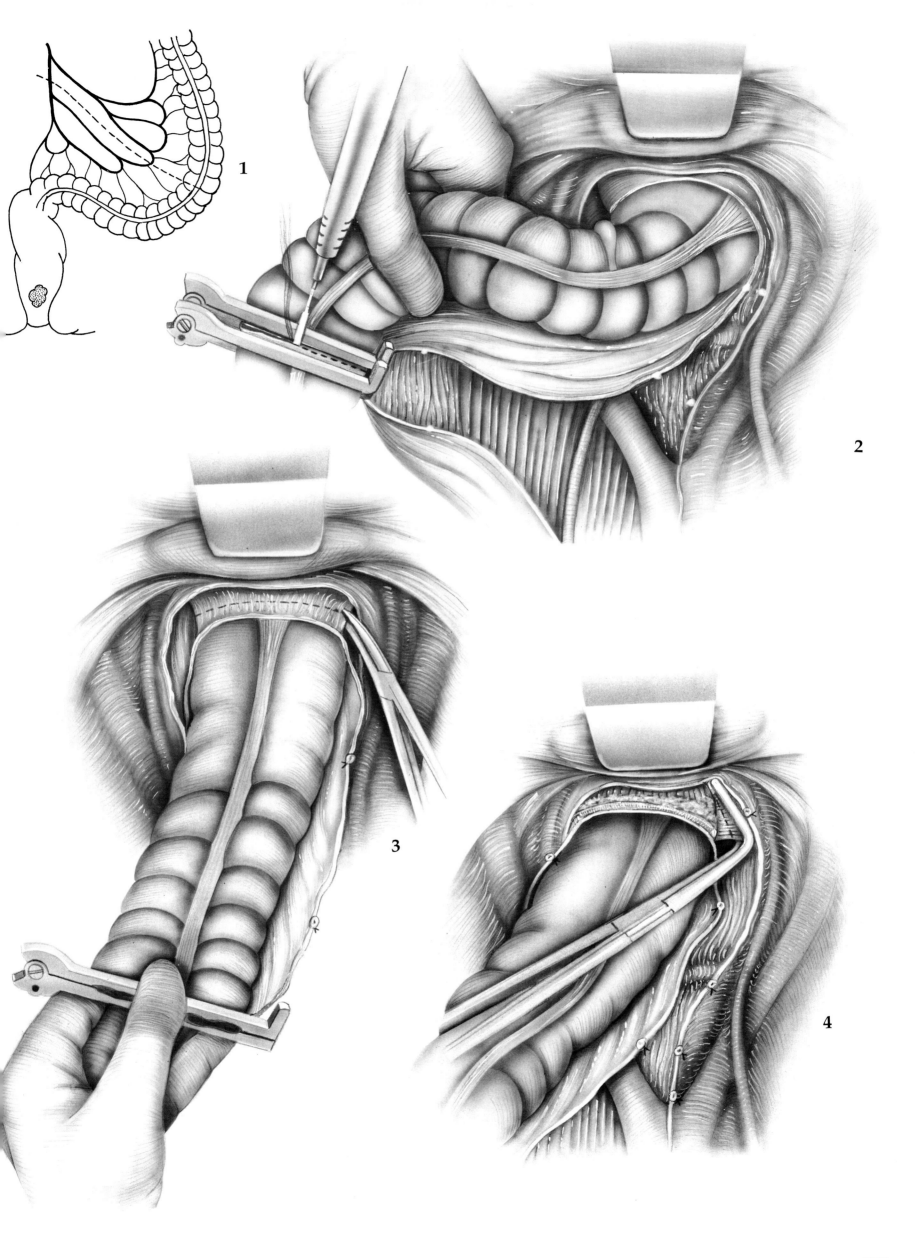

Abdominoperineal Resection (*cont.*)

5 A second glove is placed on the surgeon's left hand. The DeMartel clamp on the distal sigmoid colon is grasped with the left hand, and the second glove is pulled over the De-Martel and colon. It is then tied in place with a length of umbilical tape.

6 The distal sigmoid colon is folded into the presacral space, with the tails of the umbilical tape pushed close to the posterior distal rectum immediately above the levator muscles.

7 The floor of the pelvis is closed with several running #000 polyglycolic acid sutures. The pelvic peritoneum may be undermined to gain additional length, and the proximal sigmoid mesentery may be included in this closure. The distal sigmoid colon is passed through a separate incision in the lateral abdominal wall. The colostomy is held in place with interrupted #000 silk sutures placed into the peritoneum, surrounding the site where the colon exits the peritoneal cavity, and then into the colon in a seromuscular fashion. The colon is fixed to the skin with #000 polyglycolic acid sutures approximately 2 cm proximal to the DeMartel clamp. The abdomen is closed. The colostomy is usually matured as described previously (**Plate 159, Figs. 1–12**).

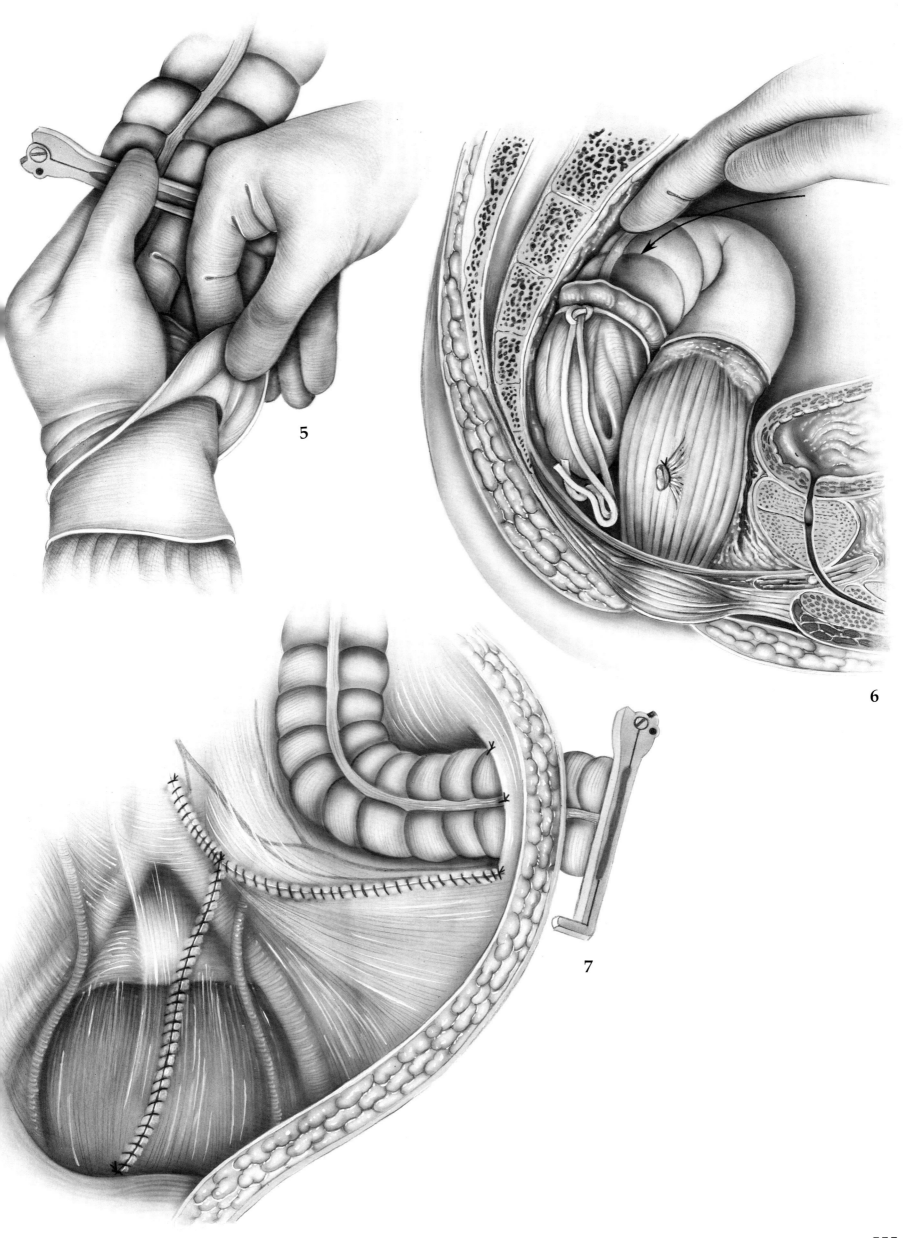

5

6

7

Abdominoperineal Resection (*cont.*)

8 The patient is then placed in the lithotomy position with the aid of stirrups. An incision is made through the skin surrounding the anus, as indicated by the broken line.

9 The lateral skin edges are approximated with a heavy running silk suture, closing the anus within the inverted skin and isolating it during the remainder of the dissection.

10 The subcutaneous tissues, deep to the incision, are divided laterally and posteriorly until the levator muscles are visualized.

11 The anococcygeal portion of the levator sling is opened posteriorly. Usually there is a gush of sanguineous fluid from the abdominal dissection through this defect.

12 The umbilical tape on the distal sigmoid is retrieved and the dissection is continued laterally, using the electrocautery.

13 When the perineal opening is large enough, the glove containing the distal sigmoid and DeMartel clamp is brought through the perineal wound. Retraction of the specimen facilitates the anterior dissection, where the specimen is fixed to the prostate. Division of these final attachments frees the specimen.

14–15 Sump drains are inserted through lateral incisions. As much of the anterior and posterior levator muscle remnants as possible is approximated with interrupted #000 polyglycolic acid sutures. The subcutaneous tissues are closed with interrupted #000 polyglycolic acid sutures. The skin is closed with interrupted #000 nylon stitches. The drains are secured with heavy silk sutures.

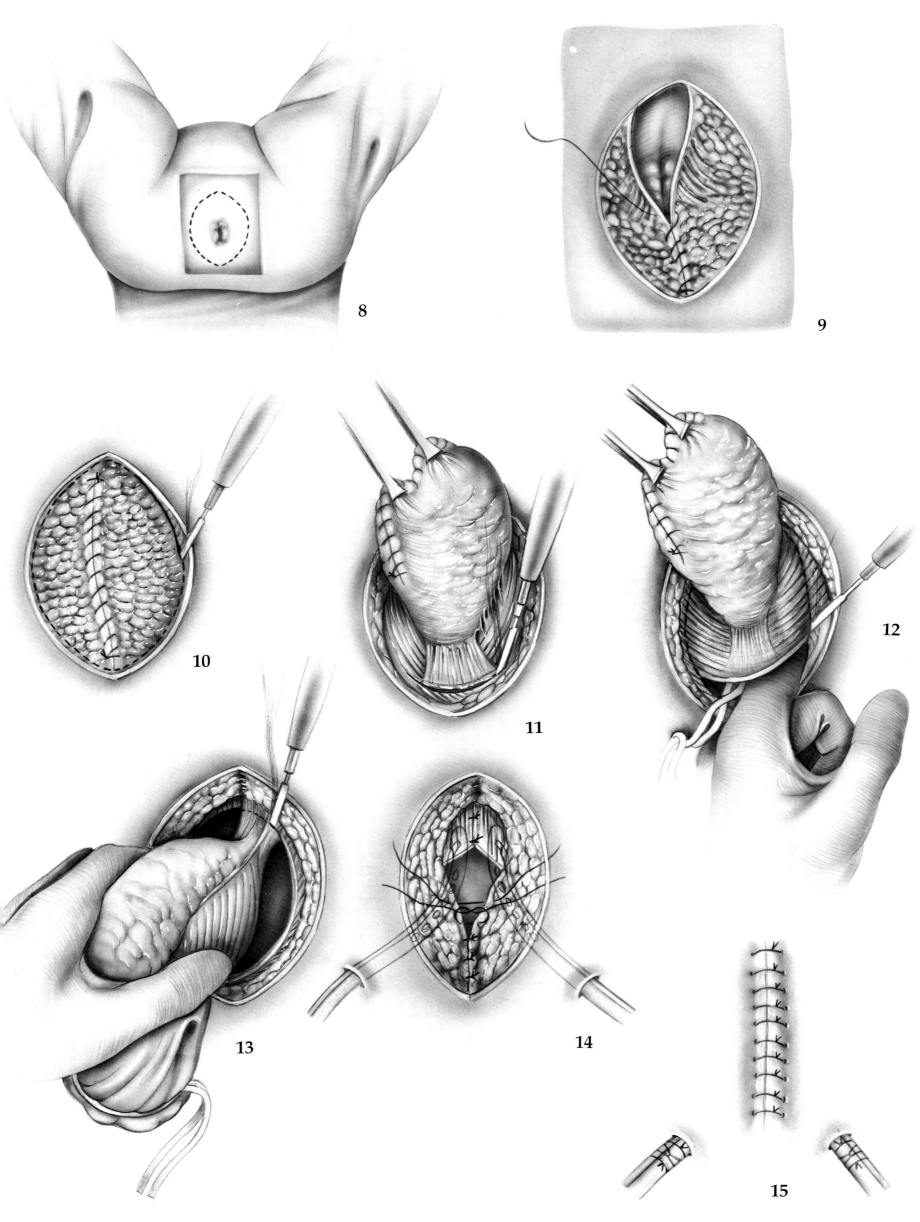

8

9

10

11

12

13

14

15

Palliative Segmental Resection

1 If the patient has a bleeding or partially obstructing colon lesion but has disseminated disease or will not tolerate a significant procedure, a segmental palliative resection may be performed. Although similar limited resections can be done for lesions of the sigmoid colon and splenic flexure, the case depicted is one of a transverse colon lesion.

2 The gastrocolic ligament is freed at a convenient point either inside or outside the gastroepiploic arcades, depending on involvement of the greater omentum by the tumor. The right colon and hepatic flexure are mobilized to bring the right transverse colon to the distal resection margin, rather than mobilizing the splenic flexure, if resection with adequate margins precludes easy reapproximation of the colon.

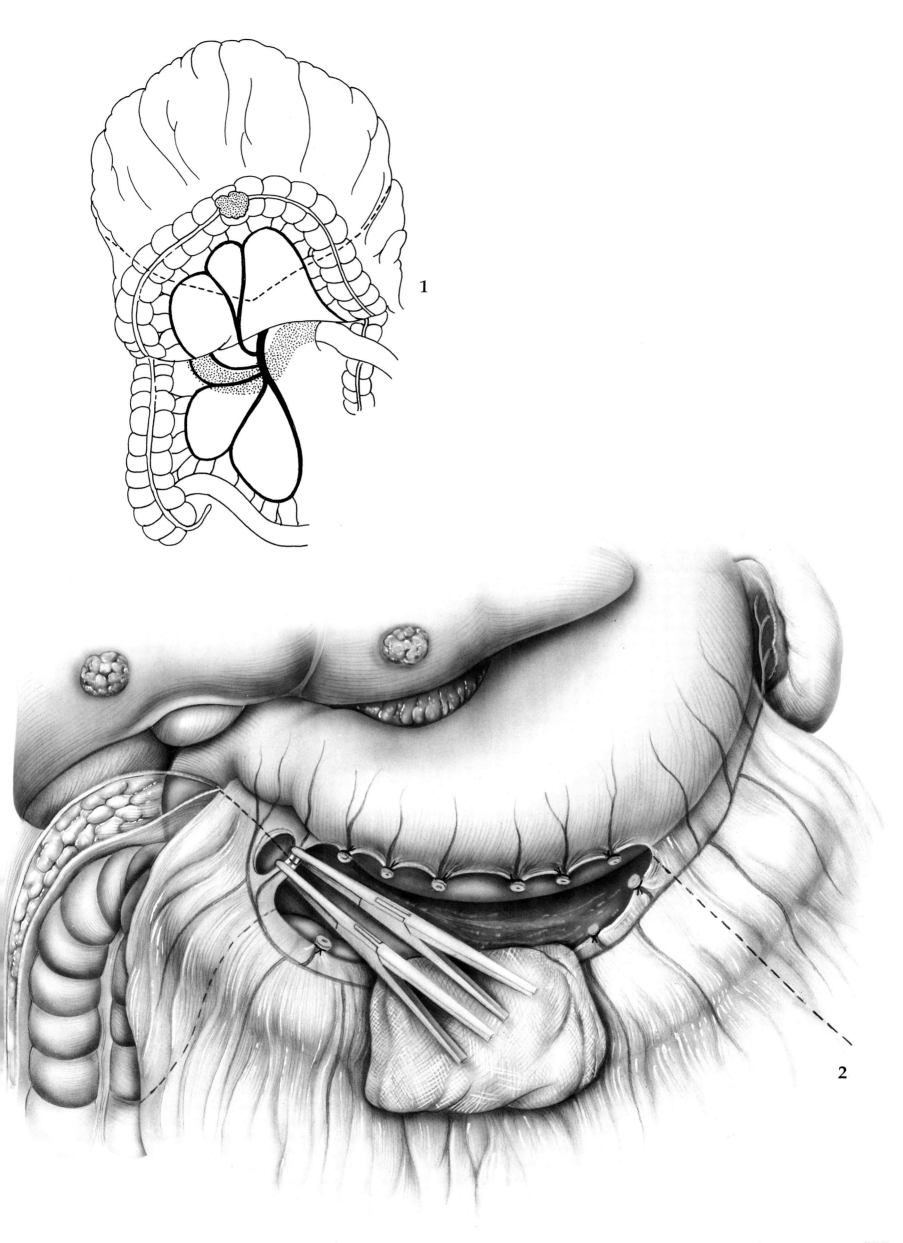

1

2

Palliative Segmental Resection (*cont.*)

3 Adequate margins in healthy and uninvolved colon are chosen. The vessels supplying the colon to be resected are divided, away from the tumor but not at their origin as in curative resections.

4 A rapid anastomosis is constructed with the gastrointestinal anastomosis stapler (see **Plate 163, Figs. 10–11** and **Plates 48–49, Figs.14–17**) after dividing the colon proximally and distally with linear stapling devices. The mesentery is closed with a continuous #000 polyglycolic acid suture. The rectum is dilated at the conclusion of the procedure, to minimize distension of the colon between the closed rectal sphincter and the competent ileocecal valve.

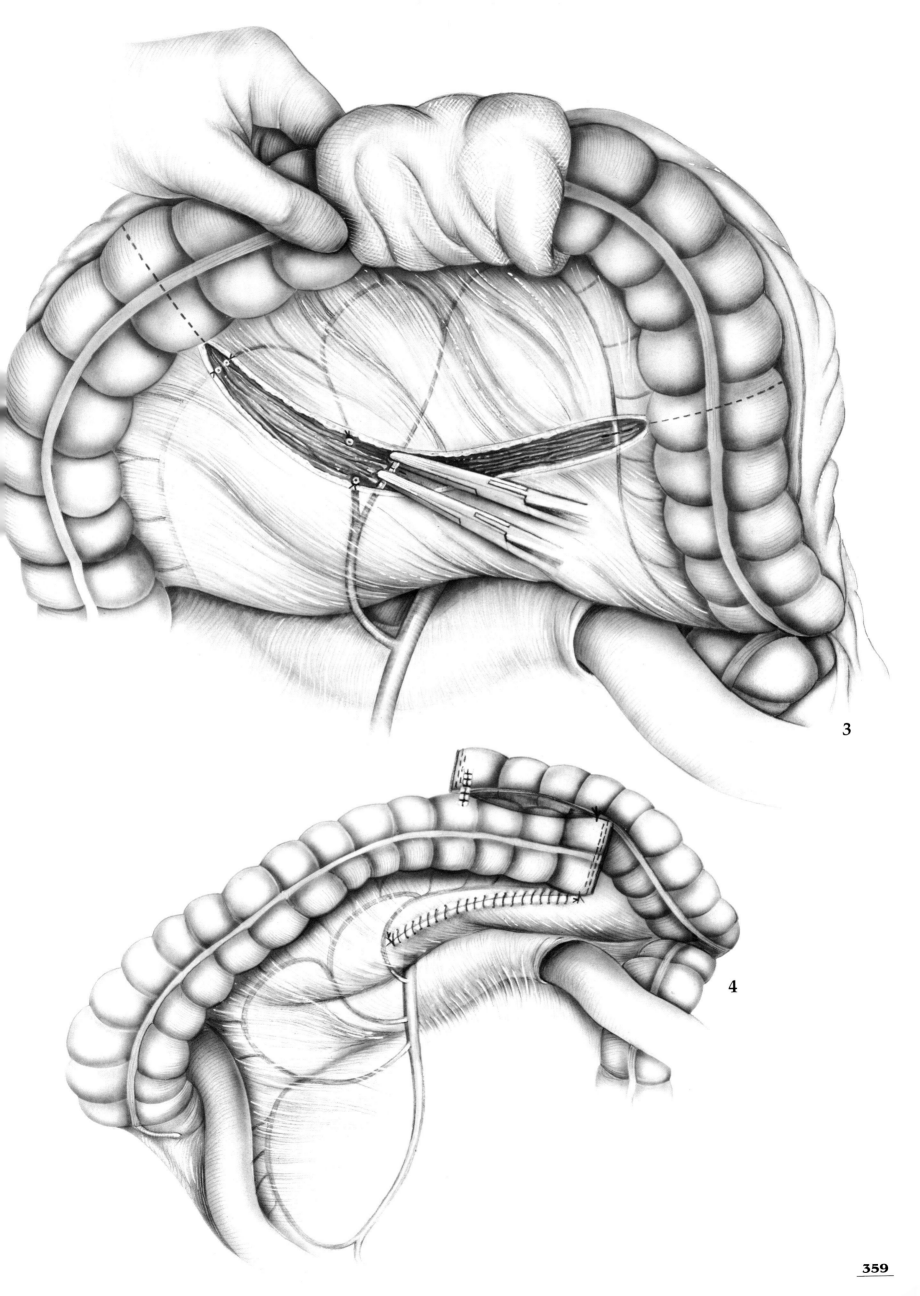

3

4

Emergency Surgery for Diverticulitis (Hartmann's Procedure for Sigmoid Resection)

1 In acute diverticulitis the abdomen is explored through a lower midline incision. The segment of acutely inflamed sigmoid colon containing the perforation into the sigmoid mesocolon is excised as indicated by the broken line. This is most easily accomplished by incising the lateral parietes and dividing the bowel between two Kocher clamps.

2 The involved sigmoid is peeled off of the retroperitoneum by blunt dissection. Better visualization of the area near the ureter is obtained by starting the dissection laterally and superiorly, where the retroperitoneum is not inflamed.

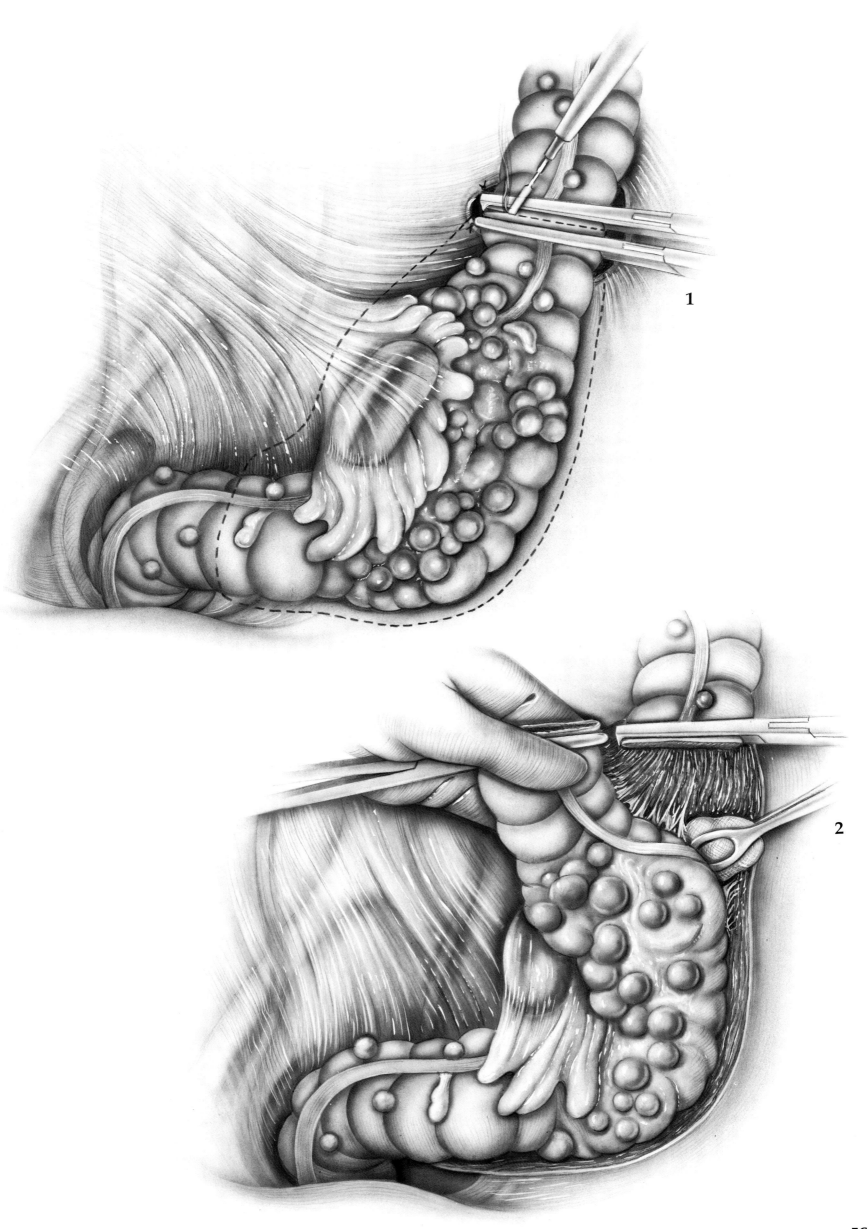

Emergency Surgery for Diverticulitis (Hartmann's Procedure for Sigmoid Resection) (*cont.*)

3 The mesentery of the sigmoid colon is divided between clamps, close to the bowel, after it is freed superiorly and laterally and after the ureter has been safely identified. The abscess within the mesocolon is excised.

4 A linear stapling device is used to close the distal sigmoid colon. The specimen is divided between the stapler and a Kocher clamp and is then removed from the operative field.

5 The distal segment is freed further if necessary, allowing it to be sutured to the lateral parietes. This is done to prevent it from retracting into the pelvis and to secure it in a position that can be verified by radiographs prior to reestablishing bowel continuity.

6 An end colostomy is fashioned (see **Plate 159, Figs. 11–12**). Often the distal segment is filled with hard stool. The segment should be manually disimpacted and the anus should be dilated at the conclusion of the operation.

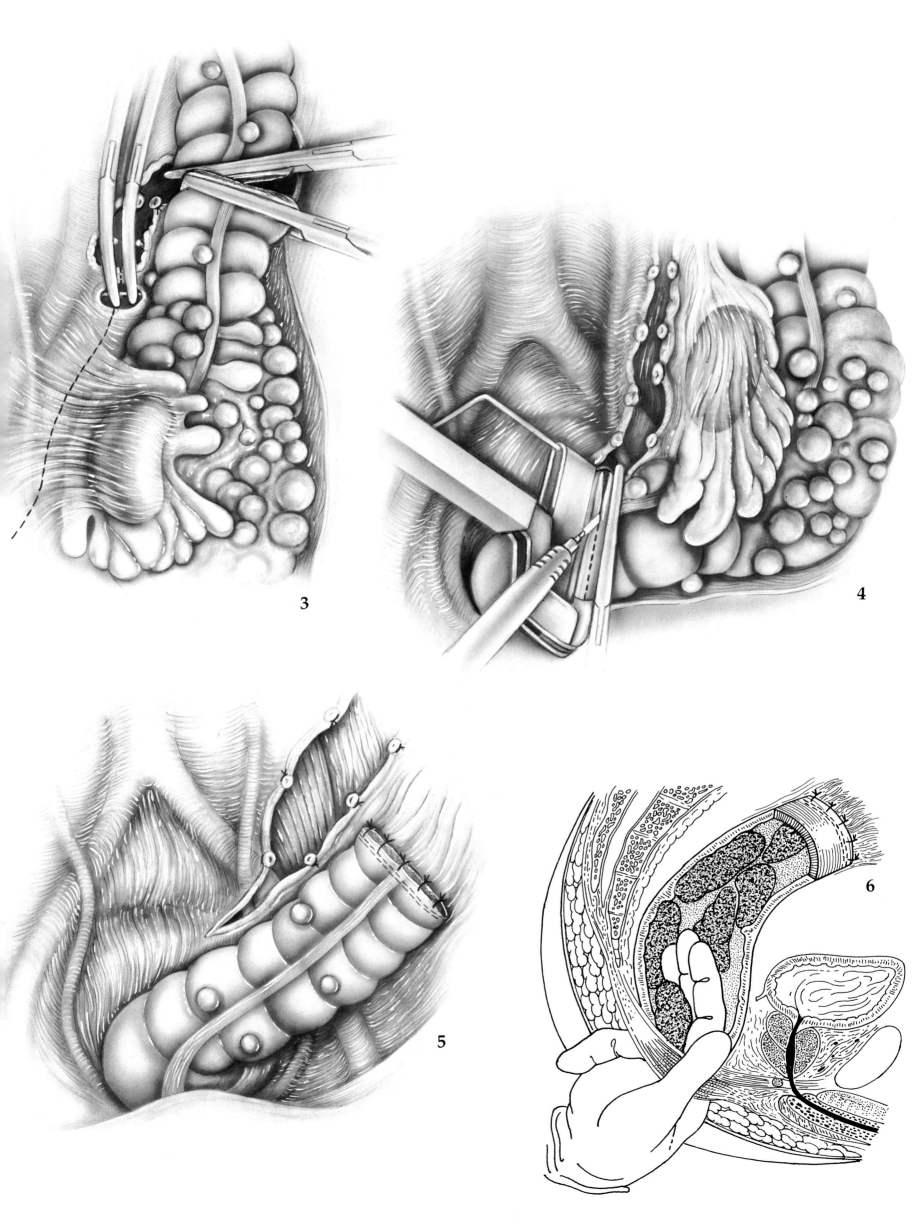

Emergency Surgery for Diverticulitis (Hartmann's Procedure for Sigmoid Resection) (*cont.*)

Repair of a Sigmoid-Vesical Fistula

7 Where there is evidence of a communication between the sigmoid and the bladder, the operation is generally made more difficult by the fixation of the sigmoid loop deep within the pelvis. The boundaries of the resection are outlined by the broken line.

8 A useful technique to facilitate this dissection is to connect the bladder catheter to a two-way bladder irrigation set. The bladder can be distended with 400 to 600 mL of saline solution, colored with dilute methylene blue, through the bladder irrigation set. This distension of the bladder elevates it out of the pelvis, allowing an easier dissection of the colon from the bladder wall. Any defects in the bladder will be easily identified by the leakage of the methylene blue.

9 The proximal sigmoid is divided, and the ureter is identified in the retroperitoneum. The segment of sigmoid attached to the bladder remains intact.

10 Traction on the sigmoid allows it to be sharply dissected from the bladder. When the fistula is reached, the methylene blue gushes through the defect, clearly identifying the hole. The irrigation bottle is then clamped, the urinary catheter is allowed to drain the bladder, and the defect is repaired with three layers of #000 polyglycolic acid sutures. The bladder is refilled to test the closure before the conclusion of the operation. Once the attachments to the bladder are freed, the distal segment is divided and closed with a stapling device and fixed to the lateral parietes as in **Figs. 4** and **5**.

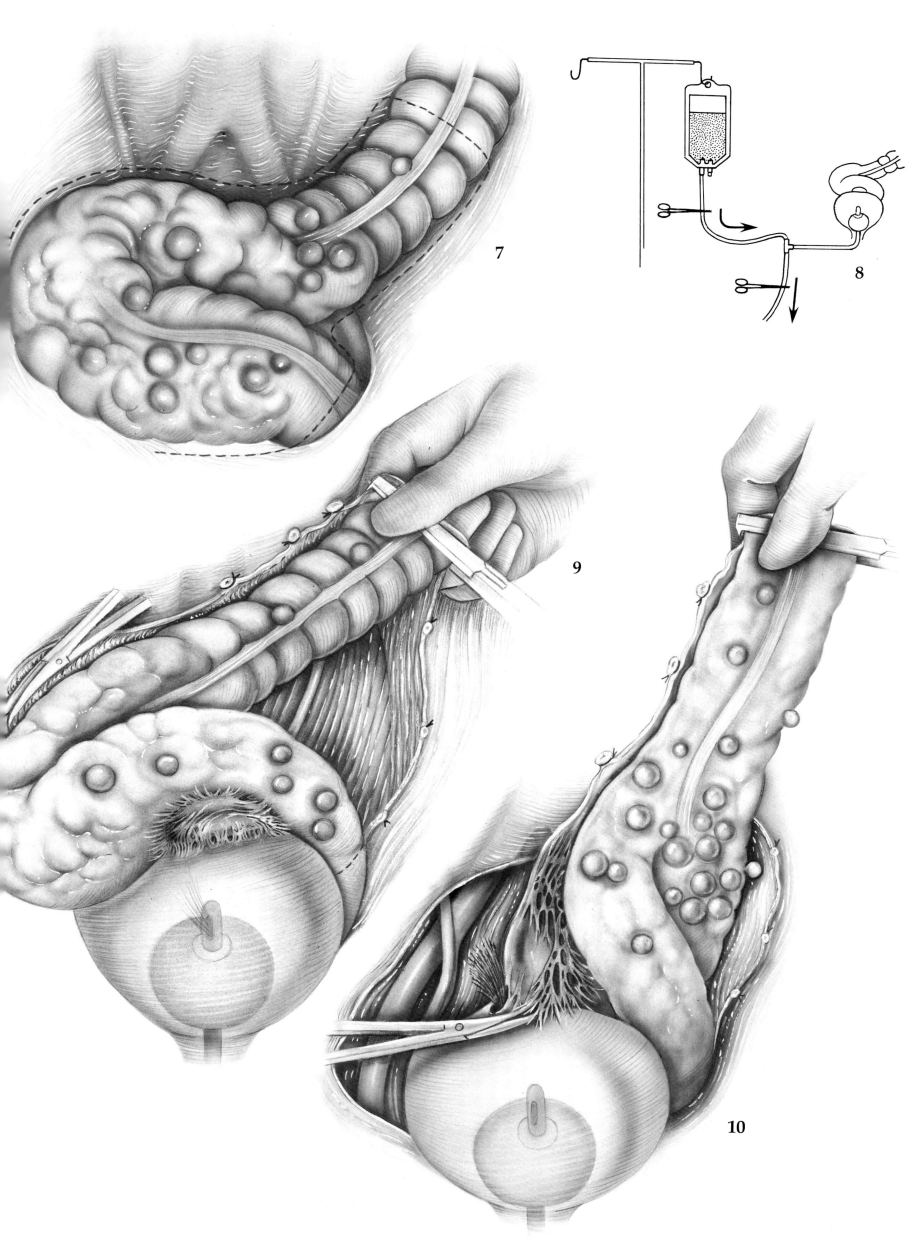

7

8

9

10

Emergency Surgery for Diverticulitis (Hartmann's Procedure for Sigmoid Resection) (*cont.*)

Reapproximation of the End Colostomy and the Closed Distal Segment

11 When the colostomy and the closed distal segment of the sigmoid are to be reapproximated, an abdominal radiograph will show the relationship between the staples on the distal segment and the colostomy. Either a transverse incision (dashed line), midway between the stoma and the staple line, or an oblique incision (dotted line) is used.

12 There are commonly many matted loops of small bowel in the pelvis, adherent to the area of prior dissection and inflammation. The approach to the distal bowel is aided by the preoperative placement of a large red Robinson catheter into the distal sigmoid via the rectum. The dissection proceeds close to the lateral peritoneal wall and is carried down to the rectal segment, which has remained fixed to the lateral parietes.

13 The anastomosis between the descending and distal sigmoid colon may be accomplished in a side-to-side fashion with the gastrointestinal anastomosis stapler, as shown.

14 Alternatively, a two-layer end-to-side anastomosis may be created. The inner layer is accomplished with a continuous #000 polyglycolic acid suture line. The interrupted, outer, seromuscular layer is performed with #000 silk, inverting the first layer. Because the defunctionalized distal colon tends to shrink with time, becoming significantly smaller than the proximal segment, the end-to-side and side-to-side anastomoses are easier. Additionally, the distal segment does not have to be extensively mobilized, which would risk injury to the ureter.

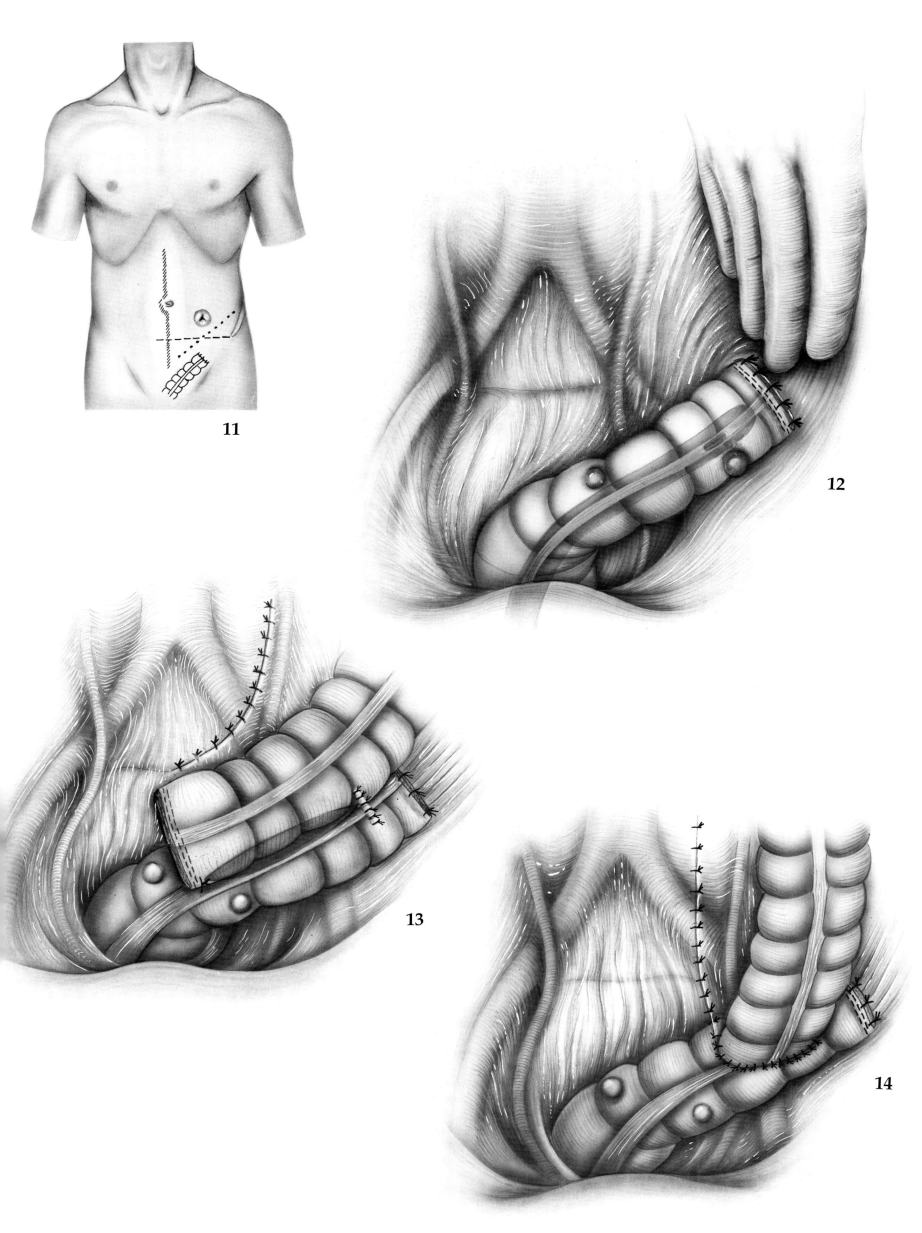

11

12

13

14

Mikulicz Resection (Volvulus of the Sigmoid Colon)

The Mikulicz technique requires long segments of free proximal and distal intestine. In addition to this description for volvulus, it may be used in the transverse colon, in the ascending colon and ileum, and with two limbs of small intestine. In these last examples a prior suture-line breakdown usually is the process that necessitates in the Mikulicz resection.

1 A generous midline incision is used, because the rotated (and possibly gangrenous) sigmoid colon often fills the entire abdomen.

2 If the sigmoid colon is infarcted, it is resected *en bloc*. If viable, however, the sigmoid colon is untwisted and the lateral peritoneal attachments of the descending colon and rectosigmoid junction incised, as indicated by the broken line. Viable proximal and distal portions of the sigmoid are identified, and vessels at the mesenteric border are divided between clamps and tied. DeMartel clamps are placed, allowing removal of the mid-sigmoid arc as indicated. The remainder of the mesentery containing the vessels to this segment of bowel is divided between clamps and the vessels are tied with #000 silk. The proximal and distal sigmoid colon is divided between the DeMartel clamps with electrocautery.

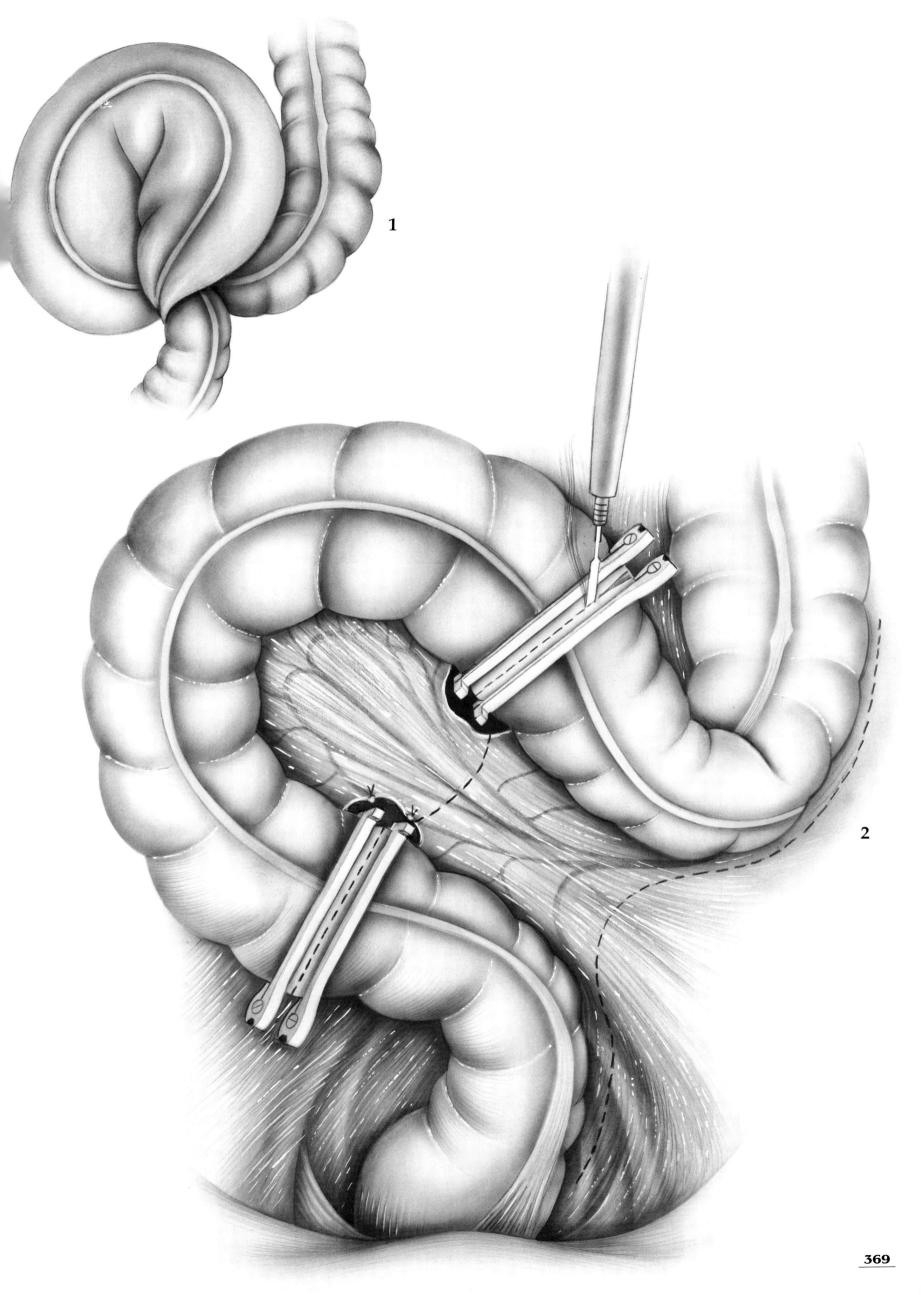

1

2

Mikulicz Resection (Volvulus of the Sigmoid Colon) (*cont.*)

3 Two rows of interrupted seromuscular #000 silk sutures are placed to fix the proximal and distal sigmoid stumps to each other in a side-to-side fashion. The first row of sutures is placed with the end of one DeMartel clamp against the end of the other. The DeMartel clamps are rotated into parallel positions, and the second row of interrupted seromuscular #000 silk sutures is placed. A wide portion of the antimesenteric sigmoid walls is contained between these two suture lines. The suture lines extend from the cut ends of the bowel to well below the fascia.

4 The attached limbs of colon are brought through a skin incision in the left lower quadrant of the abdominal wall. The bowel is fixed to the posterior abdominal fascia and the lateral parietes with #000 silk stitches. The DeMartel clamps are shown end-on and parallel to one another—as after rotation for the placement of the second row of sutures (**Fig. 3**). The DeMartel clamps are removed on the second postoperative day.

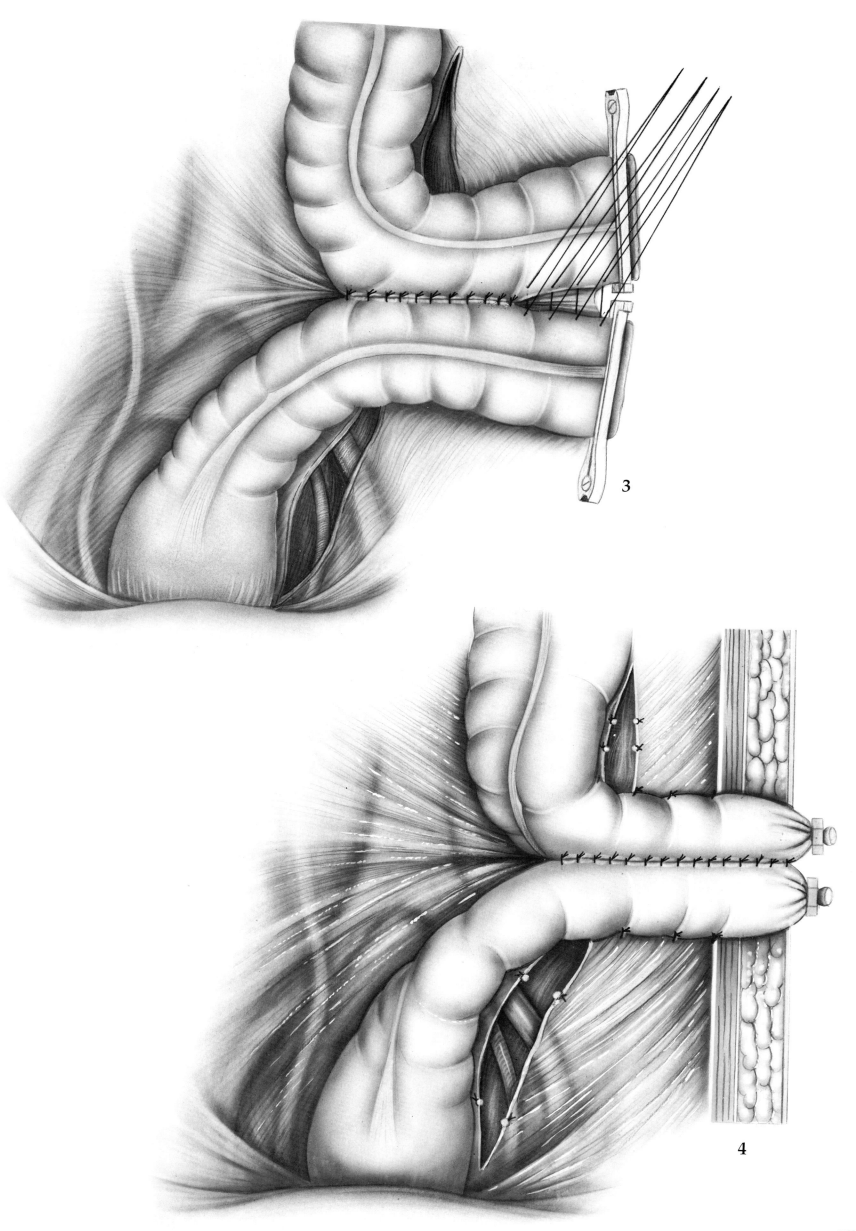

3

4

Mikulicz Resection (Volvulus of the Sigmoid Colon) (*cont.*)

5 One week after the removal of the DeMartel clamps, an intestinal anastomosis stapling instrument is inserted into the bowel through the stomas. Care is taken to position the stapler so that the previously placed suture lines, approximating the walls of the proximal and distal segments, are between the stapler blades. The stapler is fired, opening the common wall between the proximal and distal segments. Because it is essential that this wall be opened deep to the fascia, the stapler may have to be replaced and fired a second time.

6 Subsequently, under local anesthesia, the portion of bowel in the subcutaneous tissues is dissected free to below the fascial ring. No attempt is made to free the bowel segments from the lateral parietes.

7 A linear stapling device is fired across both ends of bowel protruding above the fascia. The colon extending beyond the stapler is removed with electrocautery.

8 The wound may be closed primarily or secondarily, according to the surgeon's preference.

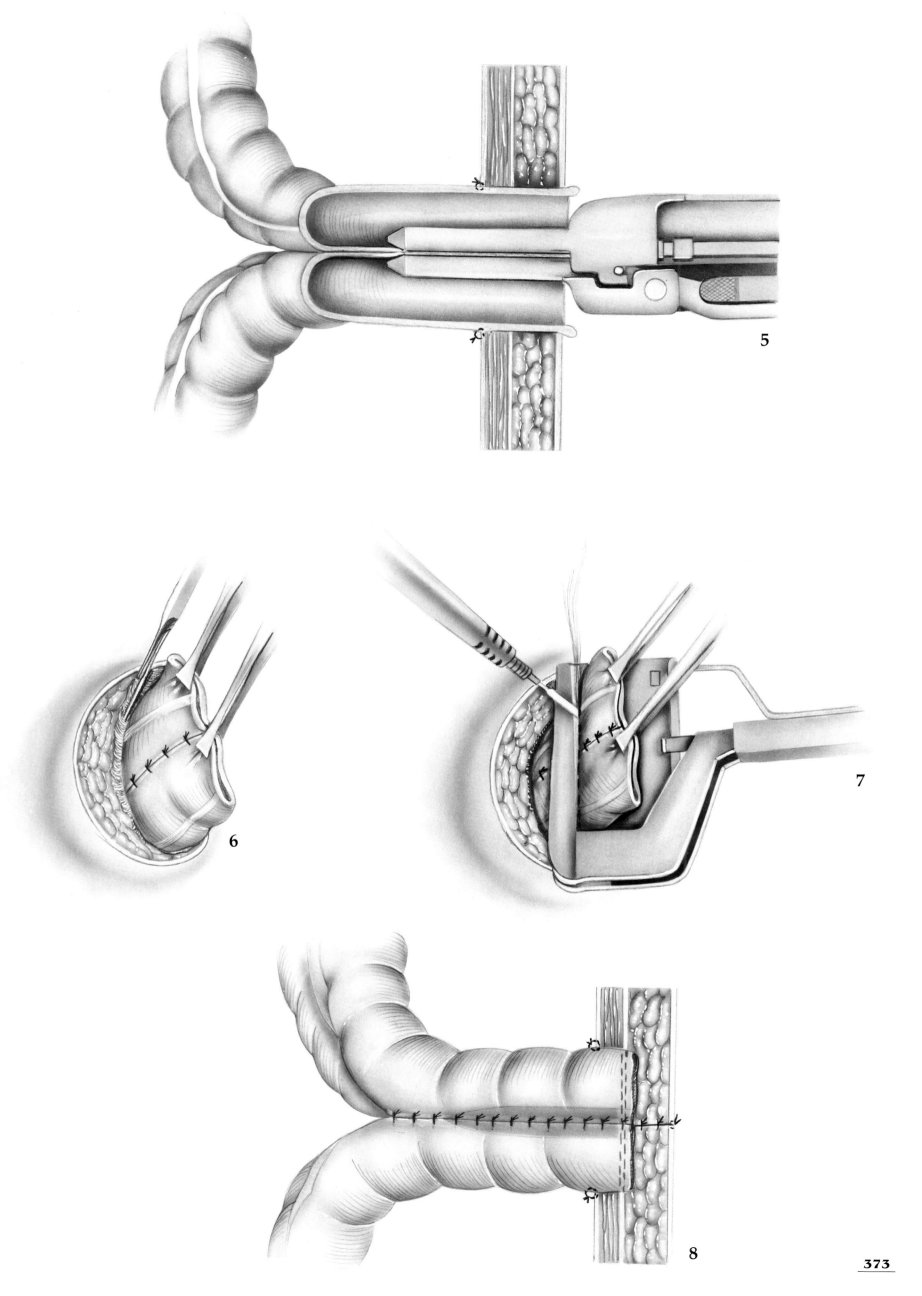

5

6

7

8

Repair of Rectal Prolapse (Ripstein Procedure)

1 The abdomen is explored through a lower midline incision. The peritoneum surrounding the rectum is incised, as is the peritoneum between the rectum and bladder, as indicated by the broken lines.

2 The rectum is retracted out of the pelvis as it is freed anteriorly and laterally.

3 The rectum is bluntly dissected from the hollow of the sacrum.

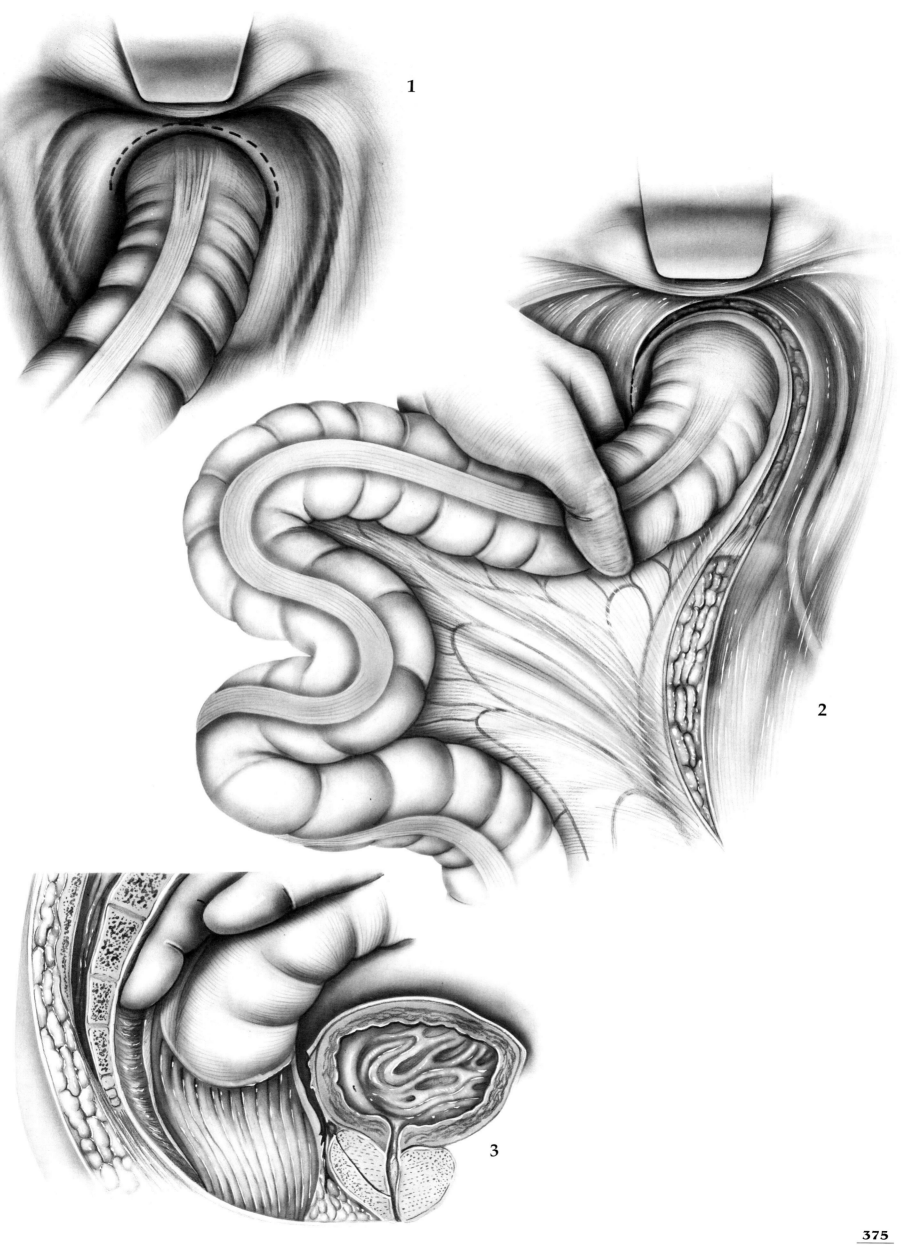

Repair of Rectal Prolapse (Ripstein Procedure) (*cont.*)

4 The anterior rectal wall is bluntly dissected from the posterior bladder, allowing the redundant and anteriorly displaced rectum to be straightened and retracted into the peritoneal cavity.

5 A 2.5-cm-wide piece of Marlex mesh is sutured to the presacral fascia overlying the first sacral vertebra with interrupted #00 silk stitches. Extreme care must be taken not to attempt this maneuver too far laterally. In addition, the stitches must not be placed through the periosteum of the sacrum, lest there be profuse bleeding from the presacral plexus of veins.

6 The colon is retracted and the mesh is placed around the rectum. It is positioned so that there is no undue pressure on the colon.

7 The opposite side of the Marlex mesh is sewn with two or three #00 silk sutures to the presacral fascia. The anterior and lateral walls of the rectum are fixed to the mesh sling with interrupted #000 silk sutures.

8 The lumen of the sling is reexamined, checking that it does not compress the rectum significantly (potentially obstructing the colon in the postoperative period). The peritoneum is closed over the mesh so that adjacent bowel will not become adherent and be eroded by the exposed mesh.

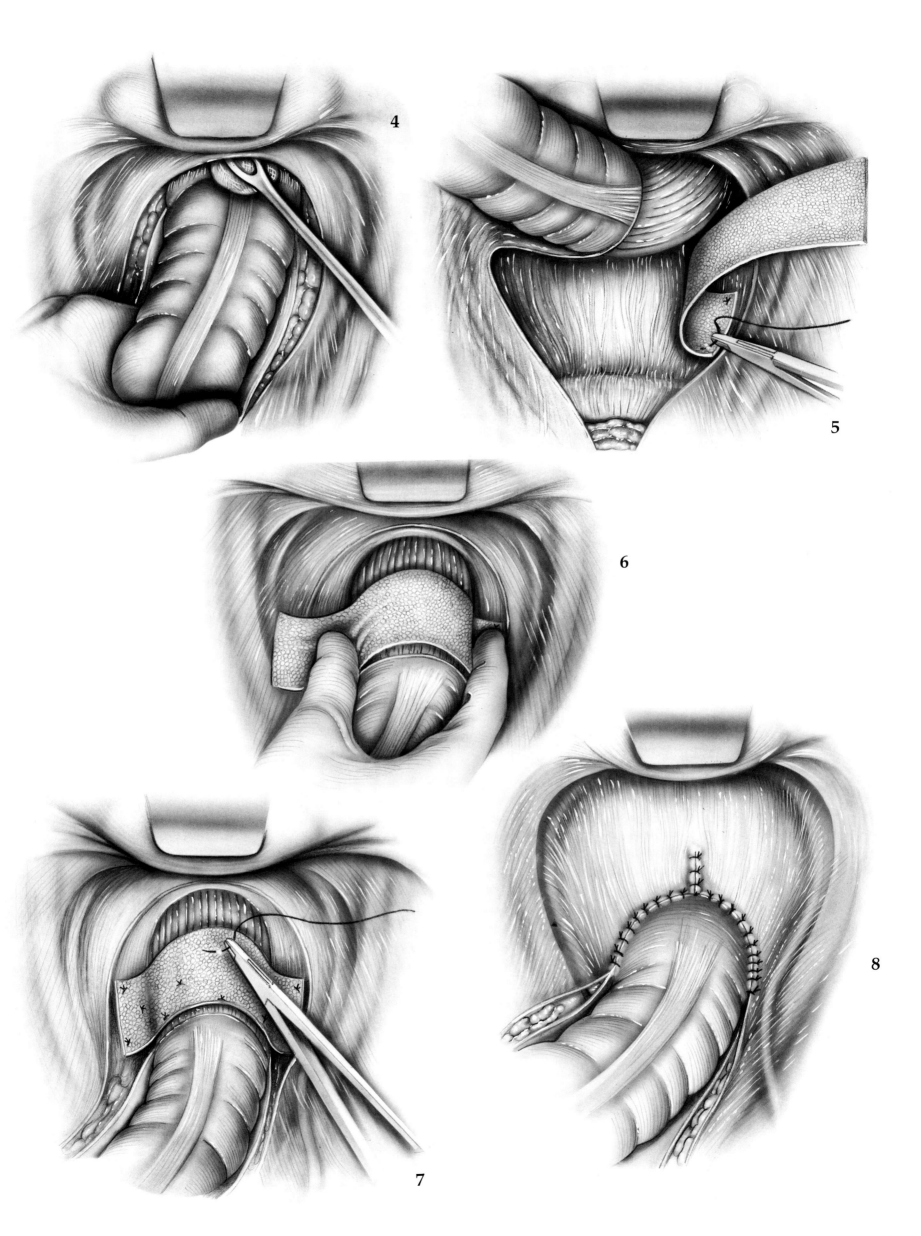

4

5

6

7

8

Total Colectomy and Proctectomy for Benign Disease

1 The patient is placed on an operating table equipped with shoulder braces. Initially the table is flat; during the pelvic dissection it is tilted steeply as shown. A urinary catheter is required for this procedure.

2 The abdomen is explored through a long midline incision extending from the xiphoid to the pubis. Because these resections are usually for benign diseases, the vessels, omentum, and lateral parietes are divided conveniently and not as would be dictated by the necessities of cancer surgery. The gastrocolic ligament is divided between clamps and the vessels are tied with #000 silk ligatures. The ascending, sigmoid, and descending colons are mobilized from their retroperitoneal positions with blunt dissection after incison of their lateral peritoneal investments. The hepatic flexure is taken down either between clamps or with the electrocautery.

3 After the division of the gastrocolic ligament and the mobilization of the proximal descending colon, the splenic flexure is taken down. The descending and distal transverse colon are retracted inferiorly, exposing the lienocolic ligament, which can be safely divided.

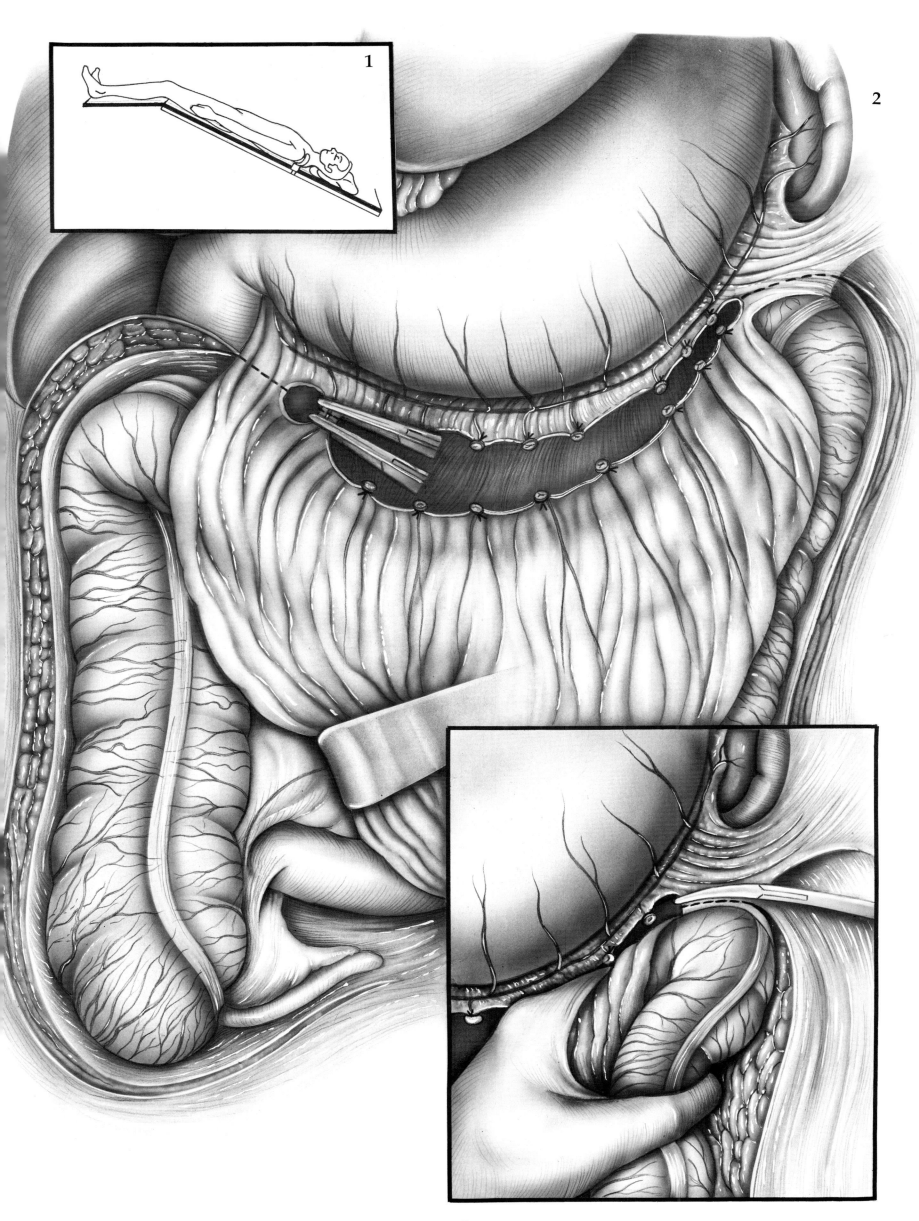

Total Colectomy and Proctectomy for Benign Disease (*cont.*)

4 After the mobilization of the colon, the blood supply is divided between clamps at convenient points in the mesentery and tied with #00 silk. The peritoneum between the rectum and the bladder, as well as that medial and lateral to the rectum, is incised as indicated by the broken line.

5 The usual line of division of the colonic mesentery is shown. By dividing the mesenteries at this level, the number of vascular arcades that require clamping and tying is minimized.

6 DeMartel clamps are placed across the proximal rectum. The middle clamp is removed and the bowel is divided with electrocautery.

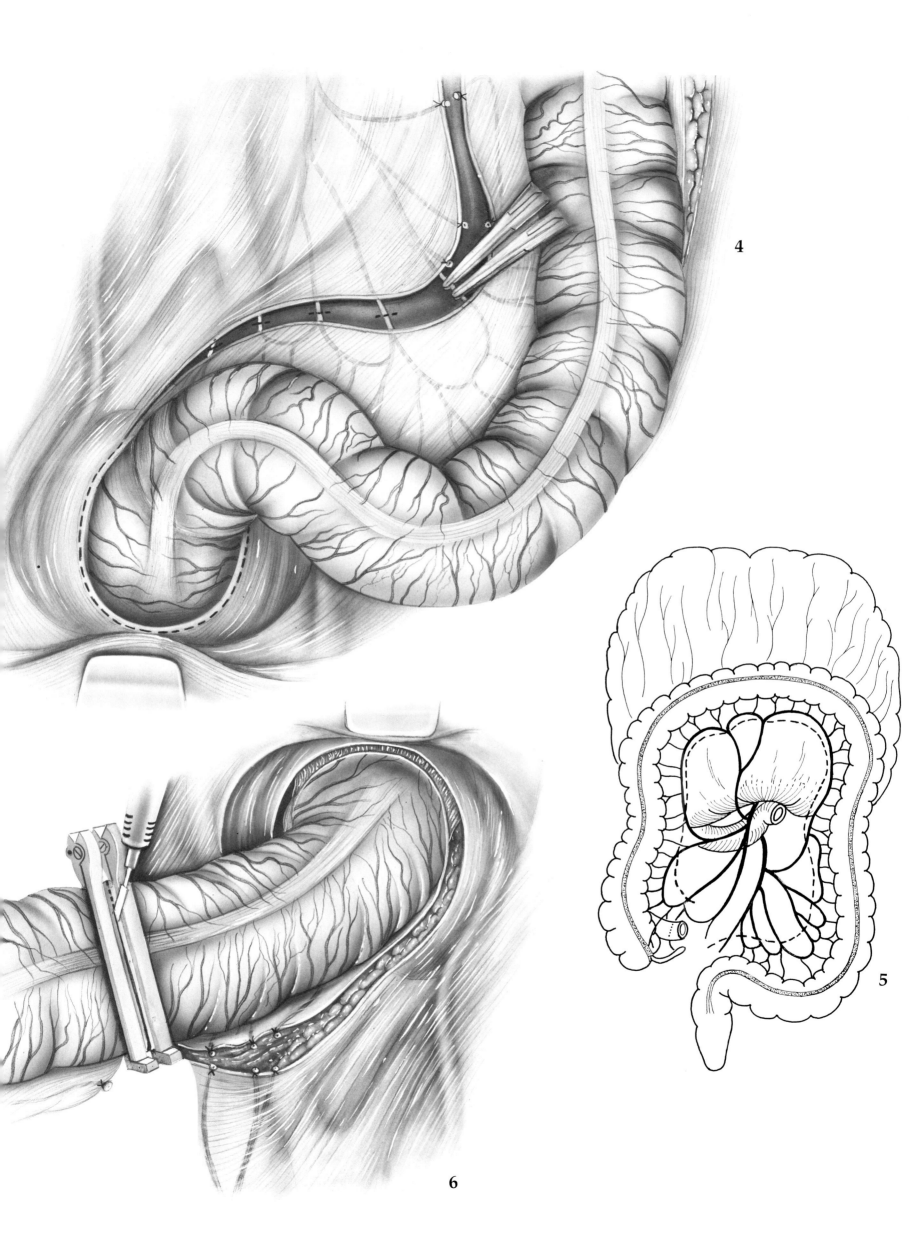

4

5

6

Total Colectomy and Proctectomy for Benign Disease (*cont.*)

7 In contrast to the dissection for malignancy of the rectum, the rectal dissection is carried out close to the bowel wall. This dissection is carried down to the levator muscles.

8 The lateral rectal stacks are divided and tied (**Plate 171, Figs. 7–9**).

9 A second glove is placed on the surgeon's left hand. Holding the DeMartel clamp on the distal rectal stump in the left hand, the glove is turned inside out over the DeMartel and rectum.

10 The glove is secured in place with a length of umbilical tape. The proximal rectum is then folded back into the hollow of the sacrum, with the umbilical tape pushed against the levators posteriorly.

11 By virtue of the small defect made for the limited dissection required to mobilize the rectum, the pelvic floor is easily closed with interrupted #000 polyglycolic acid sutures.

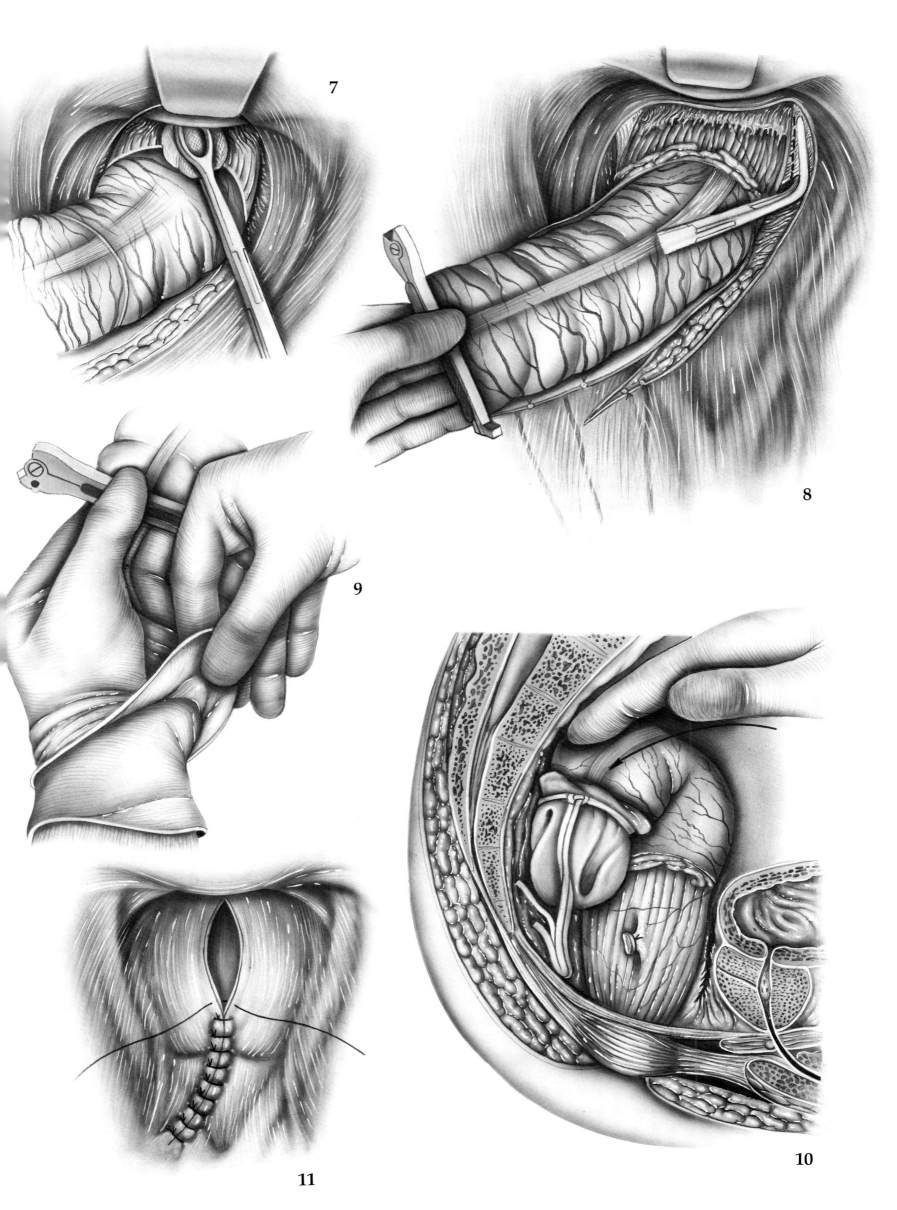

7

8

9

10

11

Total Colectomy and Proctectomy for Benign Disease (*cont.*)

12 The terminal ileum is divided immediately proximal to the ileocecal valve. The specimen is removed from the operative field.

13 For the ileostomy, the skin in the right lower quadrant of the abdomen is grasped and retracted vertically with two Allis clamps. A small ellipse of skin is excised. Normal skin tension converts the ellipse to a circular defect.

14–15 The fascia of the external oblique muscle is incised with the electrocautery in a cruciate fashion. The underlying muscle layers are split, and a wide opening is made in the peritoneum.

16 The ileum is brought through this defect and fixed to the posterior fascia of the abdominal wall with interrupted #000 silk sutures. The small bowel mesentery is fixed to the lateral parietes to prevent subsequent herniation of the proximal small intestine through this defect. The abdomen is closed.

Matured Ileostomy (Brooks' Type)

17 The ileostomy is matured using #0000 polyglycolic acid sutures. These sutures are placed at the 3, 6, 9, and 12 o'clock positions through the full thickness of the bowel stump, then through the ileum again at the level of the skin in a seromuscular fashion, and finally through the skin. When tied, these sutures cause the bowel to evert. The stoma should be constructed so that it protrudes 1.5 to 2.0 cm from the skin surface. Additional stitches are placed between each of the original sutures. These eight stitches are usually adequate to completely evert and fix the ileum to itself and to the skin.

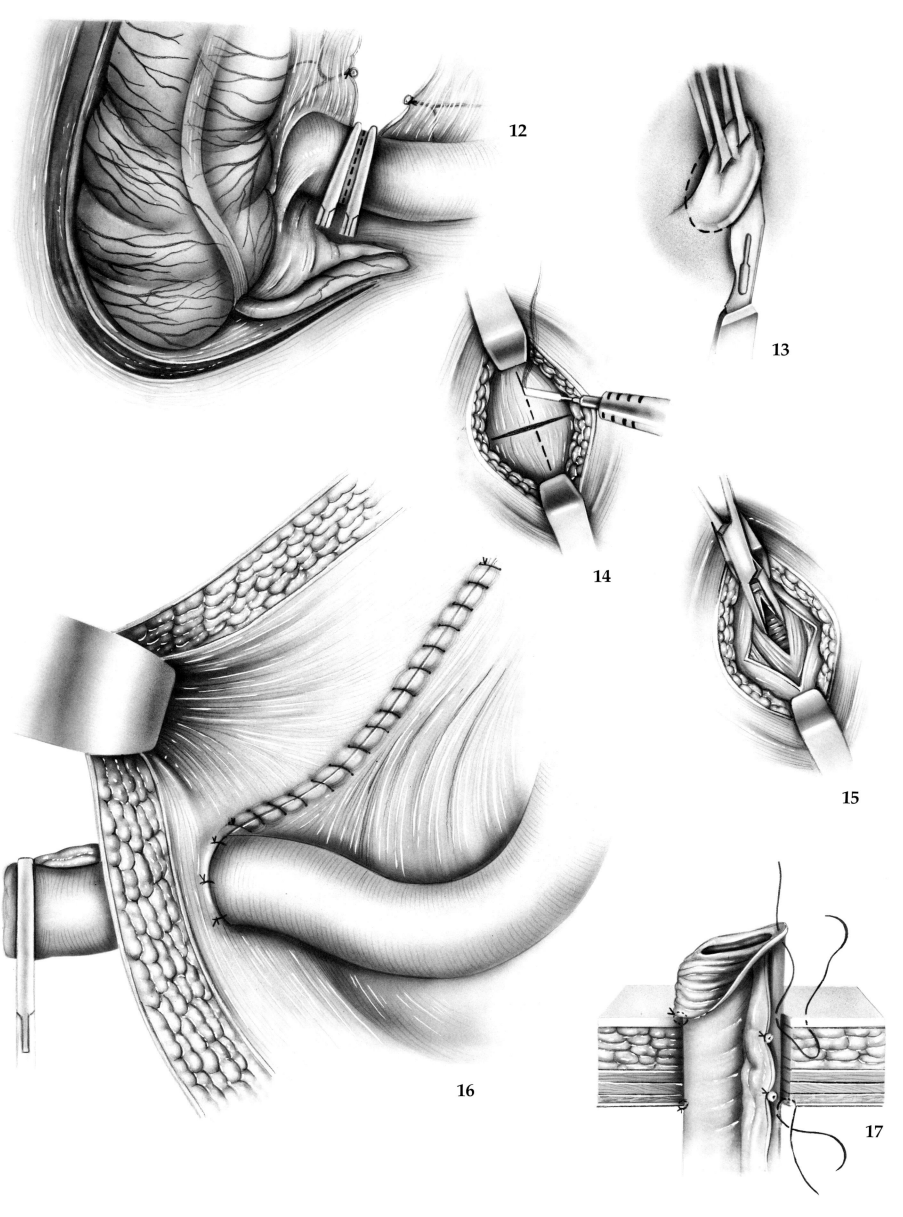

12

13

14

15

16

17

Total Colectomy and Proctectomy for Benign Disease (*cont.*)

18–23 The patient is placed in the lithotomy position as for the abdominoperineal resection (**Plate 177, Figs. 8–15**). The skin close to the anus is incised and oversewn (**Fig. 19**). Using the electrocautery, the pelvic floor is opened close to the rectal wall. The umbilical tape is retrieved from the abdominal portion of the procedure and retracted through the perineal wound (**Fig. 20**). The dissection proceeds laterally and anteriorly very close the wall of the rectum. The specimen is freed and removed (**Fig. 21**). The levator muscles are easily approximated with interrupted #00 polyglycolic acid sutures after the placement of two sump drains into the hollow of the sacrum through separate lateral incisions (**Fig. 22**). The subcutaneous tissues are closed with interrupted #000 polyglycolic acid sutures, and the skin is closed with #000 nylon stitches. The sump drains are secured to the skin with heavy silk sutures (**Fig. 23**).

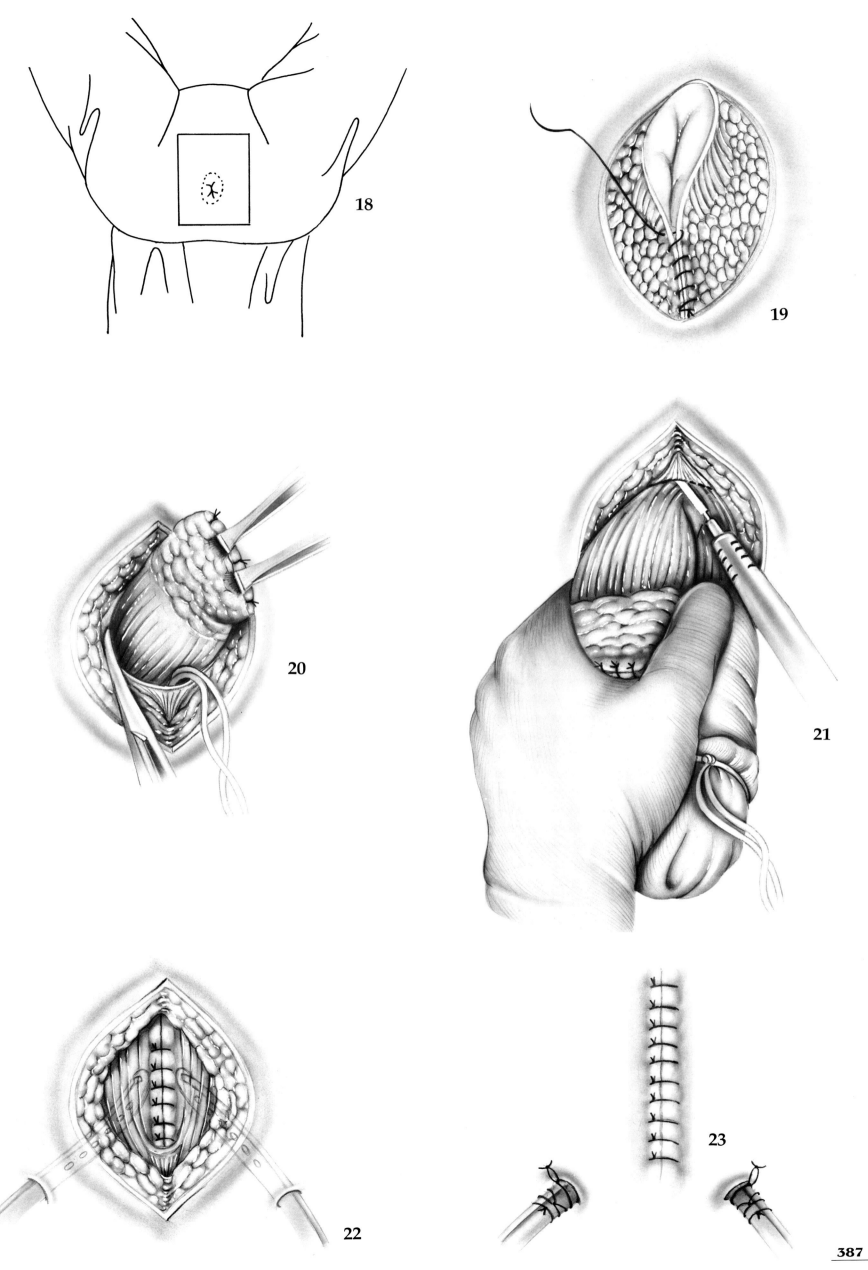

18

19

20

21

22

23

Transanal Resection of a Villous Tumor of the Rectum

Prolapsed Through the Rectum

1 For localized sessile tumors of the rectum, a transanal approach can be used. The patient is placed in the lithotomy position if the tumor is primarily on the posterior wall of the rectum, and in the jackknife position if the anterior wall is primarily involved. The rectum is widely dilated and retracted circumferentially. Four "marker" sutures are placed around the tumor, establishing the boundaries of the proposed resection.

2 Gradual but steady retraction on the lesion allows it to be brought out through the anus. This is facilitated by placing a Carmalt clamp across the "pseudo-stalk" of the tumor. When the tumor is outside the anal ring, a linear stapling device can be placed proximal to the Carmalt clamp and fired. The mucosa is divided between the clamp and stapler using electrocautery.

3 Alternatively, two Carmalt clamps can be placed across the base of the tumor. The mucosa is divided between these clamps. This technique is most applicable when the tumor is not mobile enough to be prolapsed through the anus.

4 The technique for suturing the mucosal stump is shown. A #00 polyglycolic acid stitch is run to and fro across the cut mucosa to create the hemostatic "X" suture line beyond the clamp. The clamp is released, and the rectal mucosa assumes its natural position.

Submucosal Resection

5 If the villous tumor is without a "pseudo-stalk" but rather diffusely involves the rectal wall, the next technique is helpful: Two #00 silk stay sutures are placed at the 5 and 7 o'clock positions below the tumor. Retraction on these sutures creates a fold in the mucosa. The electrocautery is then used to divide the mucosa between the stay sutures and the tumor.

6 Allis clamps are placed at the inferior margins of the specimen to provide countertraction for the subsequent dissection. A fine suction is swept back and forth under the tumor, between the submucosal and muscular coats of the rectum, elevating the lesion. The flap of mucosa and tumor may be retracted to cauterize bleeding points in the deeper layers of the bowel wall.

7 A flexible light is introduced into the submucosal space. Transillumination helps define the border between involved and normal mucosa. The tumor is totally excised with the electrocautery. Hemostasis in the bed of the excised tissue is obtained with #000 polyglycolic acid sutures or cautery.

8 The redundancy of the undermined mucosa permits even wide mucosal defects to be closed with interrupted #00 polyglycolic acid sutures.

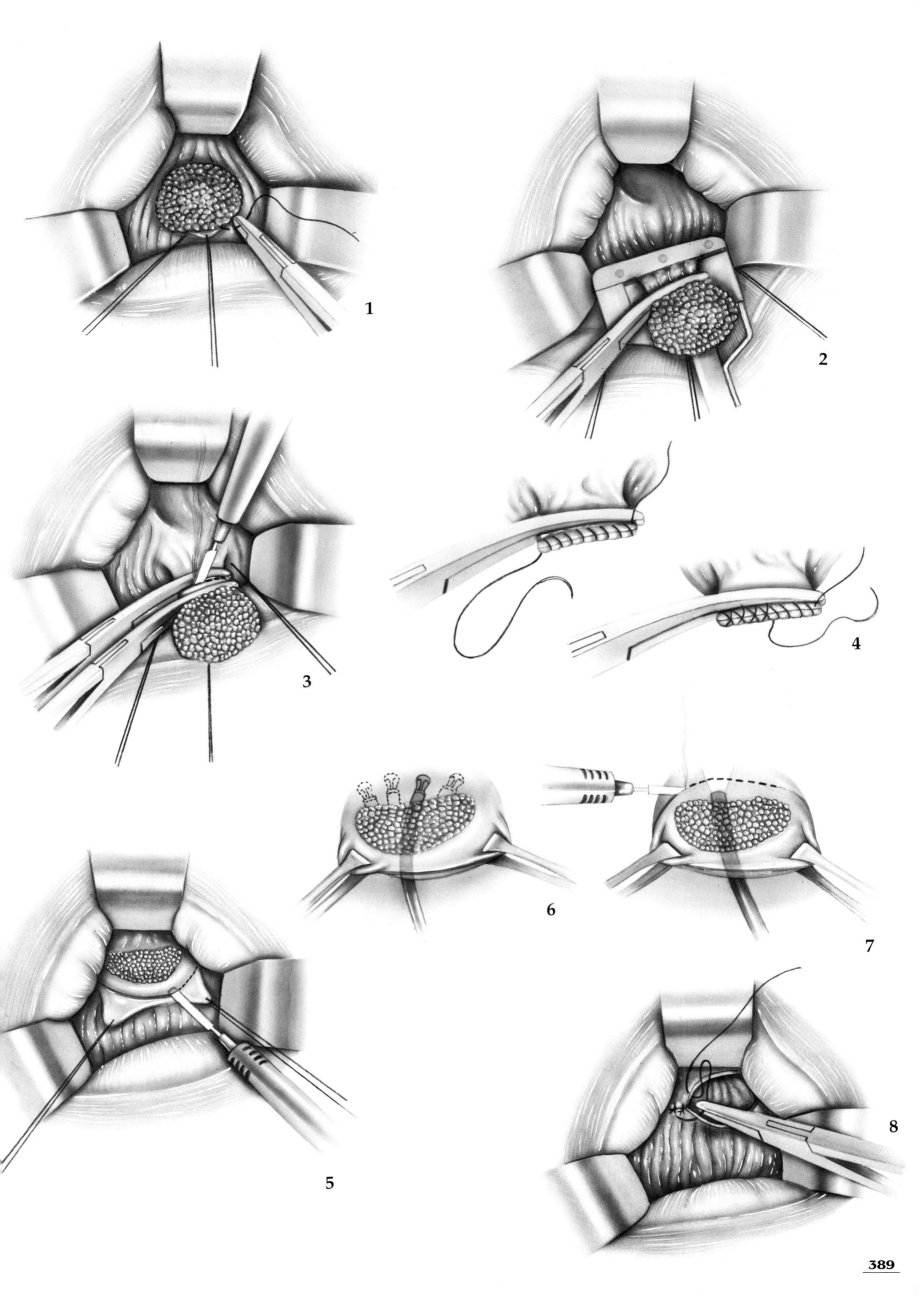

Kraske Posterior Approach for Resection of a Villous Tumor of the Rectum

1 Where a villous tumor has recurred, or where there is inadequate mobility of the lesion for resection through a transanal approach, the posterior approach, as described by Kraske, is used. While the original procedure called for the resection of the sacrum, we have only excised the coccyx. We have found this to be adequate for these lesions if the anal sphincter is retracted inferiorly. The patient is placed prone on the operating table, over bolsters. The buttocks are taped apart and an incision is made in the natal fold as indicated by the broken line.

2 The anococcygeal ligament is divided. A Kocher clamp is placed on the tip of the coccyx. The coccyx is distracted, allowing some space through which the excision can be accomplished. The coccyx is then freed and excised with the electrocautery.

3 The levator muscles are divided in the midline and retracted laterally, exposing the posterior wall of the rectum. The rectum is freed superiorly, inferiorly, and along both lateral walls. The lesion is generally palpable through the posterior rectal wall. If the lesion is located on the posterior rectal wall, stabilizing #00 silk sutures are placed circumferentially around the lesion.

4 Using the electrocautery, the lesion is excised with a full thickness of the rectal wall within the previously placed stay sutures. Once the rectum has been opened the extent of the tumor can be determined, allowing the excision to be tailored to completely excise the involved tissue. The specimen is then pinned to a sterile cork board to orient it for the pathologist.

5 The full thickness of the rectal wall is closed with either interrupted or continuous #00 polyglycolic acid sutures. If there is tension on the closure, the rectum can be further mobilized.

6 A second inverting layer of #000 silk is placed. Because there is no serosa on the rectum, these sutures should include the submucosa. If the lesion is on the anterior wall of the rectum, the posterior wall is opened transversely and the excision is carried out through the proctotomy. The anterior wall is closed in two layers from within the rectal lumen. The transverse proctotomy is then closed, as described above in **Figs. 5** and **6**.

7 The wound is closed in layers, using interrupted polyglycolic acid stitches in the levators and #00 nylon in the skin. A small Penrose drain is brought out through the inferior aspect of the wound.

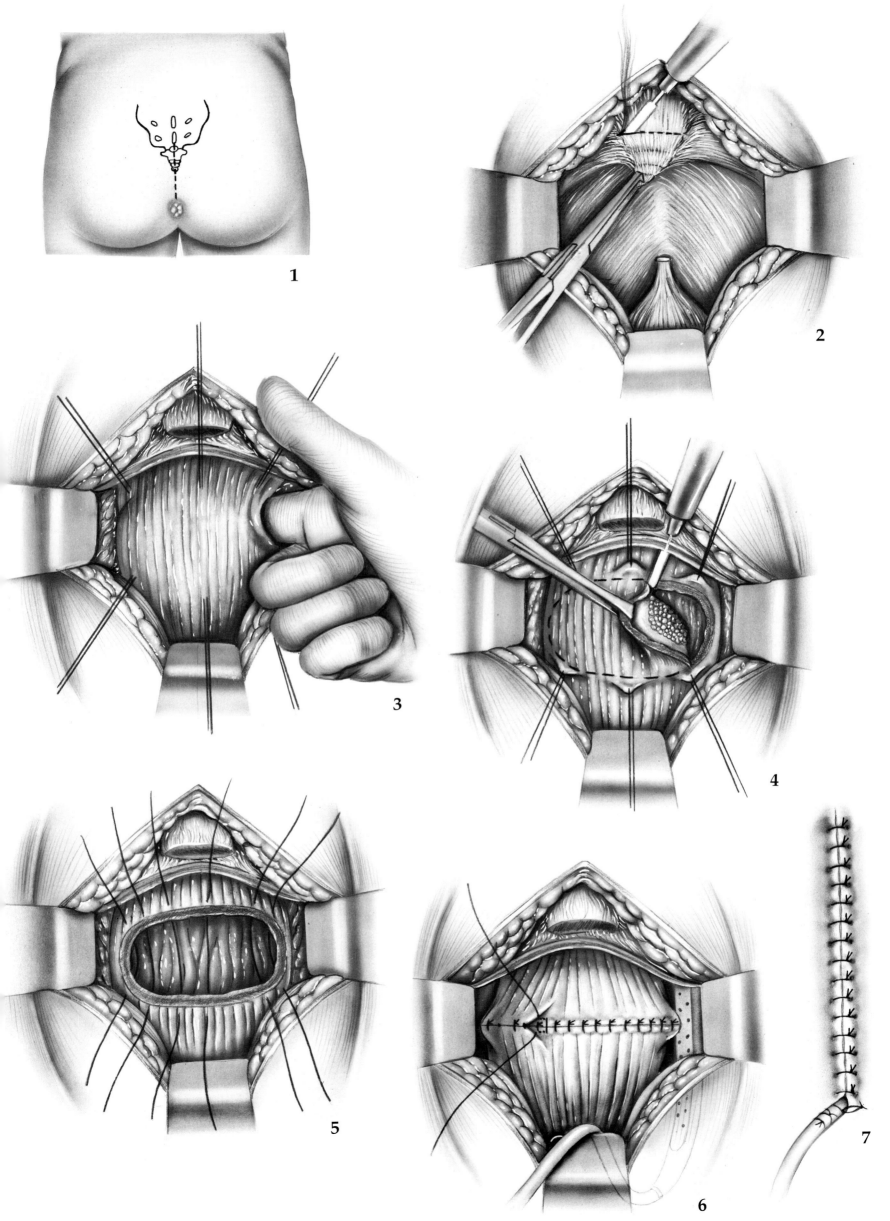

Hemorrhoidectomy

1 The patient is placed in the jackknife position on the operating table. The anus is infiltrated with 1% lidocaine with epinephrine mixed with an equal volume of 0.5% bupivacaine. A large Ferguson retractor is placed in the anus, exposing the hemorrhoid to be excised. A diamond-shaped excision, as indicated by the broken lines, is planned.

2 The hemorrhoid is grasped with an Allis clamp at the dentate line. The diamond-shaped incision is made. It is carried down to the internal sphincter muscle.

3 The hemorrhoidal plexus is elevated. A large curved clamp is placed on the base of the hemorrhoid, which is then excised distally.

4 The stump of the hemorrhoid is ligated with #00 chromic ties.

5 The wound, with the exposed internal sphincter muscle, may be left open to heal by secondary intention, or it may be closed with a running #00 chromic stitch. The anus is packed with a hemostatic gauze.

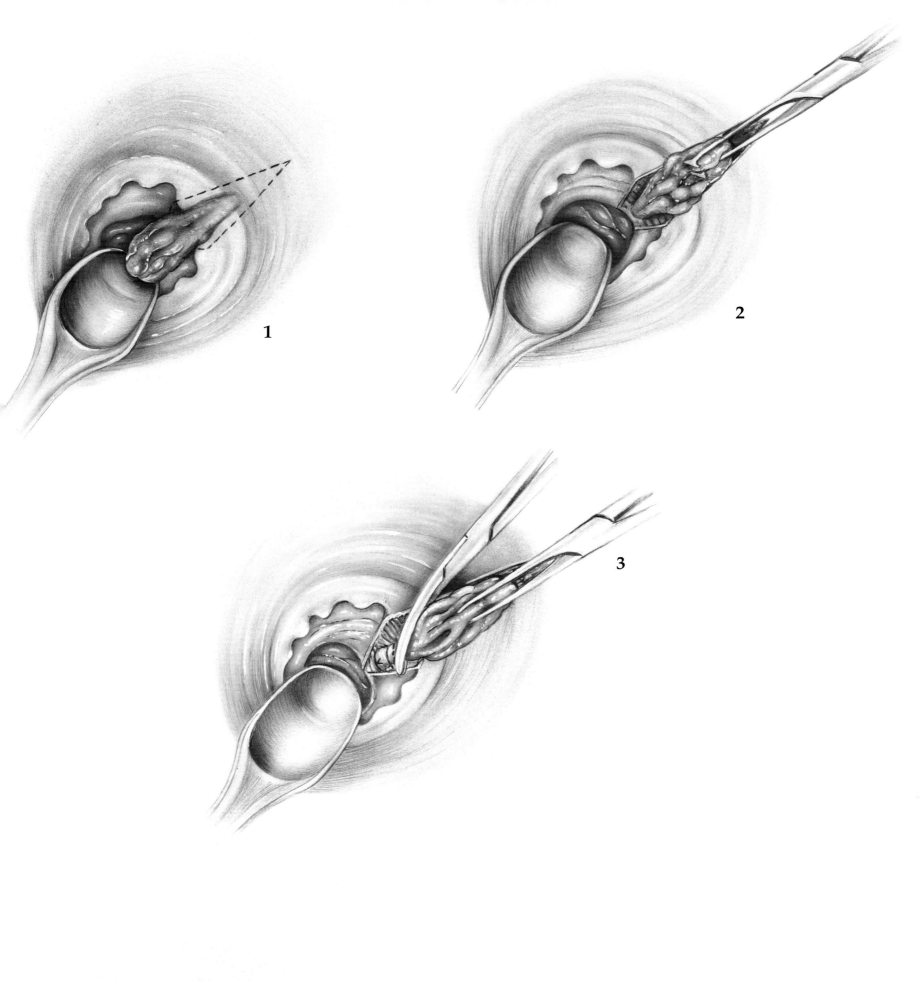

Rectal Fistula—Perirectal Abscess

RECTAL FISTULA

The patient depicted has a posterior anal fistula with an external os to the left and posterior to the anus. The operation may be performed with local, caudal, or spinal anesthesia. We prefer local infiltration of a mixture of equal parts of 1% lidocaine with epinephrine and 0.5% bupivacaine supplemented with IV sedation.

1 The patient is placed in the jackknife position on the operating table. A self-retaining retractor is placed within the anus. A blunt-tip needle attached to a syringe is used to inject saline solution into the fistula tract. Saline can be seen flowing through the internal os in the anal canal at the midline posteriorly. While this technique does not always work, it is often useful for the identification of the internal os.

2 A blunt flexible probe is passed through the external os and into the rectum.

3 The fistula tract is then opened along the probe. Once opened, the tract is examined for side tracts. If found, these are opened widely. The edges of the tracts are trimmed, and the base of the fistula tract is thoroughly destroyed with electrocautery.

4 The wound is then "saucerized." The mucosal edge is sutured with a running #000 chromic stitch. This prevents bleeding from the inflamed mucosal edge. The internal sphincter may be seen at the base of the wound; often a few of these fibers are divided during a fistula operation. Incontinence does not develop. If, however, the patient has had prior rectal surgery, the function of the sphincter must be carefully evaluated before further sphincter fibers are cut.

PERIRECTAL ABSCESS

Incision, Drainage, and Packing

5 In the case of a large ischiorectal abscess, the area is thoroughly infiltrated with 1% lidocaine with epinephrine mixed with an equal volume of 0.5% bupivacaine. An 18-gauge needle attached to a syringe is used to aspirate the abscess. A sample of the abscess fluid is sent for culture and Gram stain. In addition, the aspiration decreases the pressure within the abscess cavity, preventing a "burst" when the cavity is incised.

The abscess cavity is opened with a generous cruciate incision, as indicated by the broken lines. The cruciate incision allows the edges to retract and facilitates the drainage.

The cavity is probed manually, or with a clamp, to break up any residual collections. The cavity is packed with plain one-half-inch sterile gauze. The packing is removed the following day, and generally does not need to be replaced. Sitz baths are initiated and are continued until the abscess has resolved.

Incision, Drainage with a Malecot Catheter

6 Alternatively, the abscess may be drained with the aid of a Malecot catheter. As before, the abscess is aspirated after infiltration with local anesthesia. The cavity is opened and the contents drained. All loculations are broken either manually or with an instrument. A #16 to #18 French Malecot catheter is inserted into the cavity. The catheter is cut short and a safety pin is placed through it near the skin surface to prevent it from retracting into the cavity. Sitz baths are initiated. The abscess cavity will shrink down over the catheter as the infection resolves. The catheter is removed on the fifth to seventh postoperative day.

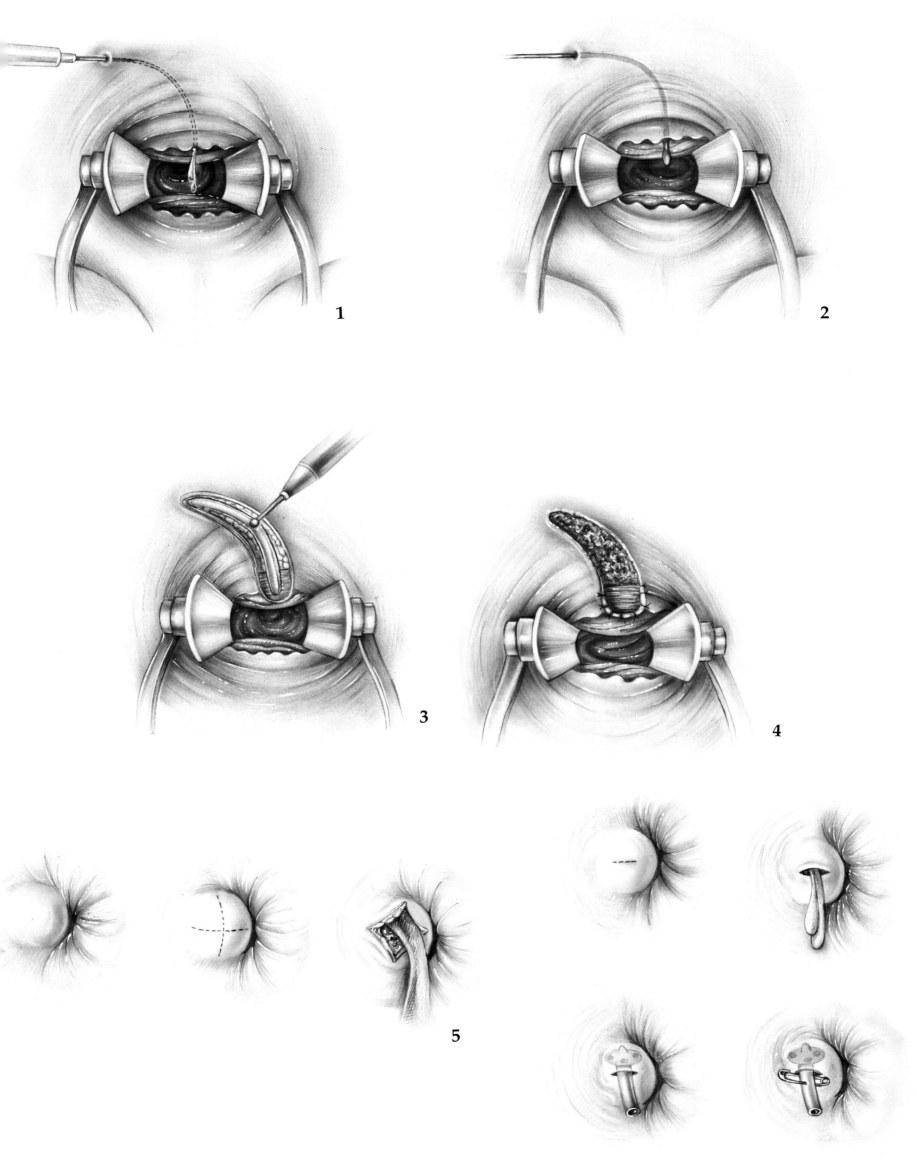

Anal Fissure with Anal Sphincterotomy

1 In the case of a large posterior chronic anal fissure, a sphincterotomy is indicated. The patient is placed on the operating table in the jackknife position. The area is infiltrated with 1% lidocaine with epinephrine mixed with an equal volume of 0.5% bupivacaine.

2 A 2-cm incision is made in the left lateral position, external to the dentate line.

3 A finger is inserted into the rectum to elevate the sphincter muscle. An Allis clamp is placed on the internal sphincter through the lateral incision. The sphincter appears as a distinctly white muscle bundle.

4 A clamp is inserted under an approximately 1-cm length of the internal sphincter. The internal sphincter muscle is then divided with electrocautery.

5 The muscle is allowed to retract into the incision. The skin is left open. If a large tag is present in association with the fissure, it may be excised and the base of the fissure cauterized.

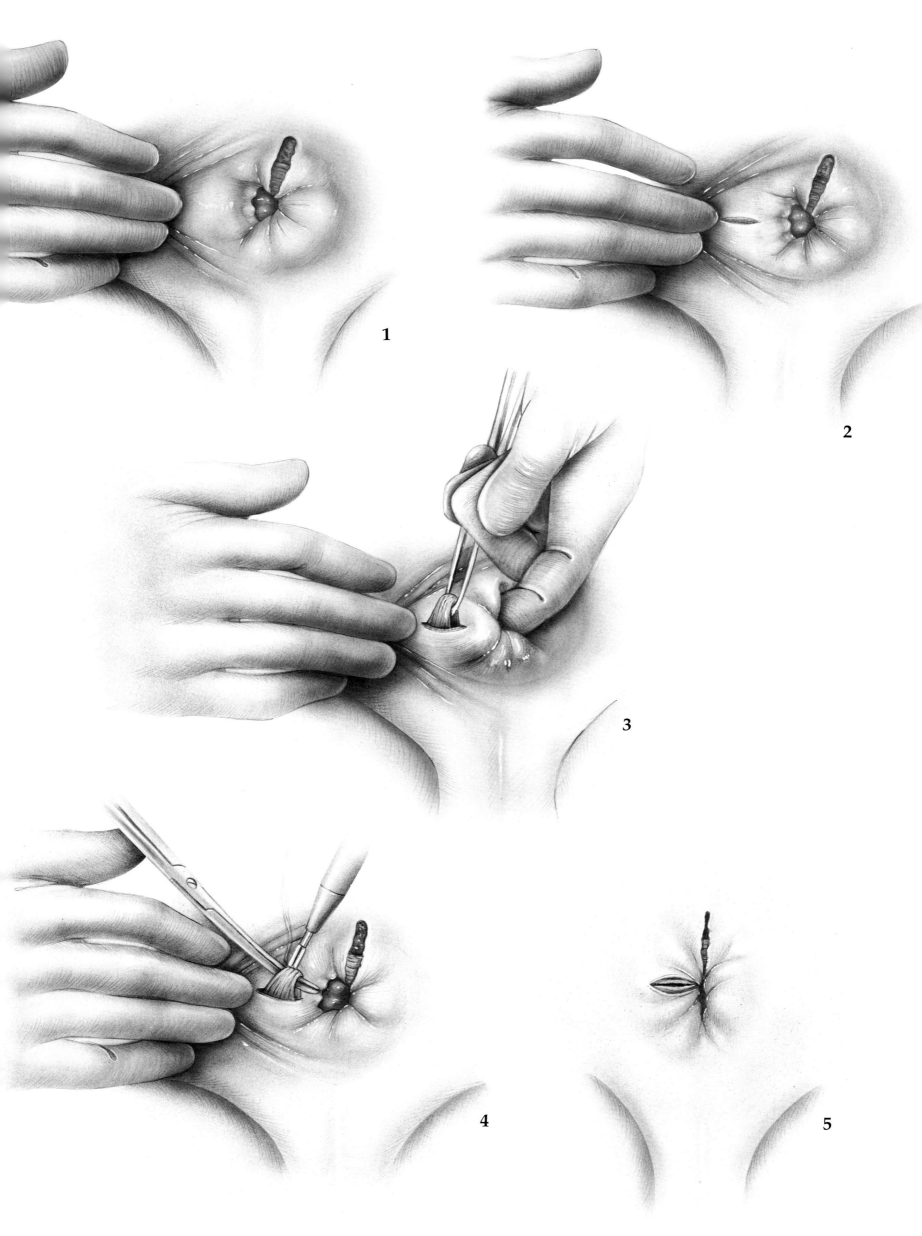

1

2

3

4

5

Oophorectomy

During any operative procedure on a postmenopausal female that allows easy access to the ovaries, and in any operation for colon cancer, we routinely obtain consent to remove the ovaries. In general, each ovary is removed with most of the fallopian tube.

1 The infundibulopelvic ligament and the suspensory ligament of the ovary, containing the ovarian vessels, are identified, divided between clamps, and tied with #00 silk ligatures.

2 The broad ligament of the uterus is divided between clamps, as indicated by the broken line, and tied with #000 silk.

3 The ovarian ligament, which suspends the ovary from the uterus, is dissected, divided between clamps, and tied. The most medial portion of the mesosalpinx between the ovarian ligament and the fallopian tube contains the tubal branches of the uterine artery. These vessels and the fallopian tube are divided between clamps and tied with #00 silk. The remaining round ligament of the uterus is divided and tied.

4 The specimen is removed. In most cases the segment of the broad ligament between the infundibulopelvic ligament and the ovarian ligament may be taken with a single clamp. This procedure is repeated on the other side.

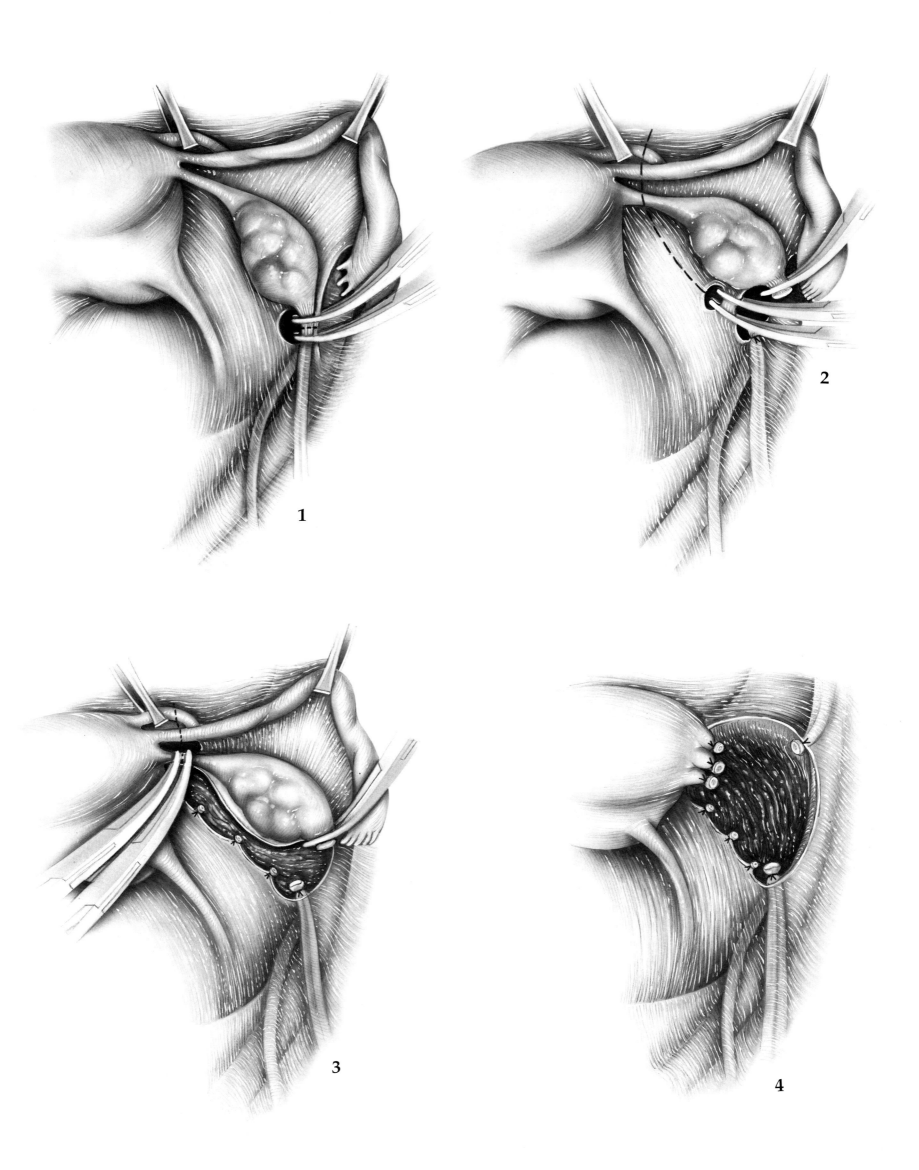

Hysterectomy

1 The abdomen is explored through a lower midline or lower abdominal transverse incision.

2 The peritoneum at the base of the broad ligament is grasped with the forceps, elevated, and incised. The ureters are identified but left *in situ* beyond the area of dissection.

3 The round ligament of the uterus and the infundibulopelvic ligament containing the ovarian vessels are divided between clamps and securely tied with #00 silk ligatures. This is done on both sides of the uterus.

4 The peritoneum between the bladder and the uterus is divided using the electrocautery over the open jaws of a right-angle clamp.

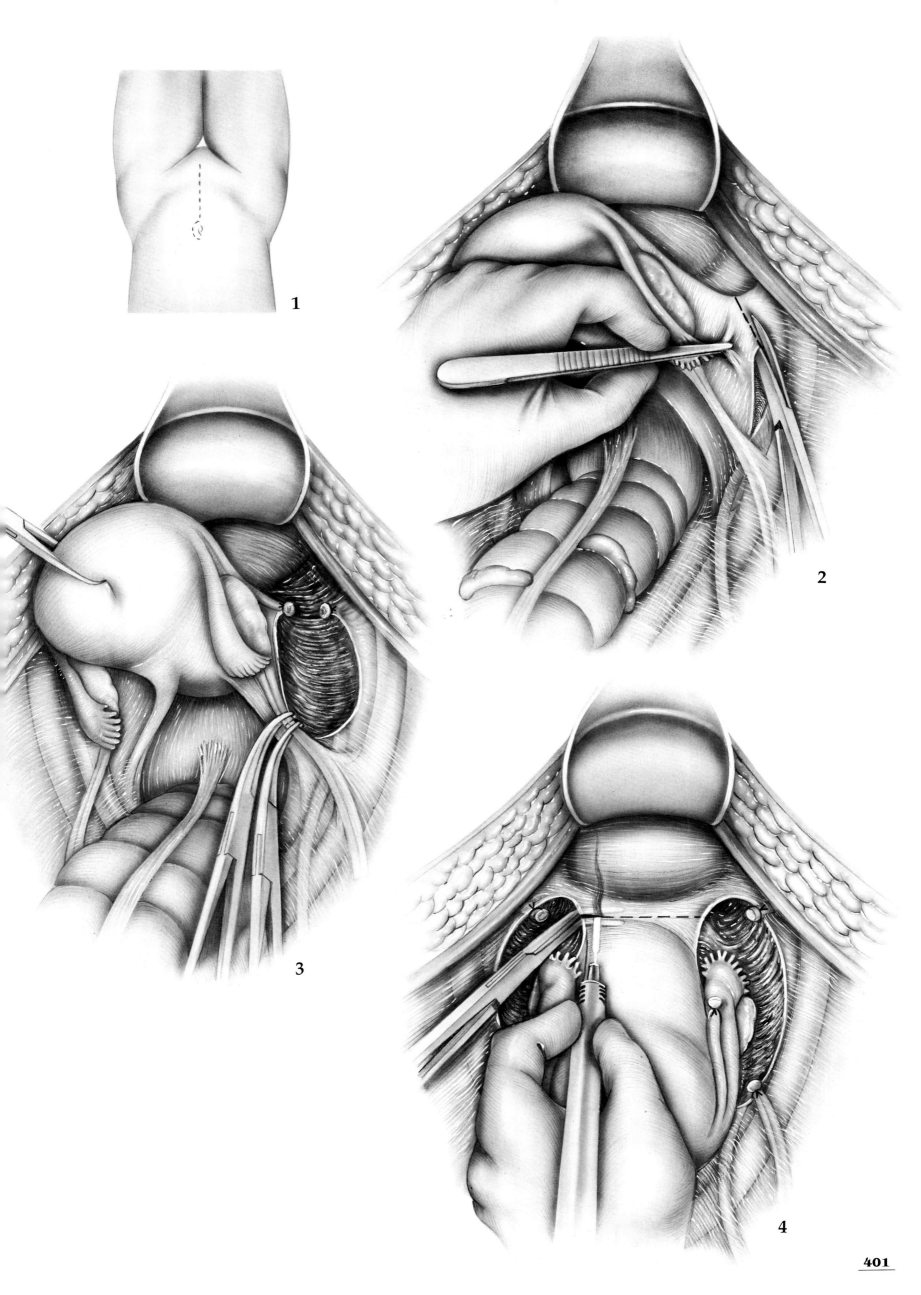

Hysterectomy (*cont.*)

5 The posterior bladder wall is bluntly freed from the anterior border of the uterus until the uppermost portion of the vaginal wall is visualized.

6 A tenaculum is placed on the fundus of the uterus and retracted anteriorly, exposing the rectouterine space. The peritoneum between the rectum and uterus is divided with electrocautery. The uterosacral ligaments are divided between clamps and tied with #00 silk ligatures.

7 The anterior rectal wall is bluntly dissected from the posterior uterus, exposing the posterior vaginal wall.

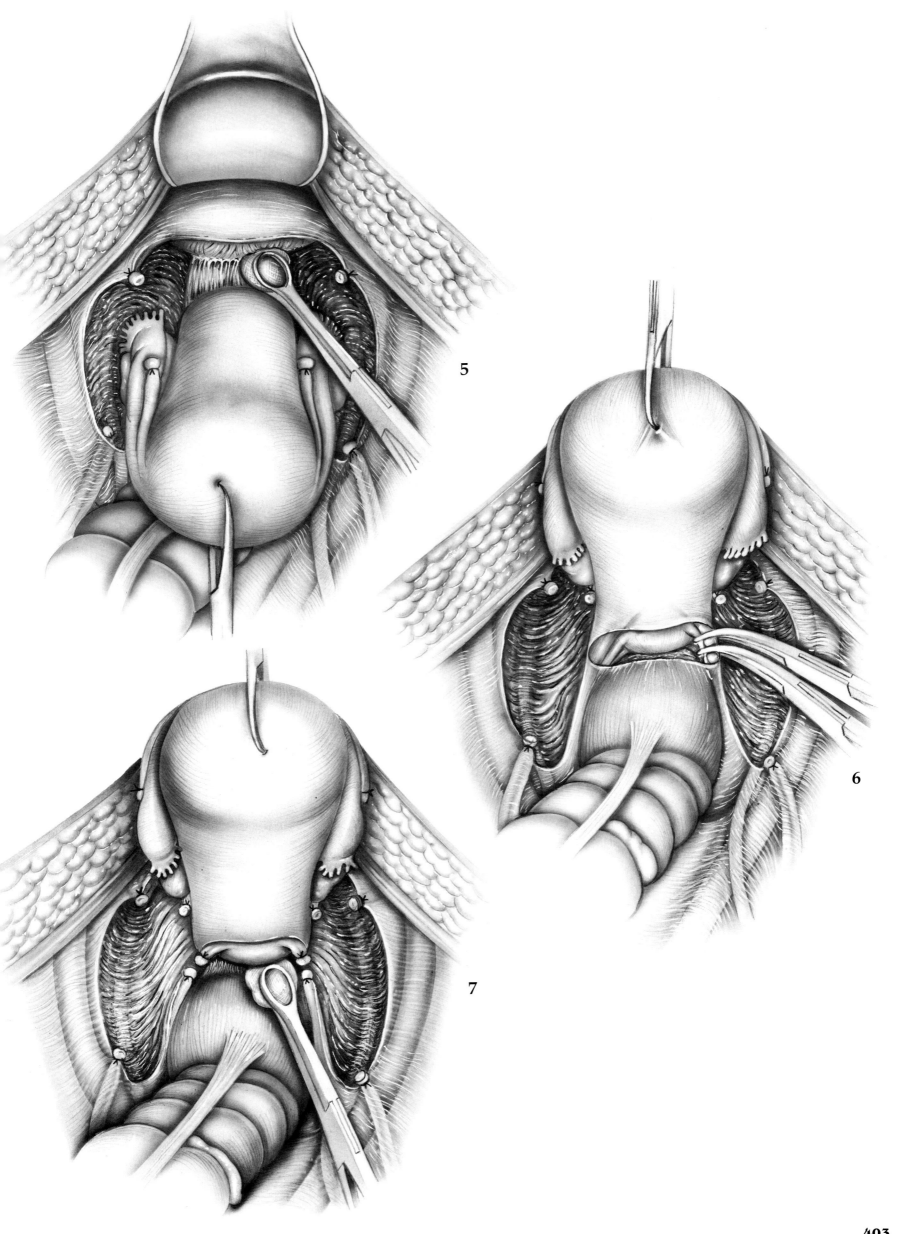

5

6

7

Hysterectomy (*cont.*)

8 While some surgeons simply clamp and cut down on the cardinal ligaments lateral to the vagina, in general it is more secure to ligate portions of these ligaments individually. The uterine artery is palpated and dissected free as it approaches the posterior aspect of the uterus, and is then divided between clamps and tied. A second suture ligature is placed on the proximal side of the vessel.

9 The residual cardinal ligaments are divided, exposing the lateral portion of the vaginal wall.

10 With the mobilization of the lateral vaginal supports, the anterolateral portion of the vagina is opened. The entire anterior vagina is divided with electrocautery.

11–12 Two tonsil clamps are placed at the corners of the anterior opening into the vagina. The posterior vaginal wall is then transected using the electrocautery, and the specimen is removed. The vaginal cuff is closed with a running #00 polyglycolic acid suture line. Tension on the tonsil clamps at the lateral margins of the vaginal cuff causes the anterior and posterior wall to come together easily, facilitating this closure.

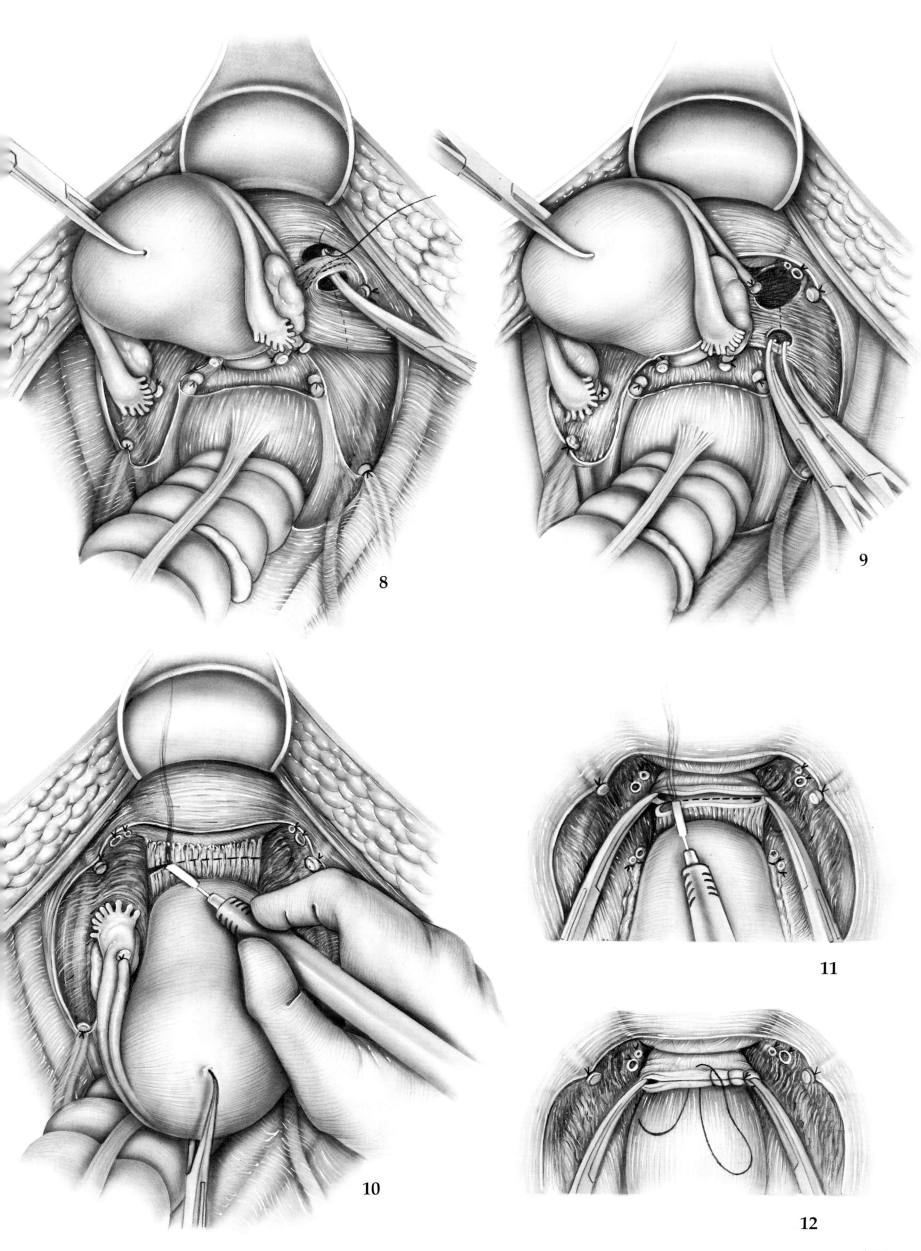

8

9

10

11

12

Direct Hernia Repair (McVay)

1 The skin incision for the repair of a direct hernia extends from a point 1 to 2 cm medial to the anterior superior iliac spine to a point 1 cm above the pubic tubercle. This line of incision parallels the inguinal ligament, 1 to 2 cm medial to it.

2 The aponeurosis of the external oblique muscle is incised along its fibers about 1 cm above the inguinal ligament. The external ring is opened by the medial extension of this incision. The ilioinguinal nerve is identified and preserved. The cord is bluntly dissected from the inguinal ligament inferiorly. It is then encircled at the pubic tubercle with a Penrose drain, and retracted from the underlying bulging direct hernia sac.

3 It is rare that anything other than the repair of the floor of the inguinal canal is necessary; however, a relaxing incision in the anterior rectus sheath is most important to achieve a tension-free repair. The length of the relaxing incision should be approximately the same as that of the proposed repair of the floor of the inguinal canal. The remnants of the transversalis fascia are incised, exposing Cooper's ligament and the iliopubic band. The iliopubic band is the deep extension of the shelving edge of the inguinal ligament. Superiorly, the conjoined tendon is visualized.

4 The repair is accomplished with interrupted #00 silk stitches, starting medially and working laterally. The first suture is passed through the periosteum of the pubic tubercle and then through the conjoined tendon. Each suture is left untied, its tails clamped and placed sequentially on an empty sponge stick holder. The subsequent sutures are taken through Cooper's ligament or the iliopubic band laterally, and then through the transversalis fascia and the conjoined tendon medially. As the repair approaches the deep femoral vessels the so-called transition stitch is placed. This stitch traverses the conjoined tendon, the transversalis fascia, Cooper's ligament, and then the shelving edge of the inguinal ligament. The stitches lateral to the transition stitch are placed through the conjoined tendon and transversalis fascia medially and the shelving edge of the inguinal ligament laterally, until the internal ring is reconstituted anterior to the inferior epigastric vessels. We do not routinely open the direct sac.

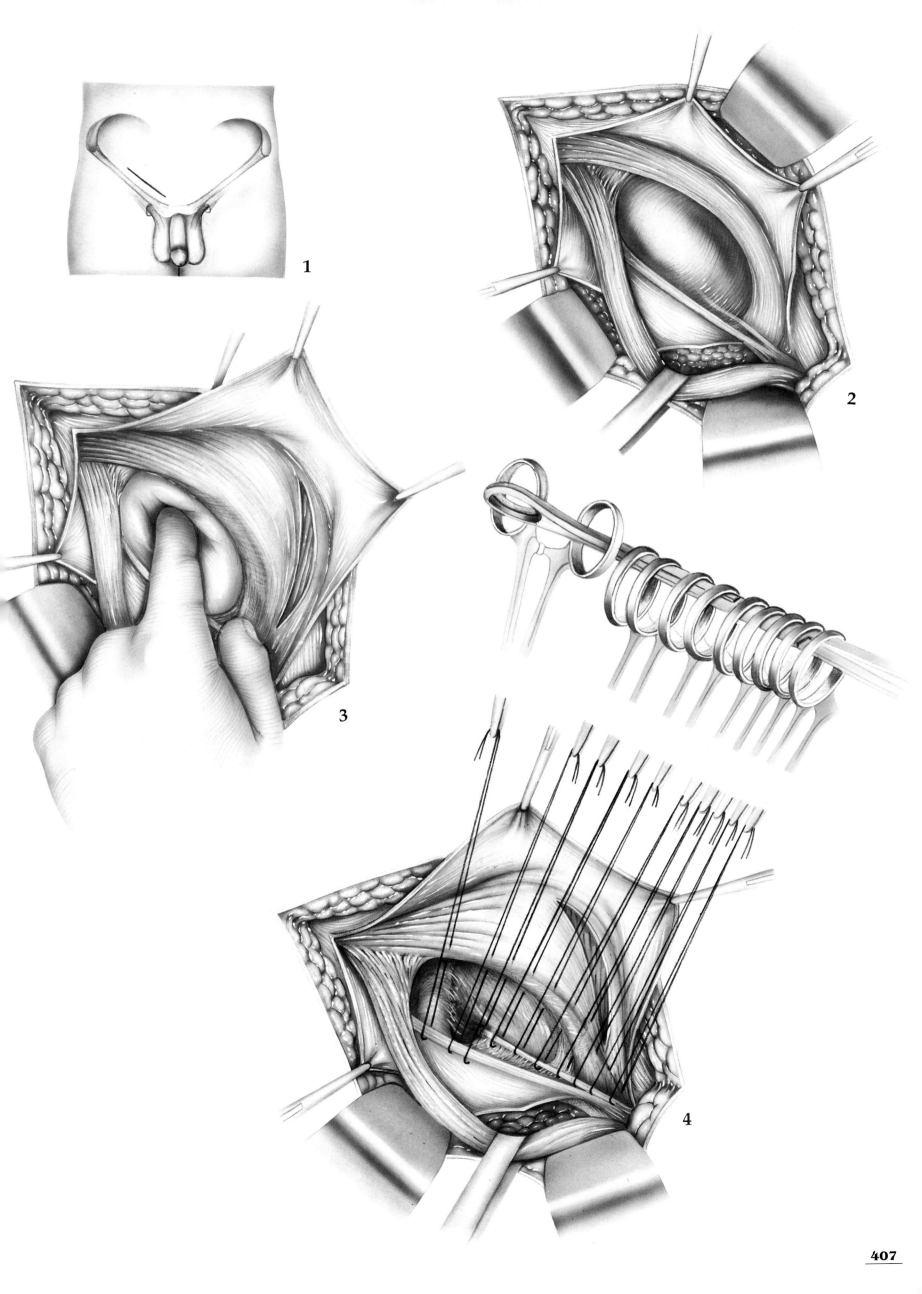

Direct Hernia Repair (McVay) (*cont.*)

5 The clamps holding the stitches are slipped onto a second empty sponge stick holder passed through the other finger hole of each clamp's handles. This allows the surgeon to tie the sutures, in order, from the pubic tubercle to the internal ring.

6 With an adequate relaxing incision in the anterior rectus sheath, the repair of the floor of the inguinal canal will be accomplished without tension. The rectus muscle, however, will gape through the relaxing incision at the conclusion of the procedure. The reconstituted internal ring should barely admit the tip of the index finger.

7 The cord is replaced in the inguinal canal, as is the ilioinguinal nerve. The aponeurosis of the external oblique muscle is approximated with interrupted #000 polyglycolic acid sutures. Medially, the external ring is reconstructed.

8 The subcutaneous tissue is closed with interrupted #000 polyglycolic acid sutures and the skin is approximated with skin staples.

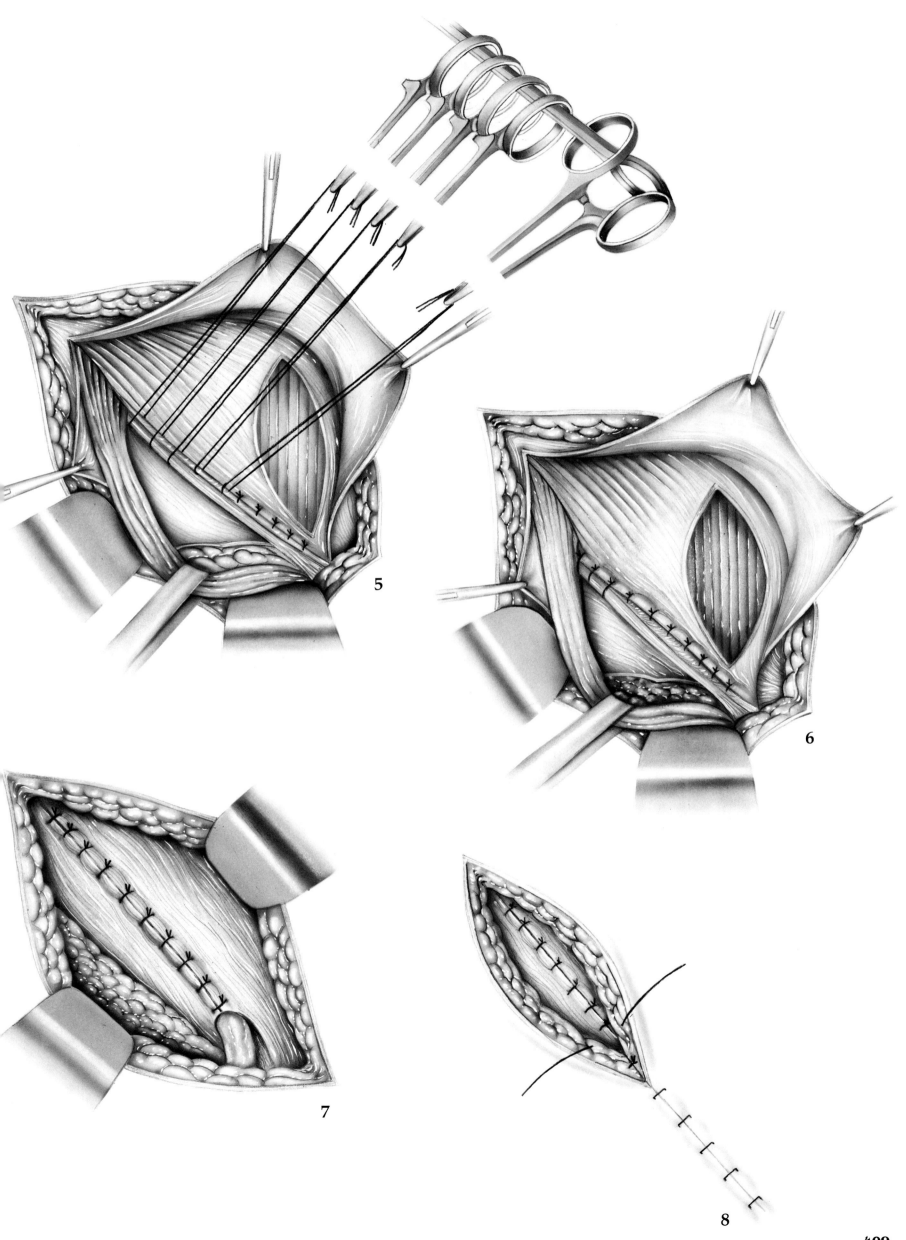

5

6

7

8

Indirect Hernia and Imbricated Repair (Shouldice)

1 The incision is made 2.5 cm medial and parallel to the inguinal ligament, beginning at a point immediately inferior and medial to the anterior superior iliac spine and ending at the pubic tubercle.

2 The aponeurosis of the external oblique muscle is divided parallel to its fibers. The medial extent of this dissection opens the external ring. The ilioinguinal nerve is identified and preserved.

3 Using blunt and sharp dissection, the cord contained within the cremaster muscle and fascia is freed from the overlying lateral portion of the aponeurosis of the external oblique muscle, the inguinal ligament inferiorly, the transversalis muscle and fascia posteriorly, and the conjoined tendon superiorly. The cord is encircled with a wide Penrose drain at the pubic tubercle. Retraction on the Penrose drain permits easier dissection of the cremaster muscle and cremasteric fascia from the contained cord structures. The cremasteric fibers are opened and dissected sharply and bluntly from the cord. This muscle and fascia are divided, tied, and excised. Extra properitoneal fat or lipomas of the cord are removed along with the cremaster muscle.

4 The distal extent of the indirect sac is usually identified on the anteromedial aspect of the cord as it exits the internal ring. Two small clamps are placed on the distal portion of the sac for traction. The sac is then dissected from the adjacent cord structures to beyond the internal epigastric vessels.

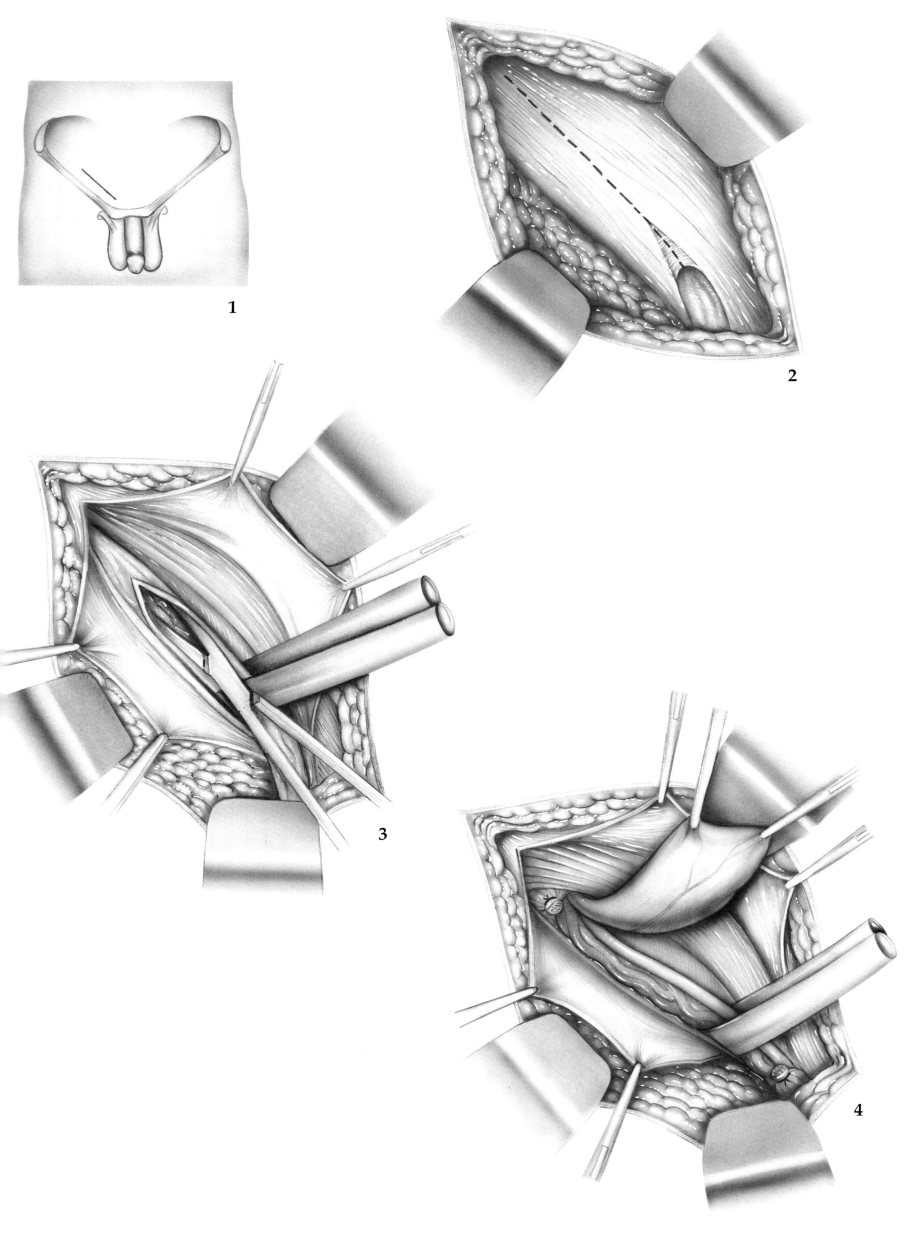

Indirect Hernia and Imbricated Repair (Shouldice) (*cont.*)

5 While some surgeons prefer to open the sac prior to reducing its contents, we prefer to reduce the contents and then twist the sac into a tight band extending from the internal ring to the clamps on the sac, without opening it.

6 The base of the twisted sac is then suture-ligated with a #00 silk stitch.

7 The sac distal to this ligature is excised. The stump of the sac is inspected for hemostasis.

8 The external spermatic vessels running along the transversalis fascia are divided between clamps and ligated. The weakened and bulging transversalis fascia is incised from the pubic tubercle to the internal epigastric vessels, as indicated by the broken line.

9 The lateral and medial edges of the transversalis fascia are elevated and freed from the underlying areolar tissue. The dissection of the transversalis is essential to this repair. The lower flap must be dissected to the line of fusion with the iliopubic band. Once the transversalis is freed, the repair is accomplished in four layers created with two continuous #000 polypropylene sutures. The repair is begun at the pubic tubercle by approximating the wide undersurface of the medial transversalis fascia to the periosteum of the pubic tubercle. The stitch is tied but is not cut. The closure is continued in a running fashion, approximating the fibrous undersurface of the medial transversalis fascia to the iliopubic band on the lateral aspect of the defect in the posterior wall of the inguinal canal. As the closure continues laterally, the internal ring is reconstituted snugly around the spermatic cord and the remnant of the indirect sac is buried behind this layer.

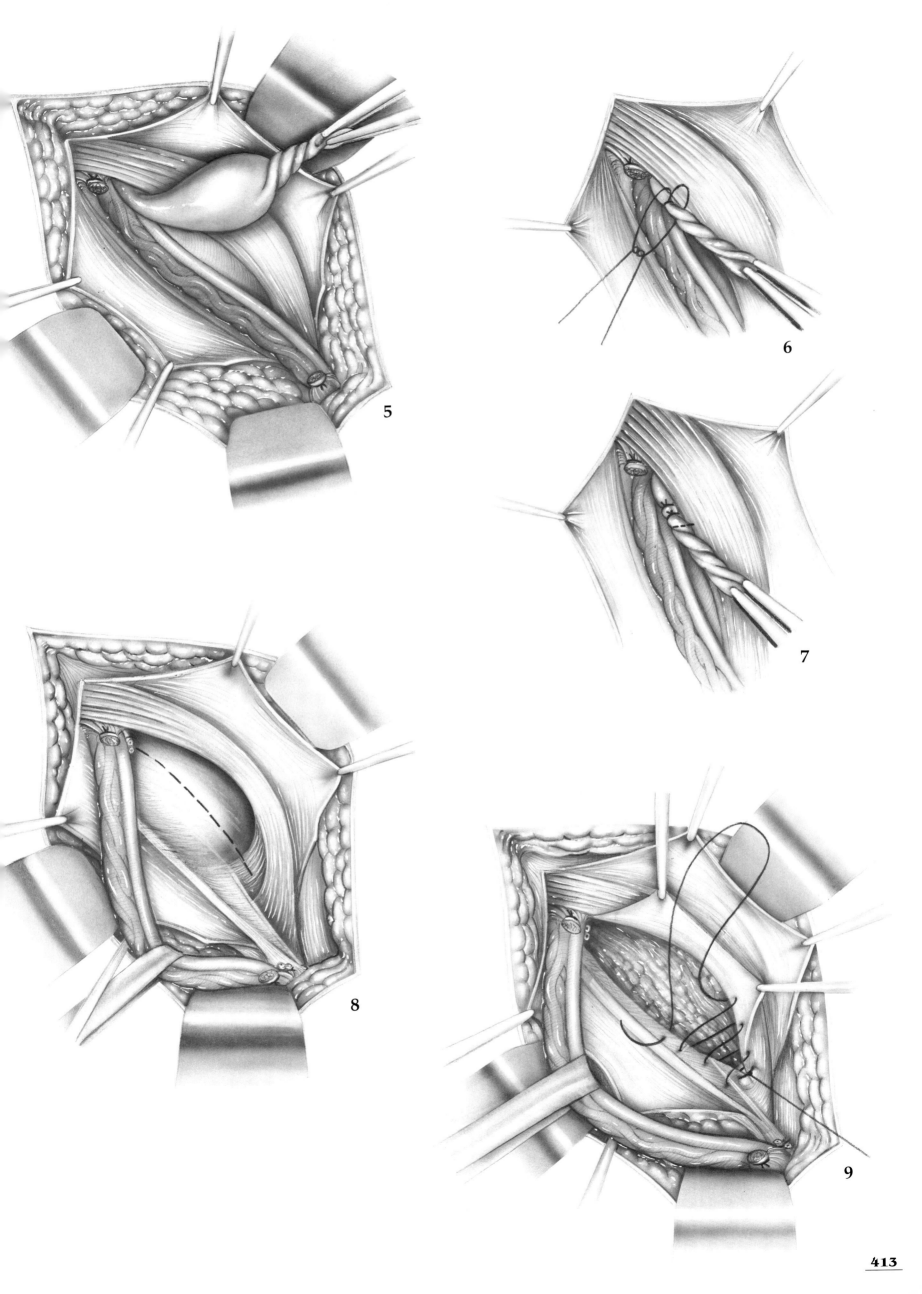

5

6

7

8

9

Indirect Hernia and Imbricated Repair
(Shouldice) (*cont.*)

10 The suturing is continued, lateral to medial, with the same stitch approximating the cut edge of the medial portion of the transversalis fascia to the line of fusion of the lower, lateral, portion of the transversalis fascia with the iliopubic band. This suture line is completed at the pubic tubercle, where the stitch is tied to the tail of the original stitch.

11 The repair is reinforced by approximating the undersurface of the conjoined tendon to the shelving edge of the inguinal ligament. This row is begun at the internal ring and run in a continuous fashion to the pubic tubercle.

12 At the pubic tubercle this suture may be tied to itself or, preferably, may be continued in the opposite direction. Medially, this fourth row approximates the anterior rectus sheath to the line where the aponeurosis of the external oblique turns to become the inguinal ligament. As this suture line is continued laterally, the internal oblique is sewn to the line where the aponeurosis of the external oblique turns to become the inguinal ligament. The suture is tied to the tail of the second polypropylene stitch snugly against the spermatic cord as it exits the reconstituted internal ring.

13 The cord and the ilioinguinal nerve are replaced in the inguinal canal. The aponeurosis of the external oblique muscle is closed with interrupted #000 polyglycolic acid sutures, reconstituting the external ring medially. The skin is closed with skin clips. At the conclusion of the surgery, the testicle is drawn back into the scrotum.

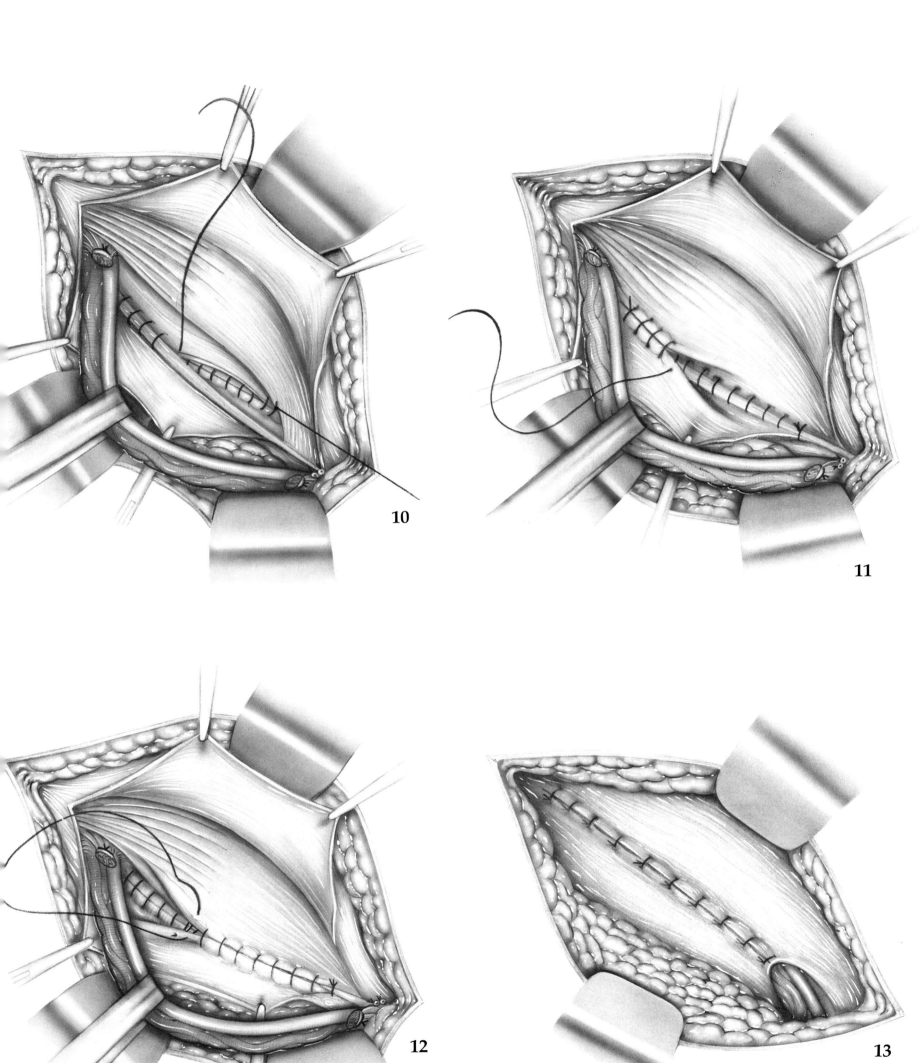

PLATE
2 0 8

Femoral Hernia Repair (Infrainguinal, Utilizing a Prosthetic Umbrella)

1 A vertical incision is made over the suspected femoral hernia. The subcutaneous tissues are dissected from the hernia sac, and the sac is opened.

2 The contents of the hernia sac are digitally reduced into the peritoneal cavity.

3 Once the contents of the sac have been reduced, the hernia sac is twisted upon itself and doubly ligated with #00 silk ligatures. The distal portion of the sac is then excised.

4 A small ellipse of PTFE graft or Marlex mesh is prepared, with a "divot" removed where the graft will abut the femoral vein. A #00 silk suture is placed in the central portion of the graft.

5 The graft is compressed as it is inserted into the hernia defect, and is then allowed to reexpand. Using the silk suture, it is drawn against the inner aspect of the hernia ring.

6 It is then sutured in place with #00 silk or PTFE stitches. The stitches are taken through the inguinal ligament above, the prosthetic graft, and then the pectineal fascia. Three sutures usually suffice. During the suturing, the central stitch steadies the graft material.

7 Upon tying the sutures, the fascia comes together without tension against the prosthetic plug.

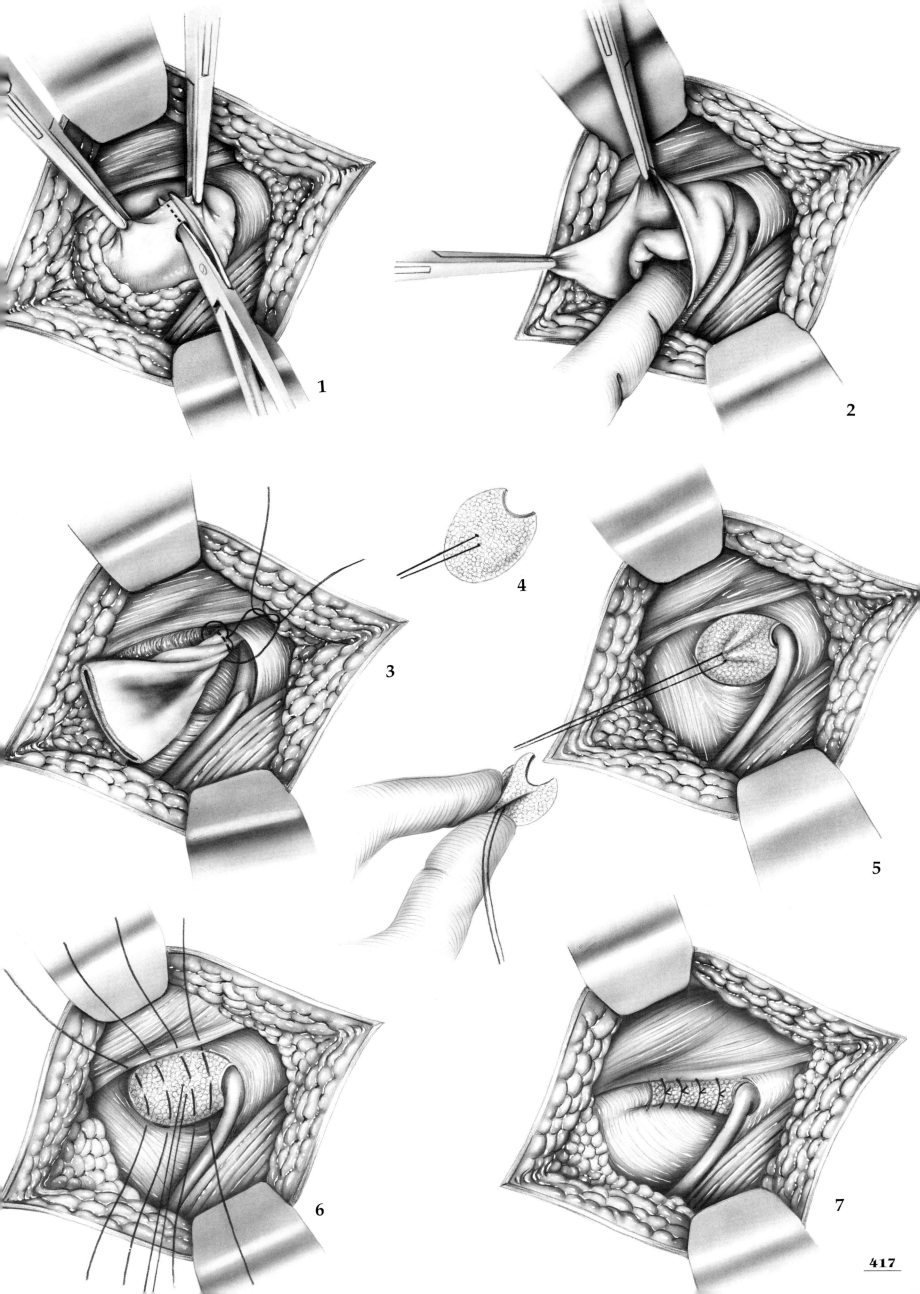

Strangulated Femoral Hernia, Transinguinal Approach with Bowel Resection (Dennis-Varco Technique)

1 The suspected femoral hernia is approached using a vertical incision. Once it is apparent that the bowel within the femoral hernia sac is strangulated, a second oblique inguinal incision is made for the repair.

2 The infrainguinal vertical incision allows the hernia sac to be explored. When nonviable bowel is encountered, the area is left covered with an antibiotic-soaked laparotomy pad. The operation then proceeds through the oblique inguinal incision.

3 The incision is brought down to the aponeurosis of the external oblique fascia. This fascia is incised along its fibers and the external ring is opened.

4 The ilioinguinal nerve is identified and preserved. The round ligament is divided proximally and distally within the inguinal canal and tied, exposing the transversalis fascia. The transversalis fascia is incised as indicated by the broken line.

5 Upon opening the transversalis fascia, the tubular hernia sac (peritoneum) is identified coursing toward the femoral vessels and into the thigh. The anterior layer of the peritoneum is opened, exposing the contained bowel.

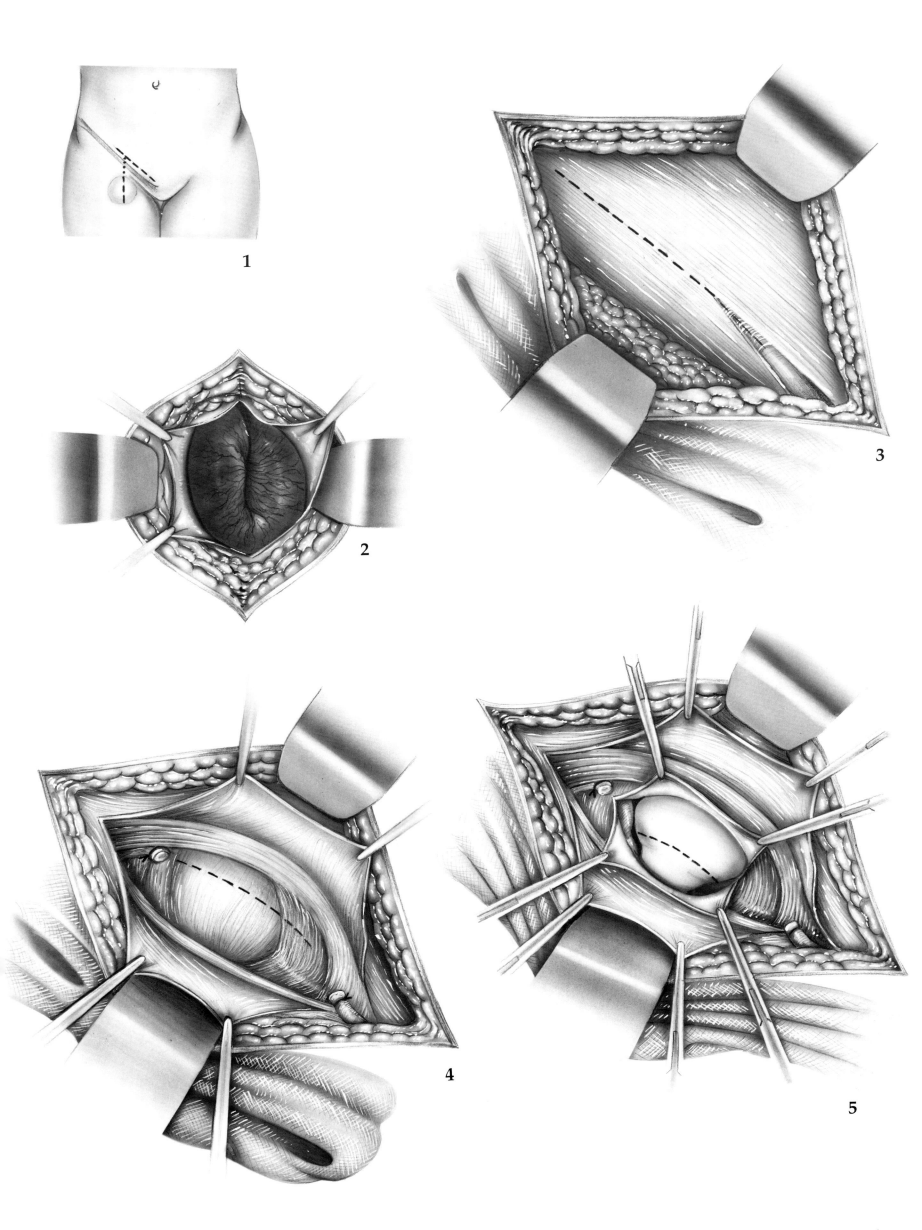

1

2

3

4

5

Strangulated Femoral Hernia, Transinguinal Approach with Bowel Resection (Dennis-Varco Technique) (*cont.*)

6 A dilated proximal limb of small bowel and a collapsed distal limb of bowel will be found within the hernia sac. Dennis intestinal anastomosis clamps are placed across the viable bowel entering and exiting the femoral ring. The bowel is divided with electrocautery.

7–8 An end-to-end closed anastomosis is constructed with #000 silk sutures in the fashion previously described (**Plate 27, Figs. 23–25**), reestablishing bowel continuity.

9 The posterior portion of the hernia sac is divided. This separates the distal sac from the peritoneum of the abdominal cavity.

10 A continuous #000 polyglycolic acid suture is used to close the peritoneal cavity above the inguinal ligament.

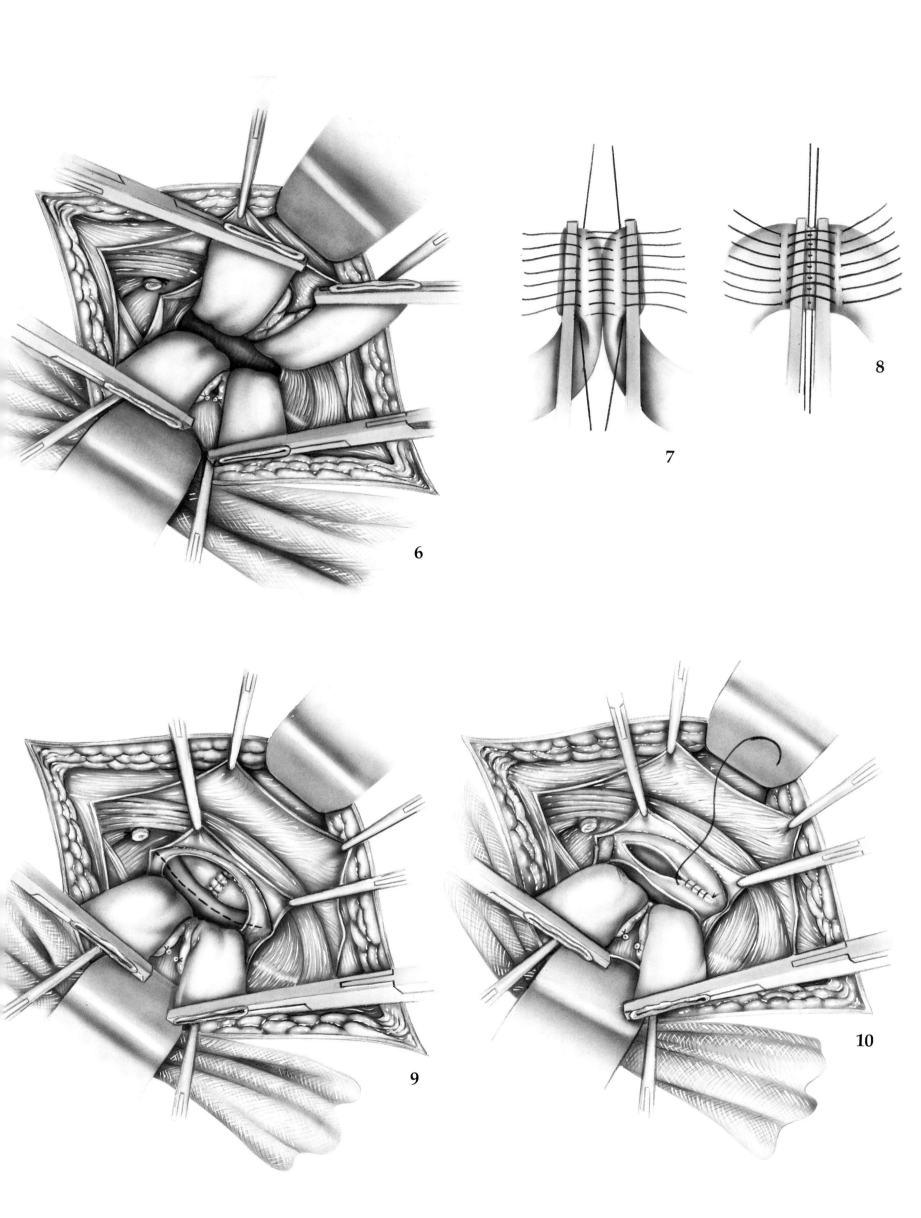

6

7

8

9

10

PLATE

2 1 1

Strangulated Femoral Hernia, Transinguinal Approach with Bowel Resection (Dennis-Varco Technique) (*cont.*)

11 The limbs of the bowel to be resected are tied with umbilical tape or stapled closed. The femoral ring, the lacunar ligament, and/or the inguinal ligament itself is cut, releasing the neck of the hernia sac. The residual hernia sac and necrotic bowel can then be removed from below, minimizing the contamination of the inguinal incision.

12 A conventional McVay repair is used to close the femoral defect (**Plates 203–204, Figs. 4–8**).

13 A long relaxing incision is made in the anterior rectus sheath to take the tension off the closure.

14 The external oblique fascia is closed with interrupted #000 polyglycolic acid sutures. The skin of both incisions is closed with skin staples.

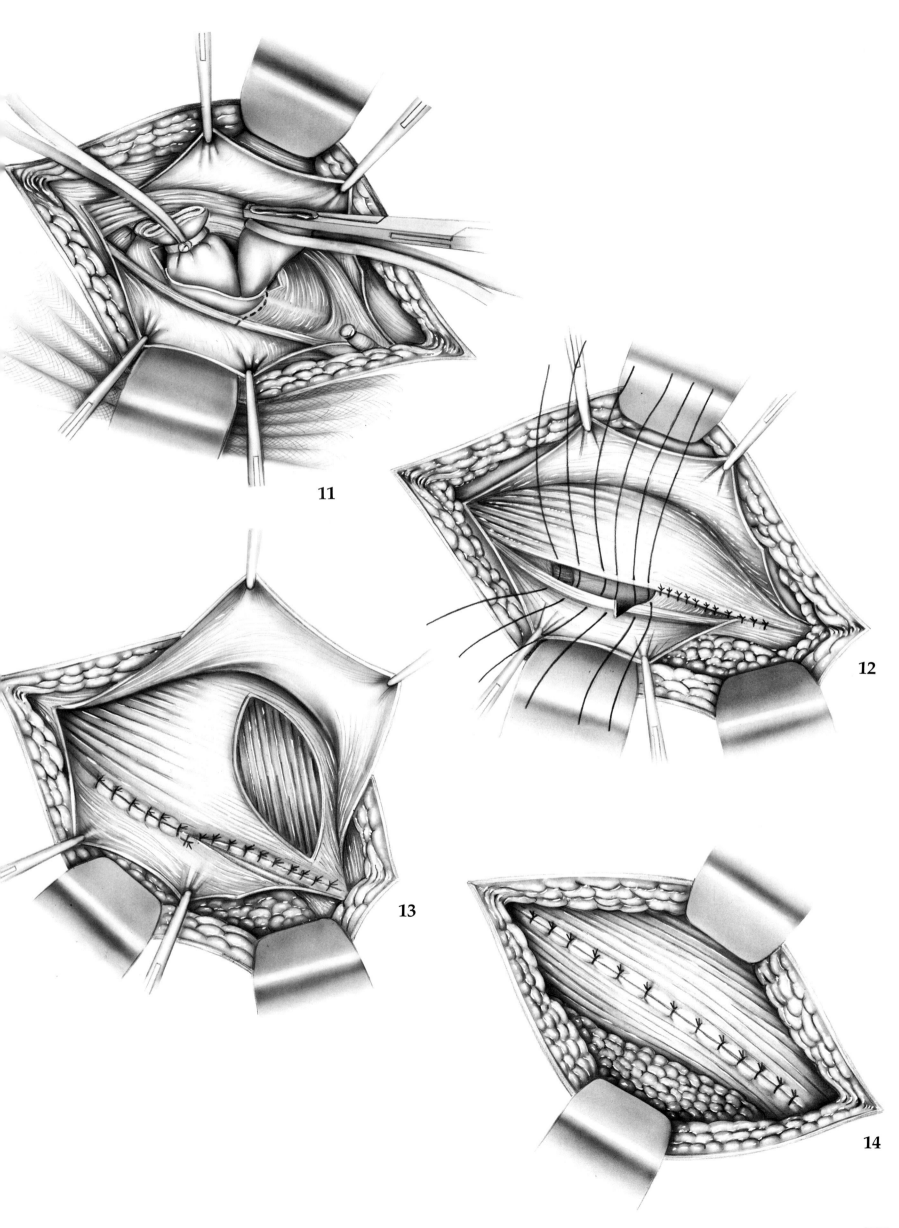

11

12

13

14

Hydrocele in a Child (Over 6 Months of Age)

1 A transverse incision in the lowermost skin crease is made, with its medial end at the point just above where the cord can be palpated overlying the pubic tubercle.

2 The Scarpa's fascia is opened, and the external oblique aponeurosis and the spermatic cord exiting through the external ring are visualized. The external oblique aponeurosis is opened lateral to, and below, the external ring, which is left intact.

3 In almost all hydroceles in older infants and children there is a communication to the peritoneal cavity through a small patent vaginalis process. In essence this is a small indirect inguinal hernia or communicating hydrocele. The small indirect hernial sac is first addressed by opening the layers of the cord longitudinally and identifying the narrow peritoneal communication.

4 The hernial sac is then freed from the cord structures by blunt dissection, peeling the adjacent tissues away from the sac up to the internal ring.

5 When the sac is completely dissected it is transected in the middle of the canal.

6 The sac is freed up to the internal ring, twisted, and suture-ligated as in a hernia repair.

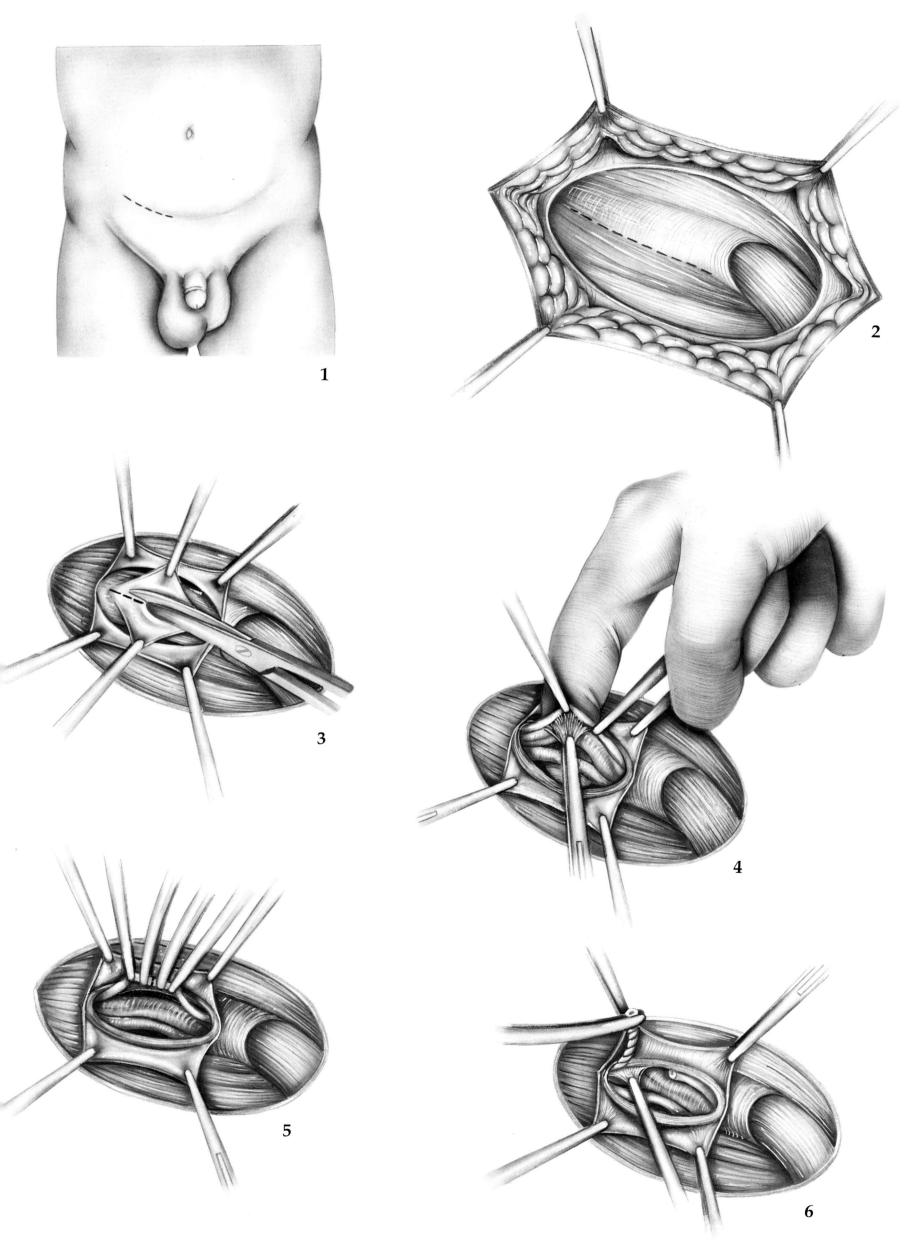

Hydrocele in a Child (Over 6 Months of Age) (*cont.*)

7 The hydrocele is then pushed up into the incision and exposed external to the external inguinal ring. The tissues over the hydrocele are opened by sharp dissection, exposing the thin translucent wall of the hydrocele.

8 A window is cut in the anterior surface of the hydrocele large enough to evacuate fluid and allow any reaccumulation of fluid to drain into the subcutaneous tissues.

9 The testicle is pulled down into its normal position in the scrotum prior to closing the incision.

10 The external oblique aponeurosis is then closed with interrupted #000 polyglycolic acid sutures, and the Scarpa's fascia and skin are closed as in a standard herniorraphy.

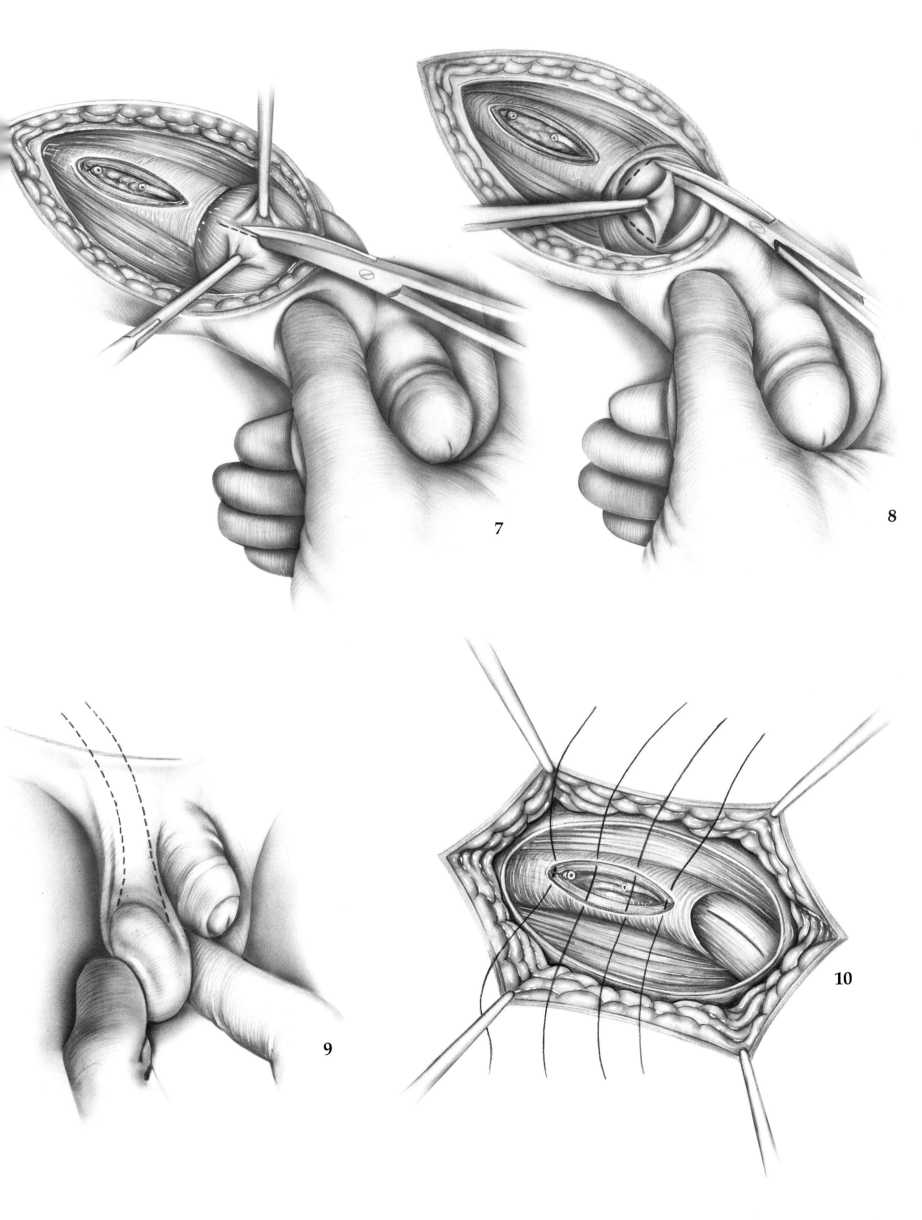

Inguinal Herniorrhaphy in a Child
(Under 6 Months of Age)

1 A skin crease incision is used, with its midpoint above where the cord can be palpated running over the pubic tubercle. This anatomic landmark will place the incision over the external ring. In infants under 6 months of age the external oblique aponeurosis need not be opened, as the internal and external rings are superimposed.

2 The Scarpa's fascia, which in infants will appear far better developed than in adults, is exposed and incised by scissor dissection. The external ring is thus exposed, with the spermatic cord coming through it.

3 The cord is freed from underlying tissues by blunt dissection, and a hemostat placed under it.

4 The layers of the spermatic cord are then opened longitudinally by blunt dissection, utilizing two forceps to grasp tissues at the same levels and to separate them from one another. In this manner the various layers of the cord are separated until the hernial sac, spermatic vessels, and vas deferens are exposed.

5 The sac is then grasped with a forceps, and tissues adherent to it are removed by blunt dissection by peeling them away with a forceps. The sac is held up by a hemostat, and the dissection is completed in a similar manner until the sac is freed up to the internal ring.

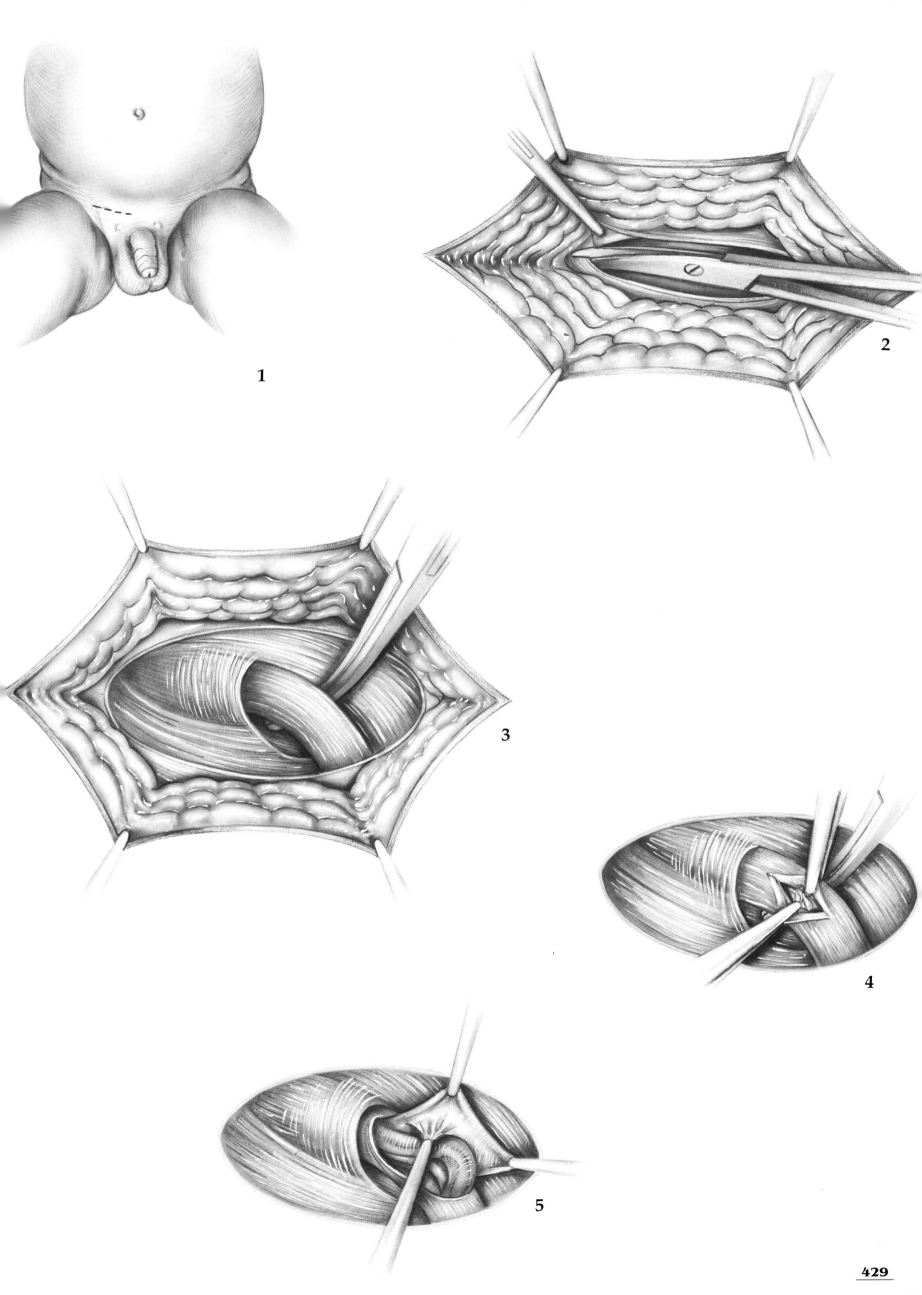

PLATE
2 1 5

Inguinal Herniorrhaphy in a Child (Under 6 Months of Age) (*cont.*)

6 A retractor is then placed into the internal ring, and the sac freed from the edges of the ring.

7 The sac is twisted to reduce any contents, to provide more substance for the ligature, and to obtain a high ligation. A ligature of #000 polyglycolic acid suture is then placed in one of the proximal twists of the sac, and the sac ligated and excised.

8 The testicle is pulled down into the scrotum to ensure that it is in normal position.

9 The Scarpa's fascia is closed with interrupted #000 polyglycolic acid sutures.

10 The skin is closed with a running subcuticular suture.

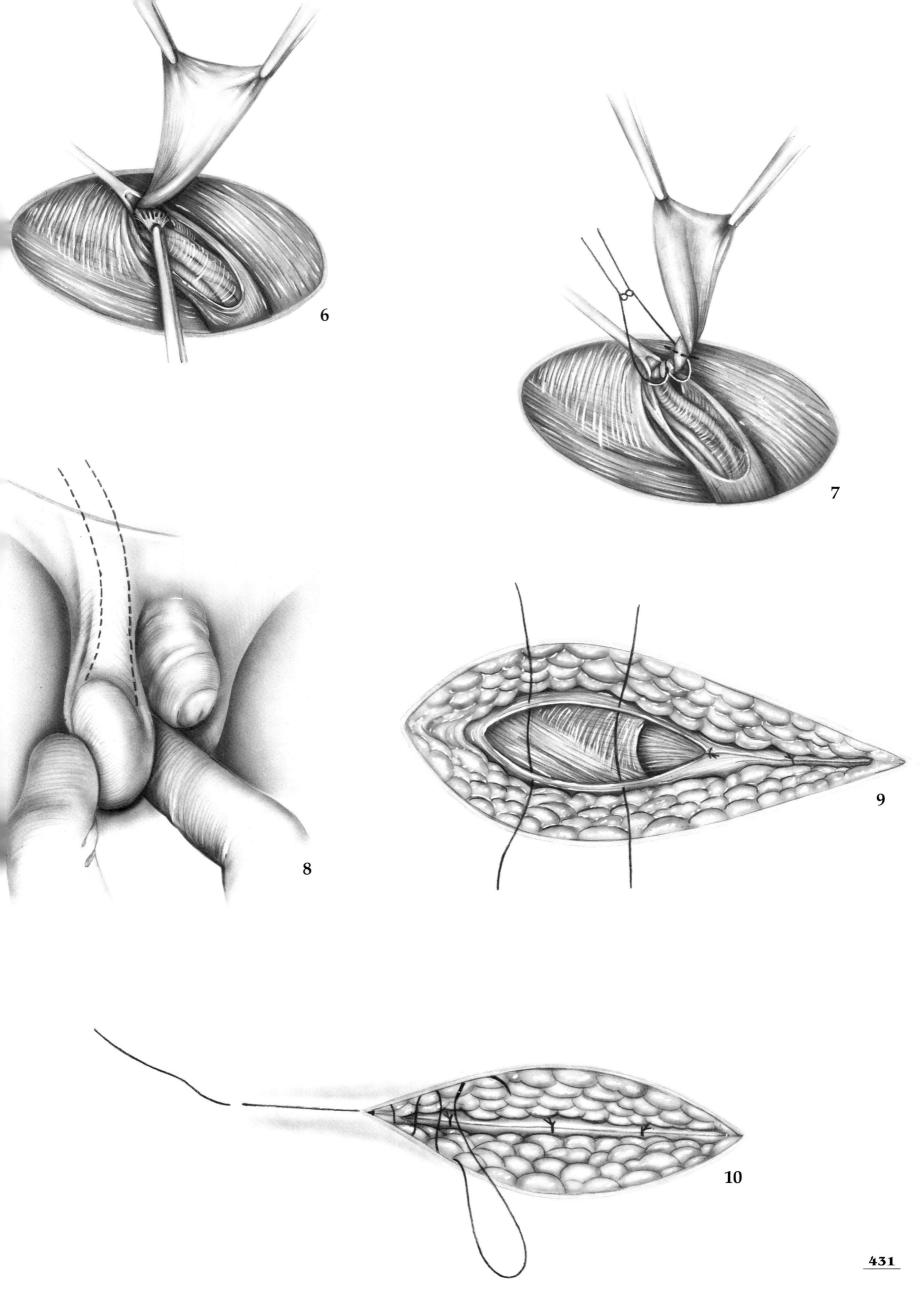

Inguinal Herniorrhaphy in a Child (Over 6 Months of Age)

1 An incision is made in the lowermost skin crease, with its medial end just above the point where the spermatic cord can be palpated over the pubic tubercle.

2 Scarpa's fascia is opened and the external oblique aponeurosis and the cord exiting through the external ring are exposed. With a hemostat in the external ring, tenting the external oblique aponeurosis upward, an incision is made in the aponeurosis lateral to, and below, the external ring—but not through it.

3 The incision is extended by spreading a scissors and splitting the aponeurosis parallel to its fibers.

4–5 The cord is exposed in the inguinal canal, and the multiple layers of the cord are opened up to the internal ring. Each layer is opened separately by sharp dissection in this procedure. Children with incarcerated hernias and those who have had several previous incarcerations do not lend themselves to the blunt dissection technique. Incarcerated hernias have friable tissue which tends to tear when one attempts to peel the tissues apart, and when multiple previous incarcerations have occurred fibrosis makes blunt dissection difficult. The sharp technique demonstrated in these drawings can be used for all hernias, and *must* be used when the blunt or "push-pull" technique cannot be employed.

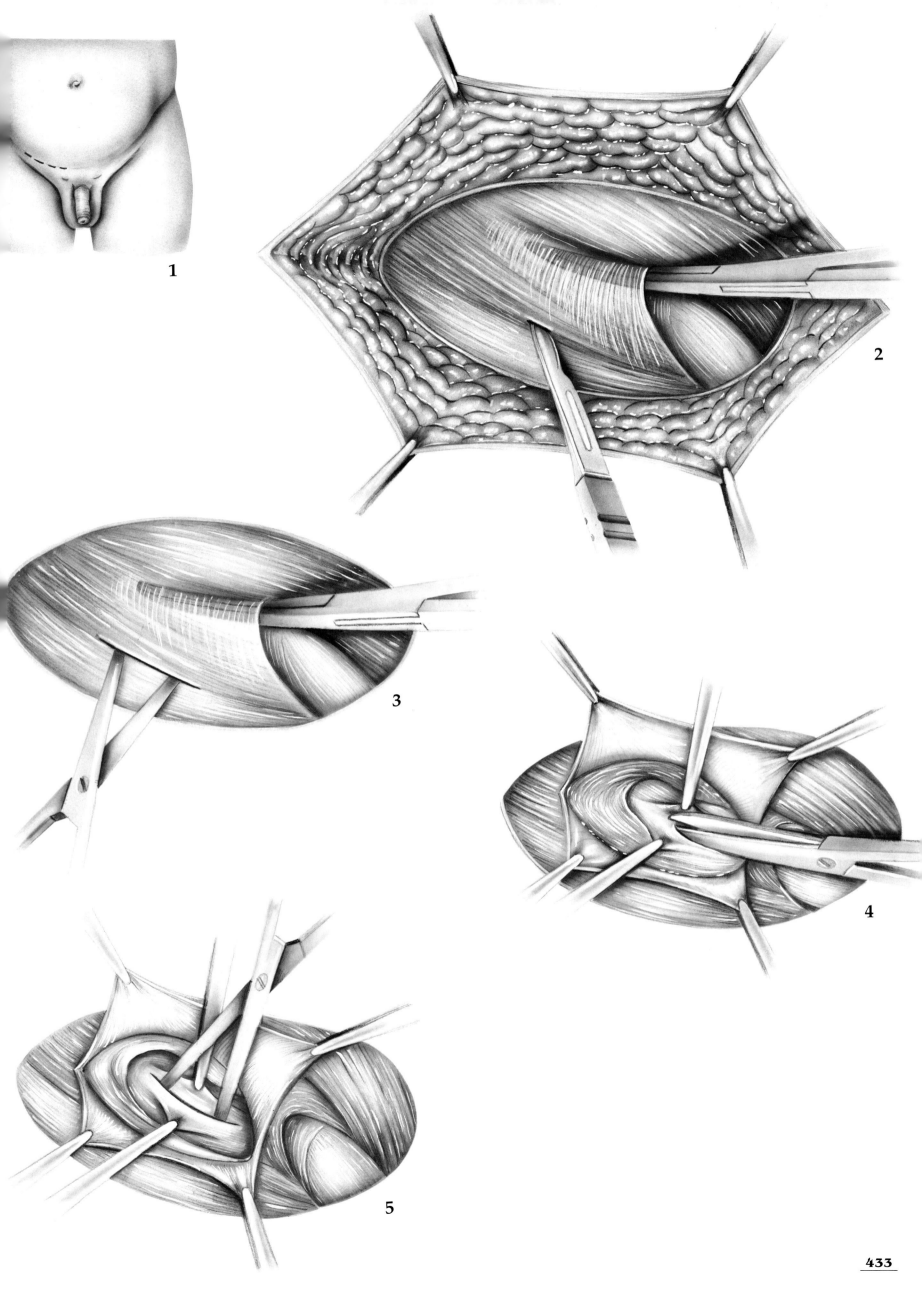

Inguinal Herniorrhaphy in a Child (Over 6 Months of Age) (*cont.*)

6–8 As the multiple layers of the cord are opened, the hernial sac, spermatic vessels, and vas deferens are identified. The sac is then dissected by holding adjacent tissues with two forceps so that, under direct vision, the sac can be sharply dissected free from the surrounding tissues.

9 When the sac is completely dissected up to the neck and around its complete circumference, it can be transected without dissecting the full extent of the distal hernial sac, which may be a completely patent tunica vaginalis processus.

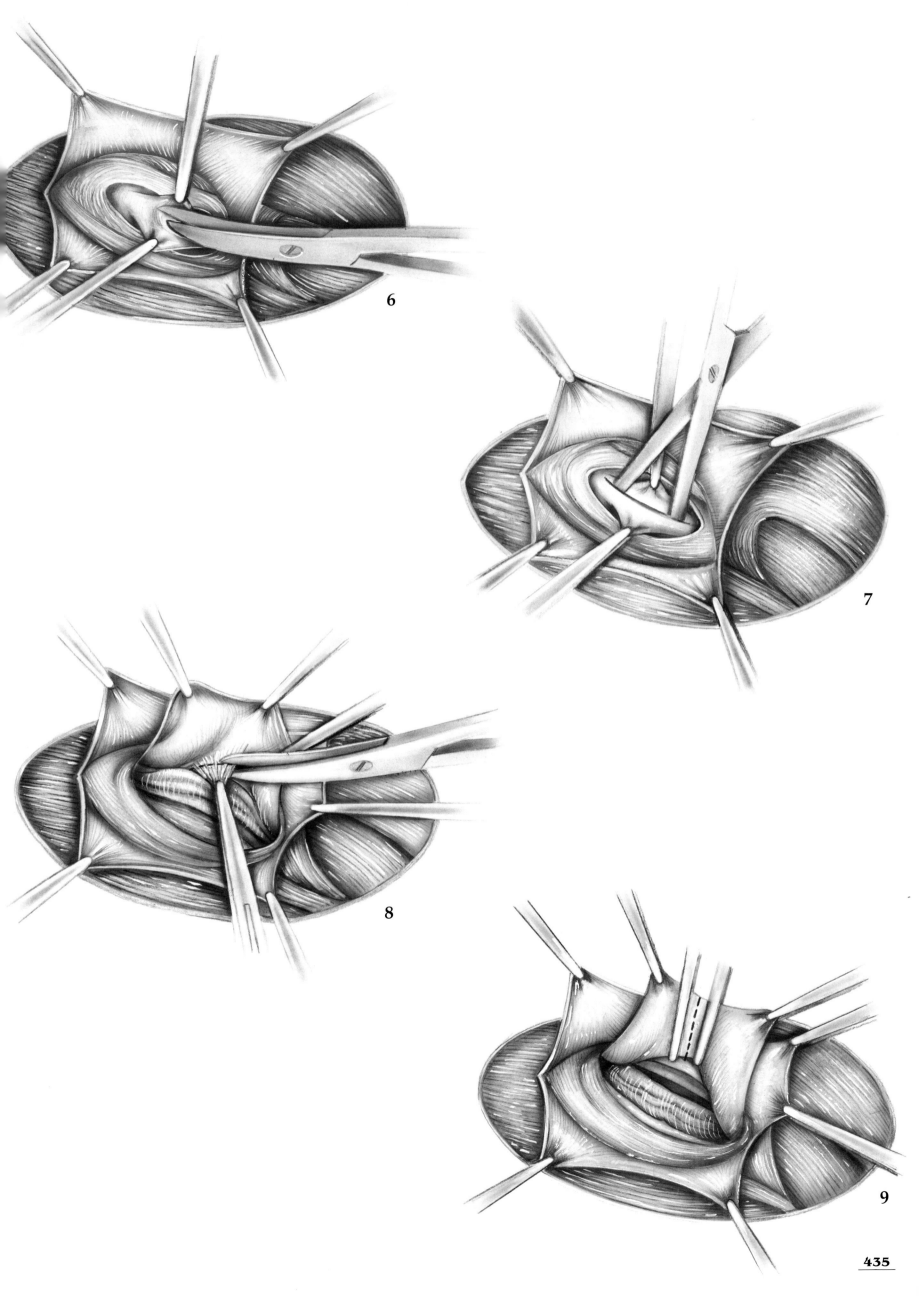

6

7

8

9

Inguinal Herniorrhaphy in a Child (Over 6 Months of Age) (*cont.*)

10 The proximal dissection is carried up to the internal ring, again by scissor dissection while visualizing the edges of the sac.

11 When the dissection is completed up to the internal ring, the latter should be evaluated. If it appears dilated a clamp is placed on the medial edge of the internal ring prior to twisting, ligating, and excising the proximal sac.

12 The internal ring can be snugged up around the cord structures with interrupted #000 polyglycolic acid sutures while traction is placed on the hemostat on the medial end of the internal ring.

13 When the ring has been reconstructed and the sac ligated, the latter retracts upward inside of the internal ring, and the external oblique is ready for closure.

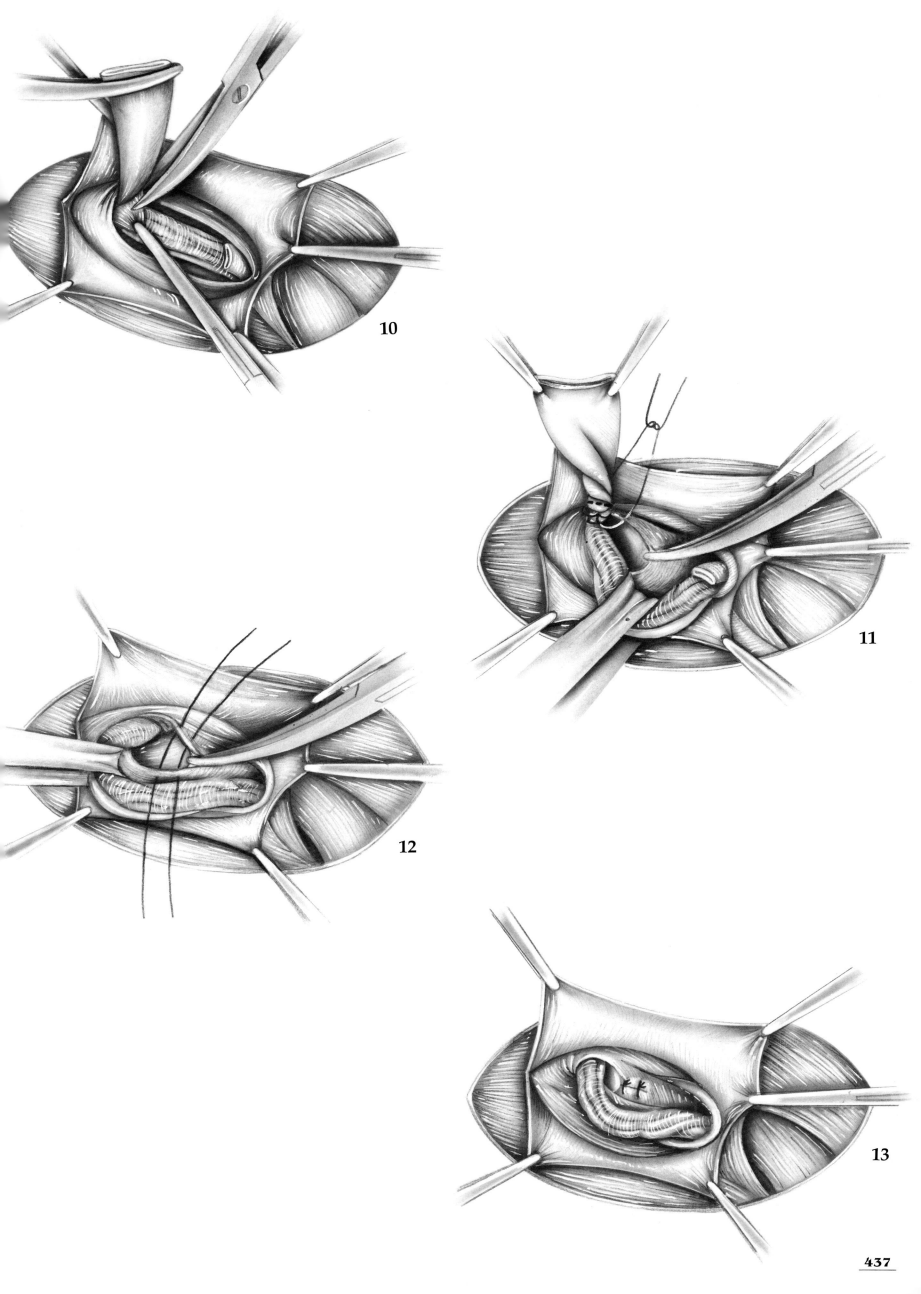

10

11

12

13

Inguinal Herniorrhaphy in a Child (Over 6 Months of Age) (*cont.*)

14 Before closing the external oblique the testicle is brought down into normal position in the scrotum, so as not to create an iatrogenic undescended testicle.

15 The opening in the external oblique aponeurosis is closed with interrupted #000 polyglycolic acid sutures. The Scarpa's fascia is similarly closed.

16 The skin is closed with a running subcuticular suture.

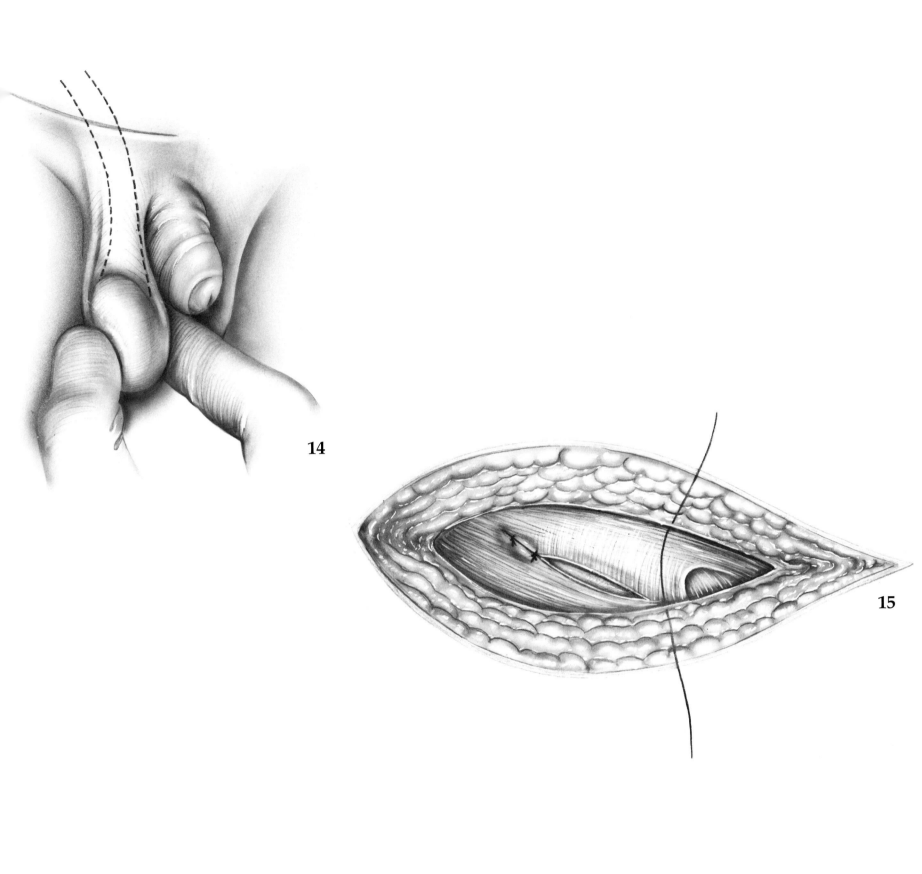

14

15

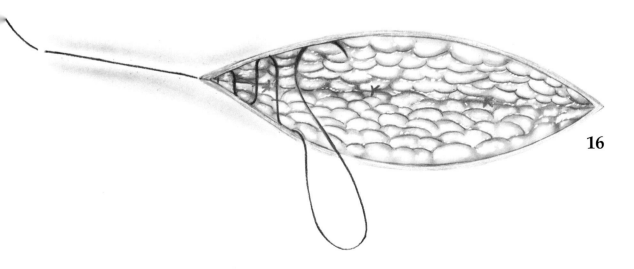

16

Orchiopexy

1 An incision is made in the lowermost abdominal skin crease, with its medial end just above the point where the spermatic cord can be palpated over the pubic tubercle. The incision is carried out farther laterally than that used for inguinal herniorraphy.

2 The Scarpa's fascia is opened and the external oblique aponeurosis and cord, exiting through the external ring, are exposed. The external oblique aponeurosis is opened through the external ring and parallel to its fibers, to the lateral edge of the incision.

3 The internal oblique and transversus abdominis muscles are then transsected for approximately 2 cm where they arch over the cord.

4 The gubernaculum is transected. Using a clamp on it for traction, the testicle and cord structures are mobilized by incising the cremaster muscle up to its origin at the internal ring.

5 At the internal ring the cremaster fibers are incised around the circumference of the cord, exposing the sac and cord structures where they go through the internal ring.

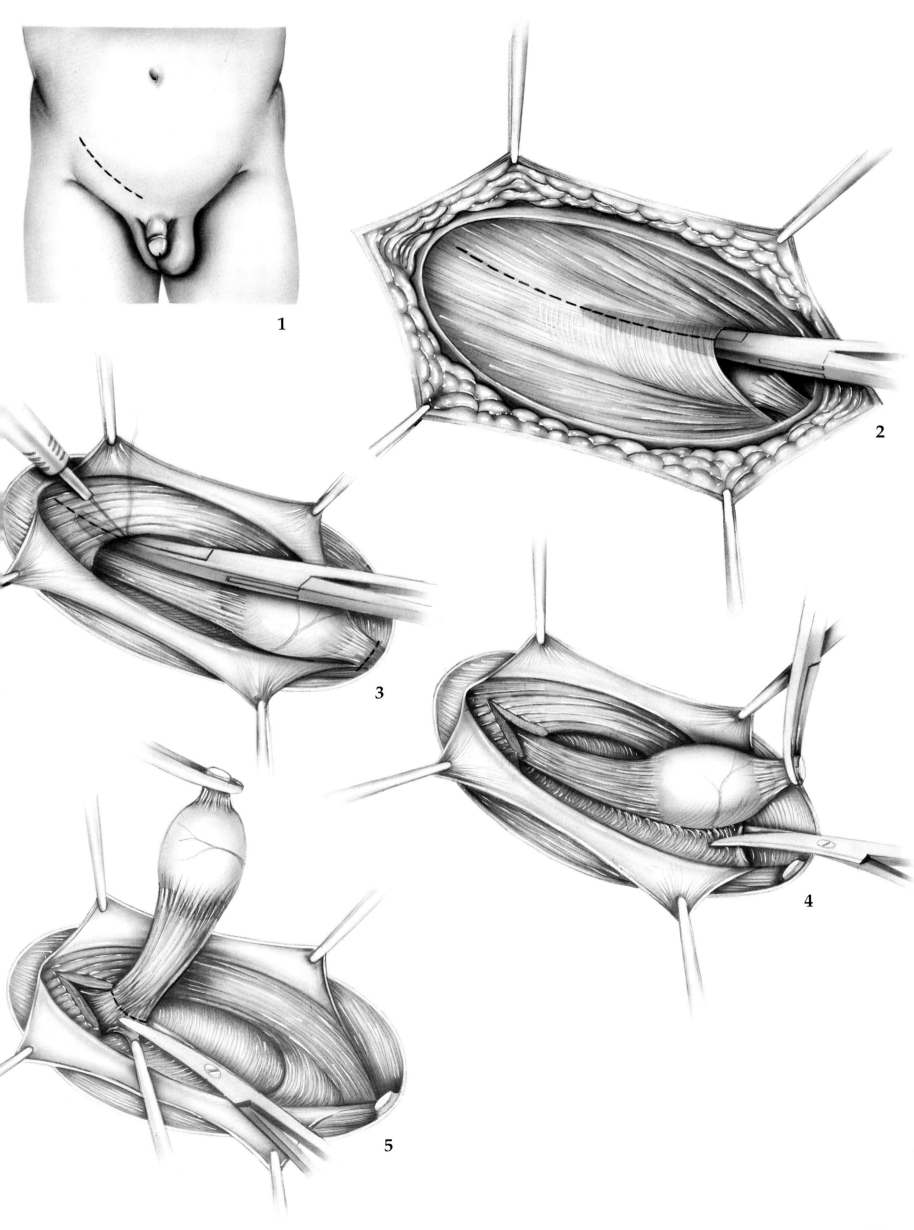

Orchiopexy (*cont.*)

6 At their uppermost end the cremaster fibers are incised longitudinally, as are the various layers of the cord, so as to expose the hernial sac, which is present in the majority of cases.

7 The sac is freed, by sharp and blunt dissection, from the other cord structures.

8 The sac is transected.

9 The sac is twisted and suture-ligated and the excess excised, leaving the distal end *in situ*.

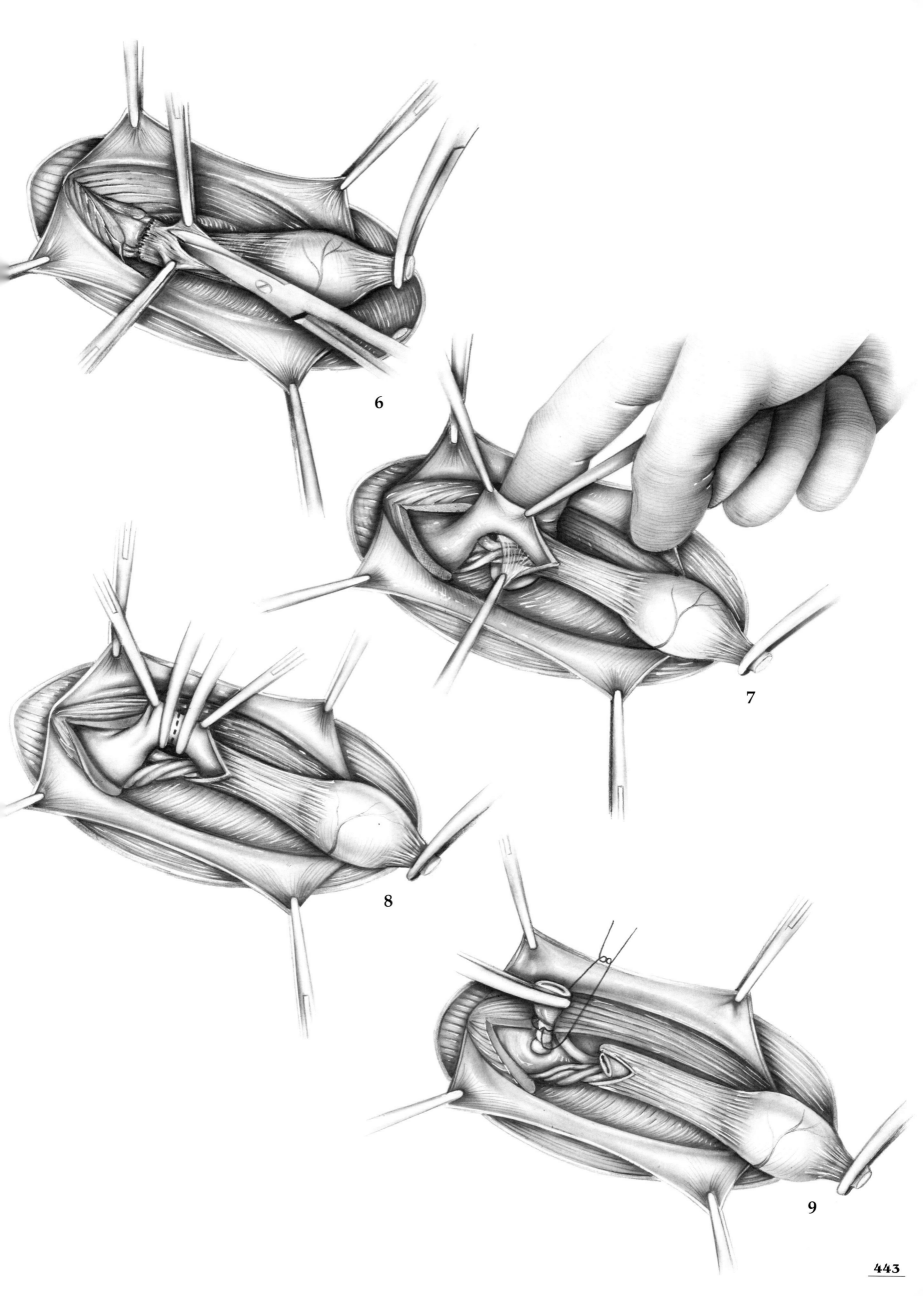

6

7

8

9

Orchiopexy (*cont.*)

10 The inadequate length of the spermatic vessels is compensated for by shortening the route that the vessels take from their origin at the vena cava, renal vein, and aorta, respectively, to the scrotum. The shorter course is achieved by changing the direction of the vessels from the two short sides to the long side of three anatomic triangles, two in the AP projection (shown here) and one in the saggital (**Fig. 13**). The normal course of the vessels is demonstrated by the shorter sides of the outer triangle where the vessels initially go out to the lateral wall of the pelvis and then move medially to the internal ring, down the inguinal canal through the external inguinal ring, and into the scrotum.

11 Length is gained initially by changing the direction of the vessels from the two shorter sides of the lateral triangle to its long side so that the vessels run directly from their origin to the internal ring. This change is accomplished by retroperitoneal dissection of the vessels to their origin.

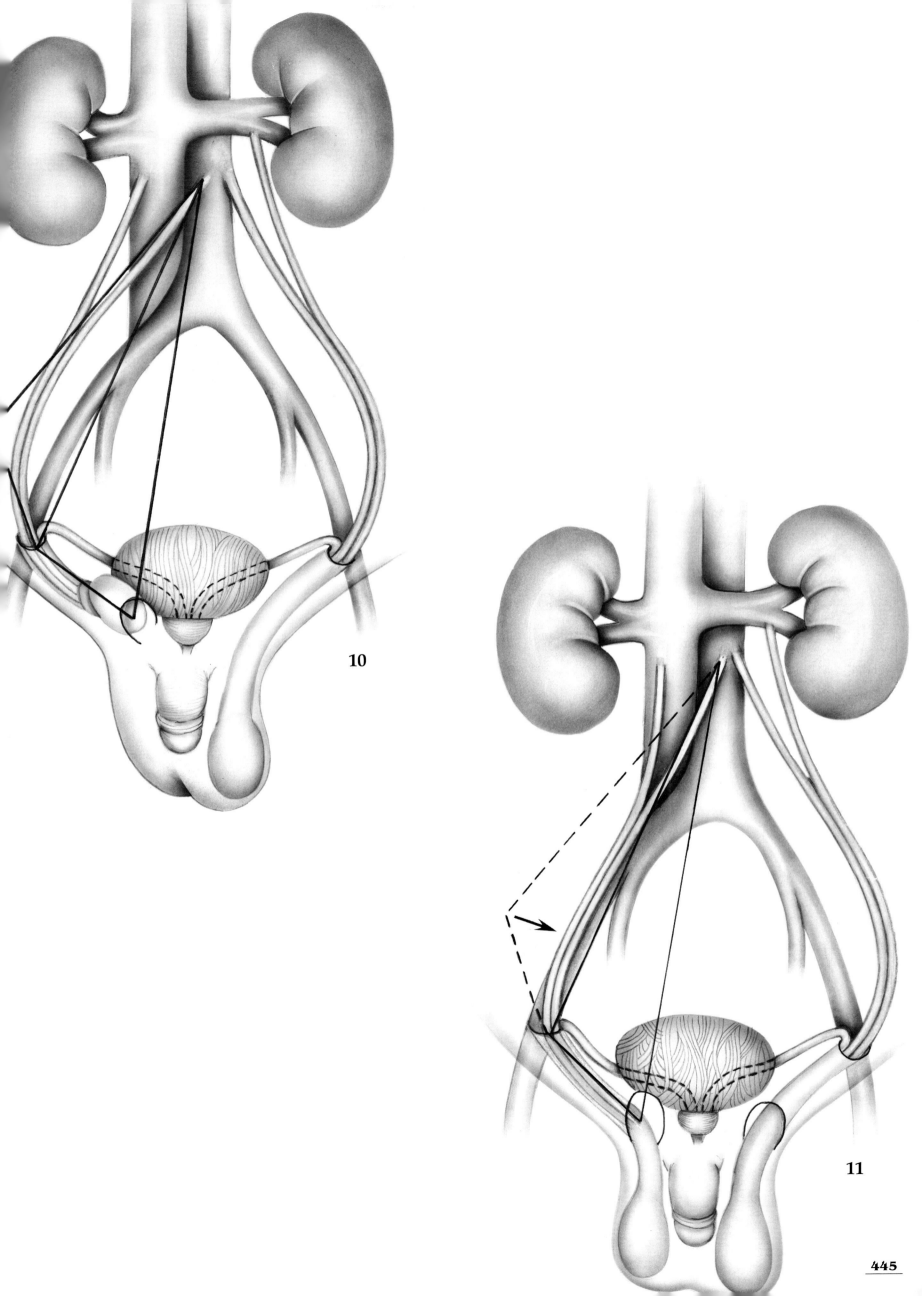

10

11

Orchiopexy (*cont.*)

12 The second change of direction is accomplished by opening the posterior wall of the inguinal canal so that the vessels go from their origin directly to the pubic tubercle, again gaining increased length by changing their path from the two short sides of the medial triangle to its long side.

13 In the saggital section, a similar change of path can be seen; the original direction of the vessels downward and around the peritoneum is altered to a direct route to the pubic tubercle, thus again changing from the two short sides of the triangle to its long one. These three alterations in the path of the vessels should provide enough length to bring the testicle into its position in the scrotum without tension.

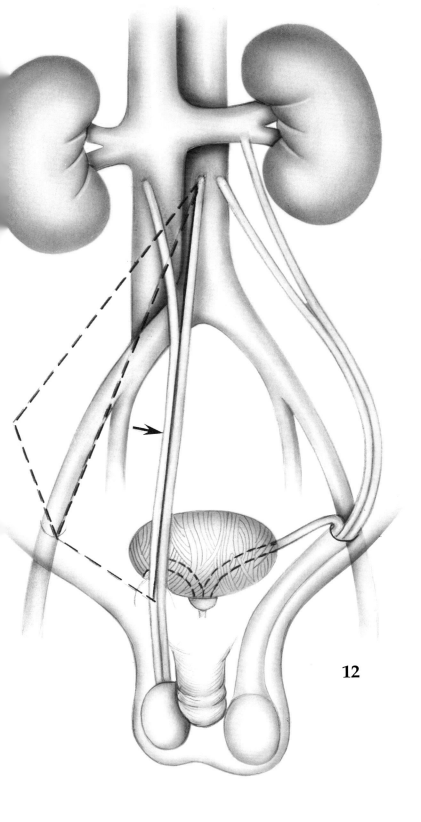

12

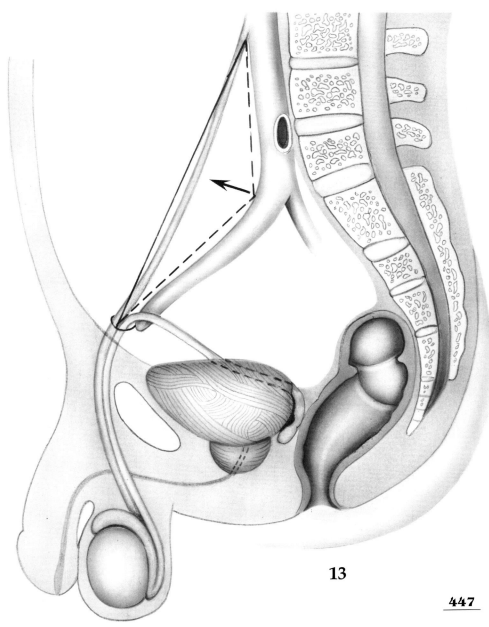

13

Orchiopexy (*cont.*)

14 The technique of changing the direction of the vessels is begun by opening the transversalis fascia, which makes up the posterior wall of the inguinal canal, from the internal ring to the pubic tubercle. The inferior epigastric artery and vein are individually isolated, doubly ligated, and divided.

15 The peritoneum is exposed and can be retracted upward to permit a retroperitoneal dissection of the vas deferens down to the base of the bladder.

16 The spermatic vessels are similarly dissected, by sharp and blunt dissection under vision, so as to mobilize them retroperitoneally up to the lower pole of the kidney, or to their origin if possible. The vessels and the vas deferens are relatively well skeletonized to allow complete mobilization.

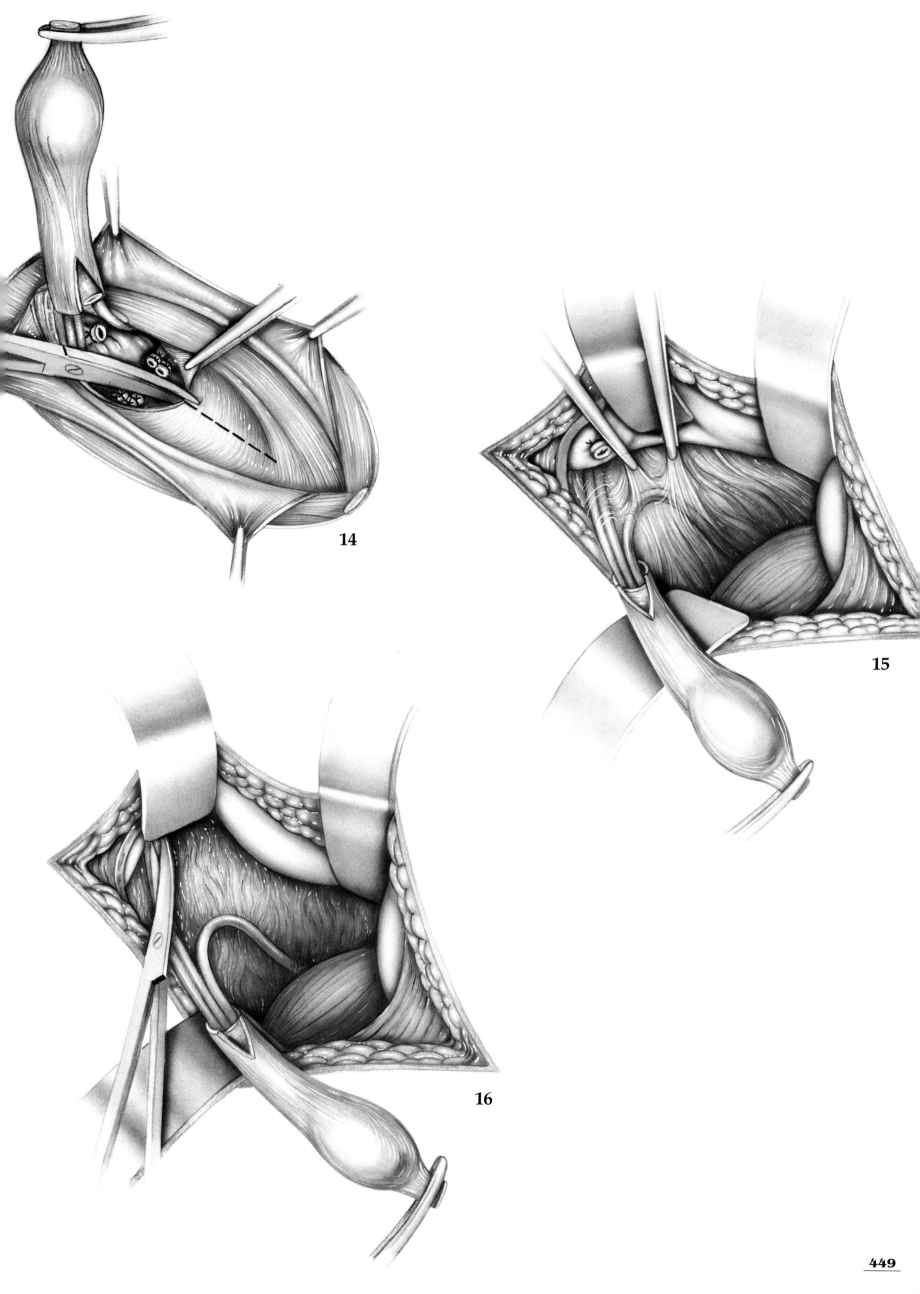

14

15

16

Orchiopexy (*cont.*)

17 The scrotum is prepared by opening up the pathway into the scrotum with the index finger and digitally dilating the atrophic scrotum. A transverse incision in the skin of the scrotum is made, carefully preserving the dartos fascia.

18 A pouch large enough for the testicle is developed between the skin and the dartos fascia, using blunt dissection by spreading a hemostat.

19 A small incision is made in the dartos fascia, just large enough to bring the testicle through it. A clamp is placed upward through this opening. The gubernaculum is grasped, and the testicle brought through the dartos fascia and skin. Interrupted polyglycolic acid sutures are then used to close the opening in the dartos fascia around the spermatic cord. The testicle is placed beneath the skin, which is closed with a subcuticular suture.

20 In this fashion the testicle is placed in a pouch between the skin and the dartos fascia. If mobilization has been adequate it should lie in this position without tension.

   The floor of the inguinal canal is closed by reapproximating the transversalis fascia with interrupted #00 or #000 polyglycolic acid sutures, including closure of the original internal ring. A new internal ring is thus created at the pubic tubercle. The external oblique aponeurosis, Scarpa's fascia, and skin are closed in the usual manner.

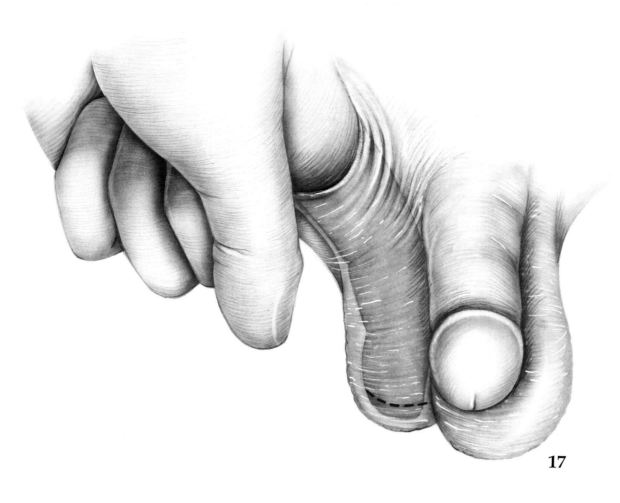

17

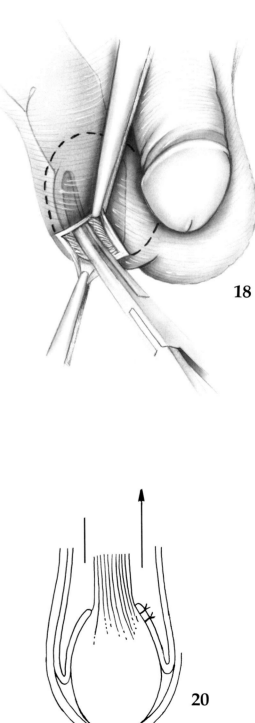

18

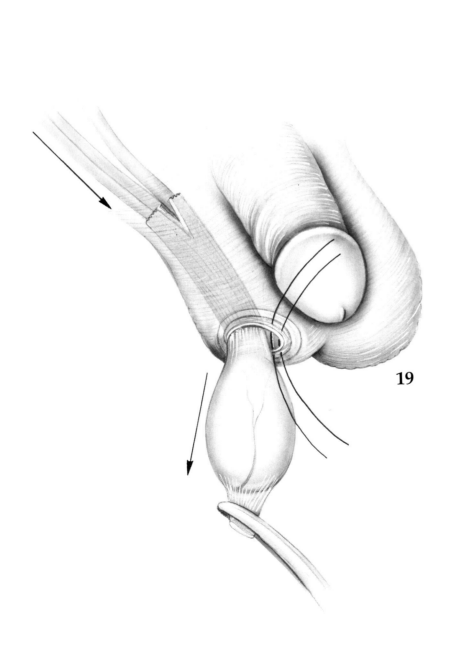

19

20

Pyloromyotomy

1–2 Various transverse incisions in the right upper quadrant are used. Muscle-splitting incisions lateral to the rectus and rectus-dividing incisions are both acceptable. Our preferred incision is a transverse incision dividing the rectus muscle high enough to be over the liver. This incision provides optimal exposure for delivering the pyloric tumor and has had minimal wound complications.

3 The skin incision is carried down through the anterior rectus sheath, after which the rectus muscle is divided transversely using the needle-point electrocautery.

4–5 The peritoneum is opened transversely, exposing the liver.

6 The liver is retracted upward and the stomach delivered through the incision by grasping the greater curvature above the pylorus. With gentle traction toward the left shoulder the pyloric tumor can be delivered into the wound. The serosa of the pyloric tumor is then incised longitudinally through the avascular area on the anterior surface between the vessels arising from the greater and lesser curvatures of the stomach, starting at the pyloric vein and extending proximally to above the palpable hypertrophied muscle.

7 The pyloric tumor is held firmly by the surgeon's index finger placed against the lower end of the pyloric tumor, inverting the duodenal wall, while the first assistant fixes the stomach proximally. A Benson spreader is pressed firmly into the hypertrophied muscle at the midpoint of the incision. With pressure, the forceps will appear to pop through the pylorus, but in fact it has only gone through the hypertrophied muscle.

8 By spreading the Benson spreader, the hypertrophied muscle is split longitudinally throughout the length of the pyloric tumor. Splitting of the distal end of the pyloric tumor can be further accomplished by repositioning the Benson spreader more distally, but *under no circumstances should the instrument be placed beyond the serosal incision.* Protrusion of the pyloric tumor into the duodenum produces a fold of duodenal mucosa superficial to the tumor at the lower end of the hypertrophied pylorus; this is where perforation most commonly occurs.

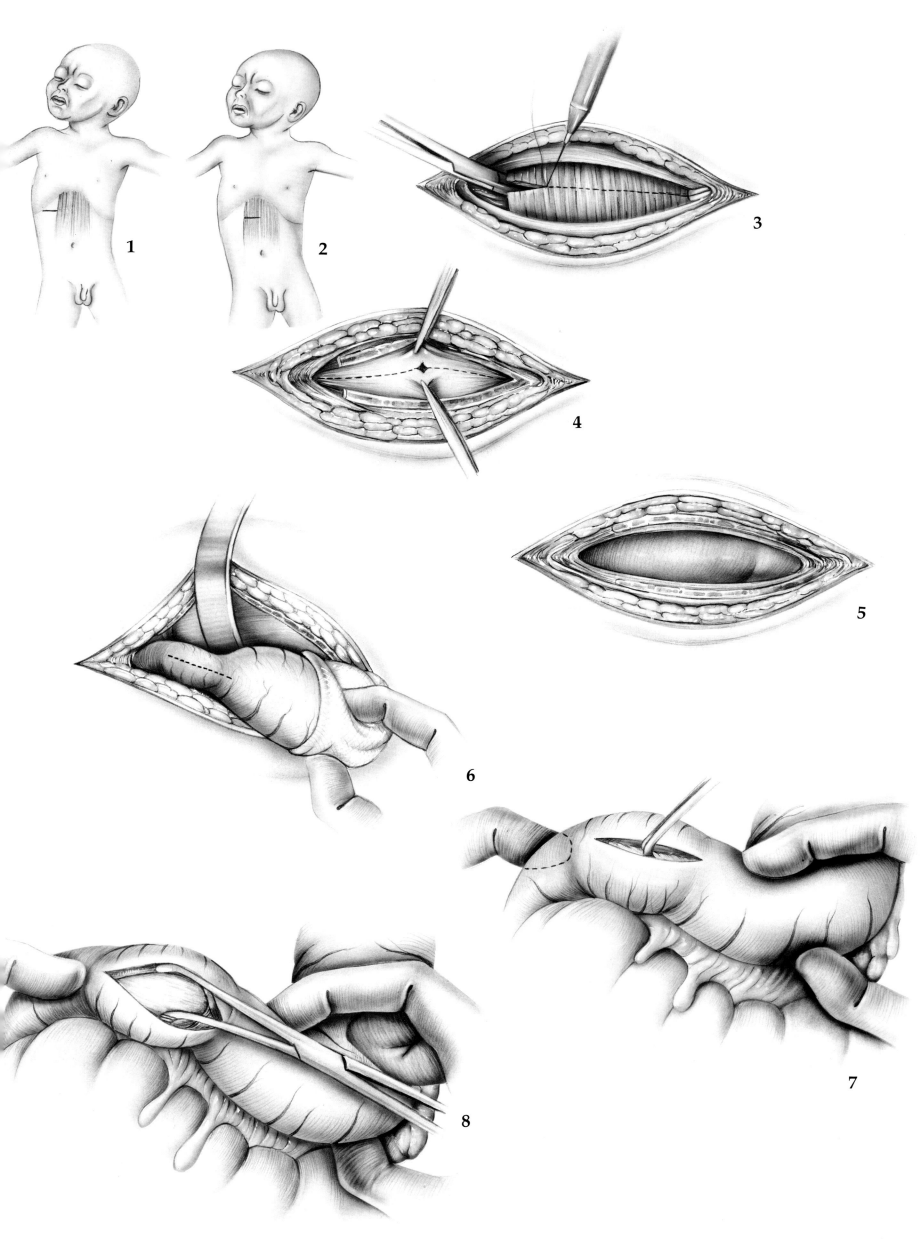

Pyloromyotomy (*cont.*)

9 After splitting the hypertrophied muscle, the proximal extent of the division is where the circular muscle no longer splits. At this point 1 cm of the intact circular muscle is divided over a clamp, ensuring an adequate proximal myotomy.

10 The adequacy of the distal extent of the myotomy is determined by feeling the overriding edges of the divided pylorus upon palpating the lower end of the pyloric tumor.

11 If the pylorotomy is incomplete, palpation of the distal end will merely indent the remaining hypertrophied circular muscle; one will not feel the overriding edges.

12 The hypertrophied pylorus as seen in cross section before the pyloromyotomy.

13 Cross section showing the completed pyloromyotomy with the mucosa protruding between the divided hypertrophied muscle.

14 With complete division of the circular muscle the mucosa can be seen to bulge between the edges of the divided muscle. Air is introduced into the stomach through the nasogastric tube and gently milked into the duodenum to check for any perforation. Most bleeding from the edges of the myotomy is due to venous congestion and stops when the pylorus is returned to the peritoneal cavity. Persistent arterial bleeding is stopped by figure-of-eight suture ligatures to the edge of the muscle.

15 The liver is allowed to fall back into position under the incision and the peritoneum is closed with a continuous #0000 polyglycolic acid suture.

16 The anterior rectus sheath is closed with interrupted #0000 polyglycolic acid sutures.

17 The skin is closed with a running subcuticular suture.

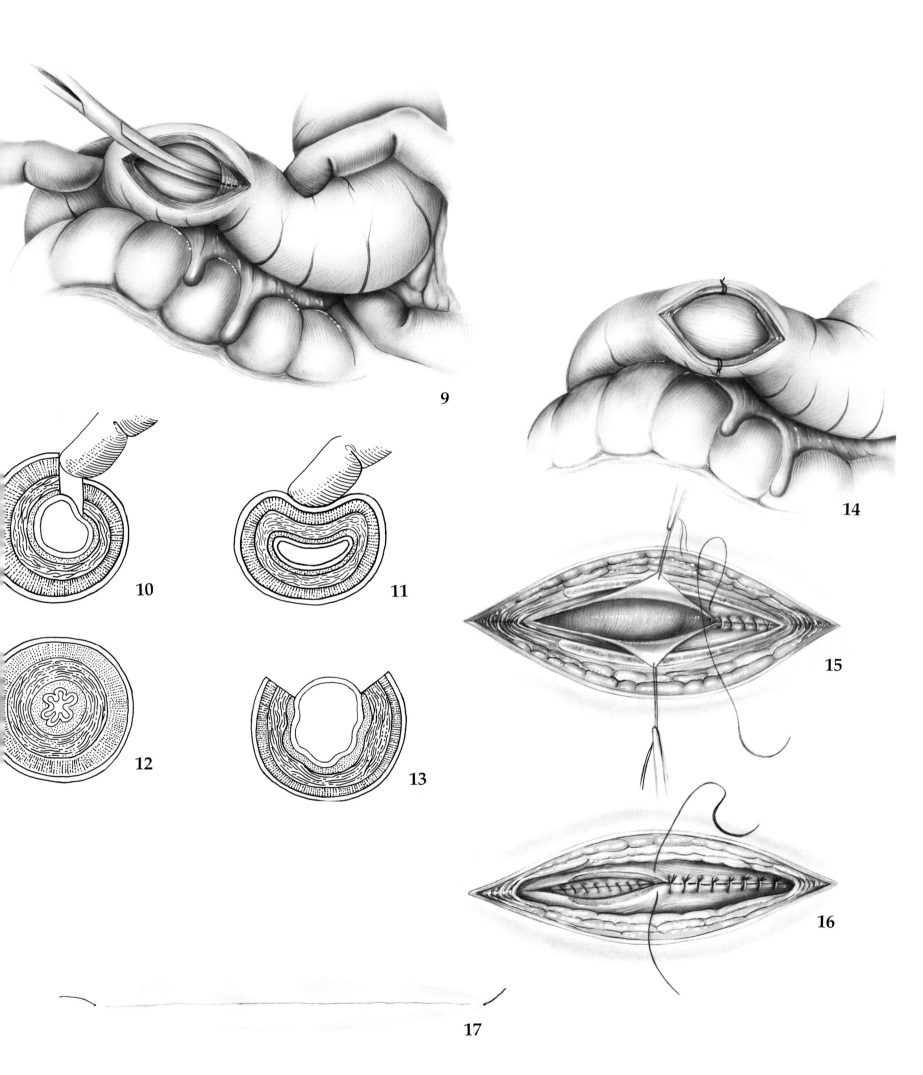

9

10

11

12

13

14

15

16

17

Diverting Transverse Colostomy in an Infant

1 A right upper abdominal transverse incision is made over the rectus muscle.

2 The anterior rectus sheath is opened transversely using the needle-point electrocautery.

3 The rectus muscle is similarly transected transversely.

4 The peritoneum is opened transversely throughout the extent of the incision.

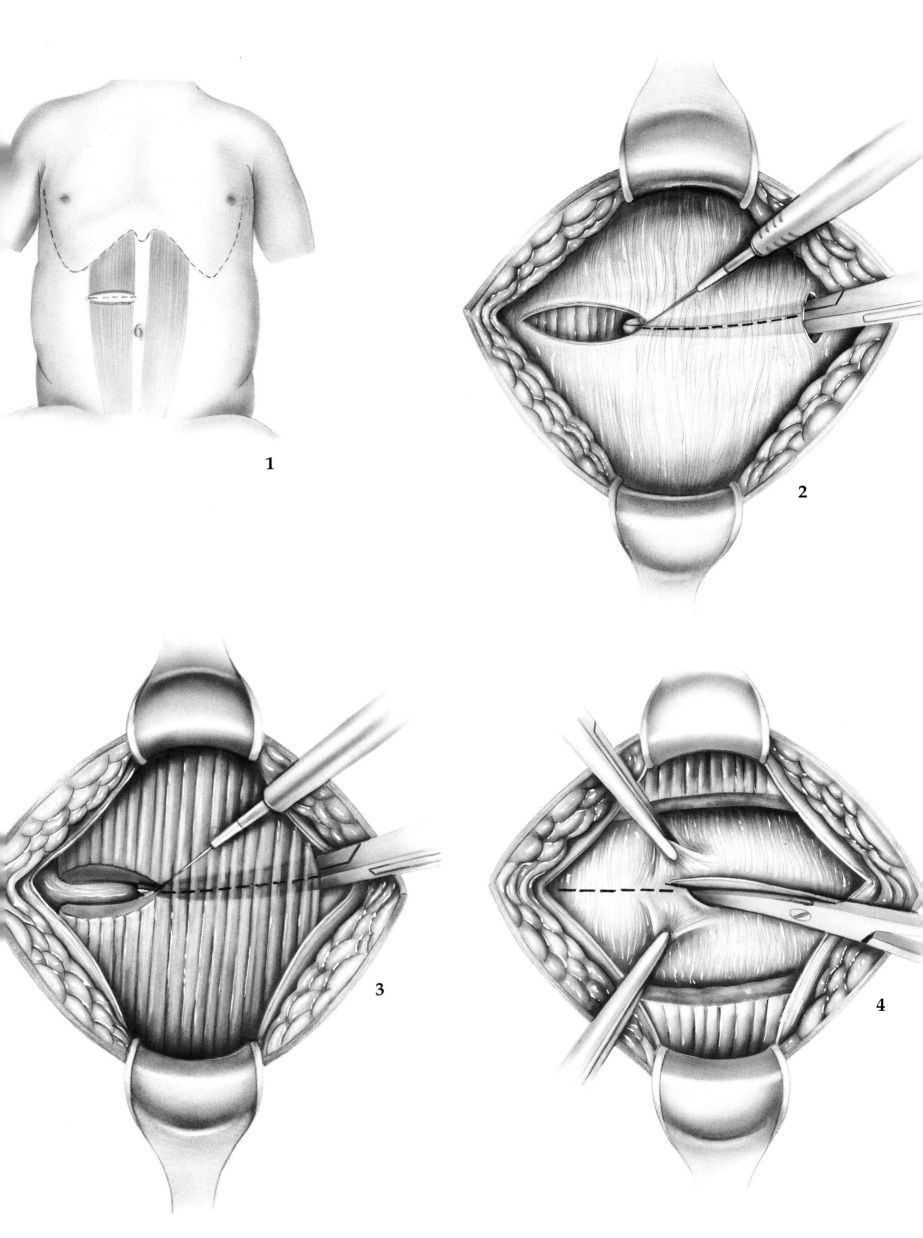

Diverting Transverse Colostomy in an Infant (*cont.*)

5–6 The right transverse colon, to the right of the middle colic artery, is delivered into the wound. The omentum is freed from the transverse colon and the colon is transected between clamps. The mesentery is similarly divided so as to permit the ends of the bowel to be brought up separately at the medial and lateral corners of the incision. The bowel is sutured to the peritoneum with interrupted 5-0 silk sutures.

7 The peritoneum is closed between the two spurs of the colostomy. The anterior rectus sheath is then similarly sewn to the two spurs of the colostomy, and to itself between them, with interrupted 5-0 silk sutures.

8 The skin is closed between the two spurs and the colostomies are matured with interrupted 4-0 polyglycolic acid sutures, everting the colon by approximating the full thickness of the end of the colon to the skin.

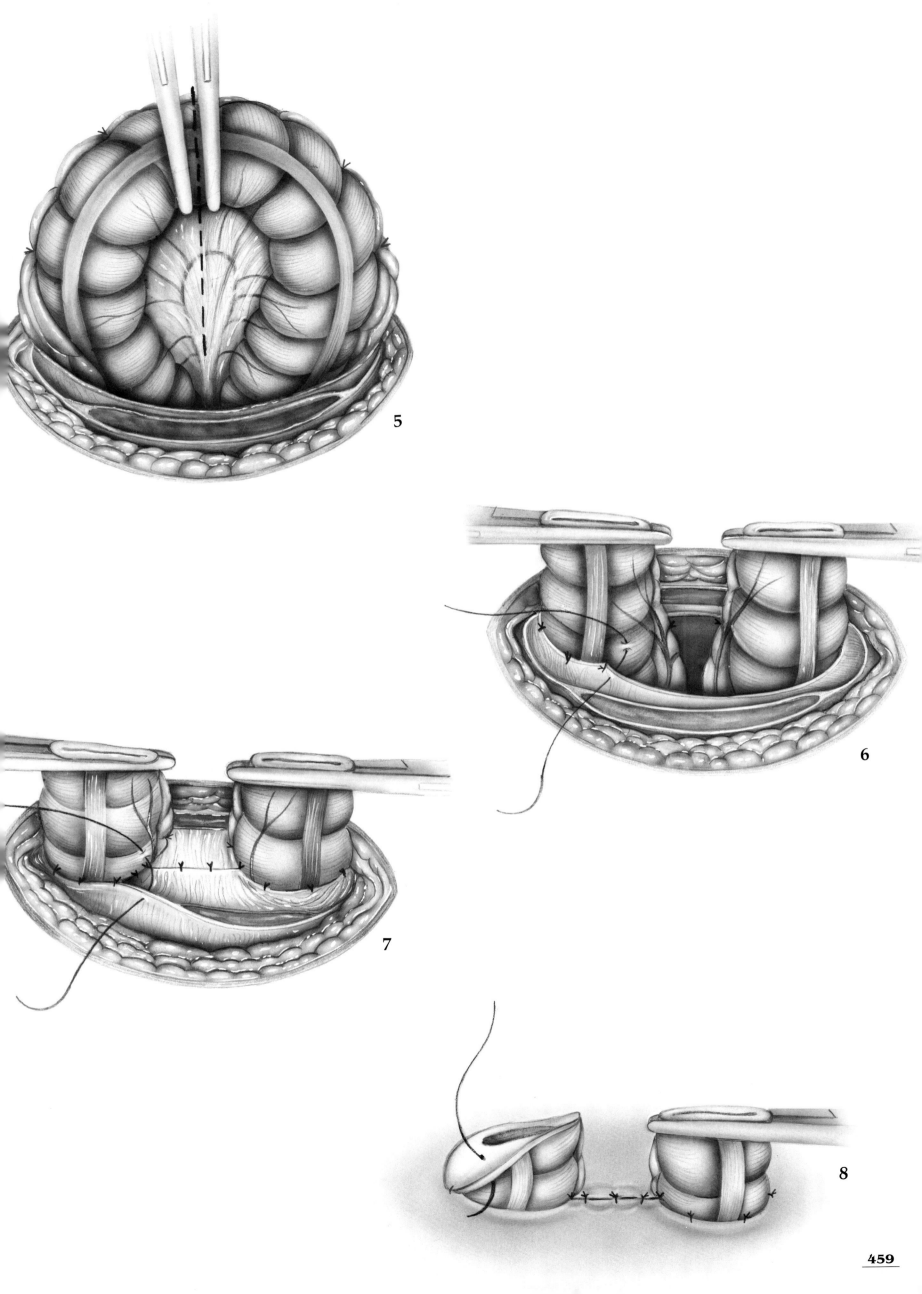

Intussusception

1 A right transverse supraumbilical or vertical paramedian incision can be used, depending on the exposure necessary to reach the apex of the intussusception.

2 In these drawings a right vertical paramedian incision has been used for an intussusception extending into the left half of the transverse colon. The muscle is retracted laterally and the peritoneum opened.

3 In an extensive intussusception a large portion of the intussuscepted bowel can be reduced before delivering any of the colon. Using the index and middle fingers, the bowel can be milked back into the ascending colon, in most instances, without difficulty.

4 The right colon is then mobilized and delivered into the wound, exposing the remaining intussusception and facilitating its reduction.

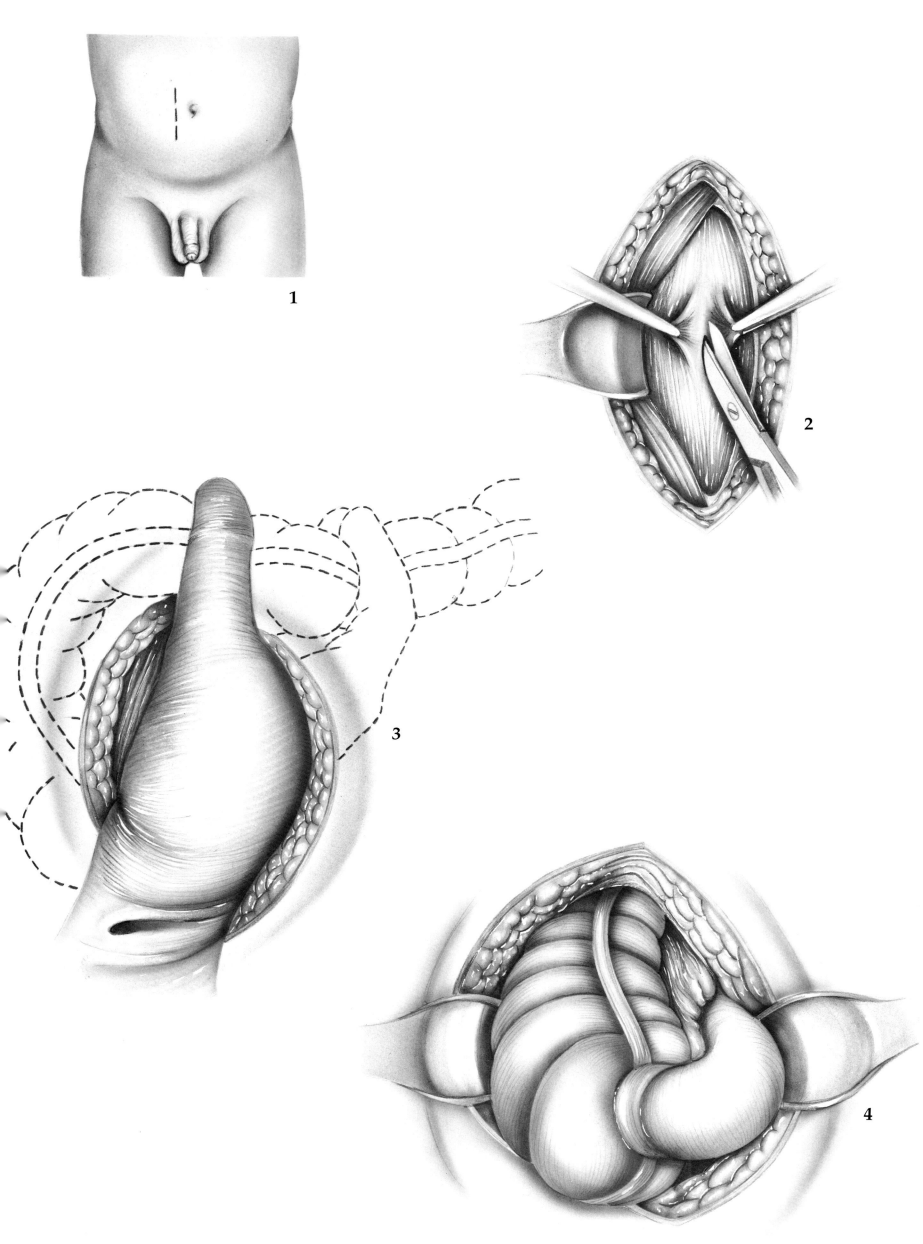

Intussusception (*cont.*)

5 The intussuscepted colon has been completely reduced (note appendix). The remaining ileocecal or ileocolic portion of the intussusceptum can be milked backward using both hands. *Traction on the intussuscepted bowel is never used.* A useful technique for reducing the last few inches of the ileocecal intussusceptum through the ileocecal valve is to use both thumbs to push on the apex while using the index fingers to pull the cecal wall back over the intussusceptum.

6 If there is an ileo-ileal component, as seen in this drawing, it is reduced by constant pressure, milking the bowel proximally.

7 Upon completion of the reduction of the intussusception, the appendix is removed and the stump inverted. The abdomen is closed in layers using continuous #000 polyglycolic acid suture for the peritoneum, interrupted #000 polyglycolic acid sutures for the anterior rectus sheath, and a running subcuticular suture for the skin.

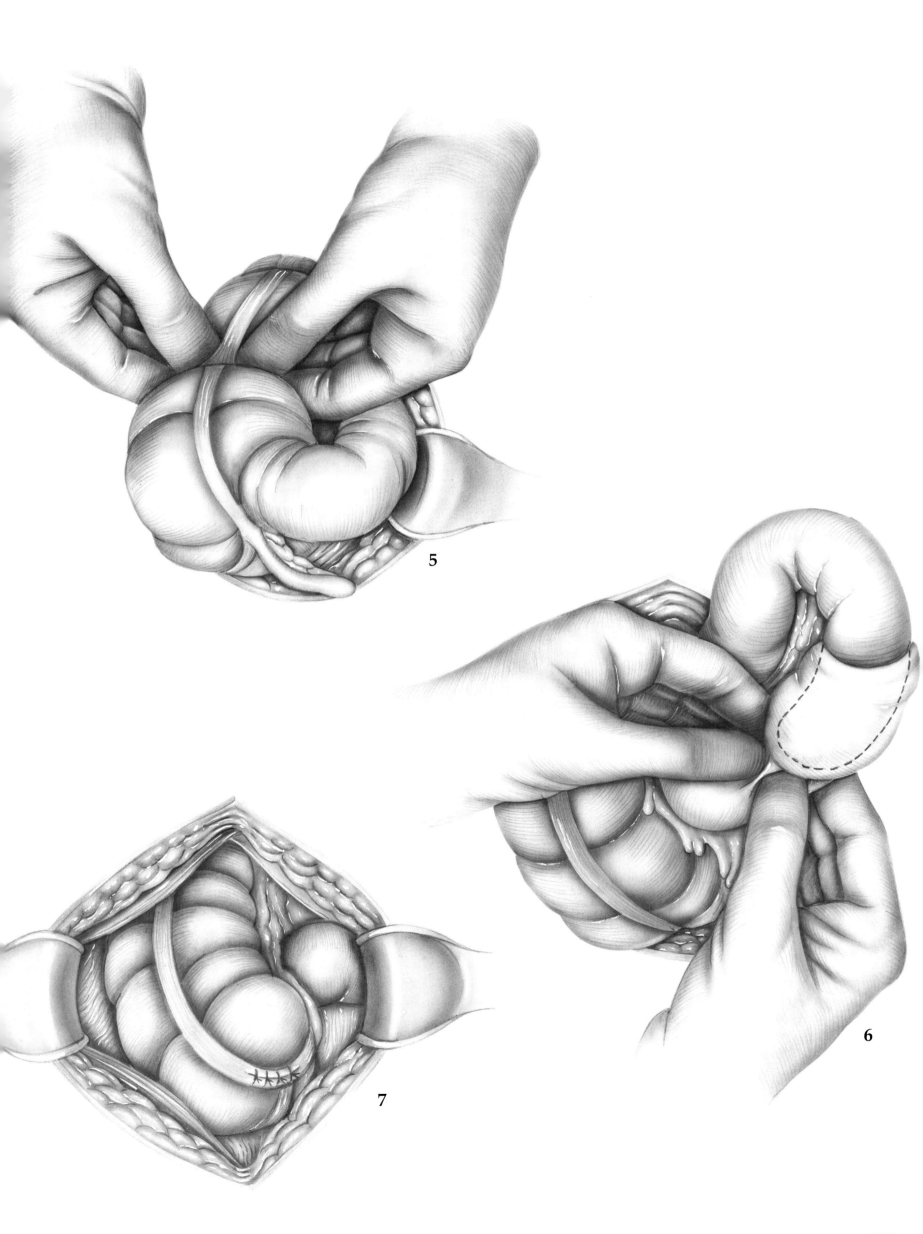

5

6

7

Loop Colostomy in an Infant

1 A right upper abdominal transverse incision is made over the rectus muscle.

2 The anterior rectus sheath is opened vertically.

3 The rectus muscle is split vertically in its middle.

4 The peritoneum is opened transversely.

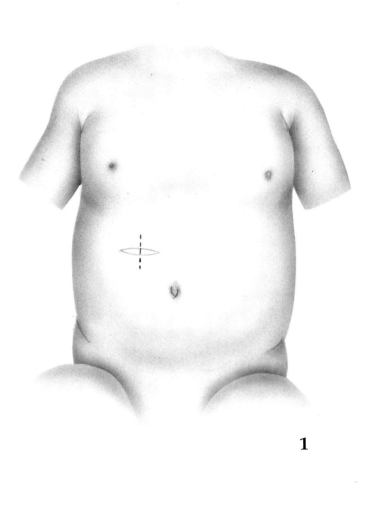

1

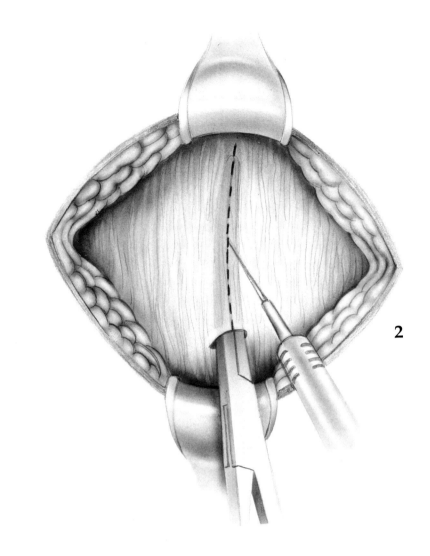

2

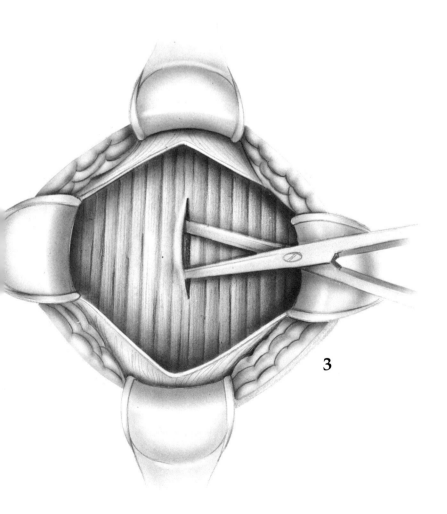

3

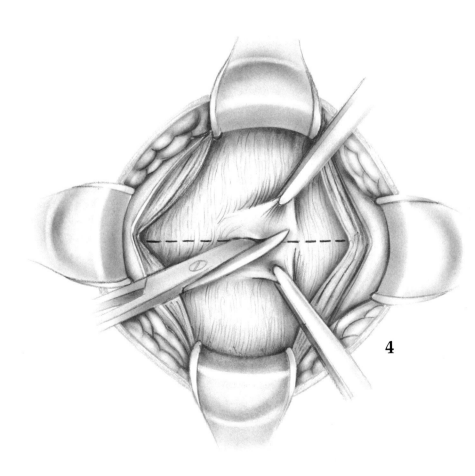

4

Loop Colostomy in an Infant (*cont.*)

5 The right transverse colon, to the right of the middle colic artery, is brought up into the wound after freeing the omentum over the portion of the colon to be used for the colostomy. A plastic or glass rod is inserted through the mesentery in an avascular area between the arterial arcades and the wall of the colon. The two limbs of the colon are approximated to each other and to the peritoneum with two U-shaped stitches, one placed superiorly and one inferiorly.

6 The colon is sutured to the peritoneum circumferentially with interrupted 5-0 silk sutures.

7 The fascia is similarly sutured to the bowel with interrupted 5-0 silk sutures.

8 The colon is opened longitudinally, with the electrocautery, through the antimesenteric taenia.

9 The colostomy is matured by suturing the full thickness of the end of the colon to the skin circumferentially with interrupted #000 or #0000 polyglycolic acid sutures.

10 The finished matured colostomy is seen with separated proximal and distal ostomies.

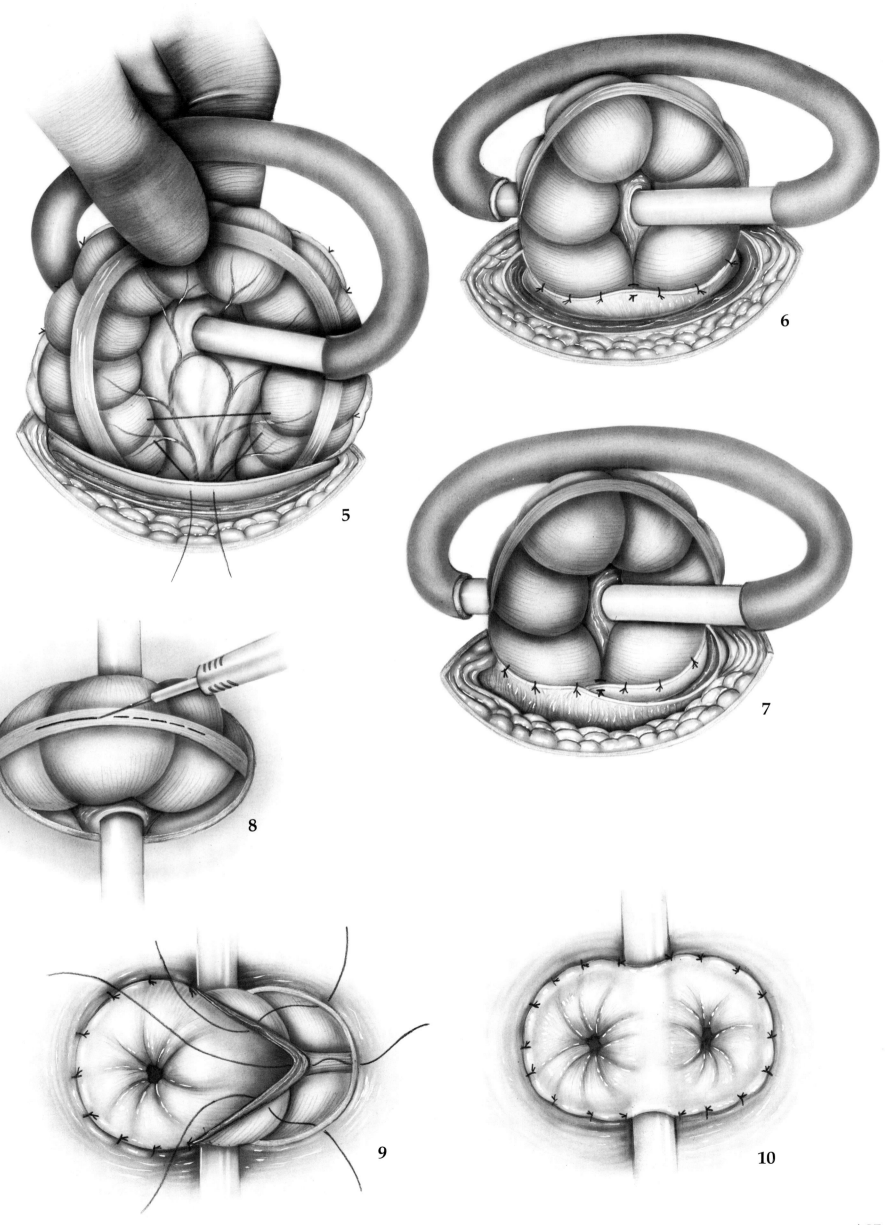

5

6

7

8

9

10

Endorectal Pull-Through for Ulcerative Colitis or Familial Polyposis

This operation is based on the same principles as that for endorectal pull-through for Hirschsprung's disease (see **Plates 239–241**), but has been modified in several ways. Although the entire operation can be performed at one time, it is usually done in two or three stages. In patients with familial polyposis, and in those with ulcerative colitis who are in good condition, we usually perform the colectomy, create the pouch, and do the pull-through at the initial operation, creating a diverting loop ileostomy at the same time. The ileostomy is closed at a later date as the second stage. However, in patients with ulcerative colitis who are in poor condition we perform a subtotal colectomy, ileostomy, and mucous fistula at the first operation; complete the resection, create the pouch, and do the pull-through at the second operation; and close the loop ileostomy at the third. The operation is depicted as it would be performed for a patient with familial polyposis.

1 The endoanal resection is performed before opening the abdomen. The patient is positioned as for the procedure done in Hirschsprung's disease. The dissection of the rectal mucosa is begun right at the dentate line, removing all rectal mucosa so as to leave no polyps or inflamed rectal mucosa. The dissection can be aided by injecting procaine solution (0.5%), with or without epinephrine, in the submucosal plane.

2 The posterior incision is then begun first so as not to have blood running over the incision, as would be the case if one started the dissection anteriorly. It is essential to establish the correct plane initially, as the tendency is to dissect too deeply and go through, or into, the smooth muscle.

3 As the mucosal tube is developed traction sutures of 4- or 5-0 silk are placed serially so that traction can be placed on the mucosal tube without tearing it.

4 The dissection is carried on by sharp and blunt dissection, also using the needle-point electrocautery to fulgurate blood vessels entering the mucosa. The circular muscle of the rectum should be visualized to ascertain that one is in the correct plane. This dissection is carried up at least 5 to 6 cm. The area is then packed with packing soaked in povidone-iodine solution, and the patient taken out of the lithotomy position.

5 The abdomen is opened and a total abdominal colectomy is performed in standard fashion.

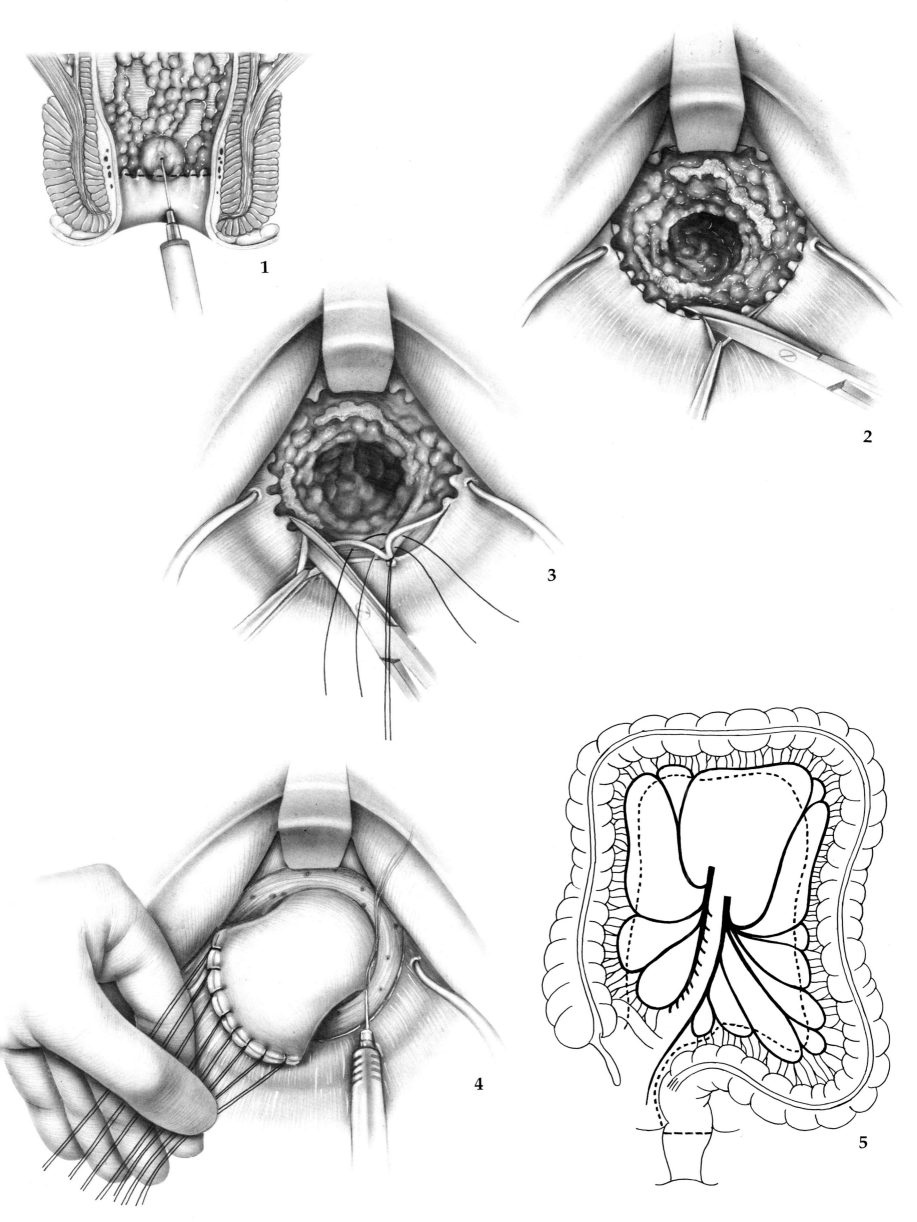

Endorectal Pull-Through for Ulcerative Colitis or Familial Polyposis (*cont.*)

6 As the colon dissection is carried down below the peritoneal reflection, it is kept right on the rectum. The rectum is dissected down to approximately 3 to 4 cm above the levator insertion.

7 At a point 3 to 4 cm above the insertion of the levators, the rectum is transected. At this point one should be at the proximal end of the previous transanal mucosal dissection.

8 This permits the entire colon and rectal mucosa to be excised *en bloc.*

9 The patient is then repositioned for a combined abdominal and perineal procedure, and the ileum and its mesentery are completely mobilized so as to permit the end of the ileum to be brought down, without tension, through the rectal muscular sleeve to the area of the dentate line.

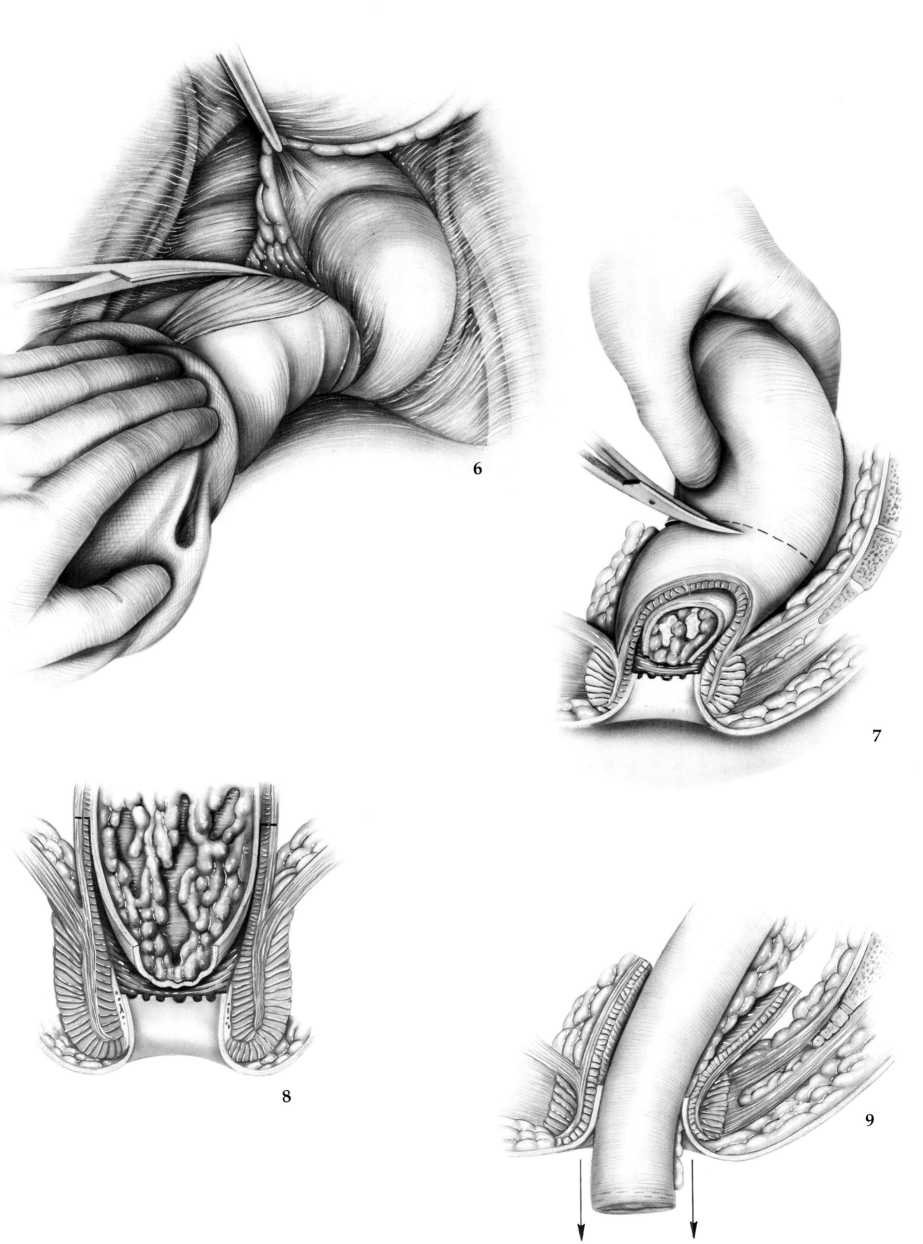

6

7

8

9

Endorectal Pull-Through for Ulcerative Colitis or Familial Polyposis (*cont.*)

10–13 One of the various types of pouches can then be created. We employ a side-to-side anastomosis of the ileum as seen in **Fig. 12**. This provides less mesentery and bowel to pull through the muscular sleeve than does the "J" pouch (**Fig. 11**), is simple to perform, and allows bringing the most mobile portion of the ileum down to the anus. This pouch is a modification of the "J" pouch in which the ileum has merely been transected and the antiperistaltic arm moves superiorly 2 to 4 cm before a side-to-side anastomosis is done. It is important, regardless of the type of pouch used, that the length of the spout going to the anal anastomosis not exceed 2 to 4 cm.

14 The ileum is then pulled through the muscular cuff. An end-to-end anastomosis of all layers of ileum and the anal mucosa is performed, after first placing four to six sutures between the seromuscular layers of the ileum and the circular muscle of the rectum. A drain is placed posteriorly, as in the operation as performed for Hirschsprung's disease.

15 Upon completion of the operation, the pouch is seen to lie in the upper end of the muscular cuff. The abdomen is then closed after first creating a loop ileostomy above the pouch. The ileostomy will be closed as the second stage of the operation.

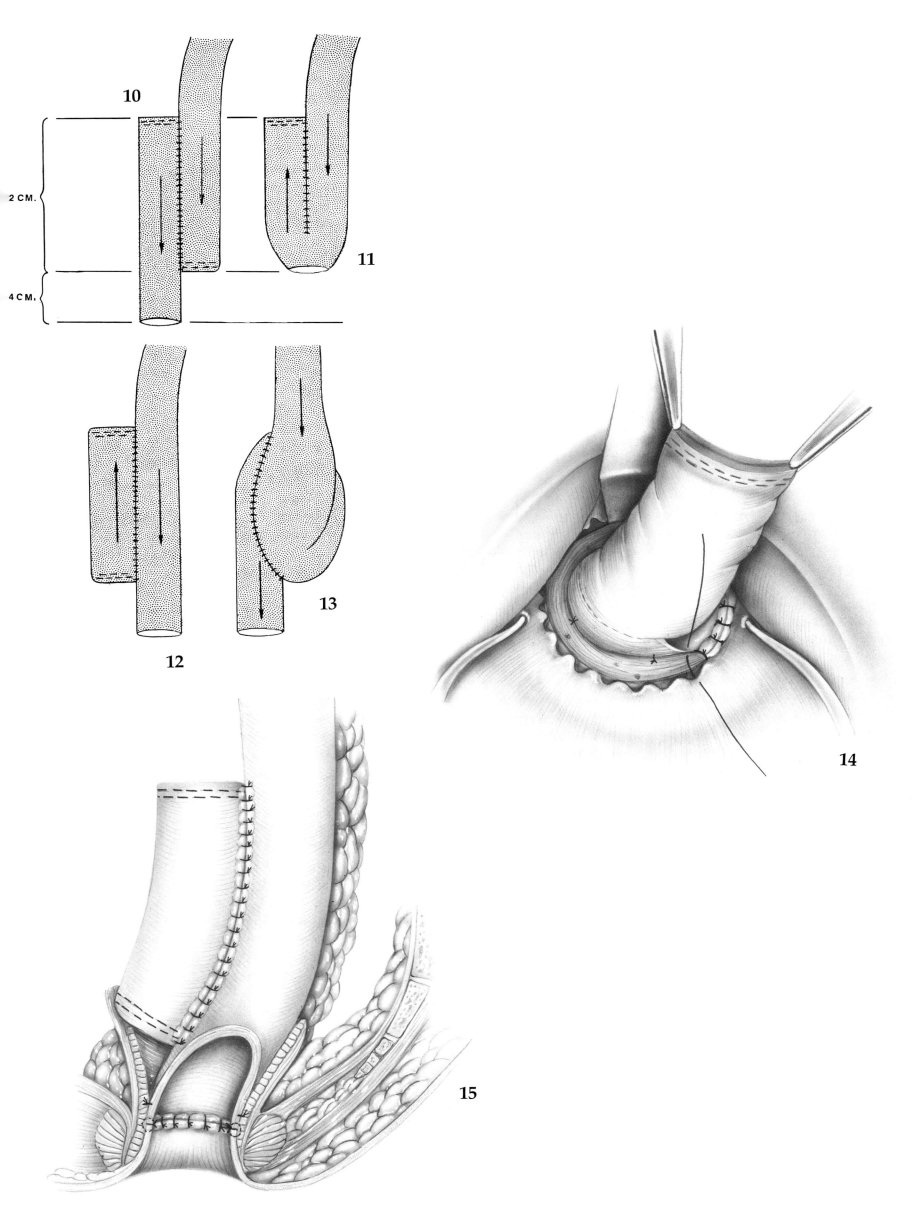

10

2 CM.

4 CM.

11

12

13

14

15

Endorectal Pull-Through for Total Aganglionosis of the Colon

1 The operation is optimally performed when the child is 6 to 12 months old. Hence, most children will already have an end ileostomy at the distal end of the normal ganglionic small intestine. A long midline or left paramedian incision is made, extending from the pubis to the upper abdomen. The ileostomy is taken down and oversewn in a standard manner. Preparatory to resection, the left colon is devascularized from the left of the middle colic artery to just above the peritoneal reflection, and the transverse colon is divided between rows of staples. The mesocolon and the vessels of the sigmoid are carefully divided close to the intestine, to preserve the communicating arcades and the blood supply to the rectum.

    The cecum and any aganglionic ileum are then carefully resected, preserving the ileocolic artery and its branches to the right colon. The ileum and mesentery of the small intestine are extensively mobilized so that there is adequate length to bring the end of the ileum to the anus without tension.

2 The remaining 15 to 20 cm of right and right-transverse colon are then opened along the antimesenteric border and anastomosed in the antiperistaltic position as an onlay graft to the distal ileum, beginning 4 to 6 cm from the end of the ileum. The caliber of the colon is usually similar to that of the ileum, since it has been decompressed by the proximal diverting ileostomy. The ends of the colon are beveled, leaving a greater mesenteric than antimesenteric length.

3–4 A two-layer anastomosis is performed using continuous #000 polyglycolic acid sutures for the inner layer and interrupted #0000 silk sutures for the outer layer.

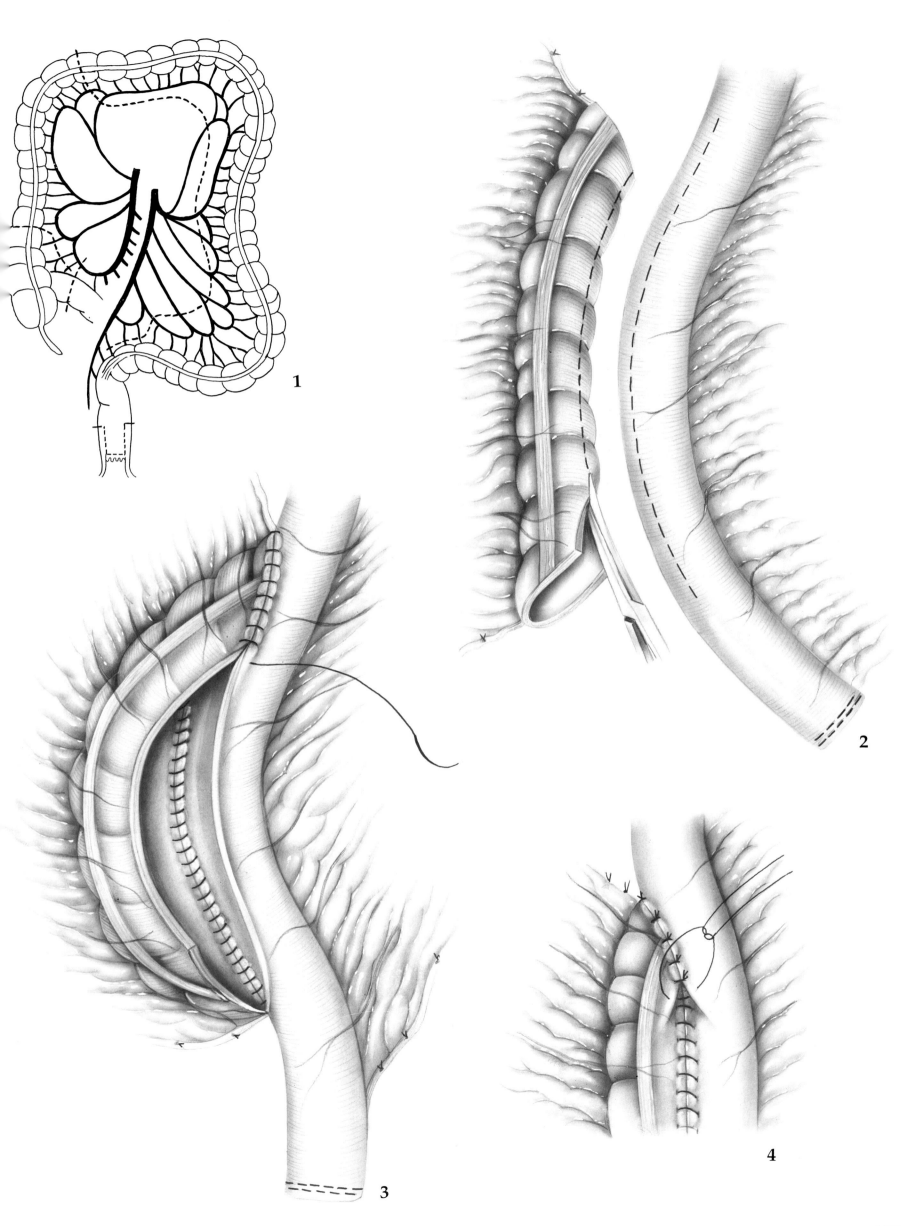

Endorectal Pull-Through for Total Aganglionosis of the Colon (*cont.*)

5 The dissection of the rectal mucosa is then performed as described below for the endorectal pull-through with primary anastomosis for Hirschsprung's disease (**Plate 240**). Approximately 6 cm of rectal muscular sleeve is left in place.

6 The child is then positioned for the perineal stage of the operation, and the mucosal dissection completed to 0.5 to 1.0 cm above the dentate line.

7 The ileum is pulled through the muscular cuff, and the upper end of the cuff trimmed, if necessary, so that the distal end of the side-to-side ileocolic anastomosis lies just within the upper end of the rectal muscular sleeve. A one-half-inch Penrose drain is placed between the ileum and the rectal muscular cuff and brought out through a stab wound posterior to the external sphincter muscle of the anus.

8 The full thickness of ileum is then anastomosed to the rectal mucosa with interrupted #000 polyglycolic acid sutures, as described below (**Plates 239–241**).

9 The patient is taken out of the lithotomy position and the abdominal phase of the operation is completed. The upper end of the rectal cuff is loosely approximated to the seromuscular layer of the ileum with four to six sutures of #0000 silk. A temporary loop ileostomy is created at a convenient point proximal to the coloileal anastomosis, using the abdominal site of the previous ileostomy. The new ileostomy can be closed in 3 to 4 weeks.

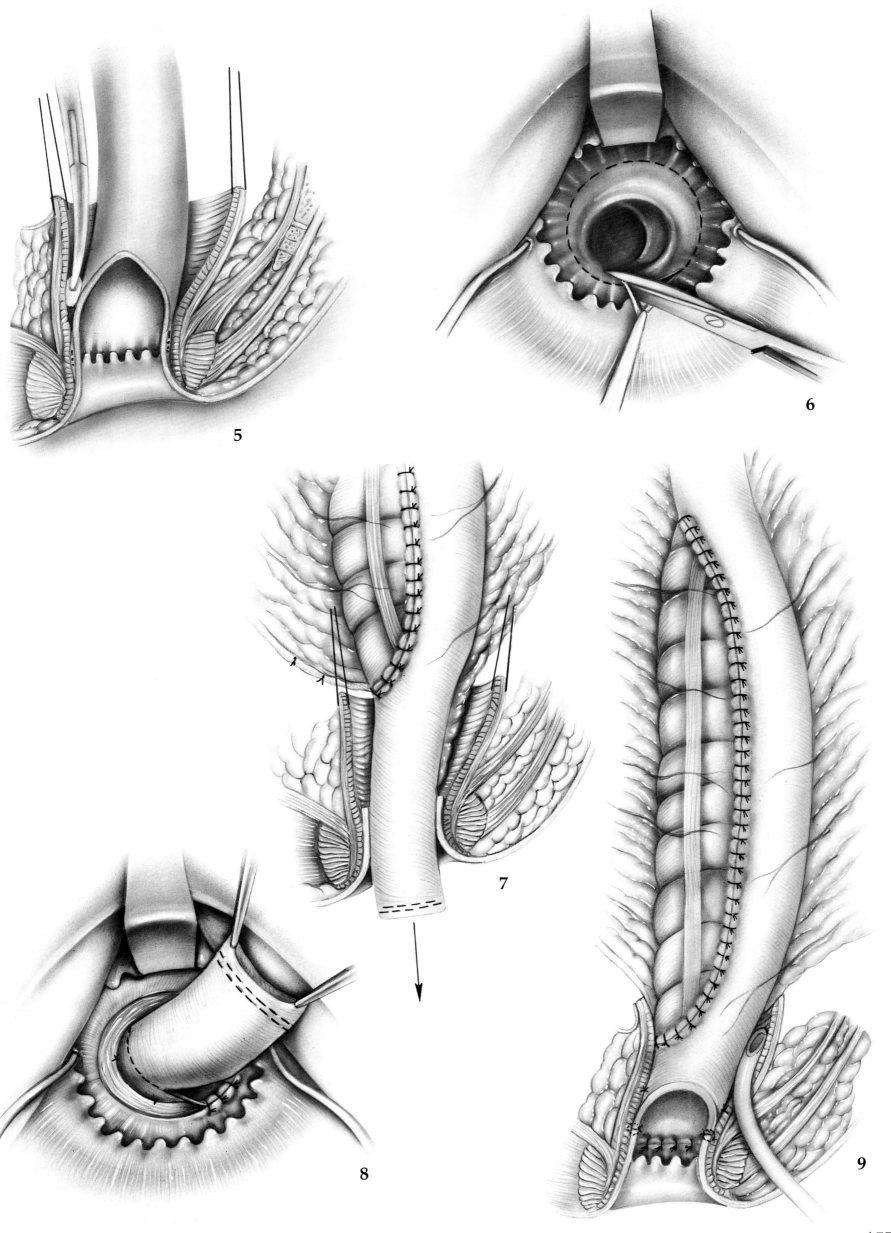

Endorectal Pull-Through with Primary Anastomosis for Hirschsprung's Disease

1 The patient is prepared and draped from the nipples down to permit positioning for the perineal stage without the necessity of redraping. The abdominal stage is performed with the pelvis dorsiflexed at least 30°. A long left paramedian incision is made, including the sigmoid colonic stoma if one is present.

2 If a sigmoid colostomy is present all of the colon from the colostomy to just above the peritoneal reflection is resected. In the absence of a sigmoid colostomy the extent of the aganglionic intestine must be established by serial biopsies and frozen section examination, and all the involved colon above the rectum excised. The mesocolon and the vessels of the intestines to be resected are divided close to the bowel wall, with care taken to preserve the communicating arcades and the blood supply to the rectum. The distal portion of the resection is the site at which dissection of the rectal mucosa is begun, just above the peritoneal reflection, in an easily accessible portion of the colon.

3 A long longitudinal incision is made through a taenia of the rectosigmoid just above the peritoneal reflection. The mucosal tube is freed from the outer muscular layers by blunt dissection with gauze pushers.

4 When the mucosal tube has been completely dissected, the muscular sleeve of the rectum is transected and traction sutures are placed on the proximal edge of the distal segment.

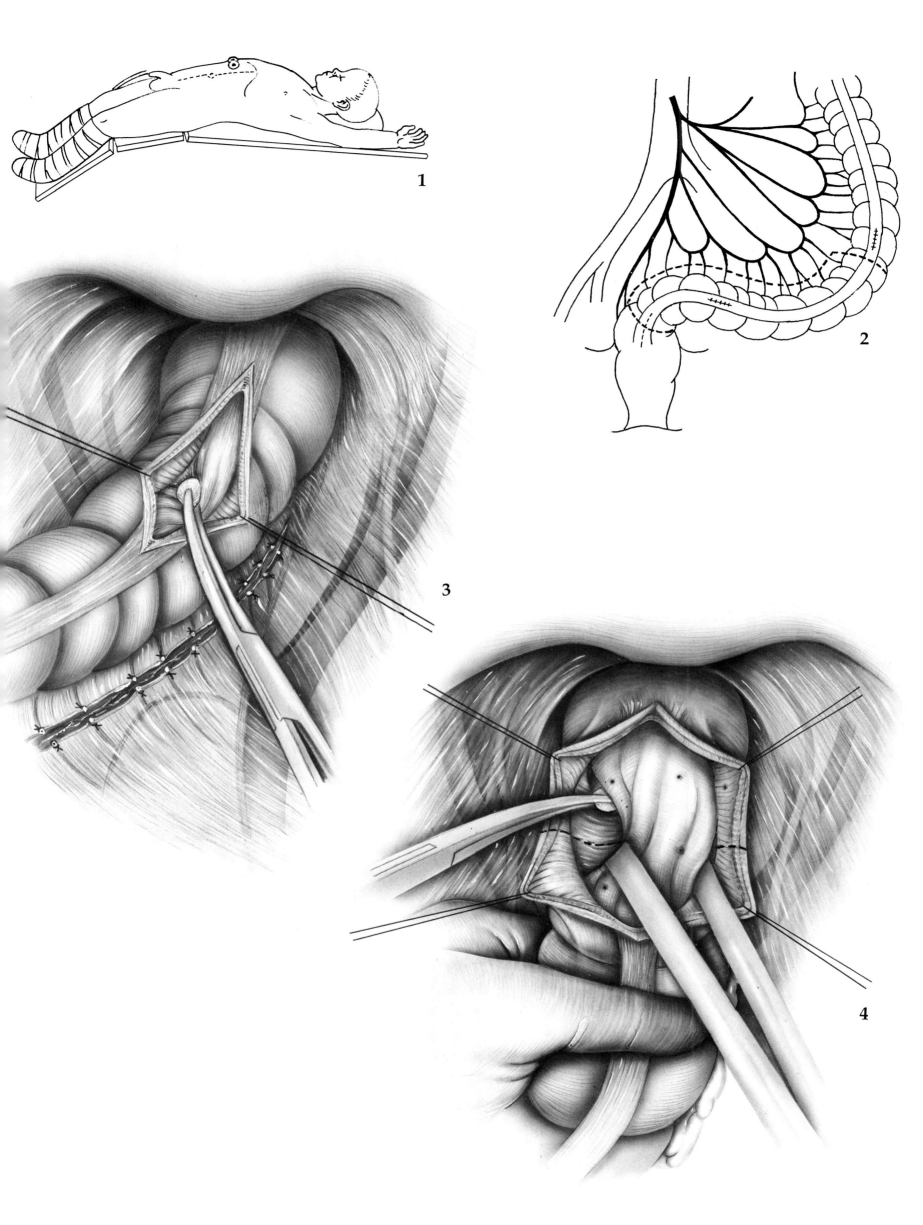

Endorectal Pull-Through with Primary Anastomosis for Hirschsprung's Disease (*cont.*)

5–6 Distal dissection of the mucosal tube is performed in a similar manner, using gauze pushers. If the colon has never been hypertrophied, the mucosa can be easily stripped down to the anus, with few if any significant blood vessels being encountered. However, if the colon has been hypertrophied, the dissection may be more difficult; numerous vessels going from the muscular coat to the mucosa must be fulgurated and transected.

7 The depth of the dissection may be checked by inserting a finger into the anus, a maneuver which also facilitates the lower dissection. The distal end of the dissection should be down to within 1 to 2 cm of the dentate line. The site of anastomosis on the normal proximal bowel is selected and prepared, and the colon is mobilized to obtain adequate length to allow this site to reach below the perineum without tension.

8 When the colon has been adequately mobilized, the child is positioned for the perineal phase of the operation. The anus is dilated and retracted with an atraumatic anal retractor.

9 Procaine solution (0.5%) is injected submucosally, just above the dentate line, to separate the layers.

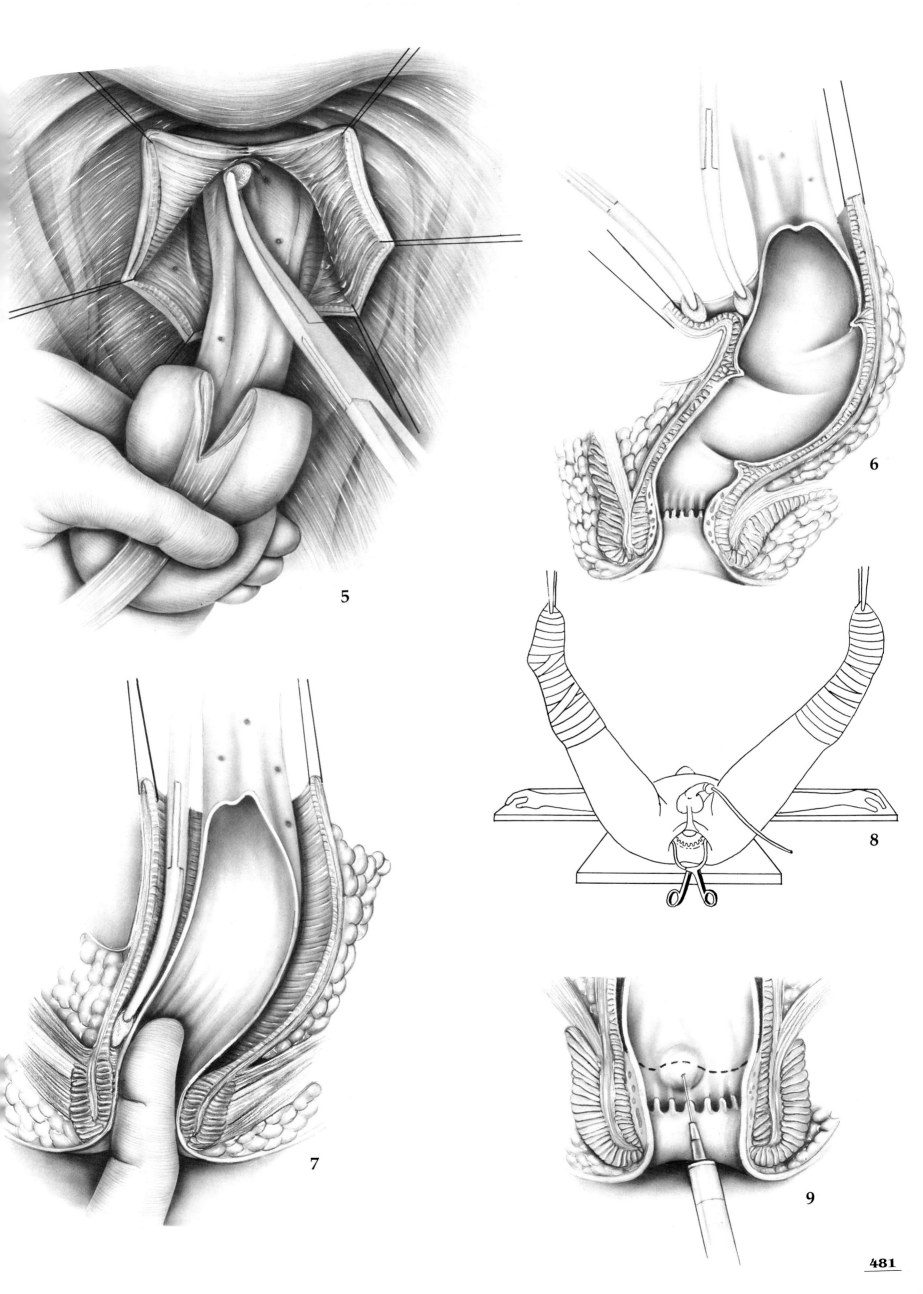

5

6

7

8

9

Endorectal Pull-Through with Primary Anastomosis for Hirschsprung's Disease (*cont.*)

10 A circumferential incision is made 1 cm proximal to the dentate line and the submucosal plane developed carefully, for the tendency is to go too deep at this point.

11 The mucosal stripping is then completed from below, joining the transanal and proximal dissections. The muscular cuff is irrigated freely with povidone-iodine solution, and hemostasis established. A one-half-inch Penrose drain is then placed into the rectal muscular cuff through a vertical stab wound posterior to the external sphincter of the anus. The drain enters the muscular cuff above the sphincter muscle and does not interfere with the anastomosis. The proximal portion of the colon is then pulled through the rectal muscular sleeve and out through the anus.

12 The previously selected and prepared site for the anastomosis is positioned without tension. Four to six #0000 polyglycolic acid sutures are placed to secure the seromuscular layers of the intussuscepted colon to the rectal muscular cuff. These sutures are placed 1 to 2 cm above the edge of the anal mucosa. The colon is transected by quadrants, and an anastomosis performed with interrupted #000 polyglycolic acid sutures placed between the anal mucosa, 0.5 to 1.0 cm from the dentate line, and all layers of the colon.

13 The legs are lowered and the abdominal phase completed by loosely approximating the proximal edge of the muscular cuff to the seromuscular layer of the colon with four to six sutures of #0000 polyglycolic acid. Any mesenteric defects are repaired, and the abdomen is closed without drainage.

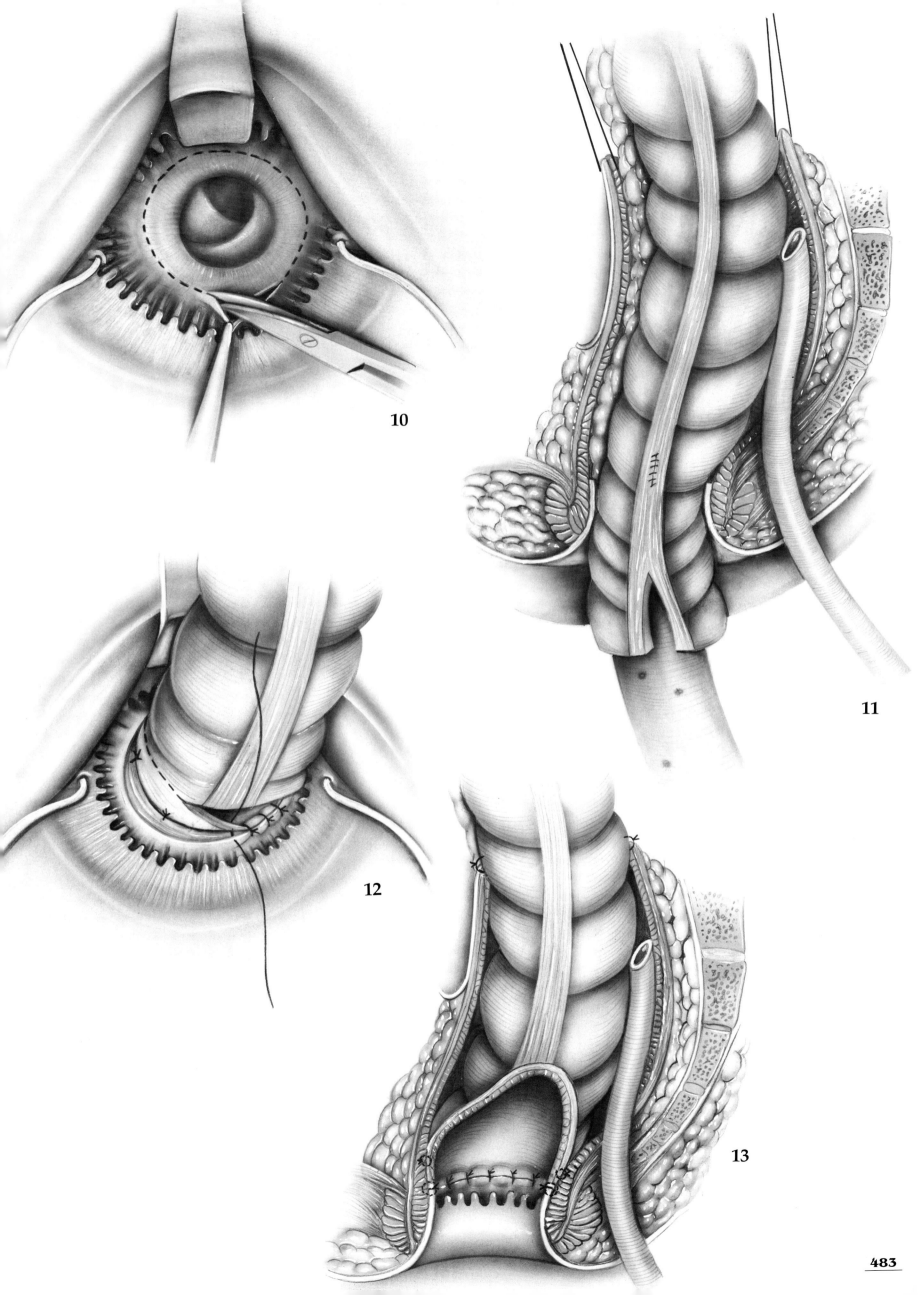

10

11

12

13

Vascular Surgical Techniques

ARTERIAL DISSECTION

1 The periadventitial tissue is grasped with forceps and incised with scissors. This may be done in several layers.

2 The artery is then freed from its surrounding areolar tissue layers using a combination of blunt and sharp dissection. Care is taken to avoid injury to all arterial branches.

3 Small crossing veins traverse some of these periadventitial layers. These are isolated, doubly ligated, and divided, as shown.

ARTERIAL INCISION

4 An arterial segment is isolated between clamps in such a way that its lumen is filled with blood. A knife is then used to make the arteriotomy. Care is taken to keep the knife-cut directly perpendicular to the lumen of the artery, so that the incision in the artery is straight and not skewed or tangential. The point of the knife is used to cut the artery, using light pressure and multiple strokes.

5 If the arterial wall is thickened with disease, a mosquito clamp is inserted into the artery to define the lumen, and the straight cut, which is perpendicular to the wall, is continued between the blades of the clamp as shown. If a scissors is used with a diseased thick-walled artery such as the one shown, then jagged, skewed openings in the artery and its various diseased layers may occur and anastomosis be rendered more difficult. The ends of the arteriotomy should be fashioned at approximately 45° angles so that there is no undermining of the media or the adventitia and so that the intimal layer can be clearly visualized for placement of stitches.

6 If the arterial wall is relatively normal, a small Pott's scissors or microscissors can be used to complete the arteriotomy.

SUTURE CLOSURE OF ARTERIOTOMY

7 Both limbs of a double-armed atraumatic monofilament suture are placed from within outward at each end of the arteriotomy and then tied. One arm of one suture is then run to the center of the incision. It should be noted that in performing the arteriotomy and suture closure, no excision of intima or endarterectomy is performed and all layers are cut evenly.

8 The suture originating at the other end of the arteriotomy is also run to the center of the incision, where it is tied to the first suture.

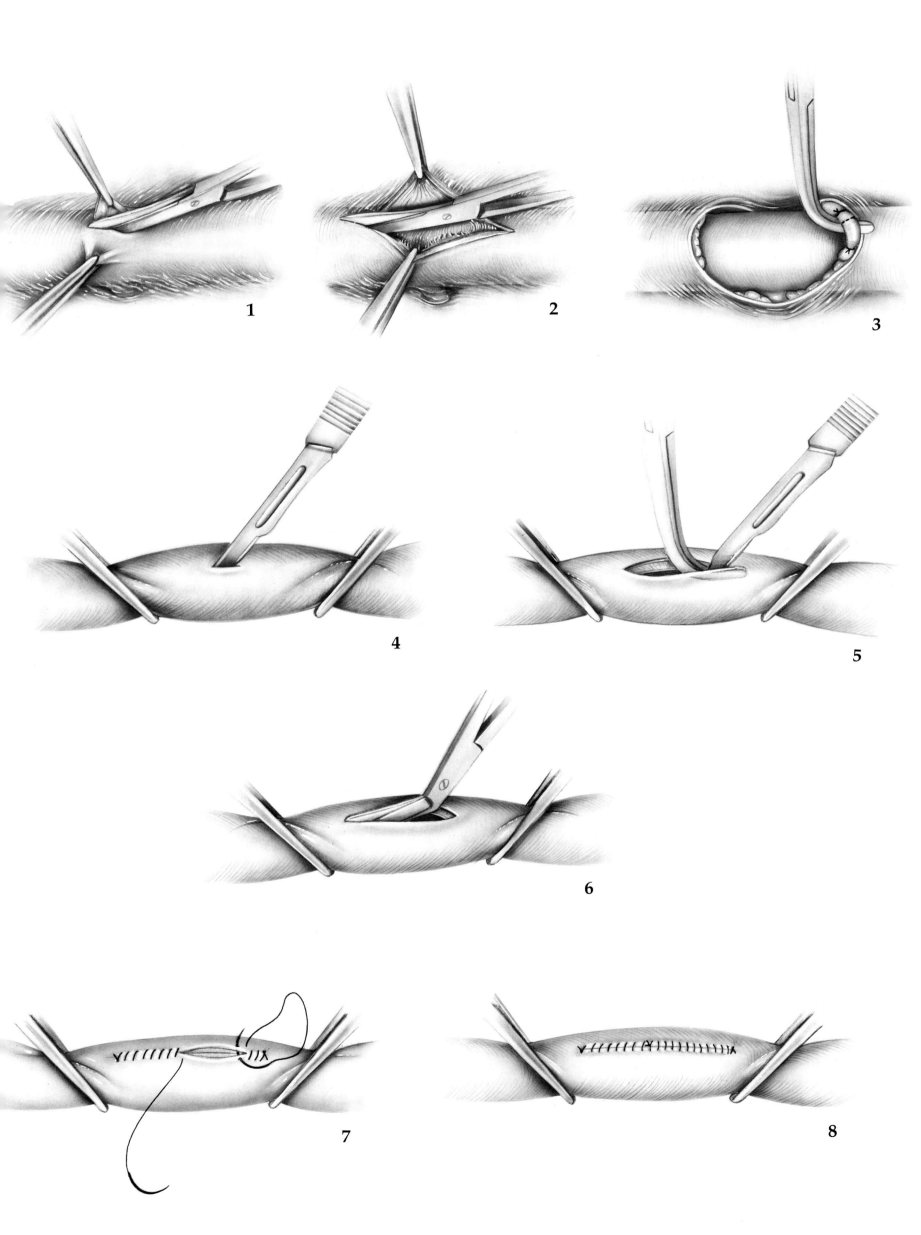

End-to-End Vascular Anastomosis

1 End-to-end anastomosis of arteries is accomplished by approximating the ends of the two arteries with occluding atraumatic clamps. A double-armed atraumatic monofilament suture is placed at either lateral side of the artery. Care is taken to include equal bites of all layers of the arterial wall in each passage of the needle. With good light and exposure, the three layers of the arterial wall can be clearly visualized.

2 The two corner stitches are tied.

3 One arm of the suture is then run along the anterior wall of the artery to the opposite corner and tied.

4 By rotating the vascular clamps and appropriately manipulating the corner sutures, the anastomosis is turned over, exposing the posterior wall. One of the sutures is then run to the opposite corner and tied to the free end of the opposite corner suture. Again, care is taken with each bite to include equal-sized portions of each layer of the arterial wall.

5 The completed anastomosis is shown.

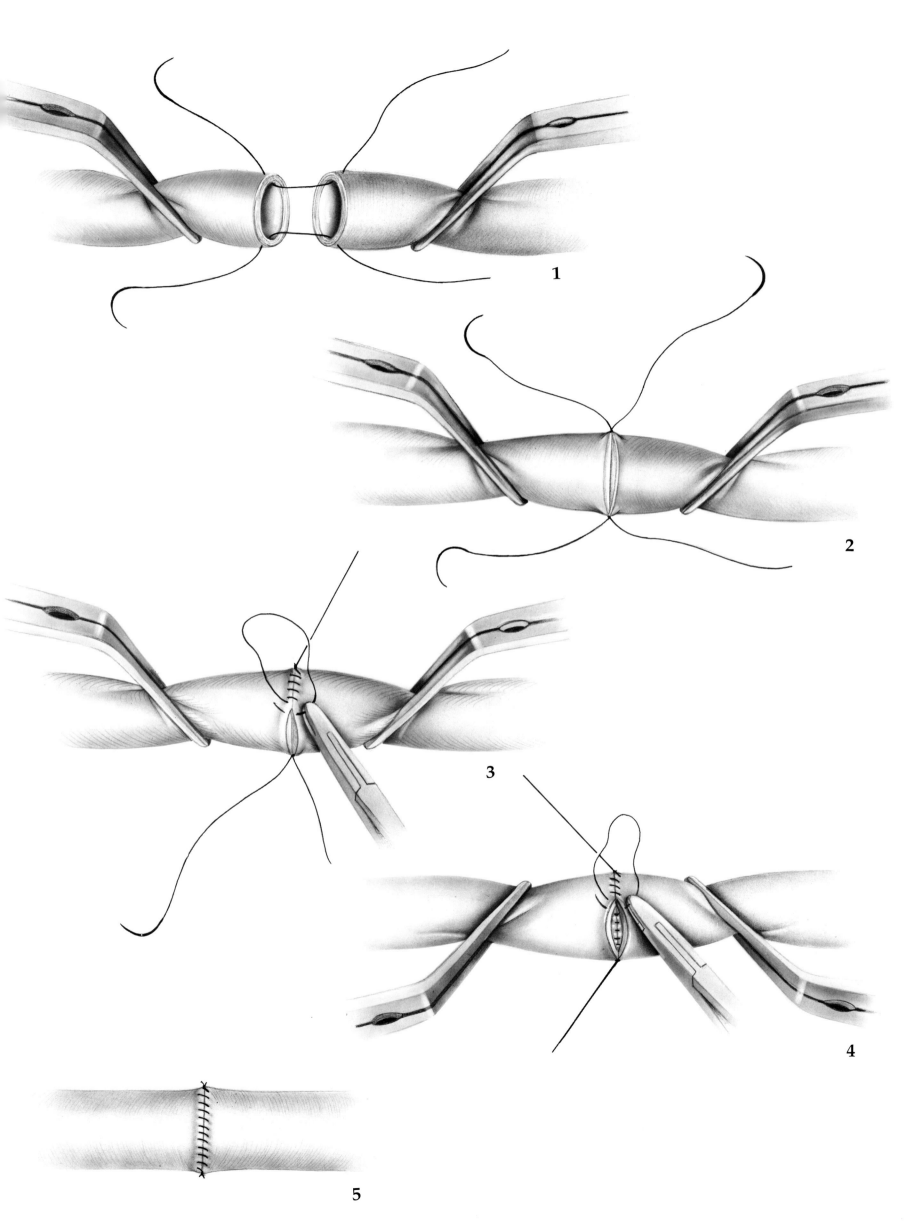

1

2

3

4

5

End-to-Side Vascular Anastomosis

1 Sutures are placed at the two ends of the planned anastomosis. Care is taken to place these stitches from within outward in each structure and to catch all layers of both the vein graft and the artery. The intimal layer is particularly important in this regard. Double-armed 6–0 polypropylene atraumatic sutures are used.

2 The apex suture is tied while the opposite-end suture is left untied.

3 One arm of the apex suture is run to the midportion of one side of the anastomosis. Small, even bites of all layers are taken with each stitch of the running suture.

4 The opposite limb of the suture is run along the opposite lateral margin of the anastomosis to its midportion.

5 The suture in the opposite end is tied and both arms of this suture are run to the midportions of the anastomosis, where they are tied to the suture from the opposite end. Good visualization of the inside and the outside of the artery must be obtained when each bite is taken so that the suture will catch and fix the intimal layer. In general the arterial wall should not be grasped with forceps but should be only pushed with the closed forceps to provide visualization. It is also important that the closed or open forceps be used to stabilize the artery as the needle is being passed through it. This can be accomplished without grasping the artery, simply by using the forceps as a pusher or foil.

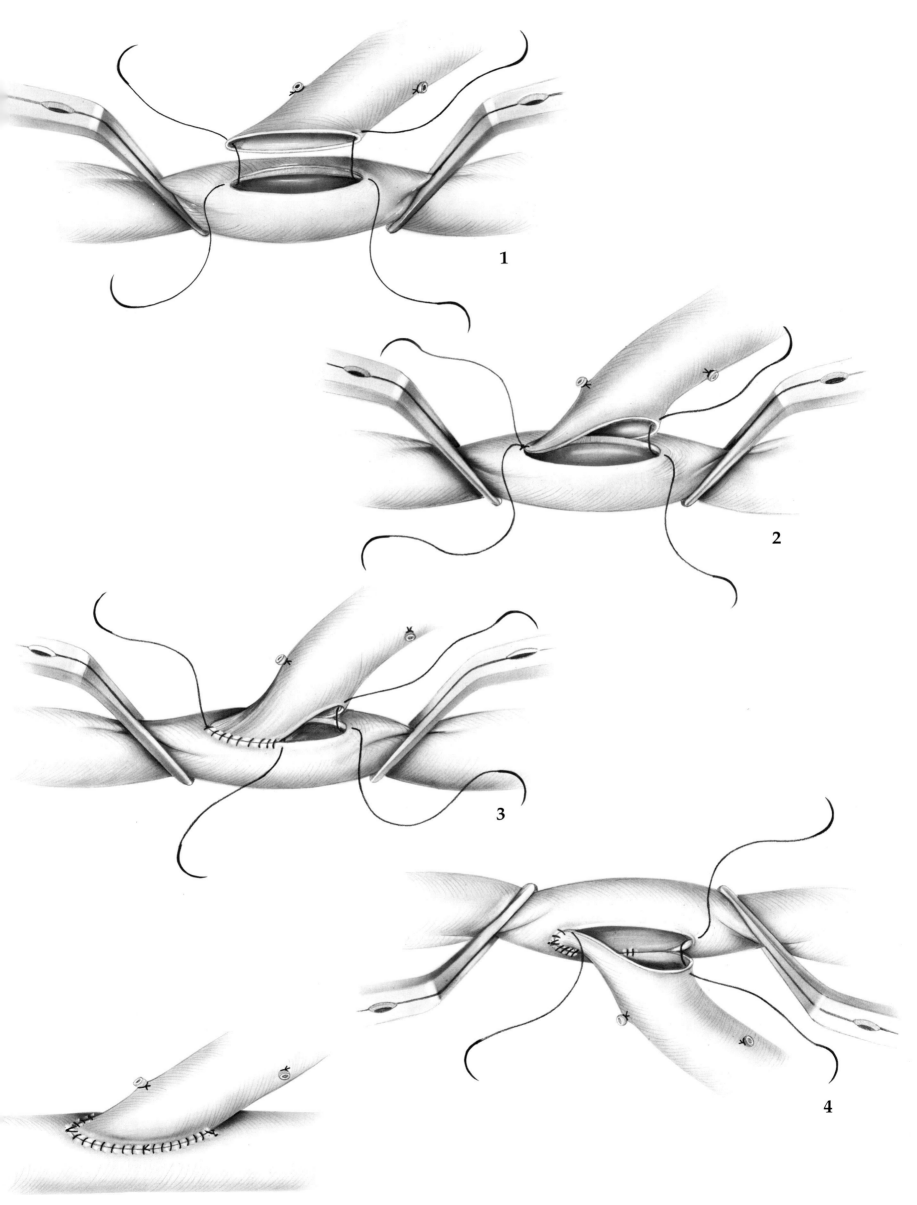

1

2

3

4

5

Repair of Lacerated Inferior Vena Cava—Repair of Lacerated Artery or Vein

REPAIR OF LACERATED INFERIOR VENA CAVA

1 A knife wound of the inferior vena cava is shown. This is controlled by emptying the segment of cava containing the laceration by sponge stick pressure proximally and distally. Finger pressure, or pressure with a tonsil sucker, is used to control bleeding from branches entering the injured venous segment. When this is done the vein may be dissected free proximally and distally and clamps applied, although this is often not necessary.

2 When the edges of the laceration can be clearly visualized and the adjacent wall of the vein is dissected from surrounding tissue, the edges of the laceration are grasped with a forceps and a Satinsky clamp is placed to isolate the laceration.

3 The laceration is then closed with a running 4–0 or 5–0 vascular polypropylene suture in a dry field precisely approximating the edges. If the laceration is through and through the inferior vena cava, the far wall must also be repaired. This can be accomplished after the inferior vena cava is emptied of blood by approximating the laceration in the far wall from within the vena cava through the laceration in the near wall. To accomplish this, one must absolutely get a dry field; it may be necessary to isolate the vessel proximal and distal to the injury and apply vascular clamps. It may also be necessary to isolate and ligate branches that drain into that segment. The temptation to grasp the bleeding vena cava in a pool of blood should be resisted, particularly before the vessel is cleanly dissected. Pressure control and emptying of the injured vein should be the theme of technical management.

REPAIR OF LACERATED ARTERY OR VEIN

Types of Vascular Injury and Methods of Repair

4 A small puncture wound or minor laceration of an artery is shown. This is frequently the type of injury encountered from an arteriographic procedure. The injury is controlled by finger pressure until the artery is controlled by the application of clamps and the injury repaired.

5 Simple interrupted sutures through all layers of the arterial wall, or the adventitia and media, are adequate to control the injury and maintain patency of the artery.

6 A more extensive and somewhat jagged, although clean, laceration is shown. This can result from a knife wound or injury with a similar sharp object. Bleeding is controlled by pressure until the artery remote from the injury is isolated and controlled with clamps. All branches entering into the intervening segment also must be isolated and controlled.

7 If the laceration is clean and there is no contusion of the adjacent edges of the laceration, it may be repaired by a simple running suture. Sutures are placed from within outward at both ends of the laceration and then run to the center, where they are tied.

8 A contused arterial wound is shown. An injury such as this can be produced by a bullet wound or other blunt trauma. In the injury depicted there is loss of arterial wall substance, and tissue adjacent to the defect is damaged. All injured artery wall must be excised by cutting the artery along the lines shown.

9 This leaves inadequate length of artery to approximate without tension.

10 Accordingly, a prosthetic graft or autologous vein graft must be used. This can be inserted as an interposition graft, as shown.

11 Alternatively, if exposure is impaired or there is excessive surrounding tissue damage or contamination, the debrided arterial ends are ligated and a remote bypass graft is carried out to restore arterial continuity.

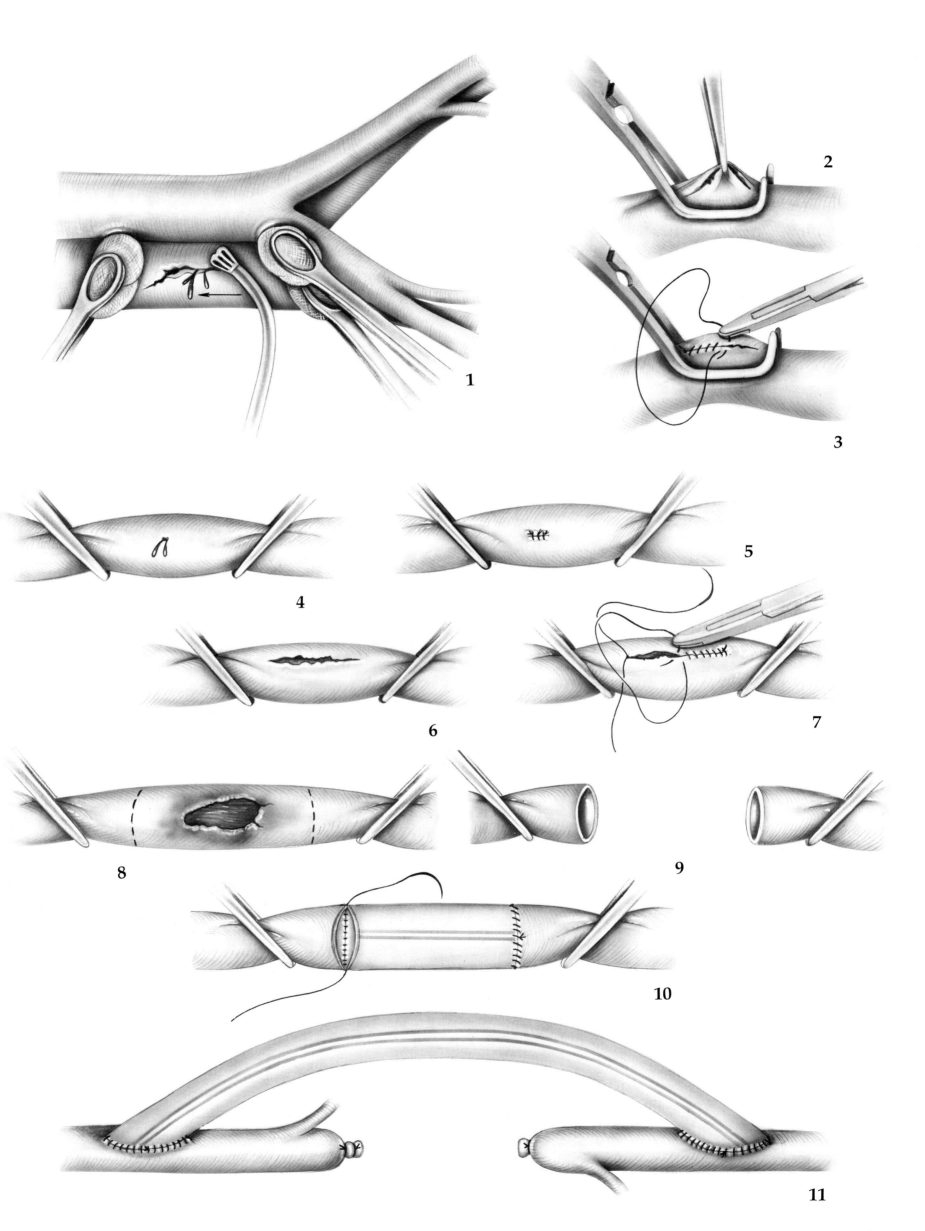

Repair of Lacerated Femoral Artery

1 If the injury is thought to be complex, proximal control of the iliac artery through a suprainguinal retroperitoneal incision is advisable. While this is rapidly being accomplished, bleeding from the femoral artery laceration is controlled with finger pressure.

2 Even with occlusion of the external iliac artery, bleeding from the groin will be brisk due to the multiple branches of the deep femoral artery. However, finger pressure can control this bleeding while the superficial femoral artery is dissected and clamped.

3 It is sometimes necessary to get clamp control of the deep femoral artery as well, so that accurate approximation of the lacerated femoral artery can be accomplished. Occasionally, if only one or two sutures are required, digital or sucker pressure will control bleeding from the deep femoral artery so that the sutures can be accurately placed. More-complex injuries require clamp control of all branches. In some instances of false aneurysm due to injury at the time of arteriography, the false aneurysm can simply be entered with a vertical incision in the groin and bleeding from the anterior wall of the femoral artery controlled with digital pressure. The artery can then be dissected proximally in the groin, and suture control of the bleeding point can be obtained. If the patient is obese or a complex injury is suspected, proximal control via the external iliac is advisable.

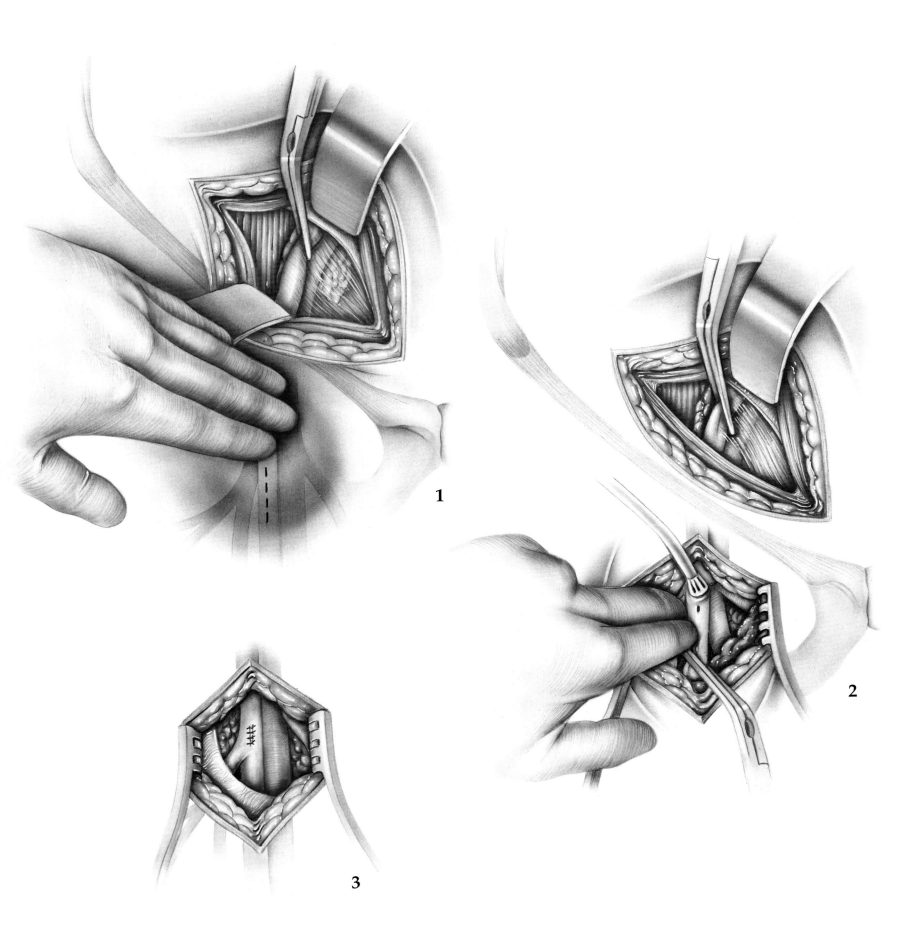

1

2

3

Inferior Vena Cava Plication

1 A retroperitoneal incision in the right flank is made at about the level of the umbilicus, or midway between the costal margin and the iliac crest. Care is taken to extend this incision across the lateral one-half to one-third of the rectus sheaths to provide better medial exposure.

2 The three oblique abdominal muscles are cut in the direction of the skin incision and the anterior and posterior rectus sheath is also incised. Rarely is it necessary to divide the rectus muscle.

3 After dividing the transversalis fascia, it is possible to enter the retroperitoneal plane and strip the peritoneum from the deeper layers of the abdominal wall. This is first accomplished superiorly, and then inferiorly.

4 Finally, the peritoneum is swept away from the posterior parietes. In the course of this the psoas muscle is visualized and serves as an important landmark.

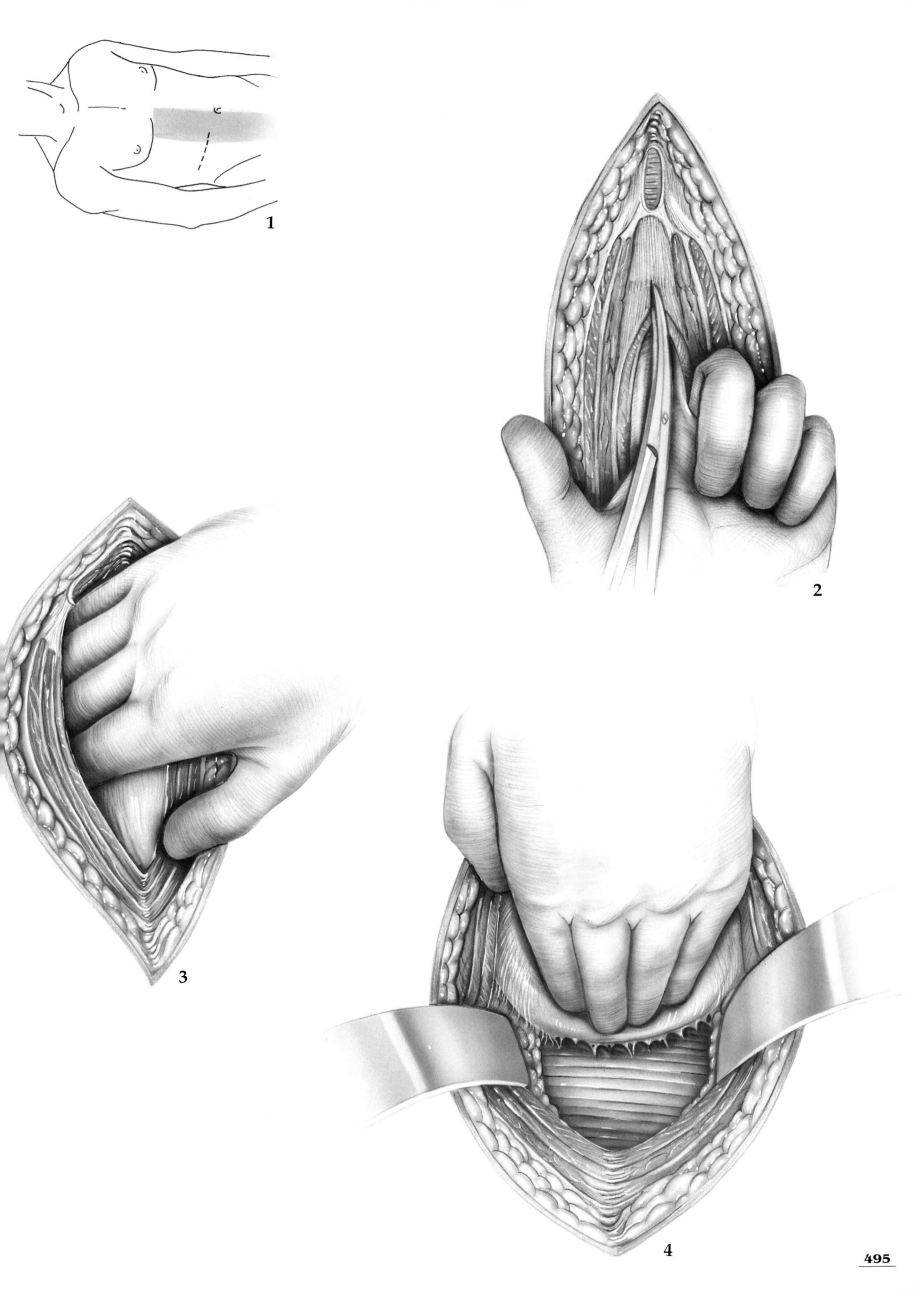

1

2

3

4

Inferior Vena Cava Plication (*cont.*)

5 By using three mechanical retractors, which are fixed to the operating table, and fitting them with appropriate one- or two-inch Deaver retractors, the retroperitoneal fatty tissue and edges of the incision can be retracted superiorly and inferiorly. The peritoneal cavity and its contents, along with the ureter, can be retracted strongly in a medial direction.

  The fatty areolar tissue overlying the inferior vena cava is then incised and dissection continued in the periadventitial plane of the inferior vena cava.

6 By pushing the inferior vena cava gently to the patient's left and putting tension on the surrounding fatty areolar tissue, the right-side lumbar veins can be visualized and protected from injury.

7 By gently holding the inferior vena cava to the patient's right, using the fingers of the surgeon's left hand, and tensioning the fatty areolar tissue to the patient's left, it is possible to visualize the left-side lumbar veins and protect them from injury.

8 Once the position of the lumbar veins is known, it is possible to compress the vena cava in the lateral plane with an atraumatic vascular forceps. A large C clamp is placed behind the vena cava to grasp a red-rubber catheter, which has been cut appropriately for the purpose. Into the other end of this catheter the posterior half of the vena caval clip is inserted so that it can be drawn around the back of the cava.

9 The clip is then closed and tied, completing the operation. The retroperitoneum is allowed to collapse over the cava. The retractors are removed and the wound is closed in layers.

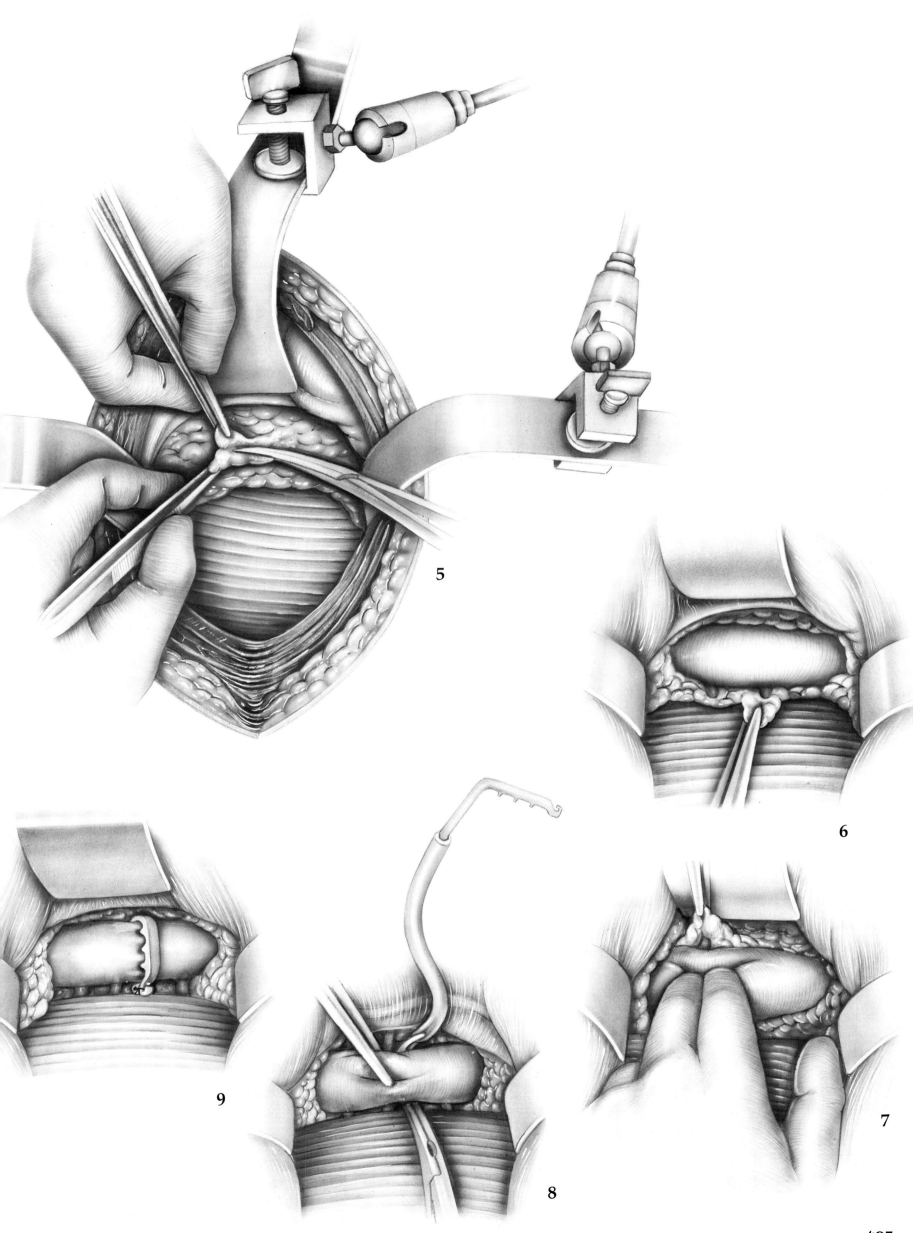

5

6

9

8

7

Saphenous Vein Ligation and Stripping

1 The anatomy of the varicose greater saphenous vein is shown, together with the three skin incisions that are typically required. The upper incision should start directly over the femoral pulse and extend medially in a diagonal fashion as shown. (All three incisions may be somewhat shorter than shown.) Additional incisions may be required if a perforator is suspected or the stripper does not pass a particular point. The position of the saphenous nerve adjacent to the vein is also shown in the ankle area. Great care must be taken to protect this from injury so as to avoid saphenous neuritis.

2 As the oblique incision in the groin is deepened in the fatty tissue, a large venous structure will be encountered. The position of the femoral artery should be carefully identified by palpating the femoral pulse; care should be taken to avoid injury to this vessel and the femoral vein. Once it has been confirmed that the first large venous structure encountered is in fact the greater saphenous vein, it can be divided between clamps as shown.

3 Both ends of the divided saphenous vein are separated and dissected free. Their branches are clamped and doubly ligated. The fossa ovalis is identified by the small arterial branch that defines its lower border. The junction of the saphenous vein with the common femoral vein is clearly identified, and the saphenous vein is clamped a few millimeters away from this junction. Without pulling firmly on the saphenous vein and tenting up the adjacent walls of the common femoral vein, the vein is ligated with #00 silk.

4 A second suture ligature is placed on the greater saphenous vein just beyond the first tie.

5 The two ligatures on the saphenous vein are shown in position, without any deformity being created in the common femoral vein.

6 A vertical incision is then made just anterior to the medial malleolus. The saphenous vein and saphenous nerve are identified and the nerve protected from injury. Branches in this area are ligated, and then the saphenous vein is divided between clamps. An opening is made in the proximal end of the distal saphenous vein so that the small end of the stripper can be inserted.

7 The remaining distal end of the saphenous vein is ligated and the stripper is tied in place. Traction is exerted in a cephalad direction.

8 As the stripper is being drawn toward the patient's head, a snug-fitting sterile elastic bandage is applied to the area from which the vein is being removed, thereby controlling avulsed tributaries. Positions of typical incisions in the leg are also shown.

9 Through these small incisions, previously marked clusters of varicosities can be removed. In the illustration, a twisting motion of a clamp avulses one such small cluster.

10 A slightly larger incision is made to remove a bigger cluster. Where possible, identifiable branches are ligated and the thin-walled varices are avulsed.

11 This shows the appearance of the veins as they are removed and the branches connecting with the deeper system are ligated.

12 This shows a larger incision, and division and ligation of a probable communicating branch. Through these incisions all major venous clusters are excised and avulsed.

13 A subcuticular absorbable suture is used to close all incisions. It provides the best cosmetic result.

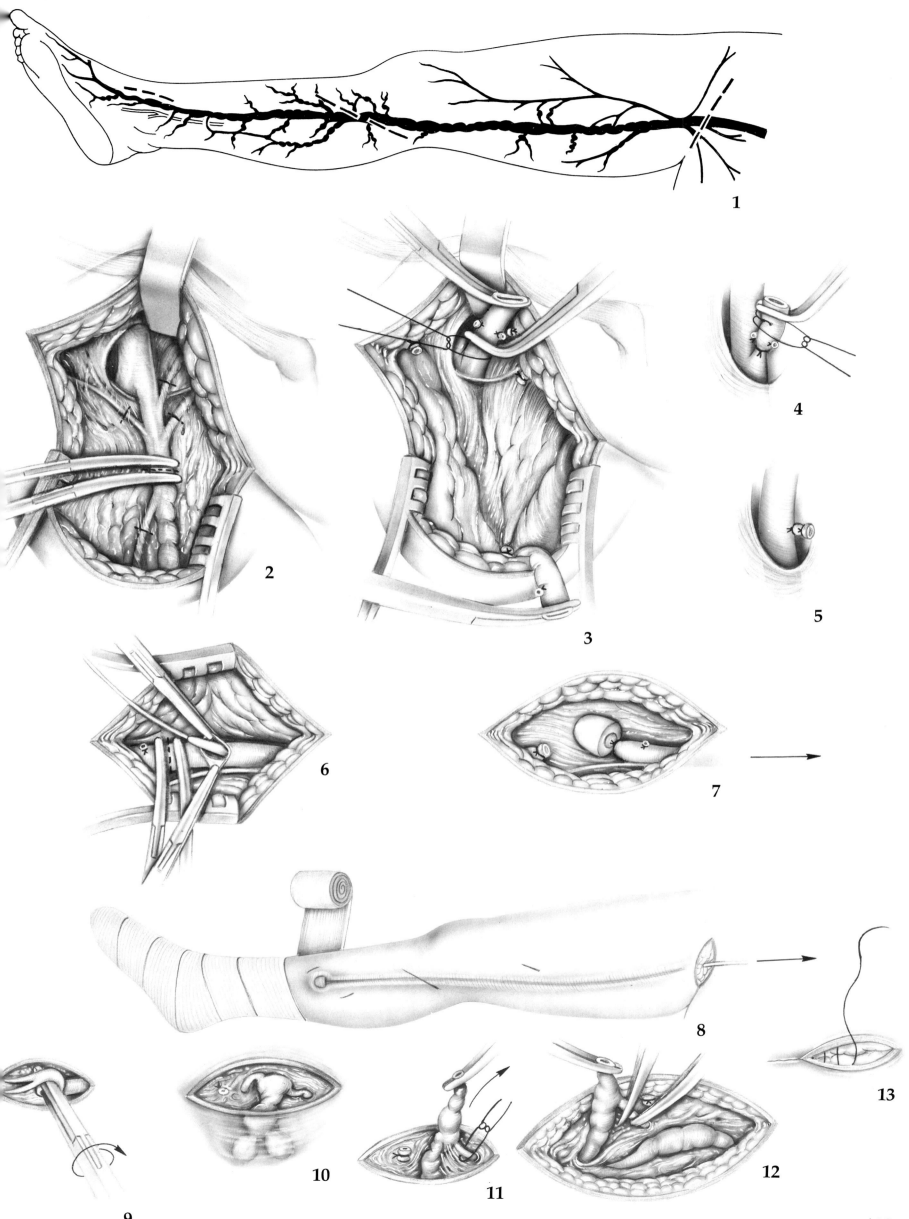

1

2

3

4

5

6

7

8

9

10

11

12

13

Carotid Endarterectomy

1 The position of the patient, with the head turned away from the side of the incision, is shown. A thyroid pillow should be placed beneath the shoulders and the head of the patient should be draped free with the anesthesiologist placed at the side of the operating table, so that the surgeon and his or her assistant can stand on either side of the table—which is rotated toward the assistant to provide equally good access to both surgeons. The incision is placed along the anterior border of the sternomastoid and curved slightly posterior in its upper portion to avoid injury to the marginal mandibular branch of the facial nerve.

2 After the incision is deepened through the subcutaneous fat and platysma, the anterior border of the sternomastoid muscle is defined and the wound edges are retracted with a self-retaining retractor. The anterior surface of the internal jugular vein is defined and the common facial branch is identified and dissected free. This vein is divided between ligatures. In the event that the vein is short, the divided ends may be oversewn.

3 Division of the common facial vein allows the internal jugular vein to be retracted laterally and posteriorly and held with the self-retaining retractor. The upper angle of the wound is then retracted with an army-navy retractor which can be held in a secure position with a robot arm, avoiding the need for a second assistant in this operation. The position of the common facial vein is a rough guide to the carotid bifurcation. The fascial investments of the carotid artery are then grasped with forceps, tensioned, and incised to expose the underlying adventitia of the carotid artery. As this incision is extended superiorly, care is taken to identify the hypoglossal nerve and protect it from injury. Once this is identified and protected, the anterior belly of the digastric muscle is identified and retracted superiorly with the army-navy retractor.

4 The common carotid artery, the superior thyroid artery, the external carotid artery, and the internal carotid artery are then dissected free in their periadventitial plane and encircled with vessel loops. Care is taken to dissect the surrounding tissue away from the carotid artery so that it will be manipulated minimally. (This is so that the risk of embolization will be minimized.) Care should be taken to dissect the internal carotid artery as far as necessary to isolate at least one centimeter distal to the palpable disease. This upper dissection of the internal carotid artery can be facilitated by isolating, ligating, and dividing small arteries and veins which hold the hypoglossal nerve posteriorly. Once these small vessels are divided, the hypoglossal nerve can be swept anteriorly and medially. This provides access to the upper reaches of the internal carotid artery. The patient is given systemic heparin [1 mg (100 I.U.) per kg]. Atraumatic vascular clamps are then placed gently across the common and external carotid arteries, and the superior thyroid artery is controlled with a doubled vessel loop. A needle is then inserted in the common carotid artery below palpable disease and the stump pressure is measured. According to the surgeon's preference, the stump pressure measurement, the EEG recordings with carotid clamping, and the patient's clinical and radiographic presentation, a decision is made regarding the need for shunt protection of the brain during endarterectomy.

5 A gently applied atraumatic clamp is placed across the internal carotid artery well distal to any palpable disease, and an incision is made in the common and internal carotid artery in a longitudinal direction. Entrance is gained into the lumen of the internal carotid artery distal to the disease, and into the common carotid artery proximal to the disease. In between, the incision in the artery is deepened to the surface of the plaque.

6 The adventitial and a portion of the medial layers of the carotid artery are grasped with fine atraumatic forceps and the appropriate endarterectomy plane defined. Ideally this is just deep to the circular muscle fibers within the media of the vessel. Using an endarterectomy spoon or dissector, this plane is further defined and the core of the diseased artery is dissected free proximally and distally.

7 This dissection is continued in circumferential fashion until it proceeds proximal to the obvious atheromatous plaque in the common carotid artery. The core of the artery is then transected through relatively normal intima and media. This frees the proximal end of the plaque, which can then be placed under tension to further facilitate the endarterectomy of the external carotid artery. This is accomplished by eversion with inferior traction on the clamp controlling the external carotid. Generally the atheroma within the external carotid separates with this eversion technique. However, it is sometimes necessary to transect the atheroma sharply to end the removal of the plaque from the external carotid. Occasionally it may be necessary to make a separate longitudinal incision in the external carotid to ensure maintenance of flow to this important vessel.

8 Following transection of the external carotid attachments of the plaque, the endarterectomy can continue up the internal carotid artery. The arteriotomy in the internal carotid artery should extend well above the upper level of the plaque, which is frequently most extensive on the posterior wall. Once the upper border of the plaque is defined, the endarterectomy may be completed by transecting the plaque through normal intima, as indicated by the dashed line in **Fig. 7**. Sometimes transection of the distal end of the plaque is unnecessary since it will feather out and come away from the distal intima as the plaque is freed under gentle tension. If any free intimal or medial edge is detected at the site of the upper limit of the endarterectomy, this free edge is secured with "U" stitches placed with the knot tied on the outside of the internal carotid artery. Although some surgeons feel that placement of these "U" stitches is almost never necessary, we employ them frequently. If placed with care they do not distort the vessel or its lumen, and they certainly may provide protection against upward dissection of an intimal flap. After all plaque is removed and the distal end of the endarterectomy secured, care is taken to examine the endarterectomized segment of the artery to remove all loose circular muscle fragments and other debris so that no material is present which could possibly embolize. This maneuver is facilitated by using fine forceps and copious amounts of saline irrigation.

9 The longitudinal arteriotomy is enclosed with fine polypropylene 6-0 sutures. These are generally begun at both ends of the arteriotomy and carried to the central portion, where they are tied. If these sutures are placed carefully and encompass small bites of the endarterectomized arterial wall, the arterial closure can be accomplished without narrowing. Although some surgeons routinely use a vein or PTFE patch, we do not use it routinely in primary cases. If a patch is necessary we favor use of an accessory saphenous vein from the thigh, or PTFE. Rupture of ankle vein has been reported in a few cases, and we would not advocate use of this material. Before flow is reestablished, both the internal and common carotid arteries are flushed to remove luminal debris. When the arteriotomy is closed, an effort is made to exclude all intraluminal air, and clamps are removed first from the external and common carotid artery so that debris will be carried up this vessel. Only after release of these two clamps is the internal carotid artery clamp removed.

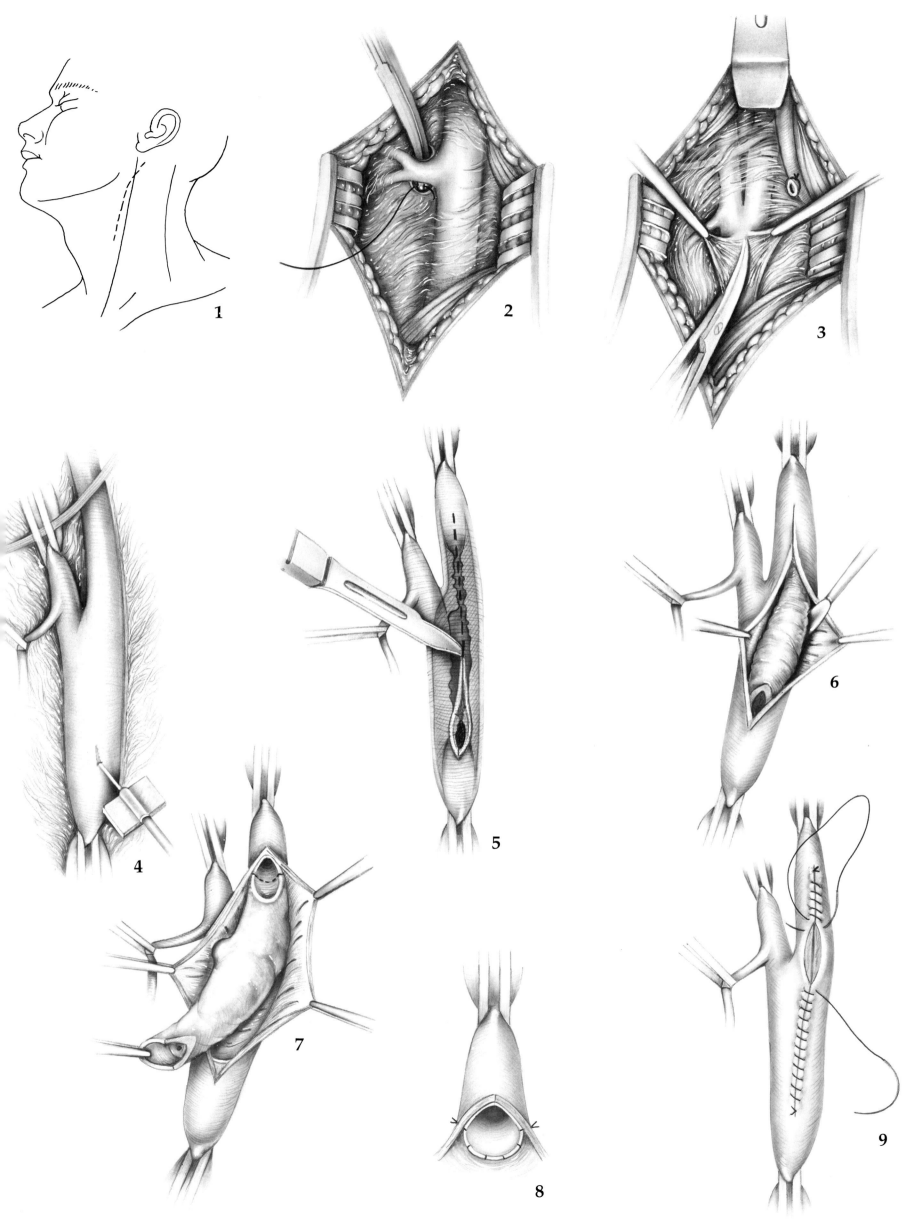

Carotid Endarterectomy (*cont.*)

10 In the event that a shunt is necessary, one possible technique for its insertion is shown. Small Rummel tourniquets are positioned around the internal carotid and common carotid arteries.

11 After the longitudinal incision is made in these arteries, the internal carotid artery vascular clamp is removed and the occluded shunt is gently inserted into a normal portion of this artery.

12 The Rummel tourniquet is gently tightened to secure the shunt in place, and the clamp occluding the shunt is released momentarily to assure adequate back-flow from the internal carotid artery and appropriate positioning of the distal end of the shunt. The clamp on the shunt is replaced.

13 After controlling the common carotid artery with finger compression, the common carotid artery clamp is removed. The common carotid artery is then flushed by a momentary release of the finger pressure, and the proximal end of the shunt is passed down the common carotid artery between the fingers.

14 The common carotid artery Rummel tourniquet is tightened and the clamp is removed from the shunt, restoring flow to the internal carotid artery. The endarterectomy is then performed in the standard fashion. This is somewhat more difficult with the shunt in place. However, it can be accomplished in an unhurried fashion with the same technical care as already described. If the dissection in the internal carotid artery has proceeded high enough, a very adequate end point can almost always be obtained and its adequacy assured by direct visual inspection.

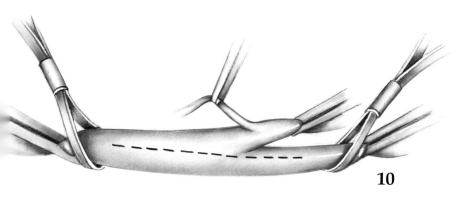

10

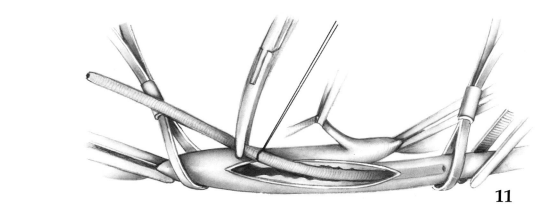

11

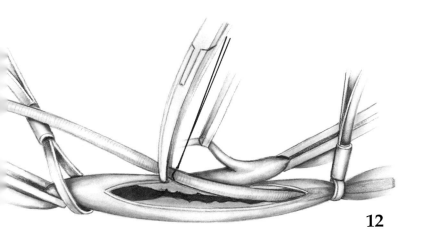

12

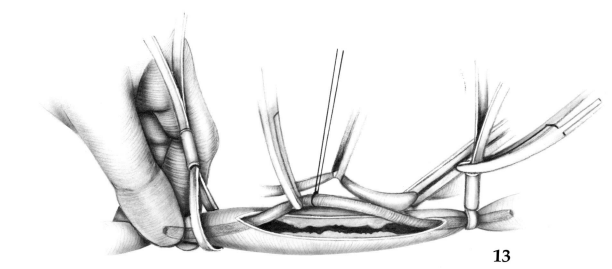

13

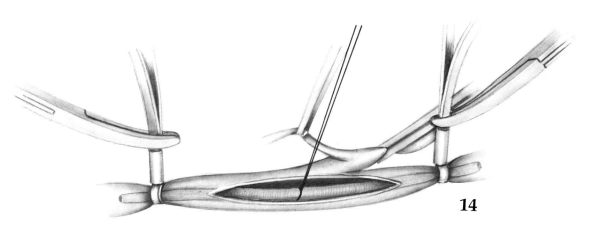

14

Carotid Endarterectomy (*cont.*)

15 To remove the shunt upon completion of the endarterectomy, the arteriotomy in the common carotid and internal carotid artery is closed for as long a distance as possible. These closures are begun at both ends of the arteriotomy and continue toward the midportion, leaving the central part of the arteriotomy open to allow removal of the shunt. The shunt is clamped in its midportion and the distal Rummel tourniquet is released. The distal end of the shunt is then carefully removed from the artery. The rush of blood aids in the removal of luminal debris. The internal carotid artery is then gently clamped.

16 With finger control of the common carotid artery again established, the proximal Rummel tourniquet on the common carotid artery is released and the shunt is removed. Clamp control of the common carotid artery is then established after flushing that vessel.

17 Traction is placed on the two suture ends defining the unclosed portion of the arteriotomy. Taking great care to avoid intraluminal air, a small partially occluding vascular clamp is placed just under the open portion of the arteriotomy. Flow is then reestablished up the external carotid artery by releasing the clamps on this vessel. After a moment of this flow the internal carotid artery clamp is released, reestablishing flow to the brain.

18 The midportion of the arteriotomy closure is then accomplished and the partially occluding clamp is removed. After securing adequate hemostasis, a few #0000 polyglycolic acid sutures are used to approximate lymphoareolar tissue over the carotid artery. The platysma and skin are then closed in layers. We generally employ a small closed suction drain for 24 hours, although this is not routinely deemed necessary.

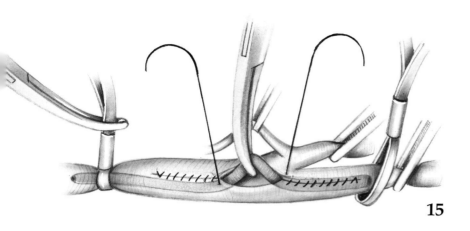

15

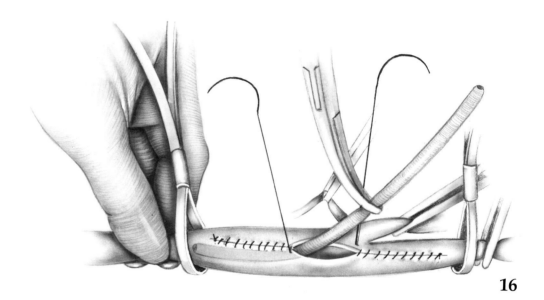

16

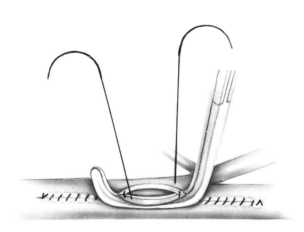

17

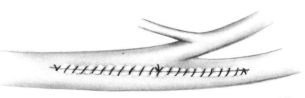

18

Aortic Aneurysm Repair

1 More than 95 percent of aortic aneurysms involve the infrarenal segment of the abdominal aorta. Aneurysms of the infrarenal aorta and iliac arteries can be approached via an anterior transperitoneal route or via a left-sided retroperitoneal route with the left side of the patient slightly elevated and the left upper extremity affixed to the ether screen. For more standard abdominal aortic and iliac aneurysms, we favor the anterior transperitoneal approach using a long midline incision which is extended superiorly above the xiphoid in the skin and fascial layers and to the pubis inferiorly. For aortic aneurysms that involve the segment of the aorta that gives rise to the renal arteries or the superior mesenteric and celiac arteries, we favor a retroperitoneal transpleural approach with the upper lateral portion of the incision extending into the 8th or 9th intercostal space.

2 After the abdomen is opened, the intraperitoneal and retroperitoneal viscera are explored thoroughly, the small bowel is retracted to the right, and the transverse colon is retracted superiorly. This exposes the posterior peritoneum overlying the segment of the aorta below the inferior mesenteric artery. Just above this area, the ascending or fourth portion of the duodenum and the ligament of Treitz can be identified. A T-shaped incision is made in the peritoneum. This begins over the lower extent of the aortic aneurysm, which in the example shown extends inferiorly only to the aortic bifurcation. The incision is extended superiorly midway between the duodenum and the inferior mesenteric vein. In its upper portion it is converted to a T-shaped incision which parallels the lower border of the pancreas. The inferior mesenteric vein is carefully identified, isolated, and divided so that the lower border of the pancreas may be freed beneath the peritoneal incision and retracted superiorly, thereby providing access to the neck of the aneurysm, the left renal vein, and the pararenal segment of the aorta if this is necessary.

3 After this incision is completed, the abdominal viscera are controlled with packs and self-retaining retraction devices. These can consist of a large ring-shaped retractor which allows retraction of the abdominal wound laterally and the transverse colon and mesocolon superiorly, as depicted. This ring retraction device must be supplemented by two deeply placed Deaver retractors, which, with appropriate packing, allow the small bowel and duodenum to be retracted to the right and craniad and the transverse and descending colon to be retracted to the left and craniad. These two Deaver retractors may be held by surgical assistants but are best held in a fixed position by robot-arm retractors which can be affixed to the operating table. This device is shaped in the form of a wishbone which is affixed securely to the operating table. The apex of this wishbone is placed over the sternum; various retracting elements may then be secured to the wishbone. Once retraction is secured, the retroperitoneal fatty areolar tissue overlying the aneurysm is incised in the midline, using a right-angle clamp and coagulating cautery to control the small arterial and venous bleeders in this layer.

4 As dissection in this plane proceeds superiorly, the left renal vein is identified and its lower border defined. It is sometimes necessary to dissect this vein circumferentially so that it can be encircled with a loop and retracted superiorly. However, this is not always necessary. To aid in the mobilization and retraction of the left renal vein it is sometimes necessary to divide the genital branch or branches and a posterior lumbar branch which is often present.

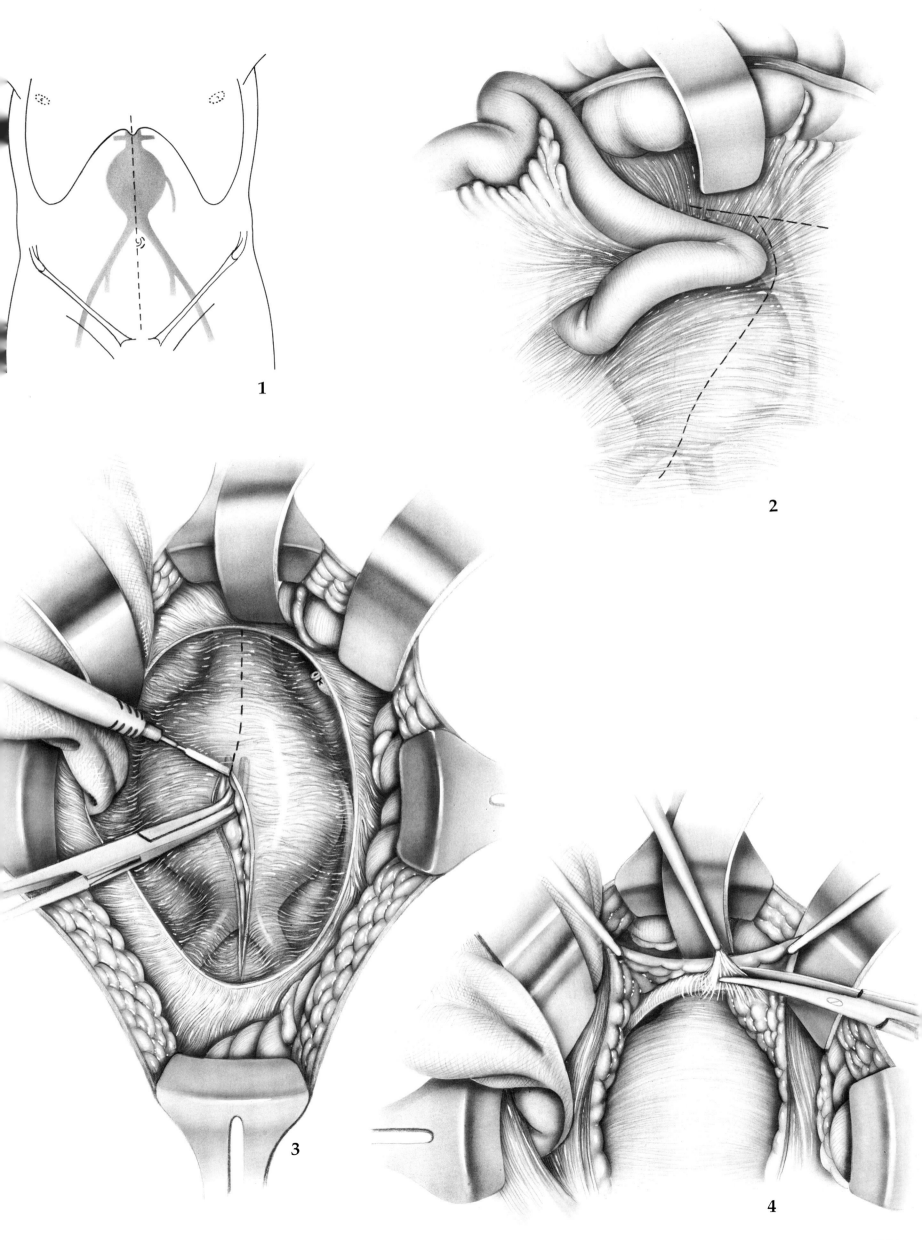

Aortic Aneurysm Repair (*cont.*)

5 With the lower border of the left renal vein identified and in some cases with it appropriately retracted in a craniad direction, the fascial investing layer just outside the adventitia of the aorta is incised after elevating this layer with forceps.

6 It is then possible in most instances to dissect the lateral walls of the aorta using a combination of blunt finger dissection and occasional sharp dissection to divide resistant bands or small branches arising from this segment of the aorta. Such small branches most often represent accessory renal arteries, and if these are less than 2 mm in diameter they may be ligated and divided to facilitate aortic mobilization. It is generally not necessary to dissect the aorta completely on its posterior aspect, although some surgeons still do so. Adequate anterior and lateral mobilization of the aorta, if it is extensive enough, will usually facilitate clamp control of the aorta proximal to the aneurysm. Circumferential aortic dissection, although it may facilitate clamp control and suturing, can also lead to bleeding. For that reason we no longer perform this dissection routinely.

7 The areolar tissue just superficial to the adventitia of the common iliac arteries is grasped with forceps, placed under tension, and sharply incised. This allows periadventitial dissection of the iliac arteries anteriorly and laterally on both sides. For reasons already mentioned we do not routinely dissect these vessels circumferentially, either.

8 After administration of systemic heparin [1 mg (100 I.U.)/kg], appropriate atraumatic vascular clamps are then applied to the proximal infrarenal aorta and distal common iliac arteries. A doubled vessel loop may be placed on the inferior mesenteric artery as it emerges from the aneurysm. Generally the application of clamps is such that the aorta and iliac arteries are compressed in a lateral direction. However, these vessels are often tortuous; compression of the vessels in an anteroposterior direction may be more easily accomplished. This is particularly true if the infrarenal aorta just proximal to the aneurysm deviates to the right. An effort is made to use vascular clamps which are shaped in such a fashion that the handles do not obscure the operative field. Some surgeons favor placement of the distal clamps first, to minimize the chance of distal embolization of clot and atheromatous material. Although this is advantageous from a theoretical perspective, the placement of distal clamps before the aneurysm is decompressed by a proximal clamp is sometimes technically difficult. This is particularly true when the aneurysm is large and involves the iliac arteries. After clamp placement in a fashion that obliterates the aneurysmal pulse is completed, the aneurysm is incised along its anterior surface and this incision is extended laterally in both directions at the superior and inferior ends of the aneurysm, as indicated by the dashed lines. This incision is generally best accomplished with the coagulating cautery to minimize bleeding from small vessels in the aneurysm wall and surrounding areolar tissue. The lumen of the aneurysm is entered. It is advantageous to utilize some form of cell-saving or autotransfusion device throughout these cases to minimize the need for homologous blood transfusion.

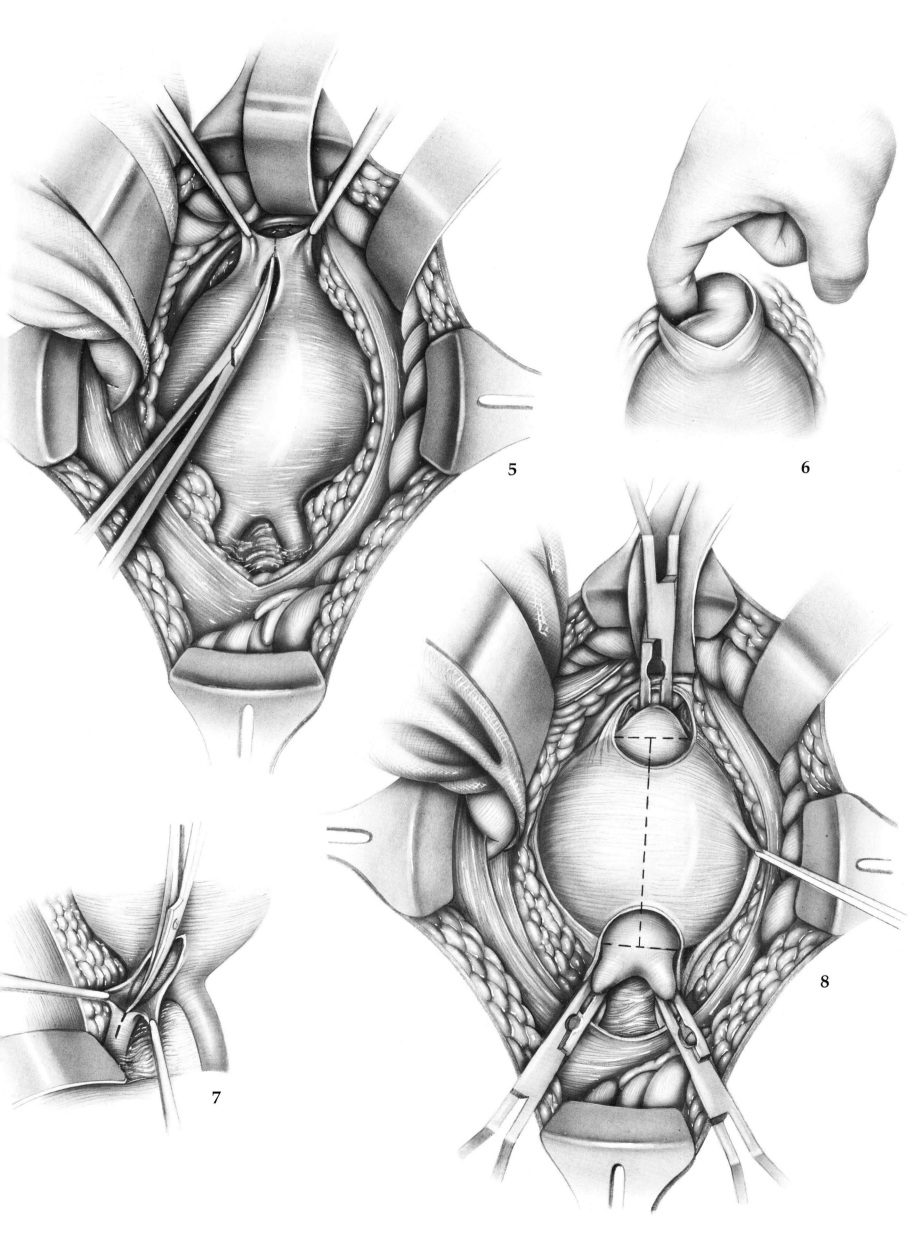

5

6

7

8

Aortic Aneurysm Repair (*cont.*)

9 Clot within the lumen of the opened aneurysm is then mobilized with finger dissection and removed.

10 This exposes the orifices of lumbar arteries and other aortic branches, which can back-bleed vigorously into the opened aneurysmal sac. This bleeding is controlled by oversewing the orifices of these branches with figure-of-eight #000 silk sutures. Although some large aneurysms have no patent arteries that require such control, other aneurysms have many branches. Bleeding from this source can be quite substantial. If bleeding from the inferior mesenteric artery is brisk and the inferior mesenteric artery is small, the orifice of this vessel may be oversewn as well. However, if this artery is large and there is only a trickle of back-bleeding from it, consideration should be given to reimplantation of this vessel into the wall of the aortic graft. This is particularly true if there is stenotic or occlusive disease involving the celiac and superior mesenteric arteries. Often, however, the orifice of the inferior mesenteric artery is occluded; no attention need be directed to this vessel as long as flow is reestablished to at least one of the internal iliac arteries.

11 An appropriate-sized aortic graft is selected for use. A variety of woven or knitted Dacron grafts or PTFE grafts may be used. If an uncoated knitted Dacron graft is employed, it must be carefully preclotted. To minimize bleeding through the graft wall, we use an albumin-coated knitted graft which bleeds minimally and is easy to handle. Suturing of the graft is best accomplished with #00 polypropylene sutures with large needles. The suture is begun posteriorly as shown. This suture is tied with two or three throws, and suturing is continued laterally in both directions. The posterior wall of the aorta need not be completely divided. Some surgeons favor the loose placement of five or six of the posterior sutures in a parachute fashion followed by tensioning of these sutures to approximate the graft to the aortic wall. This technique may favor careful placement of the sutures, but care must then be taken to assure adequate tensioning of all bites.

12 After placement of one posterolateral quadrant of sutures, the opposite posterolateral quadrant is completed.

13 The two anterior quadrants of the suture line are then completed in similar fashion. Note the large size of the suture bites, which are placed through all layers of the aortic wall. The sutures are then tied anteriorly.

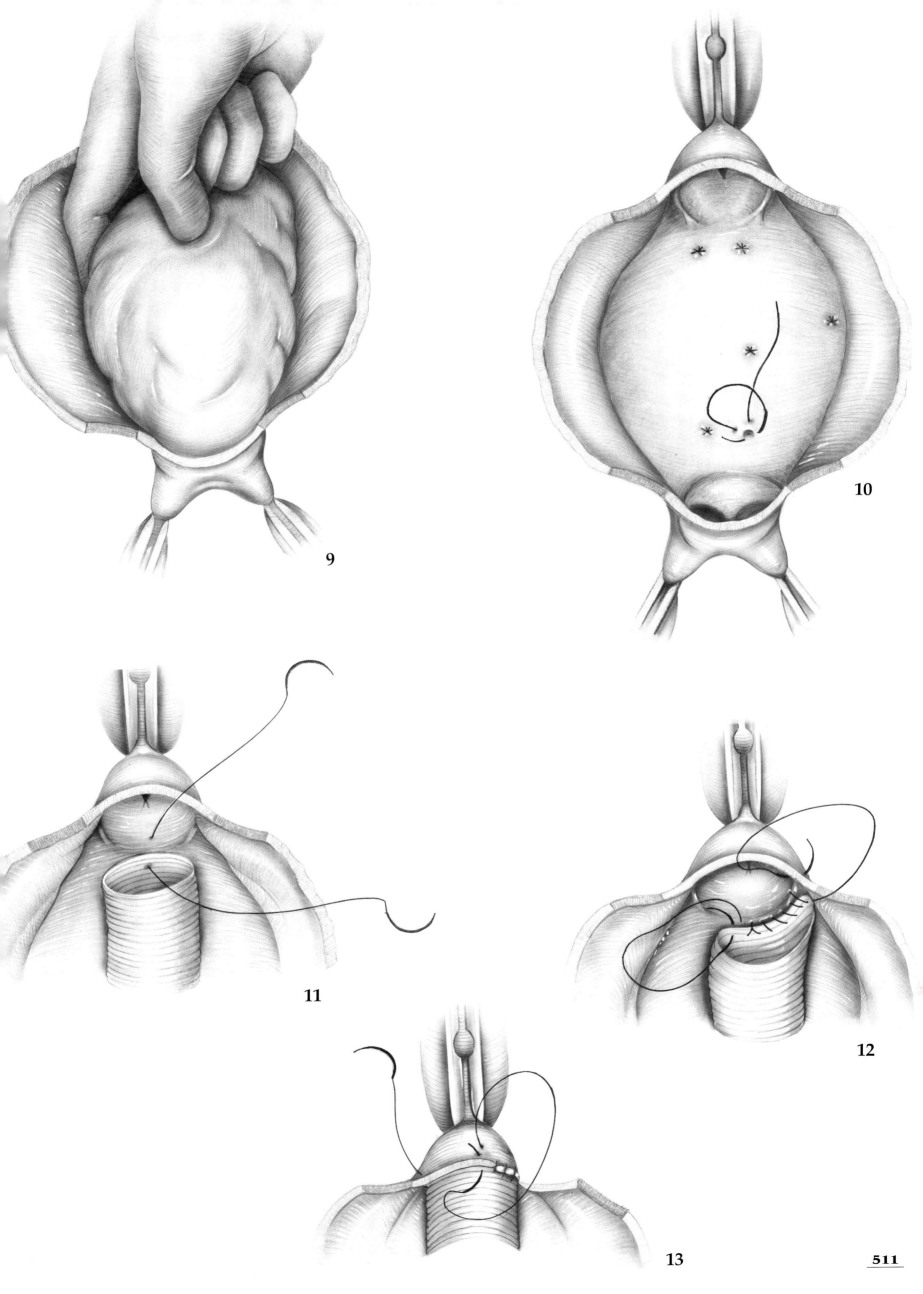

9

10

11

12

13

Aortic Aneurysm Repair (*cont.*)

14 The graft is then clamped temporarily and the proximal aortic clamp released to flush debris from the lumen and to test the suture line. Any bleeding points in the suture line are reinforced and the aorta is reclamped. After appropriate tensioning of the graft, it is transected and the distal anastomosis completed in a fashion similar to the proximal anastomosis. Just before completion of this anastomosis, the iliac clamps are released to allow flushing of debris from these vessels. After suitable volume replacement, one of the iliac clamps is removed to test the anastomoses for leaks. Once both anastomoses are found to be intact, the proximal clamp is carefully released, monitoring the patient's systemic arterial pressure and replacing blood volume as needed.

15 Heparin is reversed with protamine, and the interior of the aneurysm is again checked for bleeding. Not uncommonly a well-controlled lumbar orifice will begin to bleed again with release of the aortic and iliac clamps. Once the interior of the aneurysm is free of bleeding, the aneurysm wall is closed over the graft and, where possible, the suture lines, with #000 polyglycolic acid sutures.

16 The retroperitoneum is then reapproximated so that neither the aneurysm wall nor either suture line can come into contact with the duodenum or small bowel. Closure of the retroperitoneum is often facilitated by release of the self-retaining retraction devices. It is not necessary to completely close the upper portion of the retroperitoneal incision. (In fact, this is often impossible.) In the event that a retroperitoneal layer cannot be interposed between the graft and its suture lines, it may be necessary to use a flap of retroperitoneal fat or omentum.

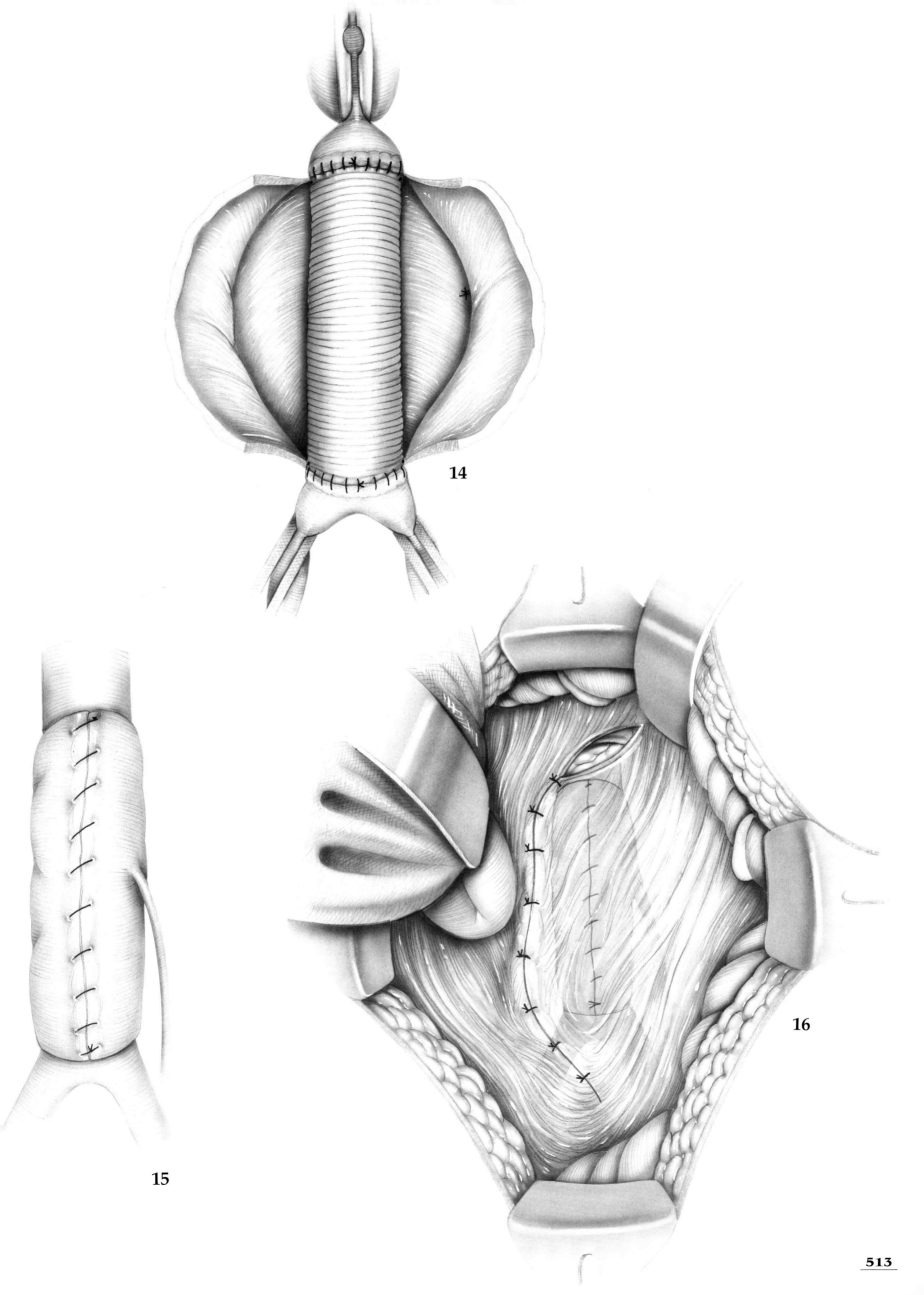

14

15

16

Aortic Aneurysm Repair (*cont.*)

17 The aneurysmal incisions for managing a large right common iliac and a small left common iliac aneurysm are shown. Clamp control on the right is at the level of the internal and external iliac arteries. Often a single Satinsky clamp can be used to accomplish the same end, particularly if the iliac aneurysm is redundant and these two branches come off posteriorly. A single atraumatic clamp is placed on the distal left common iliac artery where it is of relatively normal caliber.

18 The opened aortic and iliac aneurysms can be seen and the completed suture lines of the aortic bifurcation graft are shown. Anastomosis on the right is to the iliac bifurcation. On the left it is to the mid–common iliac artery. Similar techniques for performing these anastomoses and the aortic anastomoses are employed. Aneurysm closure and retroperitoneal closure are accomplished in the same fashion as that already outlined for a simple aortic aneurysm. Care is taken to assure adequate hemostasis before all wounds are closed.

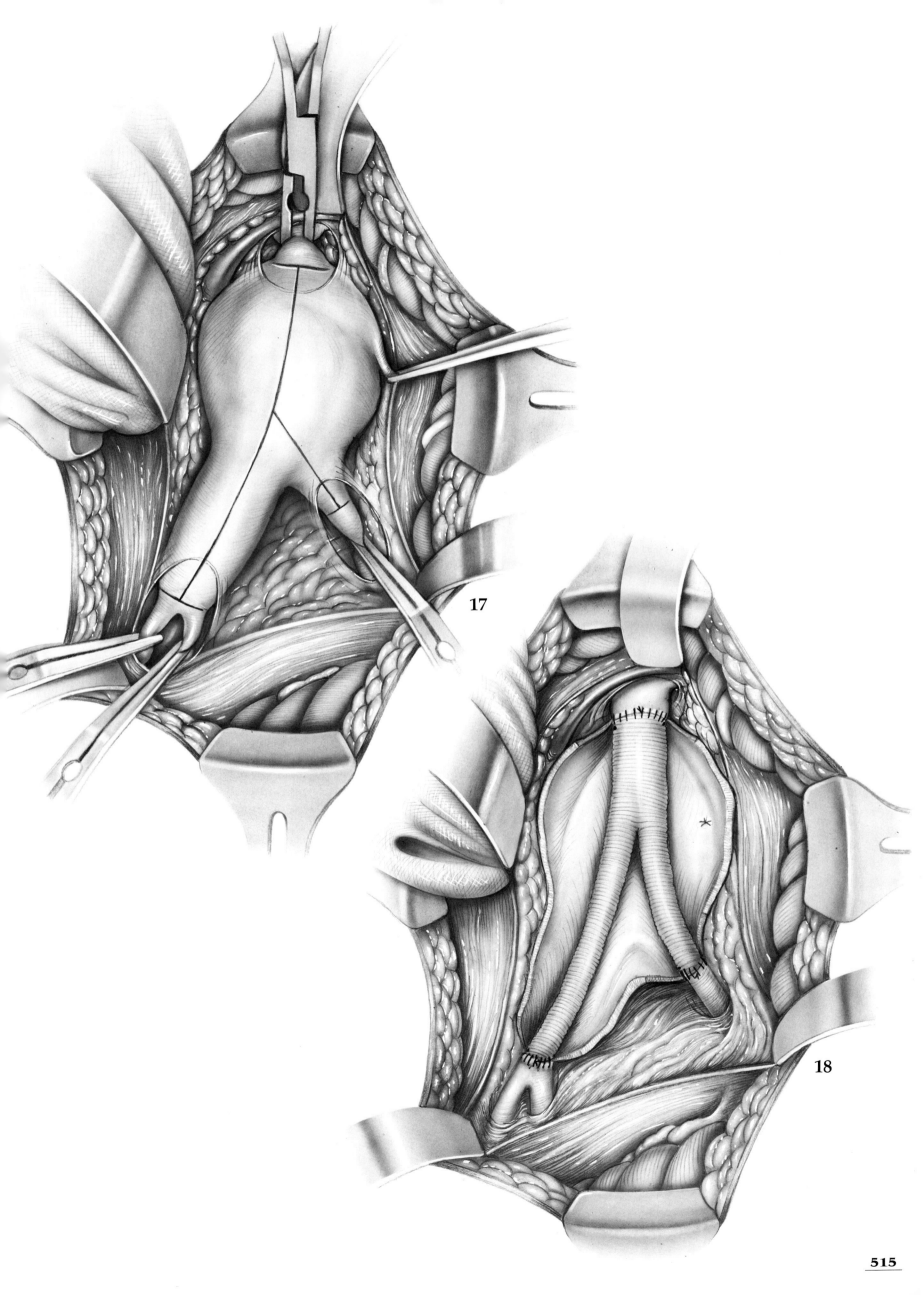

17

18

Aortofemoral Bypass for Occlusive Disease

1 Aortobifemoral bypass is performed on patients with aortic and extensive bilateral iliac disease which produces severe lower extremity ischemia. A long midline incision extending upward along the xiphoid process is made.

2 The abdomen is carefully and systematically explored. The small bowel is retracted to the right and the posterior peritoneum is incised over the aortic bifurcation. This incision is extended superiorly alongside the ascending portion of the duodenum, dividing the ligament of Treitz. This incision is placed midway between the duodenum and the inferior mesenteric vein. The retroperitoneal incision is made in the shape of a "T" superiorly along the base of the transverse mesocolon, paralleling the lower border of the pancreas.

3 After the posterior peritoneum is incised, the small bowel and other intraperitoneal viscera are packed off within the abdominal cavity and held in place with self-retaining retractors. A ring retractor and two mechanical retractors, which are affixed to the table, are shown in the illustration. Alternatively, a Stoney retractor can also be used. These self-retaining retraction devices provide steady, safe retraction and allow optimal exposure without the requirement for multiple assistants. Once the posterior peritoneum is incised and the viscera retracted, the aorta can be seen or palpated through the retroperitoneal fatty areolar tissue.

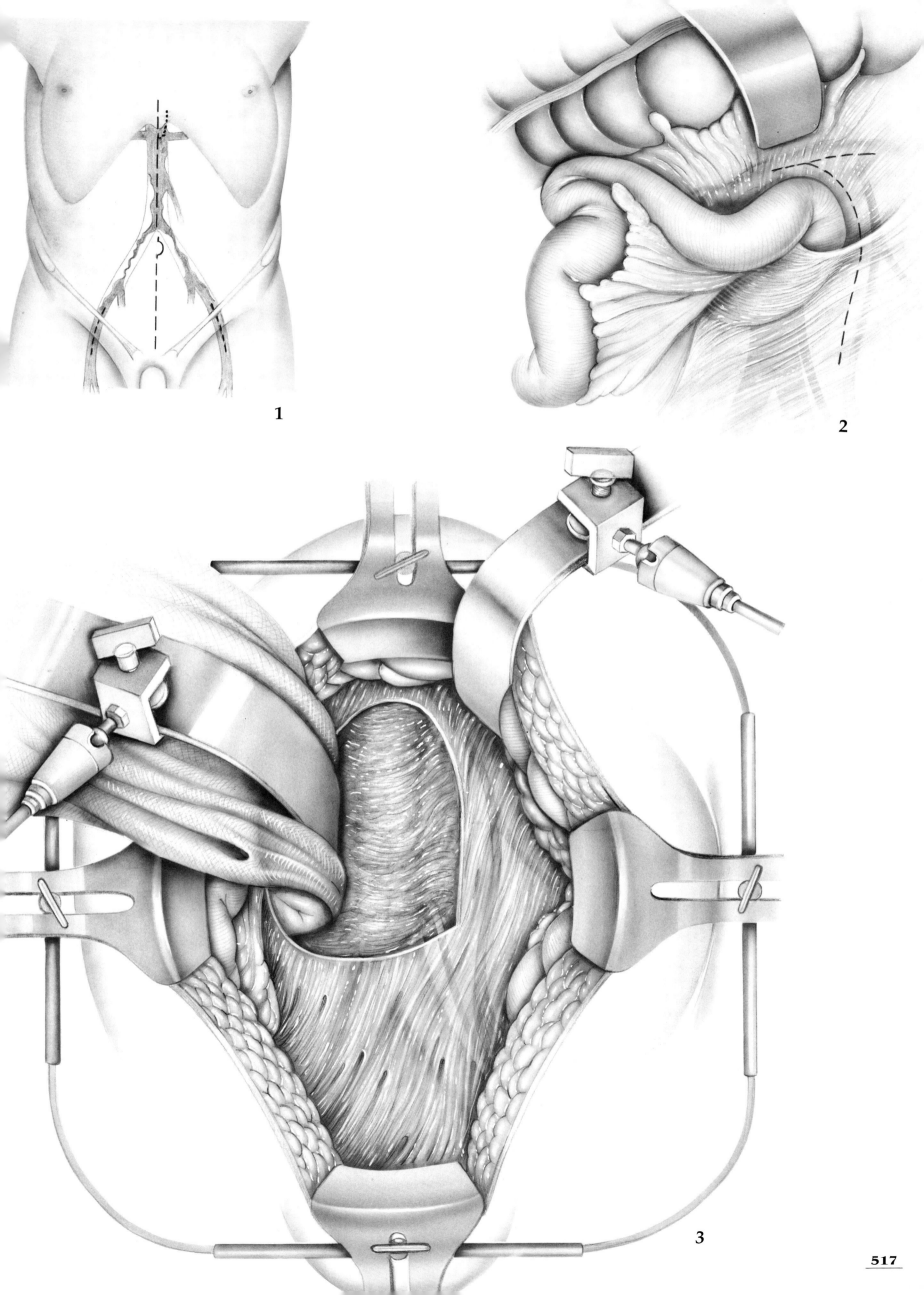

Aortofemoral Bypass for Occlusive Disease (*cont.*)

4 This retroperitoneal fatty areolar tissue contains a number of small blood vessels and is best incised with electrocautery. The incision in this tissue is begun anterior to the aorta.

5 Once the adventitia of the aorta is visualized in the midportion of the retroperitoneal incision, the opening in the retroperitoneal fatty areolar tissue is continued cephalad and caudad by elevating this tissue with a right-angle clamp and incising it with the coagulating electrocautery.

6 The aorta is then dissected free anteriorly and laterally using a combination of blunt and sharp dissection. Superiorly, this dissection extends posteromedially and posterolaterally. However, it is not necessary to free the posterior wall of the aorta completely.

7 The common femoral artery is exposed through a vertical groin incision placed over the course of the common femoral artery. If no femoral pulse can be felt, the occluded artery can usually be palpated as a firm tubular structure. If this is not possible, the incision is made midway between the pubic tubercle and the anterior superior iliac spine. This incision is deepened through the subcutaneous tissue and fascia layers. The femoral sheath is then incised, and the artery dissected free in the periadventitial plane. Care is taken to clamp and ligate all identifiable lymphatics, and lymph nodes are freed around their periphery but not transected. The skin excision extends over the groin crease. In the upper end of the wound, the inguinal ligament is identified, freed medially and laterally, and retracted superiorly. Crossing venous branches may have to be clamped and ligated. The common femoral bifurcation is identified by the decreasing diameter of the femoral artery, and the superficial and deep femoral arteries are dissected free circumferentially.

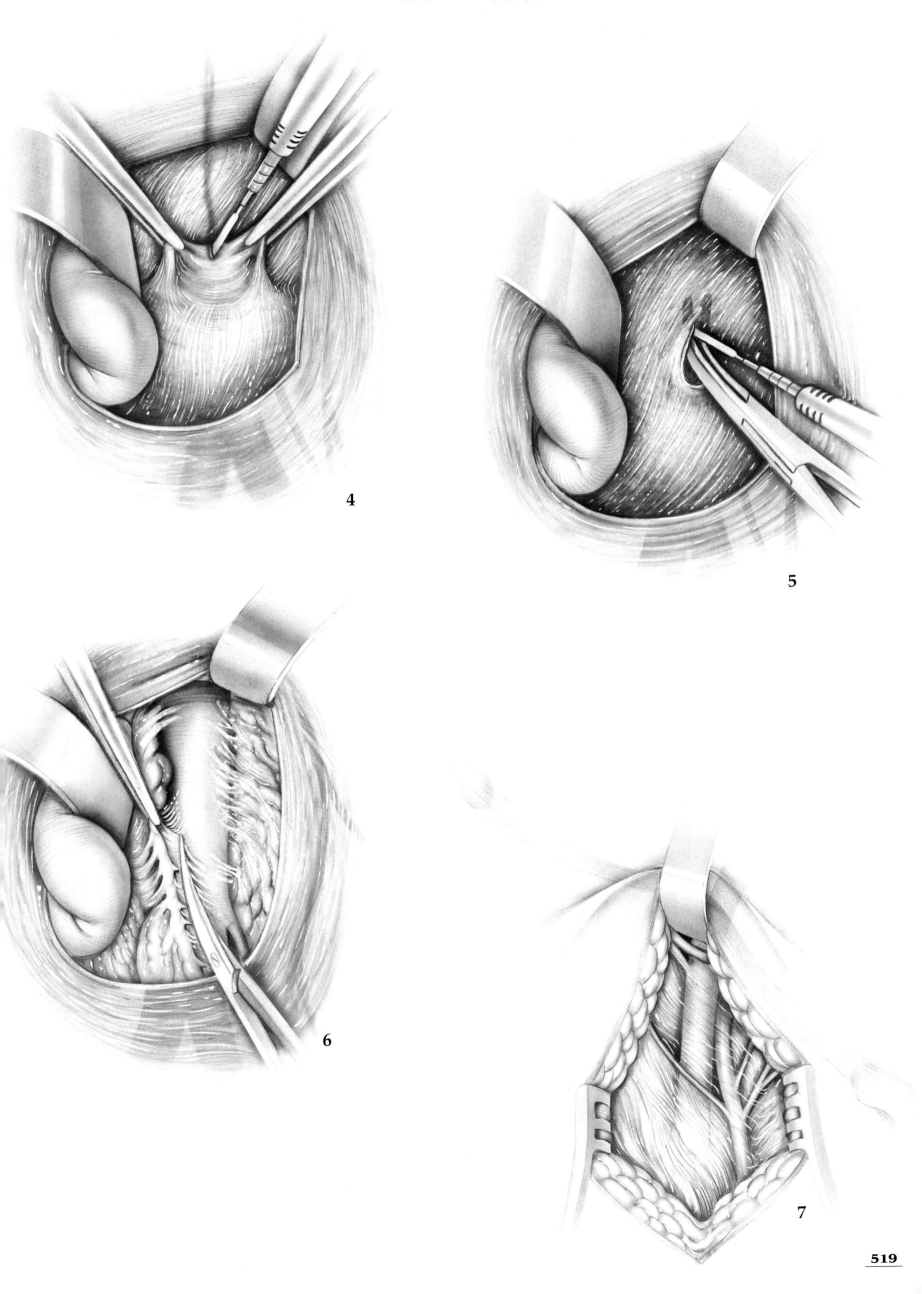

4

5

6

7

Aortofemoral Bypass for Occlusive Disease (*cont.*)

8 By elevating the inguinal ligament a tunnel between the retroperitoneal dissection within the abdomen and the groin is fashioned using primarily finger dissection, as shown in **Fig. 7**. Care is taken to avoid injury to veins which may cross over the external iliac artery. A similar tunnel is made on the left side by passing the fingers behind the sigmoid mesentery. These tunnels should parallel the course of the subjacent arteries and should be as close to their periadventitial plane as possible. In this way, damage to the ureters and other retroperitoneal vessels is minimized.

9 Prior to occlusion of any major artery, hemostasis is assured and the patient is given 1 mg (100 I.U.) per kg of intravenous heparin. A large atraumatic vascular clamp is placed entirely across the aorta just below the lower border of the renal vein, which is clearly identified. A second large curved atraumatic vascular clamp is then placed (**Figs. 9–10**) so as to occlude the distal aorta and all lumbar arteries entering the aortic segment posteriorly. The inferior mesenteric artery, if patent, is occluded by tensioning a doubled Silastic vessel loop and affixing it to the drapes with a clamp. The anterior wall of the aorta is then opened with a #15 scalpel blade. Once the aortic lumen is clearly identified, a small right-angle clamp is placed within the lumen to elevate all layers of the aortic wall and thereby facilitate a clean incision in this vessel. We favor side-to-end proximal aortic anastomoses so that all possible remaining pelvic circulation can be preserved. Some surgeons favor end-to-end proximal anastomosis with oversewing of the distal divided end of the aorta. There is, however, no convincing evidence that such a procedure is superior in any way to side-to-end proximal aortic anastomosis.

10 The position of the aortic clamps and their shape is clearly shown. The end sutures, which are usually of #00 or #000 polypropylene, have been placed through the aorta and the beveled aortic bifurcation graft. In general, large atraumatic needles (MH) facilitate this procedure. These end sutures are tied and the suture is run around from the lower and upper ends of the anastomosis and tied at the midportion on either side. Once the proximal aortic anastomosis is completed, the graft is clamped and the aortic clamps removed. Any bleeding points at the anastomosis are controlled with interrupted sutures. Removal of the aortic clamps at this time is advisable, to test the proximal anastomosis for leaks and to restore any remaining pelvic circulation. In general, smaller-sized grafts appear to perform better than larger grafts. Most patients can be treated with a 16×8 or 14×7 mm graft. We favor the use of albumin-coated knitted Dacron grafts when larger grafts are required, and the use of PTFE bifurcation grafts when smaller grafts are required. In almost every instance the proximal anastomosis is placed in the portion of the aorta between the renal arteries and the inferior mesenteric artery since the aorta below that level is so commonly involved with disease. Although one might be tempted to use a partially occluding clamp on the aorta, this is not advisable. In almost all of these patients, the aorta is thick-walled and cross-clamping is necessary to allow easy access to the lumen and adequate suture placement. When the occlusion in the aorta extends up to the renal arteries, no distal clamp is necessary. The anastomosis can still be carried out to the infrarenal aortic segment after the thrombus is removed. This is facilitated by digital control of the suprarenal aorta. More recently we have been using suprarenal or supraceliac control to allow a more deliberate disobliteration of the infrarenal aorta in these cases. If the aorta is heavily calcified, this process usually stops below the renals and the immediate infrarenal segment can be safely cross-clamped. To occlude the distal vessels, the heavily calcified aorta often must be cracked; this can be accomplished if appropriate care is used.

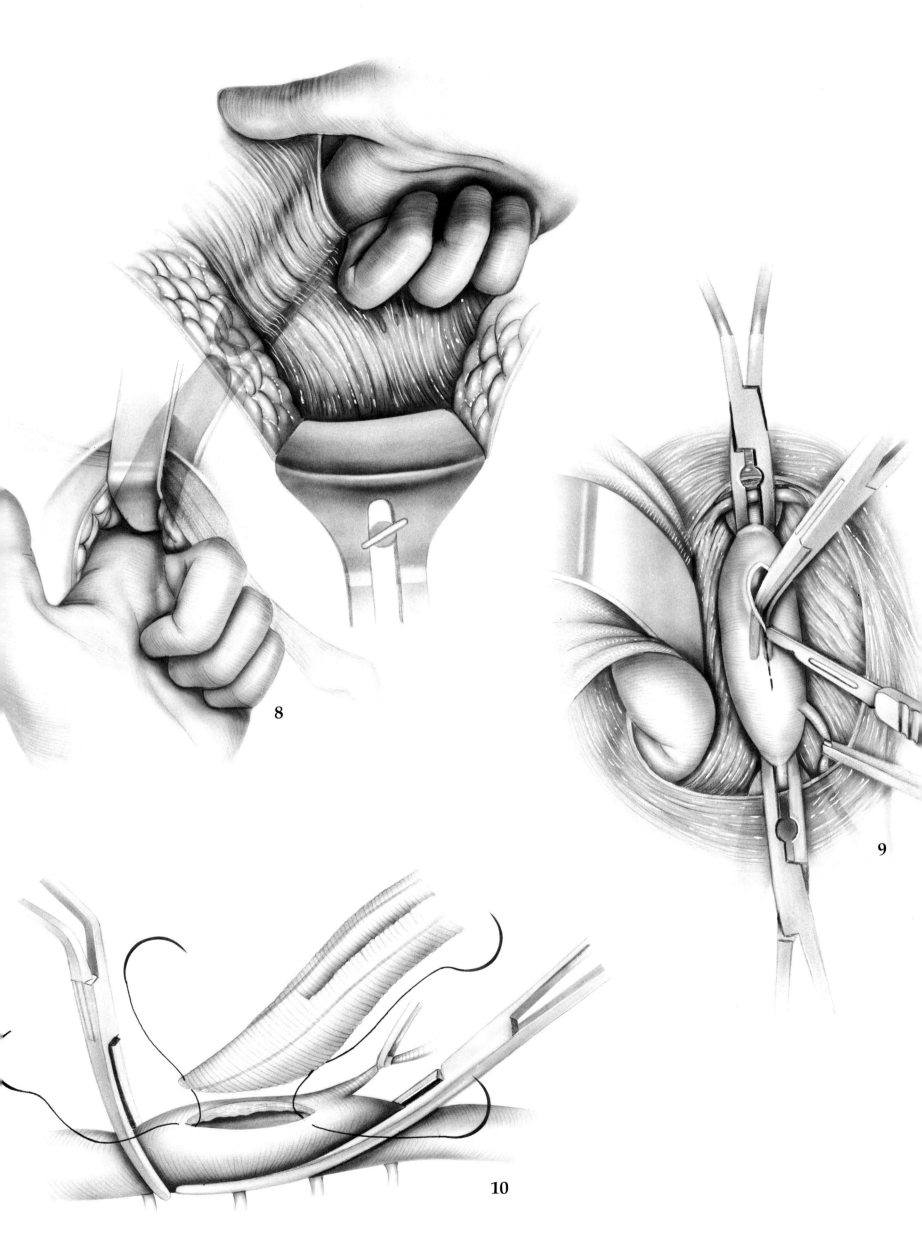

8

9

10

Aortofemoral Bypass for
Occlusive Disease (*cont.*)

11 Note that the single barrel of the bifurcation graft is kept short to avoid kinking of the limbs. The proximal end of the graft is cut at approximately 45° so that it will lie flush on the aorta without kinking.

12 A long, gently curved clamp is then passed, under finger control, through the previously dissected tunnels from the groin to the retroperitoneal incisions with the limbs of the graft carefully grasped within the point of the clamp so that there are no projecting stumps of the graft to catch on retroperitoneal soft tissue. The grafts are then pulled inferiorly through the tunnel and subjected to mild tension.

13 Angled atraumatic vascular clamps are then placed to occlude the common femoral, deep femoral, and superficial femoral arteries. A linear arteriotomy in the common femoral artery is made to expose the origin of the deep femoral artery. If this is undiseased a standard end-to-side anastomosis is carried out in the same fashion as shown for the proximal aortic anastomosis. However, the suture bites are much smaller and require placement with greater care so that even bites of all layers are taken and so that there is no narrowing of the outflow artery lumen. Particular care is taken to be sure that all sutures catch adequate bites of intima, so that no distal flaps are left. Each stitch must be placed under direct vision.

14 If there is significant disease at the origin of the deep femoral artery, as shown in the inset, the arteriotomy is extended across this disease and the graft placed over the opened lumen. We do not favor performing an endarterectomy in this circumstance, but rather prefer extending the arteriotomy across the disease and placing the graft as a patch over the stenotic segment. If a long deep–femoral artery occlusion or stenosis is present, this may be treated with a long vein patch and the graft may be placed into this. If endarterectomy is carried out, care must be taken to tack down the distal intima. After all clamps are removed, the heparin is reversed and hemostasis is assured. The wounds are then closed in layers. Care is taken to close one or more layers of fascia or fatty tissue over the graft and to obliterate dead space. The retroperitoneum is closed in such a way that a lateral peritoneal flap of connective tissue or peritoneum is interposed between the duodenum and the graft-to-aorta anastomosis. If this cannot be accomplished, omentum is interposed between the anastomosis and the duodenum.

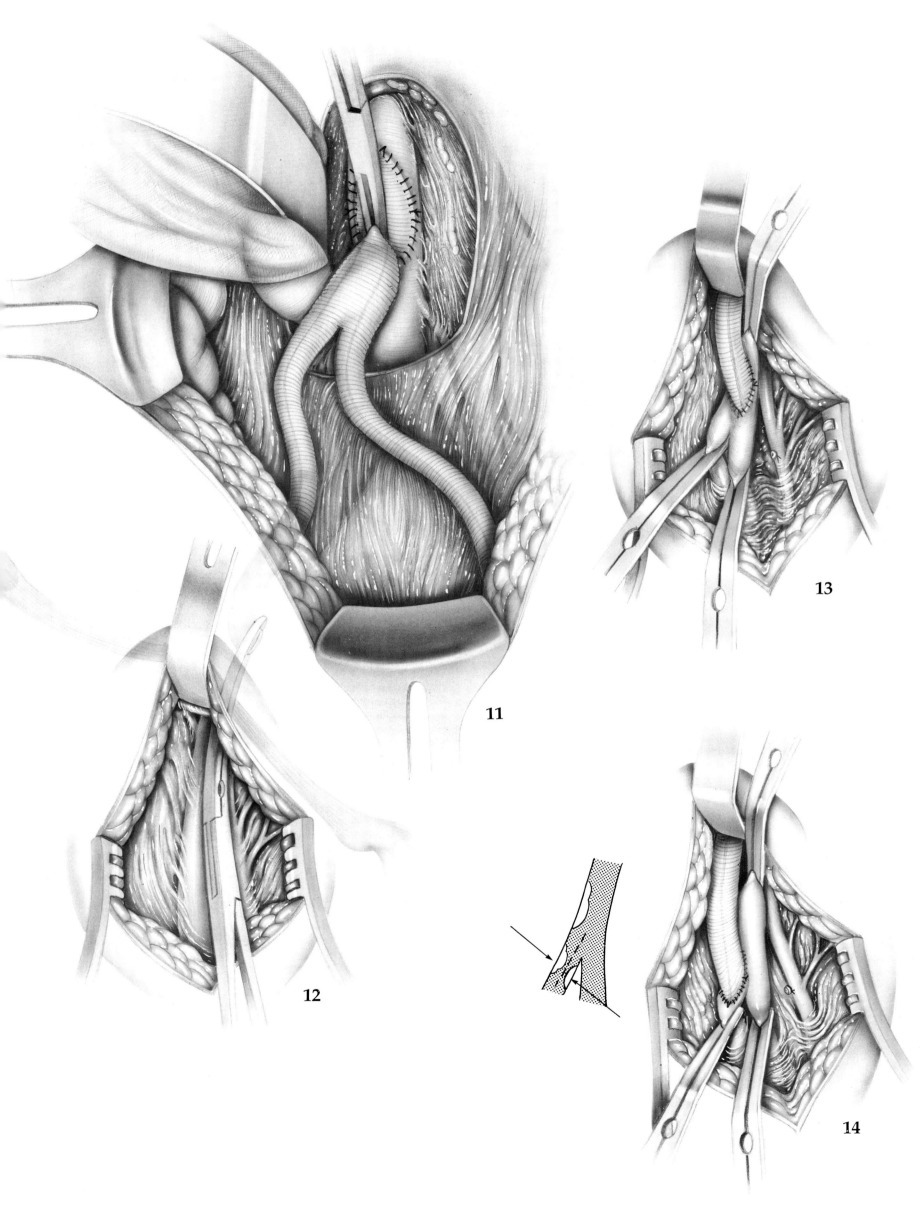

11

12

13

14

Femoropopliteal Bypass

1 The positioning of the extremity and location of the skin incisions are shown. If the greater saphenous vein in the thigh and upper leg is to be used as the graft, the skin incision is made directly over the course of that vein and deep subcutaneous flaps are raised to reach the appropriate arteries. Alternatively, if a prosthetic graft is to be used, skin and subcutaneous incisions placed directly over the appropriate arteries are employed. The positions for the above-knee and below-knee access routes to the popliteal artery from a medial approach are shown. The above-knee incision is placed along the anterior border of the sartorius muscle. The below-knee incision parallels the posterior border of the tibia.

2 The above-knee access route to the popliteal artery is shown after the skin and subcutaneous tissue have been incised. The fascial incision is then made along the anterior border of the sartorius muscle, just deep to which can be felt the adductor tendon.

3 The sartorius muscle is freed from the deeper structures and retracted with a self-retaining retractor. Care is taken to avoid injury to the blood supply and nerve supply to the sartorius muscle. The deep fascia of the popliteal space is then grasped with forceps and sharply incised.

4 This exposes the popliteal fat, which is carefully separated by blunt and sharp dissection. Any crossing veins are cauterized or ligated. The popliteal neurovascular bundle can then be palpated as it emerges from the adductor muscle. By grasping the outer tissues of this bundle with forceps and elevating it, its superficial fascial investments can be incised.

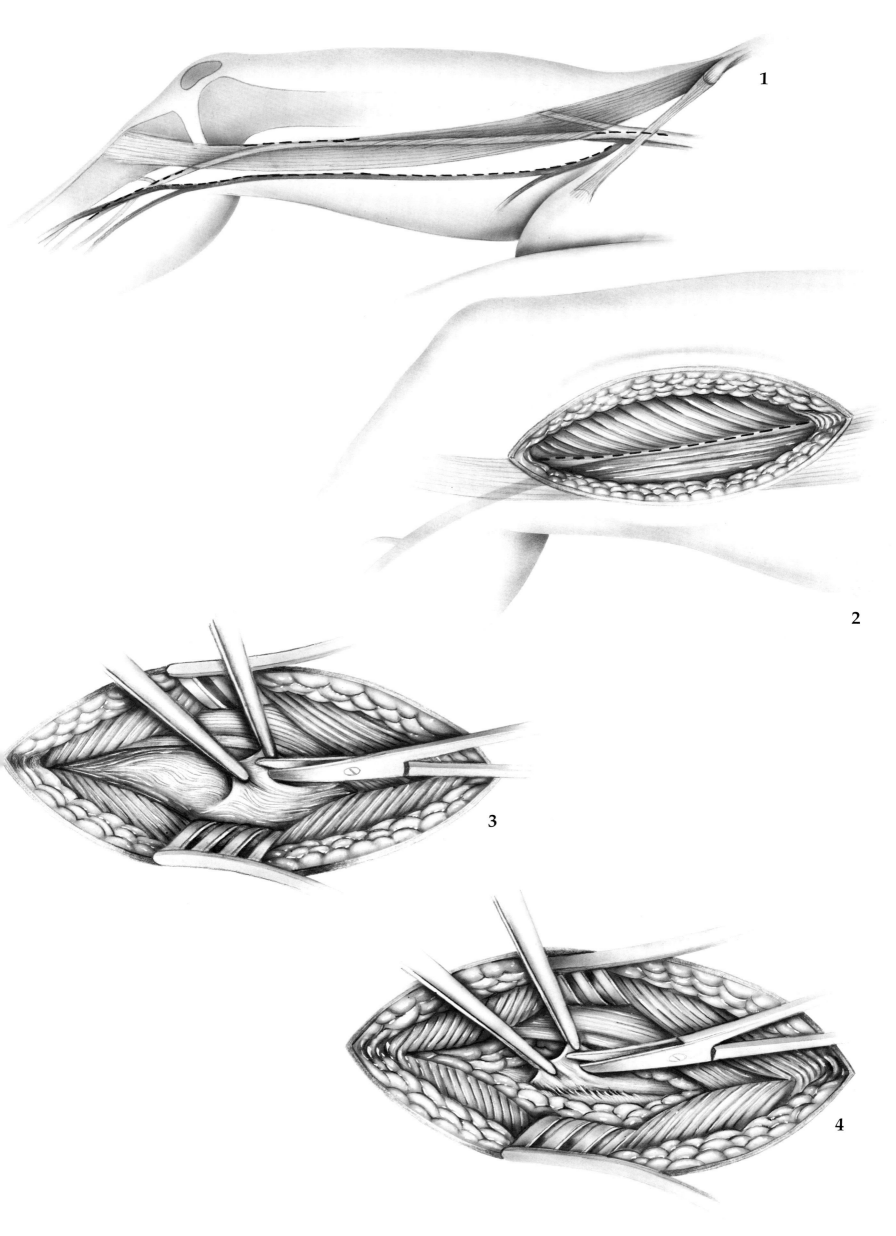

Femoropopliteal Bypass (*cont.*)

5 Additional fascial layers overlie the periadventitial plane around the artery. In these layers course many small veins which connect the main veins that accompany the popliteal artery. By sharply dividing these fascial investments it is possible to visualize the crossing veins. These can be carefully ligated and divided to clearly define the periadventitial plane of the popliteal artery.

6 After division of these veins, the popliteal artery can be circumferentially dissected in its periadventitial plane and elevated using Silastic loops.

7 A groin incision over the common, superficial, and deep femoral arteries is made in a standard fashion. A subsartorial tunnel is then created, using blunt dissection with the fingers. If the tunnel is too long for the fingers to meet, a plastic chest-tube container can be used to complete this tunnel. Once the tunnel has been created, the backs of the fingers should be in contact with the indurated surface of the diseased artery to confirm the correct location of the tunnel.

8 The greater saphenous vein is carefully harvested by a long incision placed directly over it. All branches are carefully identified and ligated so as not to constrict the vein or prevent its free enlargement as it is gently dilated. Balanced saline solution (Hank's) or chilled heparinized blood is used to irrigate the vein and gently distend it. This process is facilitated with a long plastic catheter with a well-rounded tip passed into the vein. In a sequential fashion, 2- to 3-cm segments of the vein can be isolated by gentle finger pressure and distended to identify leaks. Passage of the catheter also identifies recanalized previously thrombophlebitic segments, which cannot be found in any other way and which, if present, make a vein unsatisfactory for use. The vein is then immersed in the chilled solution until the surgeon is ready to use it.

9 After heparin is administered systemically [1 mg (100 I.U.)/kg], the segment of popliteal artery selected for the distal anastomosis is isolated by the careful and gentle application of atraumatic vascular clamps. Care is taken to avoid excessive closing pressure on these clamps, and torsion, since a diseased popliteal artery can easily be injured. Small branches entering the selected segment are occluded by microclips. The area for the arteriotomy is selected by careful palpation of the vessel. An effort to use the least diseased portion of the artery is made. However, in many instances no segment or wall of the popliteal artery is completely free of atherosclerotic involvement. The point of a new #15 scalpel blade is used to make the arteriotomy. Once the lumen of the artery has been entered, a fine mosquito clamp is inserted and opened so that the knife cut in the arterial wall will be clean and sharp and evenly placed through all layers of the diseased artery.

10 Often the arterial incision is placed across a known stenosis in the artery to widen the stenotic area and improve outflow via the distal anastomosis. The anastomosis is then completed using 6-0 polypropylene sutures. These stitches are begun at the heel and the toe.

11 Each stitch is placed through all layers of the artery and vein, taking particular care to include even bites of the intimal layers. The suturing is continued from both ends toward the center of the anastomosis on each side. The sutures are tied at the midportion of each wall of the anastomosis.

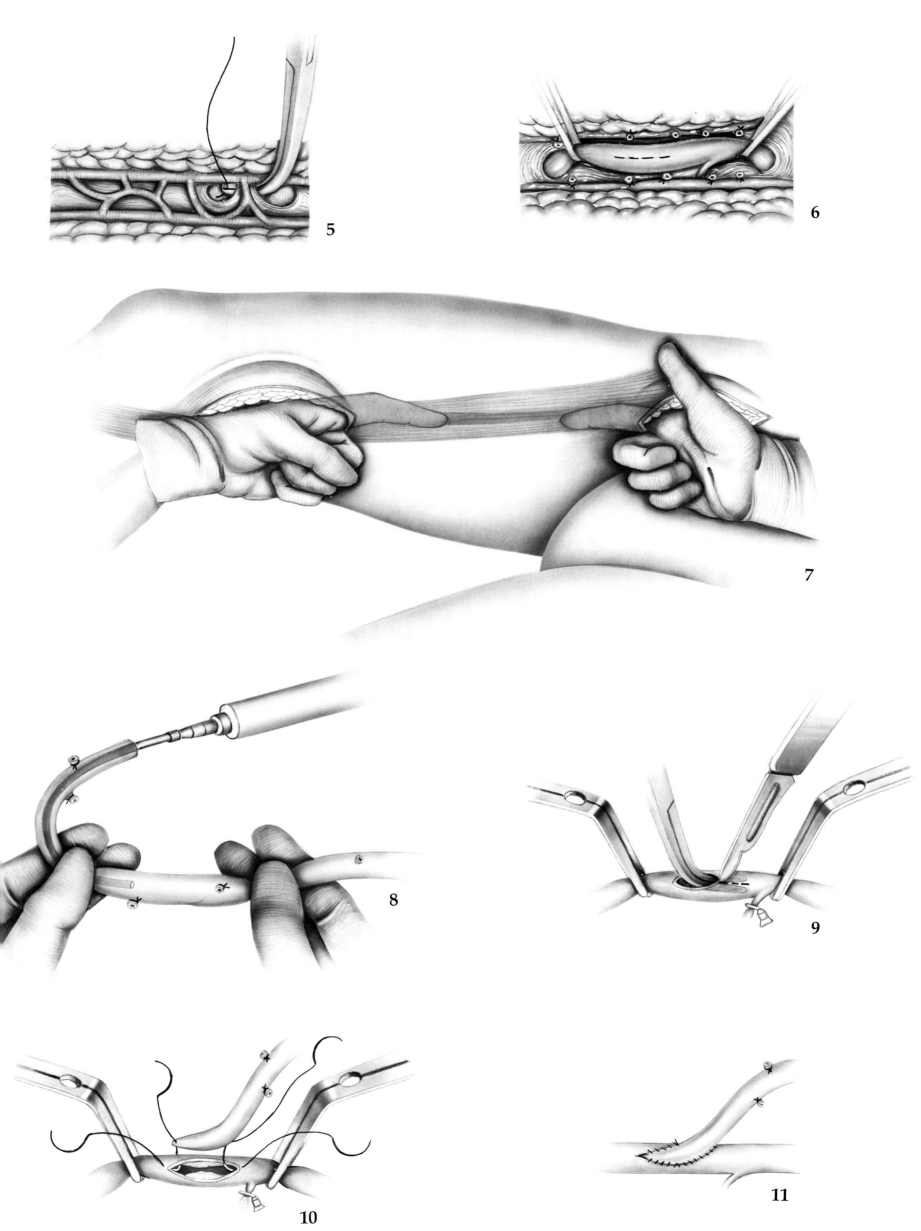

5

6

7

8

9

10

11

Femoropopliteal Bypass (*cont.*)

12 A long gently-curved aneurysm clamp is then placed through the previously defined tunnel and the graft is pulled retrograde from the popliteal incision through the tunnel to the groin incision, taking particular care to avoid twisting or kinking the graft. All occluding devices in the popliteal artery are removed and the graft and outflow tract are flushed with heparinized saline solution.

13 The proximal anastomosis to the common femoral artery is completed in a fashion similar to that already described (see **Plate 244, Figs. 1–5**).

14 If the proximal superficial femoral artery is free of atherosclerotic involvement, the proximal anastomosis may be constructed to the latter vessel. Use of this vessel minimizes the length of good autologous saphenous vein that is required. Grafts originating from the superficial femoral artery have acceptable long-term patency rates which are comparable to those of grafts originating from the common femoral artery.

15 Similarly, if vein length is limited, the proximal anastomosis may be constructed to the deep femoral artery as long as it is free of significant disease. If a marked stenosis is present at the origin of the deep femoral artery, the graft may be inserted across this stenosis.

16 If the common femoral artery is very thick-walled and diseased, the proximal anastomosis can sometimes be facilitated by sewing a vein patch into the diseased segment and then inserting the proximal end of the vein graft into this patch. This technique is particularly useful if the proximal end of the vein (which was previously the most peripheral portion of the greater saphenous vein) is small. If suitable autologous vein is not present in the ipsilateral lower extremity or if the patient has a limited life expectancy (3 to 4 years), it is perfectly acceptable to use a 6-mm PTFE graft for above-knee femoropopliteal bypass. Furthermore, if the femoropopliteal bypass is inserted into an isolated or blind popliteal artery segment, the surgeon may elect to use a PTFE graft and save the vein for a subsequent infrapopliteal bypass.

17 The position of the skin incision for access to the below-knee popliteal artery is shown. Great care must be taken to avoid injury to the greater saphenous vein, which frequently crosses the operative field. This must be carefully freed and protected from injury. The deep investing fascia of the leg is incised. As this incision extends superiorly the tendons of the gracilis muscle and the semitendinosus muscle cross the field. These may be divided to provide better exposure.

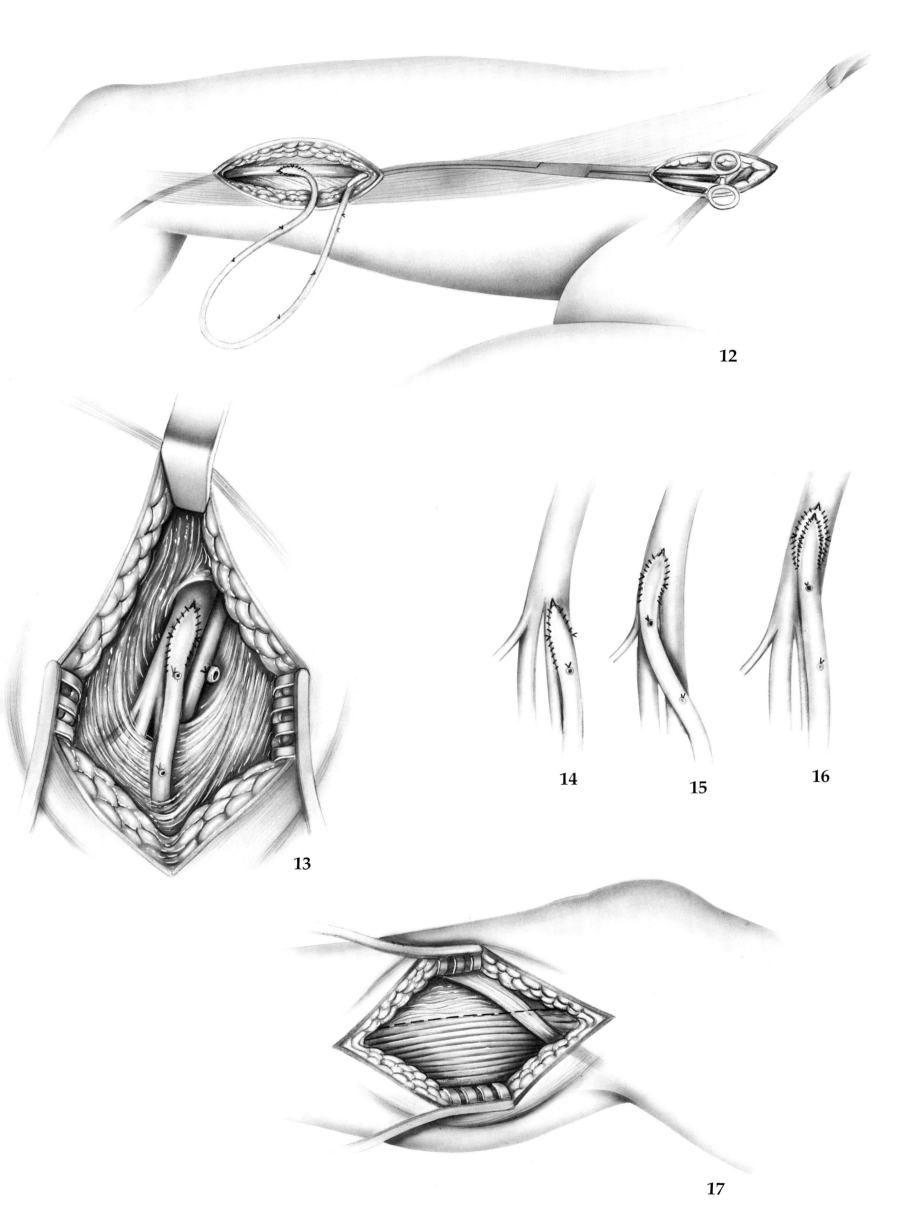

12

13

14

15

16

17

Femoropopliteal Bypass (*cont.*)

18 The popliteal space is entered and the vascular bundle palpated in the upper portion of the depths of the wound. The popliteal vein is the most superficial structure. Often dissection of the artery is facilitated by isolating the popliteal vein and retracting it with a Silastic loop. The neurovascular bundle in the inferior portion of the wound is deep to the soleus muscle. The arcing upper border of this muscle, which inserts on the posterior surface of the tibia, can clearly be seen and felt.

19 A finger or right-angle clamp can be placed deep to this muscle and it can be incised over the finger or clamp, to expose the distal popliteal artery and its trifurcation.

20 By ligating and dividing branches of the popliteal vein, this vessel can be retracted anteriorly or posteriorly to expose the underlying artery and its branches. In this view one can see the origin of the anterior tibial artery, the tibioperoneal trunk and its terminal branches, the peroneal and the posterior tibial arteries.

21 Any or all of these branches can be freed circumferentially and encircled with Silastic loops. The origin of the anterior tibial artery is best seen after ligation of one or more accompanying anterior tibial veins.

22 After administration of systemic heparin, suitable gentle clamp or clip application isolates the most disease-free portion of the artery. This is incised with a scalpel blade.

23 A meticulous anastomosis of the vein or PTFE graft to the artery is made. Great care is taken to visualize every suture bite and to be sure that equal portions of all layers of the artery and vein wall are caught in every stitch. PTFE grafts to the below-knee popliteal artery should be used only in poor-risk patients or in those in whom ipsilateral autologous vein is not available.

24 The completed distal anastomosis is shown after removal of all occluding instrumentation.

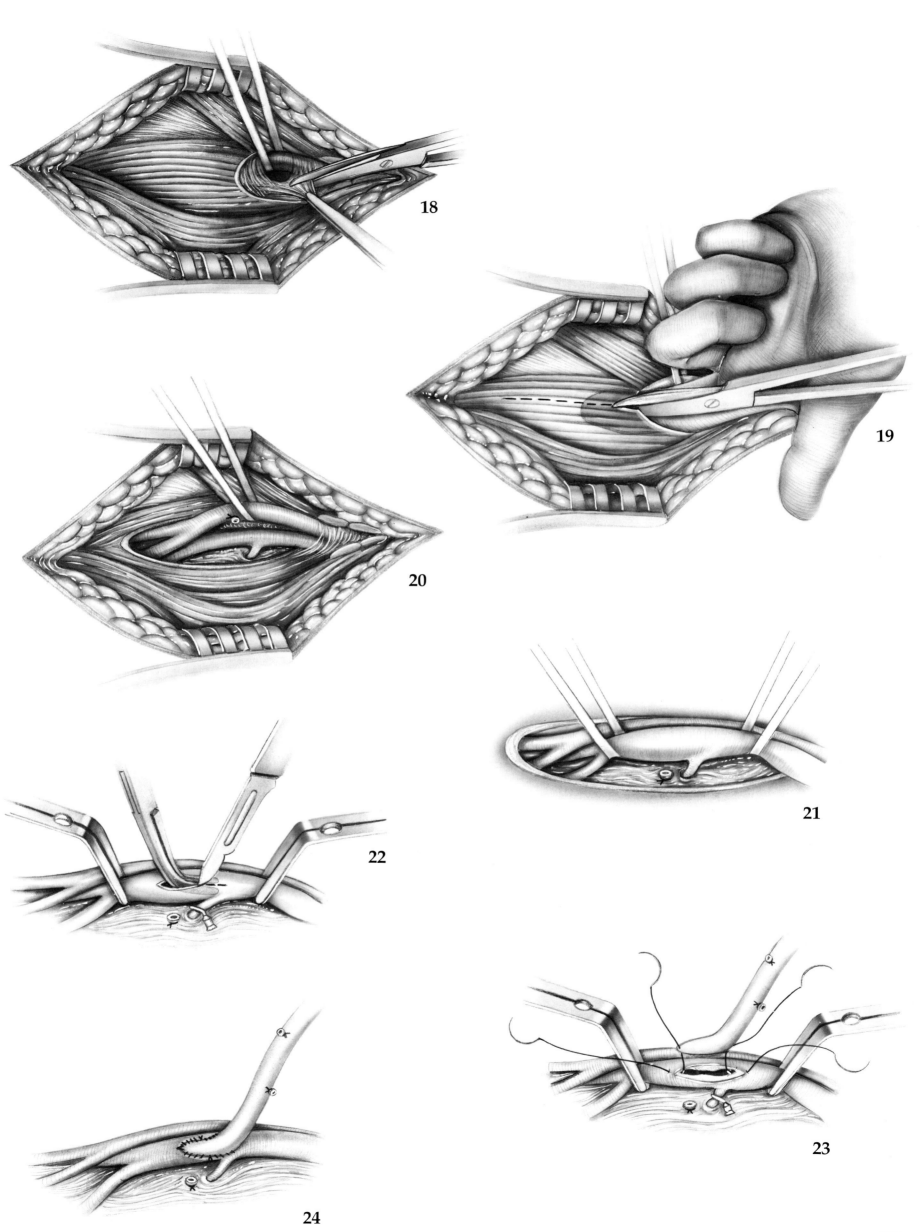

18

19

20

21

22

23

24

Femoropopliteal Bypass (*cont.*)

25 This shows the method for constructing the portion of the tunnel behind the knee. This tunneling should be carried out by blunt finger dissection, with the backs and tops of the fingers being placed against the popliteal vessels so that the graft will pass in the depths of the popliteal fossa. Usually this tunnel is constructed before the patient is given heparin.

26 The graft is then passed retrograde behind the knee, using a large curved clamp, inserted under finger guidance, to draw the vein from the below-knee incision to a small above-knee incision and then to the groin.

27 This figure shows the position of the graft in its anatomic tunnel. Before performing the proximal anastomosis, the knee should be fully extended to allow appropriate tensioning of the graft and to permit the graft to be cut at precisely the right level so that it will be neither overly taut nor redundant with the knee at full extension. Heparin is reversed with protamine and meticulous hemostasis is obtained throughout all wounds. These are then closed in layers without drainage. The *in-situ* vein graft bypass technique has received a great deal of attention recently. There is no evidence whatsoever that this technique provides superior results in femoropopliteal bypasses. Randomized, prospective comparisons of *in-situ* and reversed vein grafts in the femoropopliteal position have shown that the two grafting techniques produce comparable results; accordingly, we favor use of reversed vein grafts for femoropopliteal bypass. For tibial bypasses, many of which can be performed with short reversed vein grafts, we favor the latter procedure. However, it is possible that long bypasses from the upper thigh to the lower leg have better patency rates when they are performed with an *in-situ* graft. This remains to be proved.

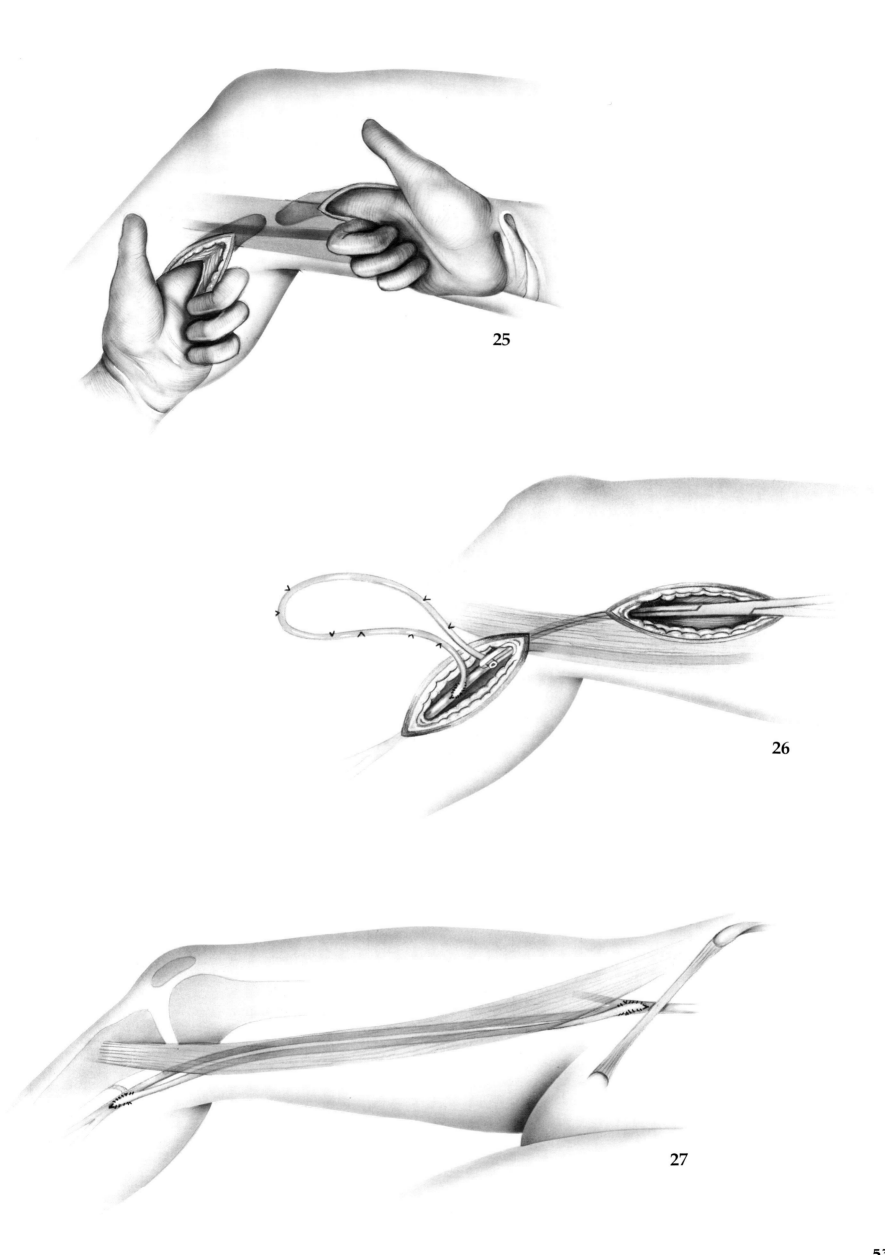

25

26

27

Axillofemoral Bypass

1 The position of the patient and locations of the incisions are shown. The right axillary artery is less likely to be involved with significant disease and is chosen preferentially to provide inflow. However, some of our recent data has shown that approximately 25 percent of candidates for axillofemoral bypass have significant unsuspected axillary or subclavian artery disease, and we presently advocate preoperative arch arteriography, via a translumbar approach, to determine the presence or absence of inflow disease and to guide the surgeon in the choice of which axillary artery to use. Although many surgeons advocate the performance of routine axillobifemoral bypass even if the symptoms are restricted to one lower extremity, we have found that axillounifemoral bypasses have patency rates similar to those of axillobifemoral bypasses. We therefore perform a unilateral procedure if a patient's predominant symptoms are restricted to only one lower extremity. The pattern of disease for which an axillofemoral bypass might be employed is shown. Severe and extensive aortic and bilateral iliac disease of a sort not suitable for percutaneous transluminal angioplasty is present. The axillary incision is placed over the proximal axillary artery and is approximately parallel to the fibers of the pectoralis major muscle.

2 The skin incision is deepened through the subcutaneous tissue and the fascia of the pectoralis major muscle. The fibers of the latter muscle are separated and retracted with a self-retaining retractor. The borders of the pectoralis minor muscle are defined. A finger is then placed beneath the muscle, and this muscle is divided as close to its insertion on the coracoid process as possible. Either scissors or cautery can be used for this maneuver.

3 The axillary artery is identified as it courses among the components of the brachial plexus. The periadventitial plane of this artery is identified and the artery is carefully dissected free in a circumferential manner. Silastic vessel loops are placed around the artery to elevate it and to facilitate circumferential dissection of a 5- to 7-cm segment of artery. Care is taken to avoid injury to the large thin-walled branches which arise from the proximal portion of the axillary artery. An effort is made to dissect the most proximal portion of the artery so that it can be used for the anastomosis.

4 After a groin incision is made with exposure of the inguinal ligament, as already described (see **Plate 259, Fig. 7**), the tunneling procedure between the two incisions is performed. This is begun by blunt finger dissection, under the pectoralis major muscle and as close to the chest wall as possible, via the axillary incision.

5 Blunt finger dissection to start the tunnel from the groin incision is also performed. This tunnel must be superficial to the inguinal ligament and aponeurosis of the external oblique muscle.

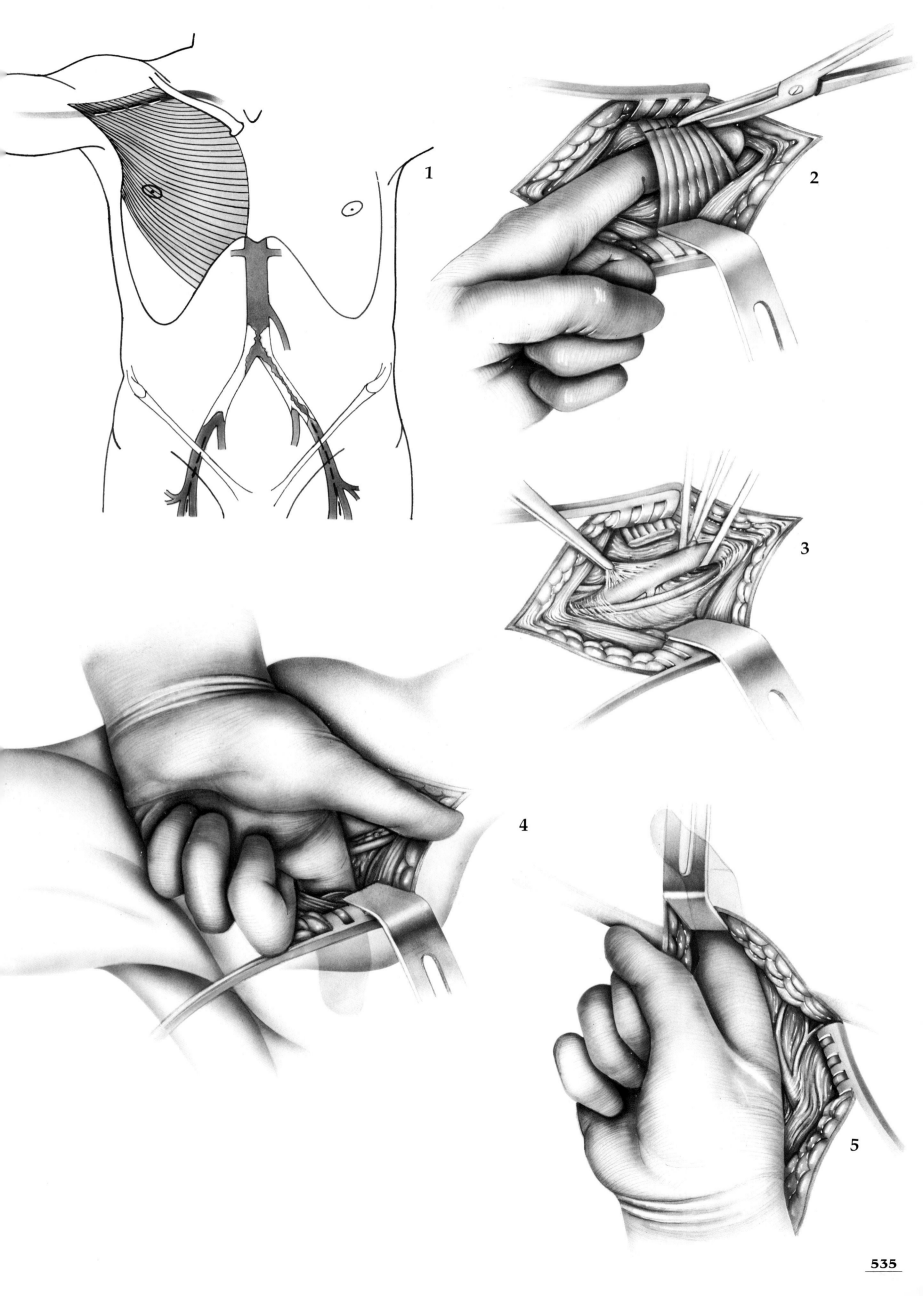

Axillofemoral Bypass (*cont.*)

6 Any of several varieties of tunneler may be used to join the axillary and femoral incisions. An intermediate skin incision midway along the tunnel is generally unnecessary. We have found that a plastic chest-tube container serves as a very effective tunneler; this is shown in the illustration. However, there are a variety of other instruments which can be used just as well. The tunneler is passed, under finger control, from below upward and retrieved from the axillary incision, taking care to guide the tunneler away from the axillary neurovascular structures. The closed tip of the plastic tube is then cut off with heavy scissors, as shown by the short broken line. If a bilateral femoral procedure is to be employed the opposite groin is also opened, the femoral arteries dissected circumferentially, and a tunnel created in the subcutaneous plane between the two groin incisions. Care is taken to place this tunnel superficial to the inguinal ligaments and abdominal musculature and just above the pubic symphysis. The tunneler is left in place but withdrawn slightly (2–4 cm) so that it can later be retrieved for use.

7 The patient is given intravenous heparin [1 mg (100 I.U.)/kg]. The axillary artery is carefully elevated and occluded with gently applied atraumatic vascular clamps. The axillary artery is a very thin-walled structure that is easily damaged; these clamps should be placed with extreme care. Microclips are used to occlude the smaller branches of the axillary artery, and tensioned double-looped Silastic loops affixed to the drapes are used to occlude the larger branches.

8 The vascular clamps are rotated slightly to expose the anteroinferior portion of the axillary artery, and a longitudinal incision is made in that artery using the techniques already shown. If the artery is perfectly normal, as it often is, a scissors may be used to create the incision or extend it to its ends. If, on the other hand, the artery is diseased, the knife-and-clamp technique already illustrated (**Plate 265, Fig. 22**) should be used. Double-armed 5-0 or 6-0 polypropylene sutures are placed in the corners of the arteriotomy.

9 A 6-mm PTFE graft is anastomosed to the artery using careful suturing technique as already described for other anastomoses. The opened end of the tunneler is then pushed into the wound.

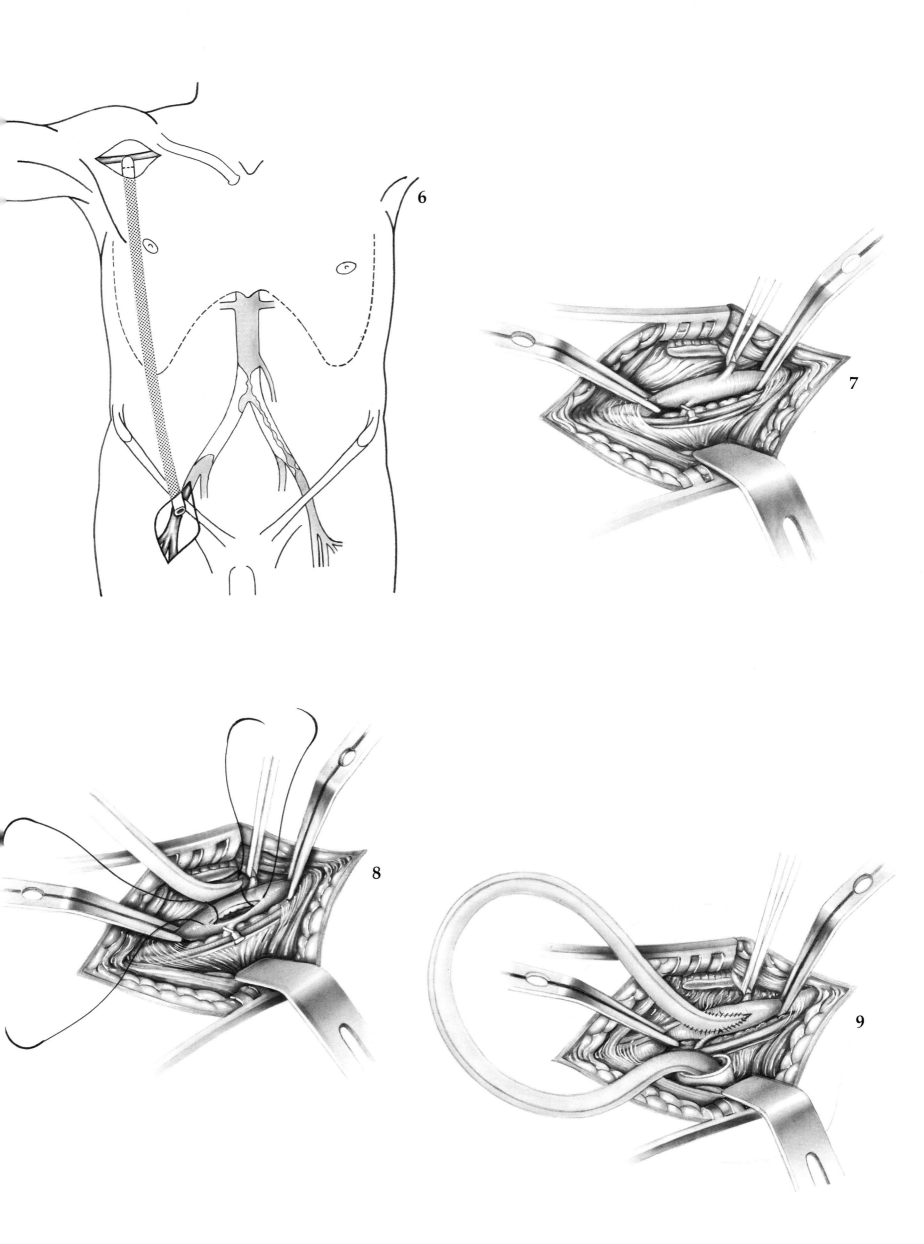

10 A long bronchoscopy grasping forceps is then placed through the tunneler, and the graft drawn from above downward (**Figs. 9–10**).

11 The right femoral anastomosis is then completed in a standard fashion. This anastomosis can be either in the common femoral artery or extended across the origin of the deep femoral artery, if there is disease at that site. Alternatively, the anastomosis can be entirely into the deep femoral artery if the proximal portion of that artery is extensively diseased. The left femoral anastomosis is completed in a similar way. Finally, the femorofemoral graft is anastomosed to the axillary limb.

12 The positions of these anastomoses are clearly shown. The nature and location of the disease in the femoral arteries determines the exact location of the graft-to-artery femoral anastomoses. If disease is present at the origin of the deep femoral artery, as on the left side of the patient illustrated, the arteriotomy is placed across this disease and the graft used to enlarge the orifice. Heparin is reversed with protamine, hemostasis is obtained, and the wounds are closed in layers, making an effort to close as much soft tissue over the anastomotic areas as is possible. This is particularly important in the groin, since the anastomosis is not deep to any muscular layers.

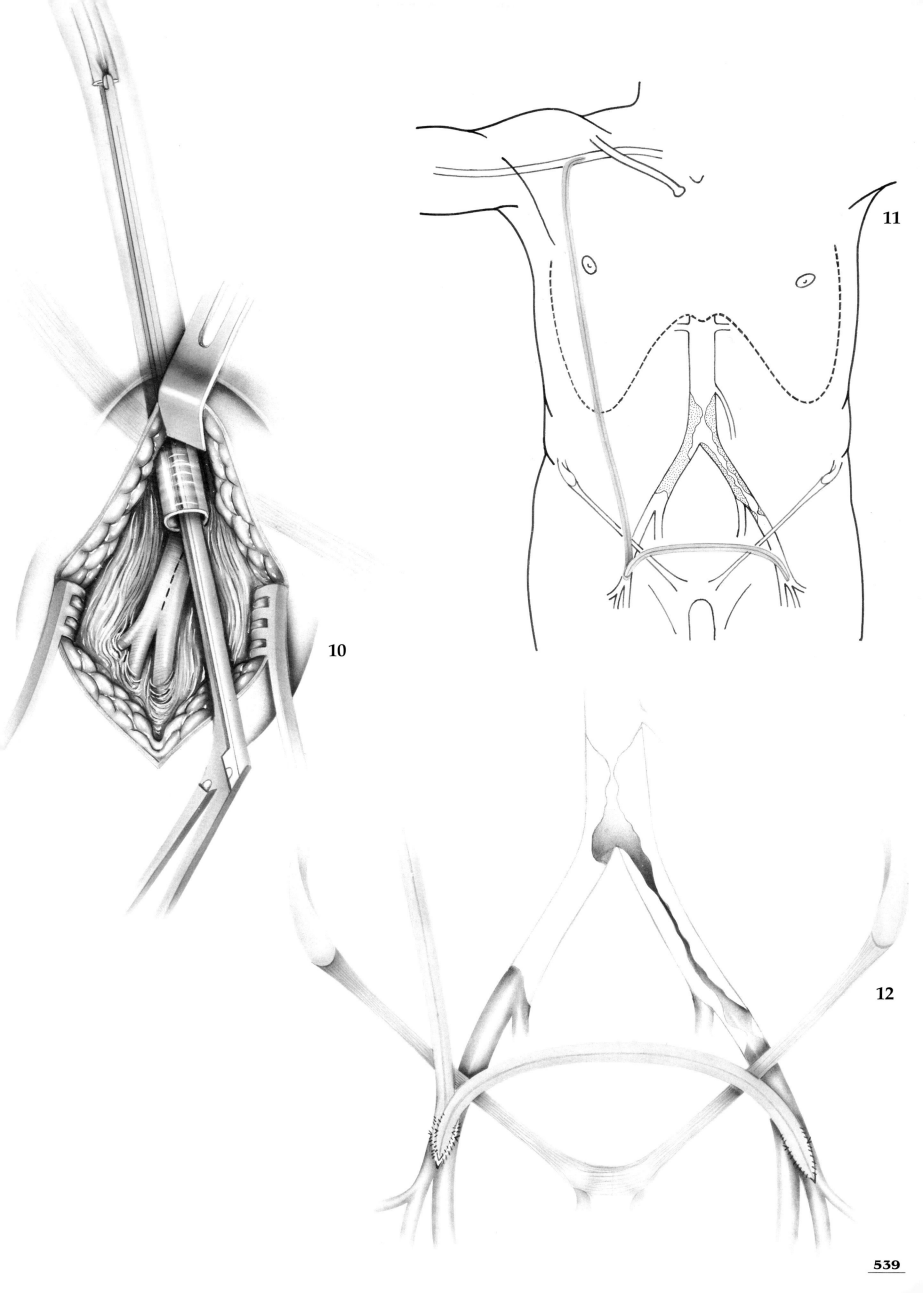

10

11

12

Femorofemoral Bypass

1 This figure shows the typical pattern of disease for which femorofemoral bypass is an effective operative treatment. Unilateral iliac occlusive disease is present, with minimal involvement of the aorta and contralateral iliac arteries. Incisions over both femoral arteries are made and extended upward over the inguinal ligament.

2 These incisions are deepened to expose the inguinal ligaments. Once these have been identified, finger dissection is used to create a tunnel superficial to the external oblique and above the symphysis of the pubis. Care is taken to avoid dissecting deep to the inguinal ligament.

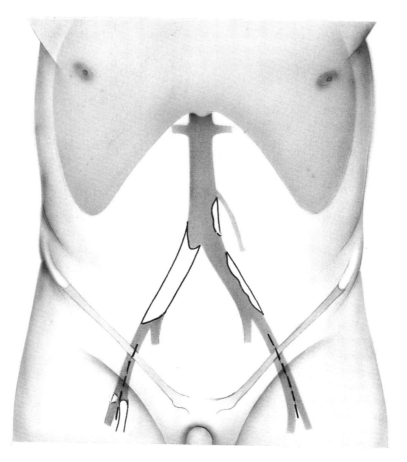

1

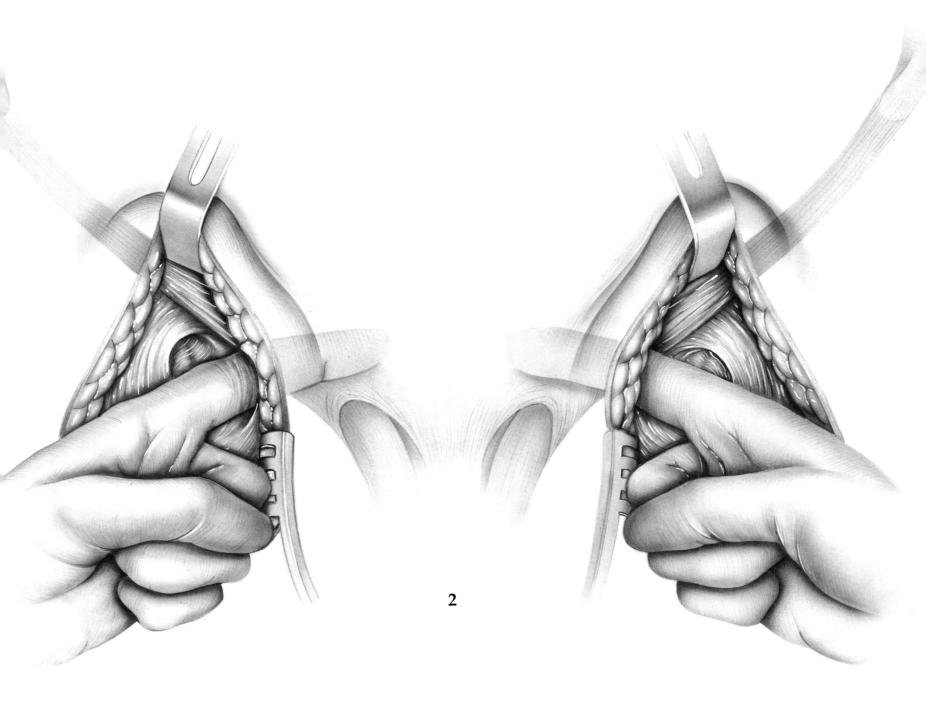

2

Femorofemoral Bypass (*cont.*)

3 Self-retaining retractors are placed to hold the edges of the wound apart and to elevate the inguinal ligament. To accomplish the latter maneuver, a robot arm and an army-navy retractor can be used. After isolating the common, deep, and superficial femoral arteries, control of patent arteries is obtained with atraumatic vascular clamps gently applied so as not to injure the vessels. No clamp is necessary for the occluded superficial femoral artery. Small microclips are used to occlude branch vessels without injuring them. After administration of intravenous heparin, the arteriotomy is made as already described (see **Plate 260, Fig. 9**). In the instance shown a stenosis is present at the origin of the deep femoral artery; accordingly, the incision in the artery is made across this stenosis. No endarterectomy is carried out.

4 After the anastomosis of the 6-mm PTFE tubular graft to the right common and deep femoral artery is completed, the right-side vascular clamps are removed and the graft is clamped. It is then drawn through the tunnel, and an arteriotomy in the left common femoral artery is made along the line indicated.

5 Both anastomoses have now been completed. The position of the graft, in a gentle C-shaped arc, is shown.

After hemostasis is assured and the heparin reversed, the wounds are carefully closed in layers, so that as many soft tissue layers as possible cover the graft and dead space is eliminated.

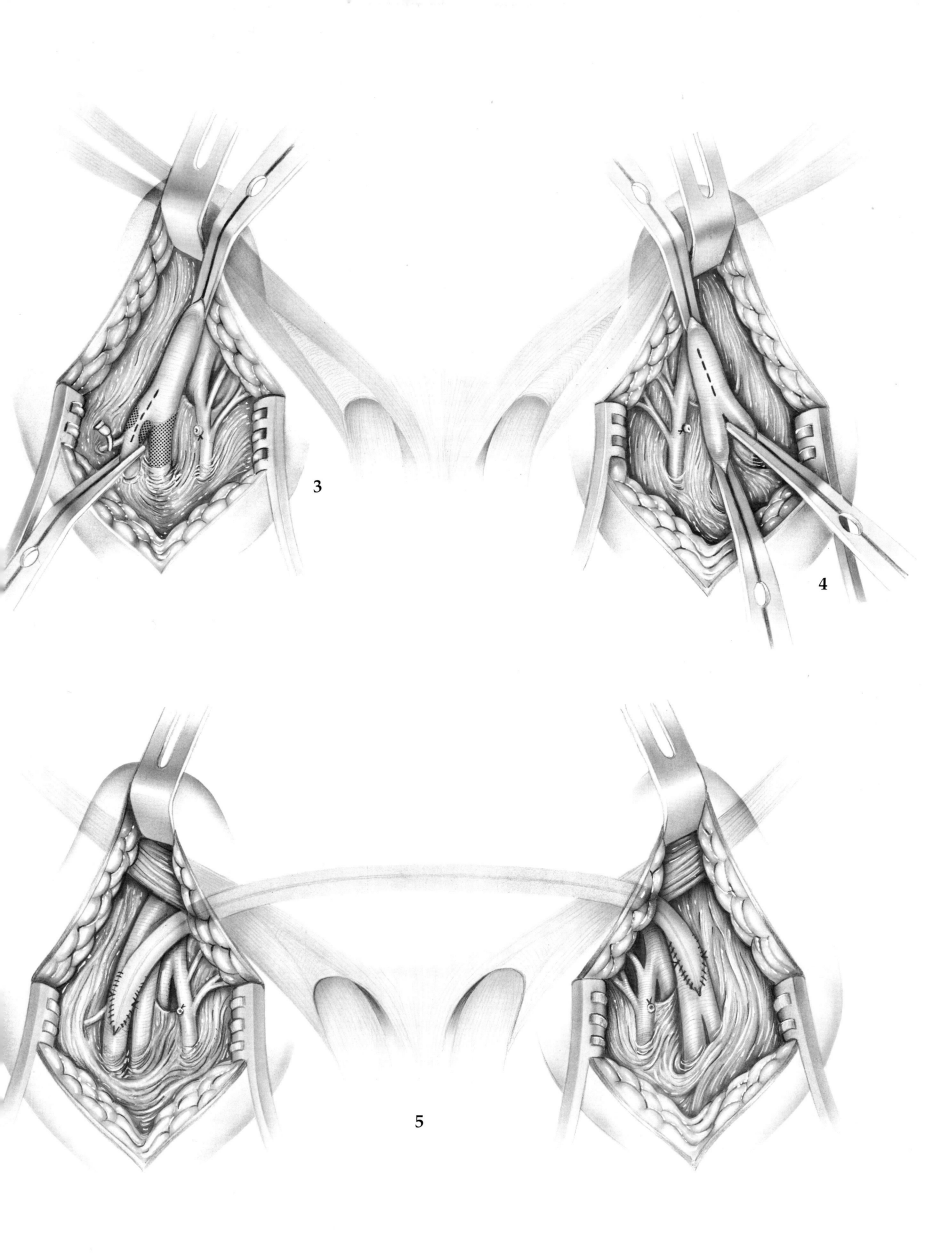

3

4

5